Robert S. Miller
July 2002

COMPASSION'S WAY

*A Doctor's Quest
into the Soul of Medicine*

COMPASSION'S WAY

*A Doctor's Quest
into the Soul of Medicine*

RALPH CRAWSHAW

Copyright © 2002 MEDI-ED PRESS

Printed in the United States of America. All rights reserved.
ISBN 0-936741-15-5

Cover design by Douglas Lynch, Portland, Oregon

Library of Congress Cataloging-in-Publication Data
Crawshaw, Ralph, 1921-
    Compassion's way : a doctor's quest into the soul of medicine/
      Ralph Crawshaw. p. cm.
    Includes bibliographical references and index.
    ISBN 0-936741-15-5
     1. Physicians--United States--Biography. 2. Medicine.
      3. Compassion. 1. Title.

R153 .C73 2001
610'.92---dc21
[B]　　　　　　　　　　　　　　　　　　2001044469

MEDI-ED PRESS
#5 White Place
Bloomington, IL 61701

Tollfree: 1-800-500-8205
Email: Medi.EdPress@verizon.net
Website: www.Medi-EdPress.com

Study Guide available by mail or on website

*To countless patients
who make possible, through trust, forbearance, and forgiveness,
for me and the reader to become wiser and more compassionate
in understanding the universal presence of human suffering
as more than a challenge to medical skill.
With the courage to willfully penetrate the obvious,
they reveal, as only shared suffering can,
the full dimension in becoming a caring human being.*

Contents

Acknowledgments 10
Foreword by Robert J. Glaser, M.D. 11
Dear Reader 13
The Author as a Person 17
Part 1 – Compassion Wakened 37
    In Defense of Fellini's *Satyricon* — *A Film Review* 43
    Oh, Where Is the Balm of Gilead? 47
    The Other Side of Charity 53
    Leprosy, A Disease of the Heart 62
    The Quality of Mercy 72
Part 2 – The Human Condition 77
    The Yammering Grandmother 83
    Humanism in Medicine, The Rudimentary Process 87
    On the Sounds of Death 93
    Who Is Saving Private Ryan? — *A Non-Review* 96
    The Value of Suffering in Medical Practice 100
Part 3 – Compassion's Necessary Courage 109
    On the Psychology of the Hippocratic Oath 115
    Hello, Hippocrates, Are You There? 118
    A Medical Code for Me 122
    Betrayal — *A Film Review* 127
    The Corrupted Land — *A Book Review* 130
    The Awareness of Courage 138
    In the Belly of the Soviet Beast 143
    Humble Pie 154
Part 4 – The Many Languages of Compassion 159
    Listening over God's Shoulder 165
    The Necessary Samaritan 167
    Going to the Movies in China 172
    A Fairy Tale for a South African Grandchild 179
    Compassion Is Where You Find It 196

Part 5 - The Compassionate Patient-Doctor Relationship 201
Nicholas and Alexandra — A Film Review 207
Patient-Doctor Bonding 213
Lasting Impressions 215
The Foley Catheter 219
The Bedpan Factor 225
Professional Diplopia 229
A Lesson from Chinese Medicine 233
The Importance of a Name 240
You Can't Kill Hope 244

Part 6 - Medical Practitioners of Compassion 249
Gandhi — A Film Review 255
Stories, Poems Look at the Heart of Medicine — *A Book Review* .. 259
A Visit to Maimonides' Grave 261
A Rose for Chekhov's Grave 265
José Rizal 272
Witness to War — A Book Review 275
Obituary: Carroll Dean Henry Behrhorst, M.D. 278
Undrained Brains 281
Dr. Karl's Finest Colloquium 285
A Psychiatrist for a Troubled World — A Book Review 290

Part 7 - Compassion in Shadow 295
Welfare — A Film Review 303
The Tattletape Tale 308
Marketplace of Pain and Suffering 311
Computerized Medicine 319
Who Is Calling the Shots? 325
Community Mental Health and Psychological Pollution 330
Reflections of a Director
    on Resigning from a Mental Health Clinic 338
They All Laughed When I Spoke of Greedy Doctors 346
Fee for Service from the Poor 348
The Cost of Caring: A View of Britain's Delivery of Health Care . 351

Part 8 - Compassion's Cruel Companions 361
African Slavery and Western Medicine 369
Shoah — A Film Review 383
An Epidemic of Suicide among Physicians on Probation 389

CONTENTS

Stalinization of Health Care 395
Academic Sanction 397
The New Custodians 411
Is There a Doctor in the Nation? 420
A Modest Policy Proposal:
    The National Health Selective Disservice 437
Nurturing Hate in Psychotherapy — *Address* 442

Part 9 - Manifest Tragedy 449
3 Women — *A Film Review* 455
Technological Zeal or Therapeutic Purpose? 466
St. Paul and Medical Technology — *Address* 472
My Brother and His Keepers 480
Requiem for an Unknown Leper 486

Part 10 - Compassion's Challenge 493
Civic Medicine 499
Mini-Internships: An Experience in Health Care Delivery
    for Community Leaders 503
The Better Health Business Bureau 508
Breaking Out of Gridlock 517
Grass Roots Participation in Health Care Reform 521
Lying 532
Intellectual Nemesis 544
Medicine, A Challenged Profession — *Lecture* 551

Part 11 - Compassion Pursued 563
The Great Santini — *A Film Review* 569
What to Do with the Bean from the Patient's Ear 579
Fraternizing with the Enemy 583
Powerless Groups 592
Friends of Medicine 598
The Patient-Physician Covenant 603
The Soul of Medicine 604
The Humanitarian Imperative and the Practice
    of Medicine 617

Epiview 623
Chartres and the Accidental Pilgrim 629
Index 641

Acknowledgments

Nothing of merit is accomplished in this complex world of ours without the help of others. Should this volume deserve merit it is due to the unstinting support of many caring people. Carol, my loving wife, who each day sustains my body, heart, and soul. Susan Page York, who so patiently and wisely has borne the heavy burden of making a coherent tale of these many disparate experiences.

My gratitude to Dr. Helen Glaser and Dr. Robert Glaser, the editorial team at *The Pharos,* is profound. Bob for his firm hand on my shoulder while pointing to what needed to be said and Helen for her seventeen-year unsuccessful attempt to teach me how to spell while turning my reflections on the movies into readable sense. Together they provided confidence and foundation for turning the inchoate into readable sense. Dr. Peter E. Dans, who graciously continues "our" movie column, for his bright collegiality, sustaining friendship, and knowledgeable insights into the art of writing. Patty H. Davies, Reference Librarian, Oregon Health Sciences Library, who unfailingly opened the literature of medicine to my easy review and lasting enlightenment.

The "A" team that did the work of making the manuscript publishable demands special recognition. Susan Page York, who lavished so many hours on developing a usable index, Douglas Lynch who magically wove ancient Celtic knots of the human heart into a dust jacket and book cover of living art. Linny Stovall who opened the door to informed marketing and Sherlyn Hogenson who ventured publication of this different kind of book. These and others unnamed are thanked. Especially to be recognized are the unnamed, the patients who, with generous trust and merciful forgiveness taught me the power of compassion by intimately sharing their vulnerable, suffering lives. To these caring people I owe more than can be repaid.

Foreword

Compassion's Way: A Doctor's Quest into the Soul of Medicine is an interesting, informative and enlightening chronicle, focused on Compassion but much broader in terms of its content than that subject, important though it is. Ralph Crawshaw, the author of this opus, is a man of many talents, and the contents of this delightful book bear clear witness to the validity of that statement. He is, of course, a highly respected psychiatrist, who has taken care of a multitude of patients in the many years he has practiced in Portland and has earned the devotion of those who have benefited from his wise counsel. On that basis alone, he would merit the fine reputation he has earned. But, above and beyond that accolade, he has been a teacher of medical students and residents in training, and his concern for his fellow men has led him to travel widely and to observe at first hand the magnitude of the need for better care in other parts of the world, notably where poverty and ignorance abound.

In the more than thirty years I have had the privilege of knowing Crawshaw, I have been continually amazed by his ability to use his talents on a wide scale without diminishing the quality of his contributions. I remember with pleasure my first contact with him, which came in the form of a review of the film, *Hospital*, with the great actor George Scott, which he submitted for publication in *The Pharos*, the Journal of Alpha Omega Alpha Honor Medical Society. I was editor of the journal, which published nontechnical articles pertinent to medicine, for example, history, ethics, and education. In truth, I had never thought about the possibility of having such a piece in *The Pharos*, but Crawshaw's paper was impressive, and my late wife, Dr. Helen Glaser, who was the managing editor of the publication, was also impressed and we accepted it. We invited him to do reviews on a regular schedule and he accepted. As Crawshaw notes in his acknowledgment, his reviews lent themselves to considerable editing, but they were enormously popular with our readers and became a key feature of each issue. Crawshaw has interwoven some of his reviews in the text of the book. After many years as "The Physician at the Movies," he passed the torch to Dr. Peter Dans, who carries on the feature.

Over the years, Crawshaw has been widely recognized for his efforts to direct attention to many important areas of medicine and medical care. In his home state of Oregon, he has been an influential force in supporting measures that address critical ethical issues, such as terminal care and the rights of individuals to participate in decisions that directly affect them. He has enlisted the participation of leaders in medicine and related professions in addressing such matters, and his views have contributed to the deliberations of key national bodies such as the Institute of Medicine of which he is a member.

Compassion's Way is an important addition to the literature of Medicine in the broadest sense, and its readers will find it an enriching experience.

Robert J. Glaser, M.D.

Dear Reader

'Tis the good reader who makes the good book.
—Ralph Waldo Emerson (1803-1882)
Success

How to read this book is for you to discover. Some may begin with the first page and read, word for word, page by page, from start to finish, a plod unlikely to ignite the imagination. What quest ever traveled a straight path to its grail?

This story has been many years in the living, weaving its record in its own natural way while serving greater ends and lesser contingencies. Reading is best pursued as an easygoing exploration of the text. I encourage you to engage with the contents as you might some prospect of nature, here human nature. Come to this fragment of the world as you might a forest glade of an autumn afternoon, alert for signs of life, the whirring of unseen wings, prepared to pause and pluck away tenacious nettles of doubt, observing yet avoiding, sprigs of poison ivy, all the while consciously alive to the least possibility of authentic thought. As in any forest, narrow byways may be left for future exploration. Never hurry, rather savor the fragrance of your own fermenting sloughs of reflection. Herein lies a way to read, keen-eyed as an Audubon, seeking the fullest pallet for addressing your most personal work of art, your life. It is my wish that our shared experience becomes a sacrament of spirit.

You, dear reader, are encouraged to enter this book with as many companionable elements of imagination as you can muster, for you are anticipated in the pages not as a passive spectator but as an engaged friend, a fellow explorer of the human condition.

Compassion's Way should be read aloud, shared, as the tales read to Havana's cigar makers in a large airy room surrounded by fellow workers, each at a bench fashioning select panatelas or corona coronas, listening while grading, selecting, and rolling aromatic fermented tobacco leaves,

The words flow from an experienced reader, paid by the workers for a clear voice and lively style. He sits on a raised platform before the attentive audience, articulating each word fully from a text selected by the workers. As they industriously pursue their work, none is too busy to pause and share thoughts and reflections. Should a misunderstanding or conflict arise with the telling of the tale, the workshop floor opens to comment and discussion. It is not a coincidence that a famous brand of cigars bears the romantic name, Romeo and Juliet.

Short of a one-on-one reader-writer relationship, you may, pen in hand, underline, star, check, comment, and annotate directly on the receptive page before you. As blossoms seek sunlight, the passages crave active dialogue in order to live.

Despite it being up front, I suggest holding off reading the autobiographical introduction, "The Author as a Person." Wait until you have dipped into the contents to establish in your own mind whether it is worth your while to pursue our friendship. There is little sense in becoming acquainted with the vintner should you fail to savor the wine.

Overviews of the eleven parts of the book are included as points of reference for our dialogue. The overviews serve as boundaries surveyed without confirmation of received custom or coda of scholarly research. Remain alert, with notes and questions, for any benchmarks missed or dislocated from your experience as we enter a world which, for me, has proven stranger than Gulliver's Lilliput.

The stories, each one exploring the human condition, take different form—lectures, journal articles, essays, thought experiments, even reviews of films. Some films you may have seen; if not, with the exception of foreign films, most should be available on video. Films offer landscapes we can view side by side, the better to gauge our understanding of the presence of compassion. Those seeking a coda, a summarizing road map, can find it at the end of part 11 in "The Humanitarian Imperative and the Practice of Medicine." With or without guides the book exists for you to use as you will in your search for enhanced appreciation of compassionate encounters.

This said, a disclaimer in service of humility. It takes no stretch of the imagination to look back a thousand years to some hypothetical writer of the tenth century and, with a touch of condescending hubris, judge him and his audience as rough and ignorant barbarians of a Dark Age. How then might a thoughtful reader a thousand years hence consider us?

Can we, who live in times replete with arrogant bureaucracies, malignant dictatorships, unforgivable genocides, hived nuclear bombs, unmitigated pollution, heedless population growth, electronically trumpeted banality, profligate exploitation of natural resources, obscene financial exploitation of the powerless, be seen as anything but uncivilized savages of a Dark Age of Technological Violence?

But then, some of you may be troubled on finding yourself on what may seem to be foreign ground, the accounts that are originally intended for physicians' eyes, perspectives on the most curious landscape that is medicine. I suggest you put yourself at ease by slipping into a metaphorical white coat to accept, not that doctors are human beings capable of being understood in their shared humanity, but that it is a wise patient who can judge his physician's humanity. Bear with these papers and their sometimes obtuse goals, didactic jargon, and inconclusive conclusions. They tell a tale worth the reading as they illuminate the vast extent of suffering to be encompassed by compassion.

"Dated" contents of *Compassion's Way* reveal how much the allure of "progress" applies to the human side of medicine, health policy, pharmaceuticals, service, and medical conferences. Like any other social undertaking there is an almost willful confusion of social cause and effect— the inevitability of human suffering. If for no other reason, the account in *Compassion's Way* of experienced medical practice reveals how much we change in order to remain the same.

Granted the social/political changes are dramatic—fee-for-service health care delivery replaced by managed care, charity obliterated in the rush of Medicaid, the impaired sufferer now rehabilitated—and yet our suffering as individuals and as a nation continues, relabeled, yet largely unabated. For example, consider the paper relating the contents of the international health care "summit" at the Royal Society in 1971 ("Is There a Doctor in the Nation?" part 8). The leaders of health care in the United Kingdom and the United States, the recognized authorities for academic, organizational, and governmental medicine, had their say about what was "new," yet with a rewording of titles and a change of names, the same pronouncements are as prevalent today as they will be in another thirty years.

There is a dread logic to our leaders' rhetoric which I suspect may be the relentless voice of the bureaucracies they direct—they look forward not backward, needing only hope rather than experience in thinking about tomorrow. Or so it seems to me as I share with you yesterday's experience in struggling with the human condition.

Despite a feared judgment by posterity, we search both past and present for means to reach beyond our age's slim promise of enhanced humanity. The author's course may meander, yet it is fixed on enlightening the human condition. This is the guide star which, distant as it is, glimmers clearly, marking the way through human suffering to compassion's redeeming strength. Here is the compass setting, I profoundly hope, the reader takes on entering these pages.

To read a book, to read it carefully, calls for trust. Thus reader's trust, so anticipated by the author, binds us in exploring incipient feeling, burgeoning ideas, unspoken beliefs. Shared trust acts as the hidden magnetic field in orienting the compass needle of our course.

Lastly, I offer a sextant, as talisman to carry on our journey, for determining where you are. I encourage you to read to be yourself. Should you try to be other than who you are, you run the serious risk of becoming nobody. This book rejoices in you as you are, the good reader who can make of this a good book.

Sincerely,
The Author

The Author as a Person

I should not talk so much about myself if there were anybody else whom I knew as well....Moreover, I, on my side, require of every writer, first or last, a simple and sincere account of his own life, and not merely what he has heard of other men's lives; some such account as he would send to his kindred from a distant land; for if he has lived sincerely, it must have been a distant land to me. Perhaps these pages are more particularly addressed to poor students. As for the rest of my readers, they will accept such portions as apply to them. I trust that none will stretch the seams in putting on the coat, for it may do good service to him whom it fits.

—Henry David Thoreau (1817-1862)
Walden

Examining a life for any tenacity of purpose calls for close appreciation of motives and aspirations. What moves the seeker to seek and to what end? Where did the search begin? What was the first step? Who pointed to the horizon? How was tenacity empowered? The truest answers to these questions are discovered in experiencing a shared path, along compassion's way.

Although it follows that one person cannot know, firsthand, the experience of another, this does not say a commonality of human experience can not be shared. Without such fellowship the parts and pieces of this book could not have been written. Indeed, the book you hold in your hand, *Compassion's Way,* can only live as it shares your experiences as much as it reports of mine, for none of us are strangers to human suffering.

The question then becomes, How well do any of us know our own experience? Over time I have tried to assess why I lived as I have. Yet no clear answer surfaced. What did emerge is a muddle of hope, aspiration, discipline, and strong desire, remaining for me a curious puzzle of why I wished so to be a doctor. That is not to say the puzzle lacks recognizable patterns of similar shape or color, yet as experience shows, they fail to lock neatly together.

The Child as Father to the Author

Who as a child has not been confronted by the frivolous question, "What are you going to do when you grow up?" Few questions have such ready yet unprovable answers. The child's response, be it fireman or Indian chief, may bring a smile to the face of the questioner, yet the answer, roughly framed, anticipates the spirit that drives lifelong aspiration.

For me, the eleven-year-old adolescent that I once was on far off Long Island, New York, my life's goal dawned as love, not the romantic love of a troubadour seeking his unattainable beloved but an all encompassing, mystic love, the dedication of the knight-errant to the quest of the holy grail. My grail appeared on a movie screen. I remember the moment in the film *Arrowsmith* when I "knew" I would henceforth devote my life to medical science. Much as the ever-gracious doctor/hero, Ronald Colman, I would discover the cure for cancer. I would defeat death. Or so I believed as I pedaled home from the Little Neck movie house on my blue American Flyer bicycle. In ecstasy of revelation, I was convinced I had found the answer to my life. I would become a research doctor.

Though first defined as pursuit of scientific knowledge, my goal in life transformed into a quest for compassion through a maze of partially formed questions, shrouded attitudes, illogical lapses of thought, empty spaces in my thinking, resulting from the collision of limited knowledge, intense feelings, and inexplicable beliefs with manifest experience, the process of maturation. Understanding the force that moved me to reach beyond the scientist's skills to learn the physician's art has proved a life-long task.

Education by Mishap

As wisdom is fertilized by doubt, perception sharpened by anxiety, so pain quickens compassion, the soul of medicine. Between the ages of eighteen and twenty-three, a number of mishaps opened my mind to compassion's power.

My inadvertent education in compassion began in the summer of 1940. As an eighteen-year-old, moved by a wish to serve the "cause of democracy," coupled with a desire for adventure, I volunteered to be an ambulance driver for the British-American Ambulance Corp then operating in North Africa.

Joining the corp required a personal interview which was conducted by a bespectacled nonentity ensconced in the clutter of a tiny office high in a Lexington Avenue skyscraper. I was accepted on the spot. Apparently with the ability to drive a truck and acknowledged interest in matters medical I met the requirements. The interviewer then precipitously switched roles from recruiter to feckless bystander by asking, "Why would anyone volunteer to go into the desert to be shot at?" Lacking an answer I left musing on what I was getting into.

A week later a letter confirmed my appointment, adding that I was expected to supply my own ambulance, a point neglected during the interview. As I had little more than the carfare to the interview, the venture proved a dud. I wrote them I was broke and, consequently, missed the boat, the SS Zam Zam.

A few weeks later, in a brief wartime dispatch the *New York Times* reported that while approaching the Straits of Gibraltar, the Zam Zam had been torpedoed by a German submarine with the loss of its cargo, crew, and passengers. The news carried an unavoidable lesson in personal vulnerability, luck is central to more than success. From it I added to my small store of wisdom that I was lucky to be alive.

Caught up in the World War II wish "to do something for my country," on returning to college I registered for Selective Service. When the army organized the Mountain Troops, the prospect of mountaineering for my country proved too tempting for me to stay with college studies. I put aside ideas of becoming a medical scientist and volunteered as a private in the army, there to encounter a widening perspective on man's capacity for inhumanity.

The letter announcing my acceptance as a volunteer in the U.S. Army dispatched me to a dreary office in downtown New York City where in a motley squad of fellow recruits I was marched off to a ferryboat. The ferry bore us across New York harbor to the army base on Governor's Island. Here recruits were given a military identity, starting with a dogtag number. Mine, 12124442, proved a fine number for singing off at the top of my lungs at roll call. Army processing continued as a series of probes into the recruit's occupational, mental, and physical being. Thus a niche in the vast army was determined for each recruit, in my case the 10th Mountain Division.

During processing my military identity took form as a handful of papers to clutch during the parade in the buff for medical certification from probing station to probing station. Each invasion into my privacy was duly noted on the papers. Finally, while wearily killing time on a bench in a holding room, I noticed that my papers lacked a stamp similar to that on the papers of the fellow recruit beside me. Curious to know what the clerk had stamped on each page of his enlistment documents but omitted from mine, I asked him what it said. Without a word, my companion passed his papers over to me. Each page was boldly stamped in bright red ink, "NEGRO." Thus the U.S. Army indoctrinated me into the intolerant power of race—man's inhumanity to man.

Enlisted and in uniform, I was ordered first to Camp Upton on Long Island and then to Camp Hale, 10,000 feet high in the Colorado Rockies, the Mountain Troops. I arrived at my training base on a snowy February night in 1943 to become a private, a dogface, in Company A of the 86th Regiment of the 10th Mountain Division. There began my advanced course in the art and science of human destruction, the discipline of combat.

It did not take long on the firing line for me to discover that, as I imagined the target's bull's-eye as the head of a German soldier now in training in his country, boyhood glee at shooting up the "bad guys" gave way to a deep antipathy to drawing a killing bead on any other human being.

That insight, an extension of the lesson of racial inhumanity, was a beginning, not all, of what was learned from combat training. Another and deeper truth gradually dawned, I was being systematically trained to be a brute, albeit an obedient brute, a missionary for man's inhumanity to man.

Despite the G.I. manual's emphasis on the soldier's mission as discipline and duty, indoctrination into the army's way of life, like most elemental lessons, seeped in from around the edges of the lessons that drill instructors drummed into my head. Inevitably, as the army became part of my experience I became part of the army, which made no difference to the army but made a considerable difference to me.

Unrelieved noise, the interminable racket of barracks life, proved an unavoidable, although incidental, fragment of wartime military training. The only respite from the rush to make soldiers of recruits came on Sunday, routinely set aside for recreation, lying on our bunks to doze, read, or reflect, but even that time never belonged to us. A bleak Sunday afternoon serves as an example. Stretched out on my bunk, I tried to read, but I lost my attention to a mean-mouthed sergeant, one of those creatures that quickly rise to the summit of their ambition as a recognized bully. His penetrating voice echoed from one end of the barracks to the other, raucously recounting to a gaggle of open-mouthed recruits the conquests of his Saturday night sally into Leadville's bars and brothels. His language typified the banality of barracks "noise." Timed by my wristwatch he used "fucking" as an adjective ten times in thirty seconds of his blather.

Wartime military training indoctrinates through many ways including cruel humor and arrogant disdain. There were many examples, but two stand out: a prank of mischievous near-castration and basic training in retrieving battle casualties.

Wartime army bunks came with a mesh of crossed bare wires purporting to be a bedspring strung from the head to foot of the bed supporting a meager cotton mattress. Sitting on the side of the bed depressed the wire mesh and mattress, leaving a sizable gap between them and the stationary iron frame. Upon rising, the stretched springs returned to their original position with the precision of a steel trap.

Should a new recruit return naked from a shower and dry his feet by sitting on his bunk, there was a good chance that a significant part of his anatomy would slip through the gap. Spied by a quick-eyed prankster, the sitting recruit was fair game to sneak up behind and shout, "ATTENTION!" Springing to his feet the unsuspecting recruit inadvertently closed the trap on his dependent parts. His consequent excruciating pain afforded high amusement to bystanders. It was one of the rites of passage from civilian into wartime soldier.

A further example of the dark side of indoctrination occurred when at the completion of combat training I was assigned to a battalion aide station. We diligently learned to treat shock with skillful use of tourniquet, morphine, and blankets. Out of the classroom on the mountainside, training was different. No one volunteered to act as a token casualty for training in rappelling stretchers down the face of a cliff, as the token casualty was helplessly strapped to the stretcher. Should ropes slip or rocks give way beneath the novice stretcher bearer's feet, instinctive reflexes prevailed. Nor was it a case of the ancient sailing-ship dictum, one hand for the ship and one for the sailor; the wartime rule, "Tough Shit," meant both hands for the stretcher bearer and "Goodbye" for the "casualty." Lacking volunteers the sergeant regularly chose from among those high on his "shit list." A vivid memory remains of Private Muck's experience as a "casualty."

"Muck," a whining mama's boy from the big city, earned his title by writing home to his mother complaining how much he disliked wearing mukluks, Eskimo footgear adapted by the army for survival in deep snow. Muck's mother took his complaint, "my toes are never warm enough," to her Congressman who, in turn, had passed it to the War Department which dispatched it down the chain of command till it eventually reached our staff sergeant. At the top of his lungs in army rhetoric he conducted a three-minute investigation of cold toes in mukluks with Muck frozen at attention before him. For as long I was with the outfit the sergeant never passed up an opportunity to assign Muck the dirtiest duty.

There hangs Muck, on a bitterly cold day, terror-stricken, strapped catawampus to a dangling stretcher, swinging back and forth across the face of a cliff, clawing at passing handholds and screaming for help. Above, the sergeant, fixed like a red-faced gargoyle on the edge of a precipice, hurling down threats and obscenities conveyed to me a great lesson of army life. When push comes to shove, or slip comes to fall, the powerful are much more likely to survive than the weak, compassion turned inside out.

Though the underlying dynamics of my indelible army experiences may be unclear to me, they still serve as rough tools in understanding the "human" in medical practice. They are with me forever, called to mind with the least scent of sweat heavy wool, the rank odor of a neglected toilet, unwelcome memories of enforced barracks intimacy. To this day a serving of creamed beef on toast, the soldier's SOS, shit on a shingle, cramps my stomach.

Brighter memories of army life are treasured as well, camaraderie around a campfire in a snowy bivouac, the wild joking of comrades crawling together beneath machine gun fire, the hubris of a busman's holiday spent on a seventy-two-hour pass climbing four fourteen-thousand-foot peaks in a day. The bliss of heading out of camp with a weekend pass to Colorado Springs in my pocket, hopping a passing freight train to ride through the stunning spectacle of a Rocky Mountain springtime, atop a lurching boxcar, shouting for the sheer joy of being alive, transformed, body and soul, into a latter-day Don Quixote, a celebrant, knight-errant of the Wild West.

Combat training ended abruptly with a brief notice on the company bulletin board announcing that the Army Specialized Training Program

(ASTP) sought volunteers for training to meet the army's need for advanced medical technicians. I applied, was provisionally accepted, and again was on my way to become a physician.

Education by Caring

There has never, not for a moment, been doubt that my early experiences moved me to the practice of medicine. The bearings of my emotional compass were set by my family, poor, yet never, no matter how slim the larder, accepting charity from anyone but other family members.

I was born in 1921 which made me a child of the Great Depression (1929-1939). I knew the immediate fear and lasting confusion that accompanies foreclosure on the family home. Unmerited as that catastrophe was—my father could not find work—I came to appreciate my parents' burden of defeat, if only from their mutual recriminations. Mother, Father, and I retreated to my maternal grandparents made-over summer home in what is now suburban Long Island. My grandparents rented their Brooklyn home to join us, the better we might all survive by pooling slim resources. Concern for money clouded childhood. It hastened me through high school. At sixteen I was off on a meager scholarship to premature independence at college.

In childhood, temporary escape from grinding money worries came each July with a visit, sans parents, to the summer home of my aunt and uncle, far out on the north shore of Long Island Sound. Days of swimming, sailing, fishing, and clam digging, unstructured play with cousins exploring the endless delights of the outdoors, ignited a lasting sense of adventure which glows as an inextinguishable lust for "being in it," the confidence of lively doing. At home, it was my maternal grandmother, mother, and father, probably in that order, but not my grandfather who shaped me to my future.

Granddad

In more ways than one, my step-grandfather was a second thought in our family. He was short of both stature and manner, living in our home but not in my life. Grandmother had married him five years after the death of her first husband, my mother's father, whose abrupt departure left grandmother to support and rear her four children, a daunting responsibility fulfilled without record of complaint.

How Grandmother and Granddad worked things out between them was never clear, as he knew only how to command. He had run away to sea from his boyhood home in Nova Scotia, eventually to become a ship's captain. Once landed by my grandmother he lost his command position, leaving him so taciturn he gave the impression that there was nothing he might even wish to talk about. This was unfortunate, for his years at sea must have left him with a cargo of tales of derring-do, but as we never became either friends or enemies it is only a guess. In my hearing, his only remark on his sailing past came during a house call by a physician caring for Grandmother. Granddad was ushered from the bedroom as the doctor wished to examine Grandmother in private. Bursting with indignation, Granddad stormed out, proclaiming, "I have seen a lot more than that in the cat houses of Rio." Apparently this was his only account of thirty years at sea.

Grandmother

Grandmother was the sun, the sustaining warmth, about which the four of us, Granddad, Mother, Dad, and I revolved. We lived together, first in her Brooklyn home. Then, after my parents' misbegotten attempt at independence—they bought a house in Little Neck six months before the Market crash of 1929—we all ended up together again in Grandmother's cottage in Sea Cliff. There four of the five of us lived out the remainder of our lives.

Grandmother once, and I believe only once, openly acknowledged me the favorite of her eight grandchildren, but that is enough to convince any child. An eminently practical woman, reserved in manner, statuesque in bearing, Grandmother believed the best education was not to be found in classrooms but in the "college of hard knocks." In keeping with her practicality she felt little good would come of me unless I went into business (to work) as soon as possible for I should be "out there, making my way in the world."

Though it might not sound so, my grandmother's practicality was never narrow, governed as it was more by prudence than by particularity. Two days before I left for college, nearly penniless, she took me to a Brooklyn bank where she cashed her lifelong savings, her "sock," two shares of American Telephone and Telegraph. Straight out, without a word, she gave me the one hundred and ten dollars to which she added a hug and the blessing of a sweet smile.

My grandmother returns from deep memory accompanied by the delicious aroma of baking bread. Her kitchen was her office and here she met with her Sunshine Ladies to discuss their projects. Grandmother founded the Sunshine Society with a mission of ensuring that every pregnant woman of the impoverished immigrants in our Brooklyn neighborhood receive a quart of fresh, pasteurized milk daily until her child was delivered and weaned. For Grandmother sharing was as much a part of life as breathing. Insensibly, out of her sustained grace under chronic stress, she bestowed on me a sense of social beneficence which remains, today, a talisman of certainty in following compassion's way.

Dad

My father, without steady work for ten years, spent the Great Depression peddling Hoover vacuum cleaners door-to-door, quietly accepting the family's judgment of him as a wreck of unforgotten imagination and unfulfilled promise. His father had been a Brooklyn roofer and union organizer, who died prematurely of a heart attack during a political wrangle at union headquarters. That long departed grandfather left my father, his two brothers and sister, and my widowed paternal grandmother adrift and penniless. My father left his boyhood home, perforce at the age of seventeen, to wander.

In a burst of young man's independence my father took the train from New York City to Washington, D.C., the lifetime limit of his scope of travel. He found work as a stack boy in the Library of Congress but failed to prosper. I never knew why but the family put it down to "reading on the job."

His work record was spotty. At one time he studied to become a court stenographer. Though eventually a shorthand expert he never secured a position to use his skills, a flaw attributed by my mother to his "living with his head in the clouds." Her judgment mattered little to me for nightly he invited me to join him there in his "clouds." Far above our depressing world he read aloud from the wide world of literature. With obvious satisfaction he would say, "It does not cost a penny to read as long as you get the books back to the library on time."

His custom of reading aloud supplied the foundation for my growing imaginative understanding. Without prescription he nurtured a persistent curiosity in me for what might lie beyond immediate encounters.

Generously, he equipped me with words and vision for searching humanity's horizons.

His attention to my mind, though he did not acknowledge it as such, also endowed me with a participatory approach to learning. We had a Sunday custom, ritual is too self-conscious a word, of visiting museums at a time when museums were free. Here, without lecture or obvious direction, he drew me into knowledge as an interactive experience. My mother went along for the ride but generally waited outside on a bench while we cruised the exhibits, complaining we walked too far and too fast.

Of a Sunday evening we would line up outside New York's Museum of Natural History to peer through a telescope at the rings of Saturn or the craters of the Moon. I was too short to reach the eyepiece so Dad would boost me up, supporting me in more ways than I then realized. Quietly, perhaps unintentionally, he shaped my wish to be a scientist.

Not that my approach to education was without its social cost. As a bumptious, flaming redhead of nine I volunteered (on the basis of having listened to the record) to sing the Soldiers' Chorus from Faust to the grade-school assembly. Wisely, Miss Sears, our teacher, deflected this potentially embarrassing offer by suggesting, instead, I play the lead role of Peter Minuet in our fourth-grade production of The Purchase of Manhattan Island from the Indians. It was a smash hit.

Participatory education went into higher gear when, at the age of fourteen, I decided to enter the field of science by the back door. It was not difficult. I went to the main office of the Carnegie Institute of Research, Division of Genetics, Cold Spring Harbor, where I knew scientists worked, and asked for a job, any job. For two high-school summer vacations I worked alone in a windowless basement room, circled by a dense cloud of feral fruit flies, *Drosophila melanogaster*, the Institute's experimental animal. They were bred by *real* scientists for experiments in genetics. Occasionally when delivering clean bottles to the laboratories upstairs I would surreptitiously inspect them, awed by the shiny equipment and walls covered with diagrams of fruit fly chromosomes, breathing deeply the pervasive and delicious odor of acetone and alcohol.

My regular assignment in the basement was cleaning moldy slop of molasses and flour from the bottoms of half-pint milk bottles, the flies' "cages." As the cleanup boy, each day I collected baskets of used bottles at the doors of the laboratories upstairs, carried them down to my hole, scooped out the ripe and rotting media, soaked the bottles in tubs, scrubbed each bottle with a brush, and returned them, shiny clean, to be autoclaved in laboratories above.

It was a lonely job. No scientist, nor, for that matter, anyone but my supervisor ever spoke to me. However, I discovered a daily recreation for sustaining the spirit. As the name implies, Cold Spring Harbor has a cold spring, which bubbles up through the Institute's lawn. Each morning before descending into my fly-infested purgatory I would place a quart bottle of fresh milk in the old-fashioned wooden cooling box through which the spring was channeled. At lunch break, I ascended from my dark fetid hole and made for the spring. Then, under a great overhanging maple tree I could lean back, drink the deliciously cold milk, munch a sandwich, and survey the beautiful scene, white clouds sailing across a bright blue sky over bobbing ships in the quiet harbor. My introduction to the reality of science was a solitary, hands-on experience, young hands fixed firmly to the lowest rung. There I learned that original knowledge results from sweat as well as thought, though the thinker may not always do the sweating.

The lasting effect of my father's custom of reading aloud to me merits more detail and context. One winter we marched through the works of Charles Dickens. Nor was his selection limited to one author, or one genre. He led a parade of thinking minds and doing people through my early years, thoughtfully introducing me to them and the beauties of the English language. He would patiently pause at each word new to me to ask if I knew what it meant and if I did not, explained it in ways I understood.

The list of our disparate friends, visitors from the public library, ran from the adventurer Richard Haliburton to Peck of *Peck's Bad Boy,* a hilarious, long-forgotten account of Victorian mischief heaped by an inventive lad on an ever-suffering father. Dad delighted in comparing how Richard Haliburton had climbed the walls of the Taj Mahal to swim under the moonlight in its reflecting pools with Mark Twain's nighttime adventure of jumping ship in Piraeus harbor to sneak into forbidden Athens, clamber up the Acropolis, and visit the Parthenon by the moonlight. It was unadulterated shared enjoyment until I fell asleep and was carried off to my bed.

The physical circumstances of my father's reading reinforced the intimacy of the tales. After dinner dishes were washed, my mother and father bundled up in their bed, recognized, in retrospect, as a means of saving on the cost of heating our home. With me ensconced between them, Father would open to the place in *Pickwick Papers* or *Don Quixote* where he had stopped the night before and we would resume our worldwide journey, sharing vicariously in tragedies and triumphs of our friends. This band of gay and tragic characters joined the humor, banter, and feeling of our daily life. An affirmative answer to a pointed question could be straight from *David Copperfield,* "Barkis is willing." Though he never remarked on my difficulty with spelling, he might put an edge on his praise of a commendable report card, with a quote from Gray's *Elegy In A Country Graveyard,* "and yet the wonder grew that one small head could hold all that it knew."

My father, more a misfit than a ne'er-do-well, had an exasperating habit of allowing opportunity to slip through his fingers. His "failures," never dangerous nor obviously irresponsible, arose from his lifelong distraction from purpose, a combination of annoying absentmindedness and passive contrariness that courted the bad luck which inevitably cost him jobs, wealth, and friends.

His unreliable witnessing to the task at hand passed over me as a lad, later it roiled me. He was forever a kid among kids, sharing a bag of jelly beans, a pocketful of Tootsie Rolls, stepping up for a swing at the ball in his Sunday best. He would administer artful, unanticipated kicks in the pants by raising his leg behind him and swiveling to kick the unsuspecting bystander. The kick was intended to raise the spirits of his victim while his cry, "Pedestilcologue," his neologism, identified the assault as playful. Family members seldom laughed but voiced the common opinion that he could never come to much. Nor could any rebuttal be raised to such judgment of failed ambition in a man who defined wealth, a condition he never knew, as the ability to buy a book whenever you might desire.

His lifelong ability to heedlessly turn immediate goodwill into long-term exasperation recurred immediately after I was called to active duty. I was at Camp Upton, the army transfer center near the eastern end of Long Island. Dad had finally landed a wartime job on the assembly line at Grumman Aircraft. From the Long Island Railroad timetables, he worked out when my train west to Camp Hale would pass directly by the Bethpage factory. Sure enough, as the train whizzed by the factory there he was, accompanied by half the assembly line crew cheering and waving placards, "Good luck Ralphie." With one of his head-in-the-clouds ideas my father stopped Grumman's wartime airplane production cold for thirty minutes. The send-off gave me a magnificent lift but was probably noted in Dad's personnel file by an irate foreman as flagrant unreliability.

He remained improvident to the end of his days. As a young man I went around town after his funeral and paid off his many petty debts, his unfulfilled promises to pay. With the passage of time I have come to think of his "flaw" of character as his lack of respect for the child who was father to his man. He lived this child rather than integrating that part of himself into a wider vision of what he might accomplish with his considerable talents as a man. One of the unintentional bounties of his "childish" attitude was to leave ample room in my mind for the wonder of ideas.

Mom

Mom, unlike Dad, was ever one for sharing the workings of her heart. He never burdened me with any unfulfilled aspirations, leaving to her the construction of the engine of my ambition which has taken years, seventy, for me to understand.

My mother was an affectionate woman as well as bright. She could complete the Sunday *Times* crossword puzzle by Monday evening. She was short, yet obese enough to never be considered petite. High regard for personal appearance never permitted her to be seen in public in any shoe but spike high heels. Her character was not flawed so much as damaged. The sudden death of her father to pneumonia when she was five together with at twenty-five the horrifying death to diphtheria of her first child, my antenatal sister, left her forever fearful of impending loss, raw with unslakable anxiety.

Mom was a full caldron of discontents that daily ran over, sloshing unresolved feelings helter-skelter under dense clouds of steamy opinion. In contrast less frequent volcanic explosions were severe, prostrating her. Having blown herself apart over, to me, some insignificant matter she would call out, "Ralphie, get the witch hazel." I would fetch the bottle from the bathroom cabinet for her to wreathe her head in a doused cloth and take to her bed for days. Despite undercover activity as agent provocateur my customary role was more than aide. By supplying solace for her suffering, each recovery reaffirmed her belief that her beloved

Ralphie would make up to her all she had suffered and lost. The rest of the family distanced themselves from these episodes with cool dismissal, "That is only Grace."

Though Mother was the obvious source of my red hair, for many years I stoutly maintained that, unlike her, I lacked the fiery temper reputed to go with the color. My insistent denials sometimes led to violence. For example, when taunted by my grade-school classmate, Roy Janson, with "Red, Red, Hot head!" I went on to make the point of my personal imperturbability by bloodying his nose. Considered "spunky" by our gang, no one ever called me anything but Ralph.

My mother's well-intentioned approach to education was founded on her rock-bottom belief that what was obvious to her should be obvious to me. She had been an excellent speller in school while, in contrast, through some quirk of cerebral wiring now recognized as dyslexia, written words with "m" and "n" were interchangeable if not indistinguishable to me. At my teacher's encouragement Mother conducted make-up classes at home which invariably started with the simple explanation that written "m" had three hills and "n" had two. Despite her straightforward approach, the problem of my misaligned cortical networks left me awkwardly guessing at such words as the many-hilled "mannerism." Frequently, the lesson ended up with both of us crying, she from exasperation at my "willful defiance" and me from having my hair pulled and my head banged on the table.

The lesson learned from my hopeless encounter with spelling is neither dread of spelling nor fear of tests but the lasting conviction that it is wise to make the best peace possible with myself and others about that which I can neither know nor ever accomplish.

However, she did empower my ability to listen. My solicited and not subtly enforced support included hearing out her plaints. If feeling well she would lay out a snack of bread and strawberry jam for me after school. As I ate, she confided, sometimes by the hour, the wrongs and injustices the day had brought her.

From time to time she would seek consultation, "Ralphie, do you think my nagging has been too hard on your father?" Aware that she was as unlikely to take my advice as she was to take anyone's, I would bridge the question with another question, "Mom, is there any more jam?" It nearly always worked. However, when she got around to "I did not want to tell you yesterday but…," I knew the focus was shifting to a personal shortcoming and lit out as soon as possible. Hers was a familial third degree that taught me how to accumulate facts to my own advantage while reading nuances of body language. Unwittingly she equipped me with the means of subverting her motives and behaviors while in the pursuit of my own advantage. Paradoxically, in her eyes I could never do wrong.

My ostensible willingness to serve Mom had its rewards. What she asked for, implicitly demanded, I ran to get. Initially my obedience not only concealed my countervailing sabotage but expressed my love of her. I would run upstairs to get her glasses, or rush off with her letters, posthaste to the mailbox, go to the store to buy a pound of sugar or other item she had neglected to purchase—little chores which she might easily have done for herself. The role of dutiful son, moppet, lackey, served to weld our evolving bond. Once, exasperated by my mother's effusive call for me to break off playing with other children, to be a "good boy and come and get me the newspaper on the porch table," my Aunt Mildred muttered loud enough for all to hear, "Has a mother ever loved a son the way Grace does?" Under the burden of relentless requests for support and service my love for my mother gradually crystallized into equivocal rhetoric and habitual response.

Mom was the only family member who unfailingly reinforced my wish to be a doctor. The others, without exception, threw cold water on the idea, predicting there would never be money for me to go to college, let alone medical school. The *quid pro quo* for my mother's unflagging support did not fall due until I had graduated from medical school and my father died. Mom was left with the cottage and my father's Social Security which would not quite cover her expenses. She explained to me that though she might take job training and support herself, as she was the mother of a doctor it would be improper for her to work. She expected me to support her which I did dutifully until she died. As "Mom" turned into "Mother" we settled for a relationship in which the spontaneity of love solidified into obligatory duty.

A Child's Renunciation of Compassion

I was not an uninvolved bystander in the suffering of our family. As a child I was a prankster, regularly thinking up tricks to torment my mother. One trick was playing Tarzan, climbing into tall hickory trees that lined the street wending down to the local stores. There I would hide, high in the sunlit boughs, waiting for my mother as she returned, heavy laden, from her shopping. Once she was below I would dangle from a swaying bough, calling out in a voice of boyish innocence, "Look Mother, I am as high as Tarzan." Predictably, it prompted her immediate alarm and a pleading command, "Oh, Ralphie, come down! You are going to fall and kill yourself. Come right down!" To which I would call back, a lie, "I do not know how to get down."

As she hurried off to call the fire department for help, the end game consisted of scrambling down the tree and off through a backyard shortcut to await her breathless arrival at the front door. The denouement came with, "Thank God, you are safe," followed by a hug and, "Ralphie, you will be the death of me yet."

It was a safe game as she seemed incapable of recognizing me for what I was, straight-out malevolent devil. For her I might be mischievous, but never a tormentor of the soul that loved me best. The reward was certain as I could always count on being received again as her blessed angel rather than the provocative imp I was.

It may seem harsh to consider a nine-year-old boy's behavior as evil, but the motive condemns the act, joyful exploitation of my mother's abject anxiety at the loss of my sister. Perverse, creative imagination was at the heart of it. I plead guilty to repeated sinning against her.

Another example should make the point indelibly. My mother's brother, Uncle Ed, lived a short distance from our Little Neck home. However, unlike ours, his family lived beyond the pall of the Depression. Consequently, their home was in an upscale neighborhood blooming with new construction. One of the joys of visiting my cousins was the game of cowboys-and-Indians played in the staked-out lots, bulldozed yet unpaved streets, and the forbidden delight of tracking through partially constructed houses.

A highlight of these shenanigans came on discovering the open manhole of a new storm sewer. It was no trick for me, a slim and agile kid, to clamber down into the five-foot main and in a hunched shuffle cruise its mysterious, branching passageways. The conduits were redolent with the aroma of fresh mortar and spookily illuminated by dim sunlight filtering down through the bars of the curbside drains.

With a bit of doing, I located the curb drain nearest my uncle's home. Crouched there, I waited for my mother who was inside at one of Aunt Mildred's bridge parties. Once the party broke up, though the women coming down the steps could not be seen, I was sure of my mother's presence and let out a low moan, "Oh, Mother." It failed to do the job, so finally I shouted, "Does anyone know how to get out of here?" Closer to the truth would have been to ask if anyone besides myself knew the way out.

Her ear tuned by maternal instinct, my mother heard the cry but from where she knew not. She responded instantly, "Ralphie, where are you?"

"Here Mother, right down here."

Tracing my voice to the underground vault at her feet, she let out a cry, "Oh, my God, he is in the sewer!"

The other ladies gathered round the real victim, my mother, while I shouted up through the drain that is was just a joke and I would be out as fast as I could run. One insightful lady suggested I deserved to stay there as it was as mean a trick as she had ever seen. My mother collapsed in the front seat of the waiting car, seething with mixed feelings, lamenting, "This is why mothers grow gray."

Predictably, I was welcomed back into my mother's arms as her saved child. It came with an inadequate dollop of punishment once we returned home. Dutifully I listened as she recounted the serious consequences of the little boy who cried wolf. Her lesson passed me by, for the tales I responded to came from *Peck's Bad Boy*, so enjoyably read aloud by my tolerant father. The moral of these escapades, I fear, is that wicked malice flourishes in the breast of mankind earlier and stronger than any bud of compassion.

Compassion Revealed

Insight, the grace of wisdom unbidden, is a blessing that need never pass without gratitude. The mysterious ability of the human mind to suddenly rearrange seemingly irrelevant details into a new and encompassing concept marks the march to maturity. For me, insight seems to be the way my heart has of telling my mind what it is really thinking by insistently repeating that the whole of life is greater than the sum of its parts.

In 1944, as an army private, First Class, I was transferred to New York University–Bellevue Medical School. The first year went by in a haze of lectures, dismembered bodies, books, and drill. In the second year the introductory course in medicine was taught in the Twenty-eighth Street Building, directly across First Avenue from Bellevue Hospital. The building's brownstone facade was heavily cloaked with New York grime. Its foyer, with a scuffed marble floor, opened on the right to the dean's office; straight ahead it offered a decrepit, wire-caged elevator reluctantly promising to deliver students to lecture halls, laboratories, and the formaldehyde-reeking anatomy room above; and, to the left, a large oak door opened into the University Clinic, maintained more for teaching than for charity.

In turn the clinic's door opened into a large, dark room with lofty ceilings. Within, crowded rows of wooden benches were intentionally uncomfortable, the better to dissuade docile charity patients from loitering. There the poor waited to be examined, diagnosed, and treated by medical students. The room's dirty windows let in meager sunlight, necessitating a green-shaded reading lamp for the factotum who called out the patients' names, dispatching them to cubicles in the examining room still deeper in the building.

Second-year medical students worked under the watchful eye of teachers in the examining room, the size of an assembly hall. Its decor was typical nineteenth-century white monochrome, the floor a maze of small, white hexagonal tiles while the walls were tiled in large, rectangular, white squares, waist high. Along one wall, sinks and large basins were available for students to wash their hands and disinfect their instruments. Token privacy was afforded by cubicles of flimsy, muslin drapes, strung from overhead wires. The room was an uninviting, public space, devoid of any suggestion of intimacy or confidentiality yet pretending to be private. The ambiance, wartime frugality, intensified charity's threadbare tradition.

Here, in ill-fitting white coats pulled over full military uniforms, students were exposed to the rudiments of the art and science of medicine. We learned how to rub a cold stethoscope warm before applying it to a patient's chest, just how hard to tap a knee with a rubber hammer, how to percuss the outline of an enlarged liver, and generally to conduct ourselves so as not to drive a patient from the room in alarm or despair.

Assigned that rainy afternoon to a cubicle, I found a young woman perched tensely on a low stool beside the examining table. Uncomfortably shifting from foot to foot, I introduced myself and then sidled onto the examining table from which lofty position I took her medical history.

She explained that she was suffering from a headache. Her family had a history of similar symptoms. Centering questions on the duration of her pain and examining its site produced a host of textbook details of normal physiology and presumed pathology but did little to help me make sense of her condition. My goal, securing a passing grade, appeared in jeopardy. Consequently, intending to minimize risk I ruled out brain tumor, meningitis, and stroke as best I could and settled for the obvious diagnosis, chronic sinusitis.

Once I had my mind made up I relaxed, waiting for the instructor to part the curtains and hear me out. But then a bout of authentic curiosity set in. Somehow her condition seemed to call for more than a prescription for nose drops and advice to take aspirin for her headaches. I began wondering who she was, really was.

By now we had exchanged positions. She was sitting high on the examining table while I, on the stool, scribbled notes in the chart. The case seemed too easy. Thinking "medicine must be more than this," I asked her, "Is there something more that brought you to the clinic?"

Clutching the meager sheets over her partial nakedness she paused, blushed, and suddenly began sobbing. Startled, I said nothing. While voices from other cubicles drifted through the curtains we sat without speaking until she regained control of herself. Then she blurted out, "It's my job."

Hesitantly, a tale of fear and confusion unfolded. A few months before she had come from upstate New York seeking war work in New York City. She had no trouble finding a job sewing buttons onto army uniforms in a garment district sweatshop. Nor did she have trouble with the work itself. But she was confused by her fellow workers. "I don't know what to make of what is going on around me."

"Going on around you?" I repeated. After another sob and a pause she recounted how there were twenty other women in the loft where she worked. The line crew of women was directed by men who set quotas and collected finished uniforms. The men also solicited sexual favors which the girls on the line willingly bestowed at work and after hours. The patient had no difficulty in drawing a line with the importuning men but she did not know what to make of the pressure from the other women. She wondered if, as they said, it was her patriotic duty to "join the party."

Nothing in my clinical course had prepared me for this development in a routine history and physical. Concealing, as best I could, my confusion, I held my tongue as she continued to weep quietly. At last, aware of my silence, she wiped away her tears with the edge of the sheet and asked, "Do you think I should go along and join the crowd?"

Rather than pass judgment where it might do harm, I gently questioned her, "You said you got along well with your parents and came to work simply to help with the war effort. Why not go back upstate and find some other way to help?"

Her face brightened. "You mean I could go home?"

"It is an alternative." She rubbed her nose on the sheet and then murmured a most perplexing observation, "Oh, how you help. You should be a priest."

Our encounter had exceeded the allotted time and my mentor was at the drapes. I excused myself, stepped outside the cubicle to report, *sotto voce*, the case history and physical together with a recommended treatment of aspirin and nose drops. My teacher looked solemn, asking if I had applied digital pressure over both frontal sinuses, a way of determining the degree of inflammation. I had not, but expressed gratitude for the information. He finished up with the suggestion I should endeavor to work faster.

I never saw the young lady again. The nurse had her dressed and out before I returned. But that mattered little. What did matter, at least for me, was her diagnosis of me, better a priest than a doctor. I remain grateful to her for her heartfelt way of awakening the healing power of compassion to my consciousness.

Endowed with this lass's insight I began my lifelong journey into the world of human suffering, searching for meaning in suffering, repeatedly finding it in companions' sharing. *Compassion's Way* recounts many of these adventures but not until late in the journey did the full import of who was with me and how they shared in the work of living finally dawn upon me. I leave to the reader the possibility of discovering in what follows my unspoken mission which echoes forever in my life. At the end of these unbidden experiences, the last, "Chartres and the Accidental Pilgrim," opened my heart to who I am. Perhaps, this late adventure into soul reveals the author better than any other words might. Thus a beginning and end can be made of the author.

Part 1

Compassion Wakened

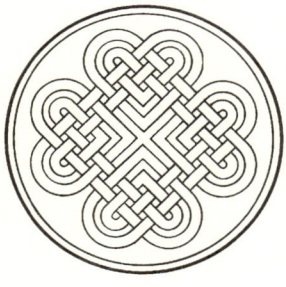

And the day-star arise in your hearts
—II Peter 1:19

Overview to Part 1

With just-around-the-corner suffering so common, accidents, losses, illness complicated by mankind's infinite proclivity to inflict heartache on others, why is the experience of compassion so uncommon? The signposts of civility, fellow feeling and forbearance are plainly posted, pointing the path to compassion. But no, as my grandmother was wont to say, there are none so blind as those who can yet will not see. An exploration of the ways in which we blind ourselves to the vast emotional world seething about us follows, starting with a review of **Fellini's *Satyricon***, useful in uncovering expert pigheadedness.

Considered awareness of possibilities opens the way, strewn with brambles and flowers, for an awakened mind. **Oh, Where Is the Balm of Gilead?** celebrates the debt physicians owe their childhood perceptions, subtle gifts which ensure physicians remain alive to the human condition. At the same time, musing about the patient's circumstances stands in stark contrast to a sharply fixed "scientific" interest, which, ironically, may handicap a doctor. The blunder of diagnosing to the doctor's satisfaction rather than for the patient's need for care may be good science but is poor treatment.

No physician should ever deny him/herself the healing power that accompanies respectfully sharing the smell, the sound, the pain of a patient's suffering. Shared suffering remains the physician's prime defense against slipping into the role of technician. For the patient, shared suffering is the bulwark against despair.

Understanding how feelings are shared is further explored in **The Other Side of Charity**. The give and take that goes with serving the needy illuminates a fearful yet hidden trade-off of varnished vanity and personal power against stifled chagrin and chronic impotence. This dynamic is inevitably at work in the hearts of caring physicians as it is in the bowels of patients.

Anomie, soul threatening, waste of the capacity to feel, is the darkest side of compassion. Physicians, repeatedly exposed to human suffering, perhaps are more vulnerable than others to atrophy of caring. Once the glory of medical school graduation subsides into routine practice, caring can become a chore rather than a continuing experiment in being. Then, with the arrival in the consulting room of dissatisfied Mrs. Querulous, yet again complaining of ill-defined symptoms, demanding ever more powerful prescriptions for tranquillity, a doctor's high dedication can wither into dry dross of unrequited duty.

Leprosy, A Disease of the Heart explores the paradox of how the pursuit of medical identity may endanger personal identity. The devastating leprosarium experience left such anguish in my heart that I fasted one day a month for the following ten years to assure time and reflection for healing that wound.

The emotion, compassion, comes with a price tag many physicians fail to examine. We practice without precise accounting of personal cost in holding fast to the care of "hopeless" patients. Like staring into the sun, there is a point beyond which the perception of suffering becomes too painful for close consideration. Who has the strength to loiter at the gates of hell?

Consequently, reflection on intense suffering is easily put out of mind as the clinician moves on to the next patient. Yet buried co-suffering can remain a nidus of professional disintegration deep in a doctor's being. During World War I, medical science diagnosed the destruction of personality wrought by overexposure to suffering as shell shock; more recently the diagnosis has become post-traumatic stress syndrome. The reverberations of intense suffering may be lifelong. Beyond a personal limit on the capacity to care, which exists for all but saints, even the kindest, wisest, most proficient of physicians dare not pass. There is no healing in a physician defeated by emotion.

The Quality of Mercy reminds us that compassion is found in the least of things, asking but a moment's reflection to awaken and refresh the spirit.

Mercy, forbearance informed by compassion, stands counterpoint to ubiquitous human suffering as it awakens caring souls to a larger meaning of service, to fully caring while effectively serving. Though mercy may not answer the "why" of suffering, it does inform human suffering through shared humanity. Here lies the succor patients desire. When nurtured by a healing, medical imagination, the patient-doctor relationship fosters merciful hearts as it does sensible minds.

Despite pain, suffering, and fatigue, patient and physician can awaken to a wider world where reward no longer is limited to curing disease but lies in discovering the grace of suffering healed.

Suffering identifies both patient and doctor. Ask someone writhing in the clutches of renal colic who they are and the answer is as complete as their pain-shrunken identity allows, "The patient." Suffering's corrosion of identity may not be clearly seen, but when in the presence of a dying patient, the caring physician perforce identifies him/herself, "I am the doctor."

In spite of any personal wish to see ourselves competent and complete against the background glow of successful accomplishment, physicians are as well defined by agony as by joy. In the grip of mortal circumstances, suffering gives deeper meaning to our lives but only when shared with a merciful, fellow human being. Co-passion in the suffering indelibly identifies the merciful and the sufferer, both. Compassion awakens our identity to what we, as human beings, may be.

In Defense of Fellini's *Satyricon*
A Film Review

Sunt bona, sunt quaedam mediocria, sunt mala plura
Quae legis hic; aliter non fit, Avite, liber.
—Martial (ca 40 A.D. - ca 103 A.D.)
Book One, Epigram XVI
(There are good things, there are some indifferent, there are more things bad that you read here. Not otherwise, Aviter, is a book produced.)

The experience of the awakening of compassion begins for us with a look at *Fellini Satyricon*, a controversial film that encompasses health and sickness and diverse aspects of mankind with all its individual variations. As compassion awakens in us, it allows a profound belief in human possibility.

A particularly glaring example of the physician as superficial art critic appeared in the movie review pages of two medical journals. Luckily I had seen Fellini's *Satyricon* before I read what the reviewers in *MD* and *Medical Aspects of Human Sexuality* had to say about the film: "…a fevered, dull, and belabored parade of degenerate passion and repetitive orgies." "The net effect is a monumental waste of time and talent…."[1] "In our opinion nothing redeems Fellini's *Satyricon* from its disjointed development and freakish atmosphere. The orgies, scourges of war and punishment… with its artificial blood and love scenes among men and boys…in the best of cases are merely disgusting."[2]

Perhaps these medics-turned-critics expected a Cecil B. deMille production of ancient Rome, a celluloid cliché which runs its course properly without offending our sensibilities. Actually Fellini's *Satyricon* was called *Fellini Satyricon* because a fly-by-night version of *Satyricon* was produced as word went out that Fellini was working on the Petronius masterpiece. The superficial *Satyricon* was produced for just this Hollywood-conditioned audience. Could the medical movie reviewers have seen the wrong picture?

Fellini's film is a picaresque tale of two ne'er-do-wells afloat in an extravagant culture. One escapes and the other goes under. But any attempt to describe the film is like trying to describe a work of art: there is always the danger of reducing the Mona Lisa to a quarter of a pound of canvas and three ounces of lead pigment. The critic's job is not to describe but to interpret.

If an honest man is to be an honest critic, he must see and think with three sets of consciousness: his own, the artist's, and the audience's. When the difficulties of understanding one's own consciousness are compounded by the need to follow the workings of an artistic mind while remaining attuned to the countless responses of his fellowmen, it is readily apparent that not many succeed as critics. We have produced few H.L. Menckens and A.J. Nocks and those that make the grade are never suffered to become national heroes. The protagonist for what is good in this culture, Eumolpo the poet, seldom speaks of morals though he talks continually of values—ah, what material for the critic—the fourth dimension of the ancient consciousness.

Symbolic: Again, as in any masterpiece, there is a story within a story and so on back into the heart of the creation. These hidden stories are there not to encumber the production nor to serve as material for some future Ph.D. thesis, but simply because artistic creation demands a wheel in a wheel, a multidimensional artistic structure completely interconnected in all its parts. That is why masterpieces can be reexamined, reread, reviewed, again and again to reveal yet sweeter humanity. The interrelatedness of their parts is not an exercise in ingeniousness but an expression of genius. Take, for example, the glass eye of Lica, the homosexual slave master. This lurid, offensive detail might very easily be glossed over as garish, but if the viewer reflects, there is a symbolism in this unblinking eye which reappears throughout Fellini's work. It is in *La Dolce Vita* centering in the vile monster that is dragged up on the beach at the end of the orgy. It is an eye that is continually intruding into the lives of the people of *La Dolce Vita,* for it is the lens of the paparazzi, photographers who live by selling their pictures of the lewd and scandalous to an insatiable public. In *Juliet of the Spirits*, this lens-eye is the detective's camera focusing in on the private life of Juliet's husband, destroying her marriage.

Lest you think this symbolism overdrawn, the director has been careful in *Satyricon* to show how close the monster is, for it reappears on Lica's pleasure ship as a great fish hoisted from the sea, ten times larger than the monster of *La Dolce Vita*, and then returns to the sea as Lica's severed head descends beneath the waves. The last that can be seen by the audience is the eye still peering up through the water. The work of Fellini is so rich in symbolism that it is difficult to choose amongst the myriad interconnections. Take swings as another instance. The unbelievable yet plausible opening of *La Dolce Vita*—a statue of Christ suspended beneath a helicopter sailing over Rome. Or the opening of *8 1/2*, a rope dangling down to a host of people sealed in their automobiles. Or that of *Juliet*, with its basket elevator to the sybaritic tree house of the sorceress. Or take *Satyricon*, with the wizard suspended in a sling for all to deride, the great swing in the garden of pleasure. Perhaps some reviewer somewhere, sometime may see these swings as a statement of man's condition, caught as we are between heaven and hell.

Musical: Ah, here is a puzzle for the reviewer to mull over. Is it just the discordant whine of ancient instruments that is the music of *Satyricon* or is it the laughter? Has there ever been a movie in which there has been so much laughter and in such variety? The orchestration of the human laugh runs from the horrid whinny of an old crone to the airy twitter of children at play, from the gladiators' bellow of glee to the giggle of a hetaera, from the sardonic chuckle of a murderer to, literally, a city roaring in worship of Mirth. But despite the suffocating impact of this most ethereal of emotional responses, no comment from previous reviewers.

Religious: Could not someone with a twig of theological interest make something of the worship scenes, the "Mother Goddess" who appears with fire and smoke again and again, or see the nativity scene as humble peasants worship? But the critics were silent.

Mythical: Perhaps some critic with an interest in Shakespeare could be moved to show the similarities of Fellini and Shakespeare in the homosexual theme of the Theseus and Ariadne myth. As the Bard says,

> Our youth got me to play the woman's part,
> And I was trimm'd in Madam Julia's gown...
> For I did play a lamentable part;
> Madam, 'twas Ariadne, passioning
> For Theseus' perjury and unjust flight[3]

But again no comment.

Literary: The theme of two men searching out their world for pleasure and stumbling on wisdom in spite of themselves has been used many times in literature. The antic chase appears in Rabelais, Fielding, and Joyce to name but a few. And should there be a wish to find a literary explanation for the scene in which the poet Eumolpo's heirs eat his body, look to the seventh circle of Dante's *Inferno* for a lurid description of men, death, and cannibalism....But again no comment from our critics....

Contemporary Cinematic: Though the movies, when considered as an art form, are generally referred to as cinema, the critic need not mince words to say that there is an expression of searching which runs through most successful modern films. By underlining the similarities between Joe Buck and Ratso of *Midnight Cowboy*, of Billy and Captain America of *Easy Rider*, with Encolpio and Ascylto in *Satyricon*, he might give more insight into our dangerous times. These people are all of the same fiber. They are the logical outgrowth of our culture which has always believed that two men riding together in search of adventure are sure to succeed, as Hopalong Cassidy and Gabby Hays, as the Cisco Kid and Poncho, as Tonto and the Lone Ranger all once came riding out of the Golden West to teach us this lesson. The wilderness our modern heroes travel through is man-made but the critics did not comment.

Archaeological: I would have appreciated an archaeological critique of *Satyricon*. Was ever a movie imbued with such a wealth of half-hidden truths, clues, and broken shards waiting to be fitted together? Perhaps *Last Year at Marienbad* or *Isabelle*, but few others. The opening shot is of man's most ancient public art form, the decorated wall. If the street was the first social organization of man, the wall may well have been his first public medium. Twenty thousand years ago the men of Lascaux and Altamira were decorating the caves of Europe with their scratchings, drawings, and signs—their hopes and fears. Their graffiti and those of every age since have been the keenest expression of uninhibited art and free speech. So Fellini starts with a Roman wall covered with the scratchings, the pleas, the graffiti of forgotten prisoners of life…and then comes full circle to end his film with crumbling walls, bearing not the earlier rude obscenities but beautiful murals of loving humans. But the significance of it all escaped our critics.

There are other facets the critics might have reflected upon—humor, philosophy, entertainment, cultural dynamics. The science fiction aspects of *Satyricon* alone merit a major essay, which could well be titled *Tom Swift and His Electric Organ*. However, the omissions noted here should make clear that we are in need of thoughtful critics, physicians or others, to give us a glimpse of the artist's majestic, though necessarily clouded, insight. To pick up a gem and say that it weighs five carats is scientifically informative but not human. To say that you do or do not like it is the beginning of insight, but to explain why with a lucidity and limpidity that enable the hearer to appreciate with his own eye and mind is Godlike. It is the soul of all teaching and leads us to grow as humans, in a world too often unnatural and inhuman.

Endnotes

Reprinted from *The Pharos* 34(Fall 1971): 154-160, with permission.
1. "Movie Review: 'Fellini Satyricon,'" *Medical Aspects of Human Sexuality* 4(5): May 1970: 33-34.
2. "Reviews of Films, Theatre, Books," *MD* 14(6): 1970: 238.
3. W. Shakespeare, *Two Gentlemen of Verona*, act 4, sc. 4.

Oh, Where Is the Balm of Gilead?

> *O thou weed,*
> *Who art so lovely fair, and smell'st so sweet,*
> *That the sense aches at thee*
> —William Shakespeare (1564-1616)
> *Othello*, Act IV, 2, 67

I expect to enter my dotage with a vengeance, devoting my final years and energies to a lost scientific cause. What Linus Pauling did for Vitamin C, I plan to do for the therapeutic effects of odors.

Yes, I believe the right smell heals. Although odor therapy is perhaps a lost cause, as neglected as the rhinencephalon itself, I plan to raise a cry among the brethren and, if nothing more, a stink upon the wards. Be forewarned, for by removing the tops of bottles, breaking the seals on packages, and squeezing the tubes of ointment, I expect to free what is left of the frail, fair fragrance of medicine, the balm imprisoned.

How slim is the chance that I will be understood! I see my pursuers now, the Disabled Doctors Committee, and worse, I smell them, odoriferous monstrosities with their poisonous antiperspirants and reeking colognes. There they are, with insensitive noses, barely able to discern between the odor of buttered popcorn and raw gasoline. I will protest to the end (at least until their tranquilizers take the final fight out of me) by proclaiming that the odor of medicine heals, and does more than simply inhibit the metabolism of some lousy microbe. But predictably the only effective odor they will acknowledge will be the one rising from my reputation.

An intolerant attitude on the part of today's "new" and "young" toward my theory is inevitable. However, when I was an intern, it was different. At that time, aberrant theories were not cause for seasoned physicians to be vacuumed off the wards. I so well remember one fine elderly physician whose ungainly gait carried him from bedside to bedside. Around the age of ninety-two, his center of gravity moved up above his center of buoyancy, leaving him in a continual state of instability, lurching and swaying like a ship without ballast. Nevertheless, he held to his practice of listening carefully to the full details of his occasional patients (who were frequently older than he), writing indecipherable notes, and prescribing what has come to be called alternative medicine.

If his patients failed to improve within a day he gave them the full bore of his pharmacopoeia—blueberry juice enemas. Apparently his patients did as well as those of the other physicians, and as the chief of the service always closely reviewed this elderly physician's work, "to learn as much as possible from such a fine clinician," there was never any question of banishing him and his theory from the hospital.

But even though there may be no hope of benign tolerance for me, quixotically I shall pursue my goal, as it moves from a passing fancy to a notion, on to a whimsy, and then, with ever-increasing acceleration, through eccentricity, to an *idée fixe*, concluding as a roaring delusion. This belief that the healing power of medicine resides in its odor was formed with my earliest exposure to curative medicine; no wonder I should expect it to remain with me to the end.

The curative power of fragrance first unfolded for me as a wee child of four. I had the usual sore throats and measles, which were sometimes severe enough to have my mother "call the doctor." I can remember hearing her at the front door anxiously awaiting his arrival, and when he drove up to the house she would put me on my best behavior by softly calling up to me, "The doctor is here."

Then would follow a murmured consultation at the foot of the stairs, followed by his presence. He would check me over, write a prescription; I would take the medicine and promptly get well.

During my convalescence, which I secretly enjoyed for its indulgences, fruit juice and ice cream at my beck and call, I dwelt on the problem of how this powerful man made me feel better. I was intent upon discovering the magic he possessed and like any prisoner, with time on his side, I picked at his secrets a grain at a time until I laid bare the source of his power. The crucial clue lay hidden in his medicine, Brown's mixture, which not only came in a brown bottle and was brown in color, but smelled brown. That was the trick, to make it *smell* brown; any fool could make it look brown, especially in a brown bottle, but to make it savor brown was wizardry.

That was it! The doctor's magic was *smell,* for the overwhelming effect that stayed with me was the unique odor of the man. The fragrance of his clean, cool hands, augmented by the brisk immaculate white odor of his starched cuffs and collar, wafted an extra draught of cleanliness into the magic brew.

Bouquet of Wool

Curiously, there was a metal twang which went with him. It arose from the silver vial for the clinical thermometer which he carried, clipped in his vest pocket next to his pen and special wallet for his prescription pad. It combined with the special piquancy of his cuff links and the gold watch chain that hung across his vest. I know metals such as silver and gold do not have odors, but I swear these did, a tangy metallic odor. Added to this smell was the bouquet of deep, rich, masculine wool, not heavy serge that has a harsh scent, but the aroma of a soft, expensive, brushed worsted, touched ever so lightly with the smoke of fine Cuban cigars.

Lastly, the essence which bore the full fragrance, the musk oil of that good physician's magic perfume, was ether. Ether was in his hair, his skin, his clothes, and carried all the other airs on its hot, sweet redolence. Ether proclaimed him an ultimate wizard in curing the sick. It made him a special man of science, a physician. Manufactured and mixed together by his daily rounds, these magic smells became the man; they announced to every patient, but especially to me, that relief from pain was not far off. The smell of the man was balm itself!

Later, my belief in the efficacy of medical essences was reinforced to final confirmation by our local drug store, an old fashioned ice cream parlour–prescription establishment. As a slip of a lad I spent my summers at the family cottage on a bluff over "the great wet barnyard of Long Island Sound." As a solo practitioner of childhood, an only child, I was given to making swords of broken laths and driving livid dragons out of their lairs among the lilac bushes. In fact, most of my summer days would have been given over to fancy but for my daily chore of walking to the village, a half mile away, to check the mail box at the local post office. My pay was a nickel a trip and with this treasure I would cross the slab, slate sidewalks and narrow, main street, which separated the post office from Schmidt's Drug Store, and enter that marble palace of bewitching smellery.

Schmidt's Drug Store was a wonder to behold. On either side of the open front door were large, curved display windows, containing vast glass vessels filled with translucent colored fluids of the purest reds, greens, and blues. In each window, between the vessels, were large cardboard cross-sections of a human being, diagraming how bile was freed as Dr. Glickam's special salts passed into the mouth, down a chute, and into the stomach. Those windows contained my first lesson in applied human anatomy.

Inside cool, dark, quiet spaciousness established Schmidt's ambiance. A floor of small, white, hexagonal, marble tiles shone at my feet. To the left was a magnificent marble soda fountain, higher than my head. On my right a series of glass cabinets, trimmed with oak, displaying straight razors and safety razors, complete with a portrait of King Camp Gillette propped up at attention, before rows of shaving brushes and leather strops—a monarch leading his troops, against a generation of beards. A far cabinet displayed rubber goods, gay bathing caps surrounded by rings of rubber enema tubing, set off against a background of icebags, hot water bottles, and douches. The wall behind the counter was covered, floor to ceiling, with oak-bound glass-faced compartments patrolled by a trolleyed ladder, easily positioned for reaching the highest, hidden, inaccessible potion.

Air circulation in this palace was uncomplicated, a large, lazy electric fan spun slowly overhead. In the back was the ice cream parlor, with its wire-back chairs and marble tables for the "swells." The back door opened out onto a little garden of tables nestling under a cherry tree.

Sorcerer's Apprentice

My conscious interest centered on the monumental soda fountain on my left for behind it lurked a hunchback who was no taller than I and consequently could only be seen after I had climbed up on a wire stool. There he would be "crouched" at full height, his crooked form in a spotless, fitted, white jacket, his long intelligent face fixed crosswise against the angle of his back—for all the world, the misbegotten attempt of some Merlin to change a white rat into a man, but to me a prince in thrall, a sorcerer's royal apprentice. He never spoke and should a customer ask a question that demanded more than a nod of his head he would scurry to the bell by the stairs and summon down the druggist, Mr. Sniffen. The hunchback's natural lair was behind the counter next to the ice cream freezer, beneath the large "chocolate sprinkles" bowl. From there he would fix his bright eyes on me and patiently wait while I did the boyish thing of slow deciding.

Strange how much thought went into the foregone decision, for no matter how I considered the different flavors of ice cream cones, with sprinkles and without, inevitably I ended up with a large, foaming, ice-cold, aromatic glass of root beer, served up in one of those old fashioned bulging glasses, ensconced in a fluted metal holder. The Russians still use these holders for glasses of hot tea but otherwise I fear that these receptacles, along with the hunchback, may have left the face of the earth.

Spices, Oils, Essences

But like the single-minded old man I predict I will become, I stray from the point—the medicinal odors of that period drug store. All the time that I was slowly sipping the sensuous taste of root beer through a single straw, I was being transfixed by a thousand essences wafting out of all those loose-fitted cabinets, those open jars, and those boxes and barrels of raw crude drugs. Think of the magnitude of the experience—no miserable whiff of burning hemp for my childhood, but rather a king's ransom of spices, oils, and essences, decadently rich oil of cloves, dark cascara sagrada, sharp alum, delightful oil of peppermint, ebullient rubbing alcohol, sweet sassafras, rose blossoms ground into exotic Parisian face powders, unsubtle ipecac, heavy lanolin, penetrating camphor, heady acetone, athletic benzoin, musty ancient arnica, herbs, and spices galore, circling my head, entering my nose, and forever fixing my belief in the essential curability of mankind, while all the time I thought it was the root beer.

So now to those modern measurers of milligrams, those deodorized skeptics of the nose, I issue my challenge, safe in the shadow of Cyrano de Bergerac, and with the certainty of Paracelsus, sure in his iconoclasm, based on the bone-deep belief that "The doctor's character can influence the patient's recovery more than any other medicine." Perhaps my science is too philosophical, too close to cabalistic knowledge and alchemy, but it is simplicity itself. Smells vile in nature make us ill. We retch over yesterday's vomitus. So, just as certainly, other smells, beneficently fragrant, make us well. Smell is the first sense, albeit primitive, yet by it we not only learn to recognize an object, but our noses teach us the object's essence as well.

Please, do not see this all as anti-intellectual humbuggery or, worse, Walt Disney sentimentality. I am no Pecksniff about smells, leading you astray with some queer emotional conviction born of mystical revelation. Neglected, the science of smell is yet a science. Some counter of mouse nasal hairs, some nose for the unique pheromone, some renegade perfume experimenter will eventually flesh out the science of smell for a waiting public. In fact, there is the makings of a Nobel prize in discovering the action of pheromones, those weirdly powerful molecules of insect secretion, capable of seducing, with an insatiable lust, male insects right out of their rudimentary minds.

Inhale to Health

Someday the science of osmology will assert itself. Meanwhile, for me it is enough to know what I know. As the world and managed care regulations become too much, I am assailed with doubt that Hippocrates even existed, then I turn to a magic elixir to refresh my inspiration. I reach across my desk for an old bottle of Sloan's Liniment, intact with the mustachioed portrait of Dr. Sloan, complete with directions in Spanish, Italian, French, Yiddish, Chinese, German, Swedish, Polish, Hungarian, Bohemian, and Portuguese. I like best the admonition, "Recommended as a counter-irritant in flatulence by applying over stomach and bowels and lay on flannel cloth," a case of fighting fire with fire. But for me, the magic need go no further than to unscrew the top and inhale a sniff of what is left of an ancient way to health; at least for me it is a way, plain as the nose on my face.

Endnotes

Reprinted from *Prism* 3 #12(1975): 8-10, with permission. Copyrighted 1975, American Medical Association

The Other Side of Charity

We are double-edged blades, and every time we whet our virtue the return strops our vice.
—Henry David Thoreau (1817-1862)
Walden

Like any human endeavor, charity has many facets, and probably the one least considered is the negative side of charity, the story of the Bad Samaritan.

The positive aspects of charity show a mutuality in the relationship between the donor and the acceptor. Though the exchange of sentiment is often tacit, sometime unconscious, both parties give and take, and both gain. The poor man's thank-you can mean as much as the rich man's dollar.

However, rather than examining the balance of benign emotions in charity, let us consider the presence of malignant feelings in any charitable exchange. Much as we are only now beginning to "see" the other side of the moon, so we are only beginning to see the other side of charity. With the combination of social pressure, technical knowledge, and man's eternal curiosity, charity is emerging as an activity not exclusively for the good. Resentment, surly demands, and curt rejection, as well as riots and taxpayer revolts now color the concept of charity. These unpleasant facts are no more news than the fact the moon has a second side, but to know the moon we must explore all of its sides and to know charity, it is wise to explore all its sides as well.

Recently a local charitable organization, The Abundant Food Program, opened its doors in a nearby community. The charity is intended to disburse surplus food to the hungry. Impelled by curiosity and by generosity to share any knowledge or encouragement which might be useful, I visited the store and consequently learned, for me, a great lesson.

It was summertime and as I pulled up in the parking place alongside two beat-up cars, I could see through the finger-stained windows a passel of children. They were fighting and squabbling in the bored, compulsive fashion typical of neglected children. My entry into The Abundant Food Program agency went unheralded by any prior phone call, nor did my nondescript short-sleeved summer shirt and slacks betray my middle-class identity. As the door closed behind me, I could barely see a low fence which marked off most of the store from public use. Behind the railing to the right was a desk where a tight-lipped, middle-aged woman clerk was pecking at a typewriter. The rear was a dusky maze of alleys and narrow passages made up of stacked boxes. To the left, in the small public area, ten women were sitting on benches along the wall. They were all women—no men—and they were dressed in the shabby style of the poor. One held a baby in a bright new white blanket, but all else was a tattered grayness. Even their skin had the same tattered grayness—the color of sick resignation. Their only expression—apathetic waiting.

The secretary had not looked up from her work. I stepped up to the railing. I waited but she continued typing what seemed an endless pile of cards. A man appeared from the back of the store, and as he made his way out of a narrow alley he gave the secretary a scowl. He passed out through the railing gate and she looked up long enough to scowl back as he disappeared out the front door. There was another wait. Soon the man came back, dragging a dolly with two boxes on it. He made his way through the door, and when I attempted to help him with the gate he scowled at me, then at the secretary, and dragged his load back into the inner recesses.

Nothing happened after he left. The secretary kept on typing. I stood there and as I did the hair gradually rose on the back of my neck. My palms quietly oozed juice, my breath became short, and fast, for into consciousness emerged the idea that I was being willfully ignored. I stiffened; nothing changed. The women on the benches continued to look into nothingness, the baby did not move, the secretary continued to type, and from the back: silence. I froze. I was speechless with rage. I flexed my hands, once, twice. I looked around. I gasped for air, whirled on my heel, and strode out.

What had happened to me? I thought of this experience many times afterwards and talked about it with friends. The most common conclusion was simply that after my years as a physician I could not tolerate the insolence that poor people bear as part of daily life. Perhaps this diagnosis is correct. It may be that direct, and vanity had once again tripped me up. But pat answers are not satisfactory and I searched my memory for more meaning than unadulterated pride leading to a fall.

In later reflection my memories went back to a time when I had once stood before such a railing. Decades before, I had experienced the same emotion, only I had not run away. World War II had begun while I was in college and by my senior year, American participation had meant so much to me that I volunteered. It seemed to me in 1942 that I could do more for my country as an infantryman than as a premedical student. I had gone off to the ski troops and, after six months as a private, learned to my complete satisfaction that my contribution as an infantryman was not going to make the difference in winning the war and that perhaps I had a greater gift to give should I become a physician.

By coincidence the army was circulating a request for all eligible enlisted men to apply to medical school as there was a pressing need for medical students. The commanding officer of my Medical detachment concurred that the application would be a good move for both the army and myself. So armed with all the properly completed forms, certified credentials, and a letter of recommendation from my commanding officer, I set out to clear the red tape necessary for transfer from the army base.

On the list of necessary signatures was the base personnel officer. His headquarters were in a rusty Quonset hut, off on a byway, to which I slogged through the mud one rainy afternoon, clutching my precious packet of papers beneath my coat. As I entered the dreary metal hut, I could make out two soldiers: a private leaning on a broom and a sergeant behind a railing sitting at a desk reading a comic book. In the back, the desks of the officers were empty and it was obvious that no work was going to be done there that day. Both the private and sergeant looked up and, having ascertained my rank of private, went back to their tasks: the private leaning on his broom and the sergeant reading his comic book.

I said nothing as the rain dripped off my coat in puddles, and the sergeant read on. I stood before the railing and he read and he read. Then I was not sophisticated enough to know the physiology of reactions, but nonetheless they were as real as any I ever had. I waited. At last he looked up at me and very slowly asked though he knew the answer as well as I, "Wadda you want?" I pulled out my packet, explained my plight, and he did nothing. Finally he drawled, "We-ell, college *boy*, throw it down over here. We ain't doin' nuthin about it today, but you can leave it." I hesitated, flushed, protested, explained the importance of the papers. He listened, closed his comic book, and said, "I said throw it down over here. Now, boy, if you wan' me to do a great big favor for you, I'll try to keep it outta dat," pointing to a wastebasket. "Get out of here, 'cause you're boddering me." I put the packet down where he pointed and left. He obviously did me that favor of not throwing it in the wastebasket, since my transfer eventually came through to medical school. No, my experience at the abundant food program was not a new one and I had not run away out of pride.

Or had I? I reflected even more on the difference between the army sergeant and the secretary and though they were different in many ways, they were really the same. The person that was different was that now I was a middle-aged man with a family and I was conscious that as I stood before the secretary, I stood there as a recipient man would stand there. I stood there not just representing myself, but also my wife and children. How many men must stand that way for their family? That is why I could not bear it. That is why I fled. If I had been a poor man with my wife on the bench and my children in the car outside and all of us hungry, perhaps I could have stayed, but at what a cost I would have suppressed my rage. My rage came from the anger of the man helpless not for himself, but for his children. How could anyone ever be grateful with such a canker gnawing on his innards? Anything coming over the railing could only be further poison to the spirit of the man. For me, that was the other side of charity.

Stepping back from the emotions of resentment and rage, I can see how the tables had inadvertently been turned during the encounter in the abundant food store. I entered as the benign donor to give encouragement and knowledge. But by the alchemy of circumstances working on my personal history, I became a hostile acceptor. My eyes were pried open by the shift. What happened had nothing to do with middle-class values versus lower-class values. I was forced to see what I shrink from—the dark side of charity—my personal dark side of charity.

Because of its uniqueness, the example of the Bad Samaritan may be of little use. It is so black and white it can lead to doubt that it really fits the shades of personal life. Actually life is frequently a matter of grays, not black and white, of possibilities, not the right and wrong conclusions. So consider another example which may be closer to personal experience.

Consider the 26th of December. The psychology of Christmas is patent, but what of the 26th of December? The reaction to having accepted? The turkey carcass, the crumpled wrappings, the dissatisfied children, the gifts to be returned, the bills to be paid? If any day should be the Devil's, it is the 26th of December. It is the farthest from Christmas. It is the day when alcoholics are most likely to go off the wagon: It is the day of the Bad Samaritan.

No, the Bad Samaritan is not just limited to the people who do nothing but lean out their apartment window watching the murder of Kathryn Genovese. I suspect that the Bad Samaritan is not limited to sergeants and secretaries either, for I feel that anyone who examines himself on the 26th of December will have little difficulty in finding the Bad Samaritan. Both of charity's sides exist in and for all of us.

Going back to the benign equation of charity, there is an equilibrium of sentiment between the donor and the acceptor. If they both agree upon the need, the donor gives the gift out of compassion, while the acceptor receives the gift out of gratitude. The material forms are the gift itself and some expression of thanks, while the emotional forms are the positive feelings of compassion and gratitude. In all natural equilibriums there is a law that for every action, there is an equal and opposite reaction. So for any donor who experiences compassion, he must also know, and possibly deal with, the opposite side of compassion, disgust, revulsion, the wish to withdraw feelings rather than share them. Though unpleasant, forgotten, or even repressed, the law is incontrovertible, if you are human.

Disgust comes in many forms. Revulsion for a leper. Disdain for the unwashed. Dispassion for the dying. Apathy for the helpless. The most pernicious, and perhaps most prevalent, form is hypocrisy. The appearance of caring to cover the disgust of involvement; giving to remain aloof. In the natural equilibrium of psychological forces within the donor, he must deal with his own lethargy, his wish to stay uninvolved. The great temptation is to see oneself as an island, to care but for one's self and for one's own, so that charity which has begun at home needs never leave. However, as the donor cares, so must he know he is able not to care.

One other example of the ugly side of the balance: whenever the news carries a report of some poor, demented mother murdering her children, the strongest reaction comes from mothers who love their children. They most shrink with fear as they cry with horror. In their secret heart the crime resonates in fearful disharmony and it is their forgiveness which counts, if forgiveness is possible. The balance in the human soul is as real as any other balance of nature. For each passion, including love, there is another side. For charity there is greed. For each gift given there is a wish to withhold.

The balance holds for the acceptor, too. Riding in the wake of the gratitude comes resentment. The acceptor's weakness is uncovered with the gift. He stands not naked but exposed. Whether it is one million dollars for research from the Rockefeller Foundation, a welfare check, or a man led across a busy street, the gift always recognizes the acceptor as in some way less than the donor. And being less, being inferior, being dependent, though the most human of situations, stirs ancient resentments in every man and woman. Begging for one's hungry child means more than resentment. It means rage.

But does all of this apply to the 26th of December? Most assuredly so. How often do parents feel depleted on the 26th of December. "Did we give enough or perhaps too much? How are we going to pay the bills? Next year we will not have a Christmas like this," is how they voice it.

And what about the receiver on the 26th of December? How does he think after all the presents are known and not a single package remains unopened? What does he feel after the initial ecstasy of his new bicycle, when he sees the lad down the block on a new bicycle with three more gears than his? He feels somehow resentful, cheated. For in all the gifts there has never been enough to gratify his wish that there might be more. The child is restless and unhappy in his failure to find the ultimate gift and in his innocence has yet to understand the natural balance of giving and accepting.

Dr. Will Menninger has made the point so clearly, not just in terms of Christmas, but in any personal giving. Everyone must at times stop to have his "tank filled." Everyone must work through a personal sense of loss or diminishment which calls for more than just the balm of gratitude. The donor must realistically know his gifts have a limit. He is not Santa Claus, who gives and never receives. He gives what he can give and though it hurts at times, it should never injure. The hurt, like most hurts, mends with personal care, and he should recognize that hurt.

Here is a look into the negative feelings of charity. But perhaps these feelings are still denied as immature, unnecessary, and charity can exist without them for the unsentimental, the mature, the strong. The donor need only recognize the need, leave his anonymous gift and steal away unobserved, a la Santa Claus. It is possible if the person is without curiosity for his fellow man. The anonymous giver of a true gift (that is, one without compulsion that fills a real need) steals away to a point where he observes anonymously. Even the man who leaves a fortune to future generations can see men and women yet unborn who will be better for his bequest. It is simply that the contract between donor and acceptor is implicit, not explicit, and calls upon each party to do the emotional work internally. It remains an emotion-stimulating encounter.

No feeling man can pass, drop out, from the emotional implications of charity. It is only possible to exchange gifts unemotionally if the encounter has been dehumanized. Every exchange between humans makes the individual more or less human, never leaves him the same. If the emotions are not worked through, they accumulate. They then seek discharge and if not discharged in a human exchange, no matter how devious or delayed, they first boil internally and then either explode to destroy the relationship, or cook the donor in his own juice, destroying spirit.

Could any example be clearer of the destructiveness of unresolved feelings than government welfare? It is a historical fact that the dole destroys the people, their villages, and their countries. Dull, emotionless animals are produced by gifts that fill no commonly felt need, given by social devices without feelings, to people beyond caring. In scientific lingo each encounter carries a positive or negative reinforcement; only by making the encounter meaningless can this inexorable truth of human involvement be avoided. So, even in the act of giving man's inhumanity to man may find expression: giving easily becomes misgiving.

We have taken a peek at the other side of charity and can take heart in the promise that with the help of psychoanalysis this other side of charity can be explored, much as science sets about exploring the other side of the moon.

When freed of the feelings of guilt and fear, the donor and the acceptor can work through the unconscious apathy and resentment which characterize all charitable exchanges. The first step is personal recognition of feelings, leading to sustained introspection. The work is done by classifying feelings, clarifying distortions, identifying sources, and freeing the mind for deep consideration of human possibilities. Insight, reflection, and study are essential, in charity, as much as any other *human* encounter.

The second step is action, the action of words as well as deeds. The first step, knowing the felt need and all its implications is followed by the act of giving and, to be complete, should whenever possible include the act of talking. More than a ritual of common courtesy is served by the poor man's "God bless you" and the rich man's "You are welcome." As the dialogue is explored, it becomes a source of growth for both. The initiative in speaking to the deeper meanings often lies with the donor, much as with the parent, responsible for clarifying, not adjusting, the implicit contract with the child. In our times, the responsibility of the donor is to talk with the poor, the sick, the enemy, and sustain the talk. The donor should encourage a dialogue with the expectation that his hand may be bitten occasionally, though it should never be extended far enough to be chewed upon.

A supreme example of the donor-acceptor dialogue was related by Dr. Alan Gregg, who for many years was the director of the Rockefeller Foundation's Division for Medical Education. He gave away millions of dollars and knew the problems of charity firsthand. In Dr. Wilder Penfield's sensitive biography, Dr. Gregg is quoted:

"A Rumanian who was returning from a year spent on one of our traveling fellowships stopped in at the Paris office on his way home. I had recommended him some two years previously for a fellowship, and he had passed a year in Boston with Walter Cannon, who had commented favorably upon his work. He came into my room with a rather tense and formal—indeed almost unfriendly—manner. The purpose of his visit, he said, was to thank the Rockefeller Foundation for the fellowship it had given him. This he proceeded to do in elaborate and ornate terms that gave the impression of having been committed to memory. As I listened and watched him, the contrast became more and more striking between the warmth of his words and the coldness of his facial expression. So I decided to make an experiment.

"After he had finished with his set speech, I thanked him for it and said I would pass on the expression of gratitude to our trustees. Then, to get his full attention, I told him that I was going to say something he would probably not understand. 'How do you think I earn my living?' I said.

"'By directing the great philanthropic activities of the Rockefeller Foundation,' he answered.

"'No,' I said, 'I earn it by betting.'

"'I beg your pardon?'

"'Betting,' I repeated, 'Two years ago I made a bet that you would do well if the Foundation was to give you a fellowship to work with Professor Cannon.'

"'Ah,' he said, catching the idea.

"'Now what,' I continued, 'do you think would happen to me if I had made a lot of bad bets?'

"'That the traveling fellowships are suppressed?' he replied.

"'No,' I said. 'I would be fired. The Foundation wants someone whose bets come true.'

"'Excuse it,' he said, 'what is fired?'

"'Demissione, separated from the foundation—mis a la porte,' I said.

"My Rumanian looked incredulous and uncomfortable and puzzled. Why was I talking to him so seriously about my own affairs?

"'I've had a letter from Dr. Cannon,' I said. 'He comments very favorably on you. So it is clear I made a good bet—or at least you have made my bet come true. So if we are speaking of gratitude this morning, let me express my gratitude to you for your part in helping me to earn my living.'

"His whole expression changed—changed completely—and all his discomfort was gone."[1]

Here it is, the perfect dialogue, but we may ask what does it have to do with us. We do not give away millions of dollars, or do we? Who is it who pays for welfare? Who is it who sends the millions into our city's ghettos? Who is it that is supporting an unwed mother with six children? Is it the government or is it you and I? Who is it who is going to work out the negative feelings of charity? Is it the government or is it you and I? Who is it that walks up to the railing in the abundant food program? That one I can answer with certainty, for it was I. I failed because I panicked, rather than with resolution and courage establish the needed dialogue.

It is impossible to expect a government to have human values and, though possible, it is presumptuous to expect the poor to express them. Can I expect the sick and poor to supply what I lack? I should set my best to understanding and speaking out for what I believe is right. The ultimate value is equality in human dignity—social and civic freedom. Equality is not to be had without testing, without an exchange, without a dialogue, and it is we who understand who must initiate the working through. The other side of charity waits to be explored by science, not the dispassionate science of cold analysis, but the science of being a human being; of accountability for ultimate values. And even in this, a form of vanity and selfishness exists, for with the ultimate value goes the ultimate gift, self-respect.

Endnotes

Reprinted from *The Pharos* 34(Spring 1971): 75-78, with permission.
1. W. Penfield, M.D., *The Difficult Art of Giving: The Epic of Alan Gregg* (New York: Little, Brown, 1967) 269-70.

Leprosy, A Disease of the Heart

> *Leprosy is a chronic, transmittable disease, due to a specific microbe, the* Mycobacterium leprae. *It is a constitutional disease, accompanied in its beginnings with fever, chills, etc. The lesion consists of either well-defined patches of macular erythema or blebs, followed by the development of anesthetic patches of cicatricial tissue with atrophy of the skin and hair; or else of nodules and tubercles which may become absorbed or atrophy. In both varieties atrophy may be followed by mutilation and deformity of the digits. Other parts other than the skin may become involved, especially the larynx, nerves, viscera and bones.*
> —*Dorland's Medical Dictionary,* 19th edition

While visiting India one summer, I was invited by Dr. Shubhada Pandya to join her at the Acworth Leprosy Hospital, Bombay, and then to accompany Dr. R. Ganapati, a public health officer, on his rounds in Bombay's Dharavi slum.

The taxicab ride to Acworth Leprosy Hospital passed through some prosperous sections of Bombay, yet the ride, as in every city of the Far East, was a battering encounter with masses of people. In addition, the ride had the eerie quality of a submarine dream, for the drenching monsoon with its oppressive humidity had me soaked in my own sweat as I peered through the cab's steamy, rain-streaked windows. The sidewalks were crowded with makeshift cardboard and plastic hovels that seemed like barnacles growing along the base of the buildings. The underwater effect was reinforced by the swirl of bicycles passing like schools of fish and clusters of umbrellas hopping up and down over curbs like scallops over a rough seabed.

The hospital itself did nothing to relieve the illusion of being underwater. It crouched behind its dilapidated walls like some inundated ruin, complete with a wavering file of patients, some clutching children, some on crutches, some with torn pieces of plastic held over their bent, cramped bodies, like a line of fiddler crabs limping and scurrying for shelter through the hospital's gate.

Inside the scarred two-story building, Dr. Pandya greeted me. A youngish woman, slim in her white coat, she obviously did not spend afternoons over tea and pastry. Her penetrating gaze conveyed a gentleness continually challenged by the violence of a world of intransigent disease. From her glowing dark eyes to her sandaled feet she is the picture of the focused intensity that uniquely marks the Indian intellectual. The formalities of greeting took but a moment, and we quickly moved through a series of rooms, meeting pharmacists, technicians, nurses, and fellow physicians, while she explained in the clipped accent of Indian English, "You must understand from the beginning that this disease is a socioeconomic one. Leprosy is on the increase in this country and should anyone tell you that it will be eliminated by the year 2000, poppycock! Our hospital treats 5,000 cases a year, and each day 250 new patients are seen, even though they may have been diagnosed elsewhere. All patients get treatment; in fact, the sulfones can be supplied for a patient in adequate doses at a cost of only 50 cents a year. However, it must be taken for a lifetime, and patient compliance here as the world over, is a sometimes thing."

We made our way out a back door onto a sheltering veranda where a small group of men and boys were busy hammering and sawing, making chairs and desks. Dr. Pandya explained that although they were not economically competitive, since it was a sheltered workshop, the state had agreed to buy the furniture made by patients with leprosy. However, as in all things connected with leprosy, arrangements are never easy. She had been unable to find anyone in the city of Bombay to supervise these young men, who in turn were reluctant to learn, since patients could make more in the established trades that support 80 percent of Bombay's patients with leprosy: prostitution and bootlegging. Only a few dedicated patients stay long enough to become carpenters.

The rain had let up, so we stepped from beneath the dripping veranda for Dr. Pandya to demonstrate the symptomatology of the young men in better light. "This lad has a rash over his lower arm and hand which could easily pass as impetigo, and yet he is in the infectious stage. He has responded well to medication and if he sticks with it, the rash will subside and he will probably suffer no serious complications. Probably, that is, but only if he sticks with the medication and cares for himself. Remember, this is a socioeconomic disease. Once he is diagnosed as a leper, he is fired from his job. The government punishes him for something he has not done. He is continually tempted to conceal his disease, both from his employer and himself, simply to make enough to eat." She directed my attention to an older man. "Here, look at the nodules around the ears. These are like the tubercles of tuberculosis, each loaded with Hansen's bacteria. With adequate treatment this will subside. We seldom see what was once the characteristic leonine face; disfigurements are not as prevalent as they used to be, though the disease is on the increase. Here is a claw hand," and she pointed out a man holding a chisel between two stumps of hands. "The ulnar nerve has been attacked. Notice how difficult it is for him to work, yet he works. The most important part of our work—and it seems like we never can accomplish it—is to have the patient learn to protect himself. He must not pick up anything hot; he must wear special shoes, but telling a patient to get special shoes is like telling him to buy a Rolls Royce. The disease causes the loss of pain fibers, so stepping on a nail, cutting a foot, or burning a finger goes unnoticed until a secondary infection produces the ulcers you smell when you enter the hospital." She called over an older man with leonine features. "Zemil has worked here for three years and is helping us teach carpentry. You see his nose has collapsed. The cartilage is gone. Incidentally, most of the transmission of leprosy is through the nose."

I asked her if she was not afraid of leprosy for herself. There was no question in my mind but that I was afraid of leprosy for me, as I hesitated to touch a patient or shake any hands even when proffered out of clean, white coats. She answered, "No, I know I've had leprosy. It's like tuberculosis. Most of us have had tuberculosis as a primary tuberculosis focus; the same is true of leprosy, a primary eruption. It is a matter of immunology, and so much of that is nutrition and as I say, this is a socioeconomic disease. It happens to the rich as well as the poor, but it happens mostly to the poor, and it will disfigure and destroy the poor who cannot protect themselves properly. Shoes, clothing, cleanliness, and food. Oh yes, I'm quite sure I've had leprosy."

We moved back to a room where female patients were being trained as seamstresses. Dr. Pandya continued, "You see, if we can get our women to make any sum of money, just the least, they will immediately be taken back by their families. However, when they have no money to contribute to their families, they are forever outcasts. It really makes little difference whether they are lepers or not; it's whether they are adding to the family's food. Incidentally, these sewing machines were given to us by a group of ladies who come regularly with a check, but you can be sure that once they give us the check, they never shake hands with anybody in the hospital and touch no one as they quickly leave. There are ancient feelings about leprosy which are unchanged today. Come, we'll go upstairs to the treatment clinic."

We made our way up a back stairway, through a crowded corridor—dark except for a lone neon tube flickering against the ceiling—and attempted to turn into a long room. In the doorway a knot of people had formed about a young doctor who was lecturing a dark-skinned, apathetic, youngish man. It was more an argument than consultation and after perfunctory introduction, the doctor turned back to the patient, explaining to me over his shoulder that the man had just been diagnosed as having Hansen's disease. "Look," he pointed to the butterfly-like configuration of inflamed skin shaded ever so lightly redder than the rest of the man's face, but distinct once pointed out, "he is telling me that he doesn't want to come back to be treated, and he is in the infectious stage. He says that if he takes the treatment his employer will find out and he will no longer be able to support himself and his family. He has to protect his job, but his disease is sure to spread, not only to him but to his children. What is there to do? How loud should I shout at him to tell him that he has to come back?" He knew there was no answer and desperately, more to reassure himself than to inform me, abruptly changed the subject, "Look over here; we have some work at hand." Anxiously, he pointed out a vial of a newly developed vaccine. A nurse was injecting it into a row of patients. "We're doing everything we can to stimulate the immunologic response. It seems strange that some people are protected and others are not. We do not understand. It is not a simple thing by any means, because leprosy produces so many different reactions." When we turned back, his patient had slipped away and disappeared into the mass of flowing patients, crowding in and out of the doors.

As though in relief to the pervasive despair, Dr. Pandya drew in a father and daughter for me to see. The short gray-haired father, in a Western three-piece suit and tie, had obviously come on important business, and his daughter, probably sixteen years old, in a shimmering blue sari, stood sullenly beside him. He was elated, as Dr. Pandya explained, "He thought his daughter had leprosy. See, look, this discoloration around the mouth, a loss of pigment, we see that at times, and I know it's not leprosy, and I told him so but he is having trouble believing. Understand that in this country marriages are arranged, and if the woman is damaged—and there is no doubt that leprosy is a damage—it will be very difficult for her father to marry her off. You can see, he has trouble believing that such good fortune could happen to him, that his daughter does not have leprosy." The man's face was alternately lighting with smiles and darkening with frowns as he looked first to one and then another doctor, hoping that each and all would concur with him in beating down the fear that his beautiful daughter was damaged property.

"Come and see our dressing station," suggested Dr. Pandya, and we elbowed our way into the center of the long room where a wall of half-open jalousies did nothing to relieve the stench of putrid flesh. Rows of disfigured patients seated on the long benches proclaimed the final stages of leprosy: arms missing, faces askew, hands clawed, stumps dripping pus from what was once an ankle. The floor was a litter of blood-soaked gauze and mud. "They are not infectious, probably; none of them are infectious at all, but they have lost most sensation in their bodies and secondary infection is killing them all," she remarked. As if in response to her attention, a creature without name or shape detached itself from the line against the back wall and like some misbegotten error of evolution snaked toward me on its belly. It had neither ears nor a nose, and what had been a face was the color and consistency of burned meat surrounding a slobbering slit lined with broken teeth. It approached close enough to grab at me, with its claw alternately outstretched and pointing to the remnants of a leg, but Dr. Pandya, staring the horror down, explained, "He is only trying to use you," which confirmed that it was a man and that he was begging for a shoe to cover the stump of his left leg. "Money, money," he screamed, at least I presumed he said money, since his Hindi was unintelligible to me. But the pleading claw eloquently expressed his whole tale of filth, disease, and ignorance. He was begging for a share of my strength and knowledge. My blunt "No," turned him away cursing. No one took heed, for the other patients busily continued dressing their own wounds, searching among the piles on the floor for cleaner rags than the ones they had torn off. Behind me, he cursed again and again, but his cries eventually were lost in the turmoil.

Leading me downstairs and back to the entrance, Dr. Pandya explained, "Now, I'll turn you over to Dr. Ganapati who will take you into the field." As she spoke, an attendant rushed up with a note that caused her face to light up. "See, we are having some effect. Here is a referral from a doctor. For so long doctors have not even referred patients to us for treatment for leprosy," and then with a sobering second thought, "but perhaps it is that some doctors are willing to recognize leprosy now simply to rid their practice of lepers."

Dr. Pandya pointed out the microbus. Thanking her, I climbed in and met Dr. Ganapati, who proved to be an unprepossessing middle-aged man, with a short-sleeved white shirt open at the neck, neat slacks, thick horn-rimmed glasses, receding hairline, and gray about the temples—the type of man who might have been class treasurer throughout medical school, collecting dues, yet never expecting and always surprised by any recognition for a lifetime devoted to hard work. As we lurched along, he shouted over the unmuffled roar of our microbus that we were headed for the Dharavi slums, where the Bombay Leprosy Project had one of its stations in case detection, treatment, and public education. The leprosy project, which is supported by funds from the German Leprosy Relief Society, is staffed by two doctors, fifteen paraprofessionals, and a few support personnel. It focuses on the million people living in Bombay's wards "H" and "G." Today we were delivering drugs and other supplies to the Dharavi middle school, where the principal had generously allowed the project to undertake a health survey.

Before we reached the turnoff, Dr. Ganapati explained that this slum was reputed to be one of the worst; the inhabitants lived in degradation, eating, sleeping, defecating, urinating, and copulating in the open. The dangers for children are fierce; many drown in open septic tanks, while the most common source of child abuse and murder is frantic mothers who break into uncontrollable fury at the unrelieved cries of their starving children to beat them, sometimes to death.

Unexpectedly, we veered off the viaduct onto a side road that became a byway straggling down to a lane, which contracted to a passageway barely wide enough to allow our microbus to squeeze through as it rubbed against improvised shops and splashed the bystanders with the filthy mud of the Dharavi. Up close, poverty is a gigantic, socially propelled slime mold, without form, yet an inexorable force that defiles everything it touches with malignant degeneration. Poverty's essence is trash, and with the exception of a very few faces lighted with dignity despite a life of suffering, everything else in the slum was broken, torn, marred, grimy, and filthy. There are not even rocks as such, for a rock would have had wet moss or at least some surface of clean rain-washed sheen. Everything was besmirched, mismatched, or worn: pieces of glass, rusted cans, piles of offal, garbage, shattered barrels, crushed plastic bottles, sickly chickens, thin pigs seeking to eat the chickens, small, weak children, shreds of human beings, yet beating the pigs with sticks. Everywhere a trash of expressions: scowls, threatening stares, disgust, and surprised hostility at the presence of an invading "European." As though expressing the ultimate example of trash, a garbage pile was pointed out in which a live, discarded baby had been uncovered the week before.

Slowly we made our way to the school, which could be heard before it was seen, since this one massive building in the Dharavi was filled to bursting with screaming students (school attendance is discouraged, since there are more children than seats and a high dropout rate—which might better be called a force-out rate—is necessary). It was filled to overflowing with a trash of discordant noise.

Dr. Ganapati led me up to the roof and then to the final crest of the water tank, from which the rusty tin roofs and infinite squalor of the Dharavi could be seen in every direction. Directly below, a woman was squatting, defecating, at the edge of the school grounds. Further off, the people were less distinct, and Dr. Ganapati pointed out narrow chimneys belching steam and smoke, explaining that these illicit distilleries were the main support of the people.

Convinced that I had had the broad view, Dr. Ganapati led me back down the ladder of the water tower, through the door, down the stairway, to an airless room on the third floor—Bombay Leprosy Project's station. The windows were closed to lessen the piercing racket of the classes. The doctor gave me a "close" view of the project, complete with slides—again, photographs of leprosy and, inadvertently, a picture of a physician who is fighting leprosy. When one slide announced "leprosy can be cured," I did not confront the doctor with my doubts. Perhaps it may be arrested, but it cannot be cured, particularly as it is a socioeconomic disease. The doctor accentuated repeatedly the paradox of Hansen's disease, the undamaged infectious nose disseminates, while the disfigured but noninfectious face repels; the carrier easily passes in society as simply having scabies or an innocuous red rash, while the burned-out noninfectious patient causes the people to shrink. Slide after slide, some showing how symptoms can be contained, some showing how prevention can work; statistics showing how the sheer mass of people makes contagion inevitable. It is madness to think the disease could be eliminated in fifteen years; instead, it will continue to spread. If I had needed convincing, which I did not, the slide showing the yearly incidence of new cases—fifty-five a year—among children in the school we sat in was the clincher.

When the lecture ended, we made our way out of the school, and our talk turned to the role of the medical profession in fighting leprosy. Dr. Ganapati's voice, although not penetrating, had a clarity of understated conviction that carried through rather than over the turmoil. "I do not hold it against medical students who seek to become surgeons. They are taken up with the glamour of the specialty and realistically want to enter a field where they can make money. Like it or not, medical schools teach what is important to a successful career. A bright student does not take long to see where the profession gives recognition and know that with the recognition goes freedom from the insecurity of living on state budgets which are always endangered by political whim. No, I can understand why medical students are not attracted to working with a disease that lacks glamour and continually threatens your own health."

His explanation continued as our bus moved out of the Dharavi and into the wider streets of Bombay, but my eyes were open to a different matter, for when the bus stopped at an intersection, or a traffic light, and I saw those countless hands shoved in through the half-open window—the begging hands of children and adults, all imploring money—I was now alert to the leper's claw, the subtle rash of Hansen's disease, and the meaning of stumps for fingers. Despite this distraction, I listened closely to the doctor, trying hard to understand his forgiveness of medical students, hoping it included traveling physicians such as myself.

The microbus eventually wended its way back to my five-star hotel. I gratefully thanked my guide and the driver, who cheerfully waved me up the marble steps as the doorman, a formidable uniformed Sikh, threw open the door to my immaculate, air-conditioned palace. I turned to wave back only to see them merging into the flow of traffic milling about the "Gateway of India." Few would question why I immediately made for the hotel pharmacy to purchase a bottle of methyl alcohol. The bored clerk informed me that medicinal alcohol was illegal in India; however, when I explained I had just returned from a leprosy hospital and wanted to disinfect my camera and myself, he instantaneously called the manager and after considerable rummaging the two of them produced a bottle of Listerine. I said, "No thanks," and went to my room, where I removed my shoes before entering. Balancing my camera carefully on the edge of the bathroom sink, I stripped naked, rolled all my clothes into a tight bundle, placed them in a plastic laundry bag, and plunged beneath a hot, soapy shower, where I remained for thirty minutes.

Once my body was cleansed as only a scrubbing with soap and hot water can do, I slipped into a fresh robe, retired to the sitting room of my suite, and in the silence of the dark room, I slumped into a large chair, chin on chest, arms splayed, staring straight ahead into the cool shaded dimness, the picture of a defeated Roman general sorting through a lost campaign. All I had were thoughts, thoughts to be arranged and rearranged and rearranged yet again, until at last the diagnosis of leprosy, that grim socioeconomic disease, would make sense to me.

What did I think? I thought my eye sharp enough to see the lesions, the loss of pigment, the fine macular quality of the infected skin, the nodules around the ears that would never again go unrecognized by me, but those were niggardly clinician's thoughts. What did I think? I thought it curious that there is no physical pain connected with this disease. There is no squeezing chill or overbearing fever as in malaria, just the faintest touch—so easily denied—of dread death. What a strange psychology for an illness. Diabolically, leprosy preserves the illusion of health by destroying the pain fibers that lead to the brain. Only those fibers that run to the heart remain intact. The pain of leprosy originates in the eye of the beholder and becomes pain for the patient as he is shunned and ostracized, as he loses the humanness he once possessed. The pain of leprosy is not inflicted by the bacillus but by his fellow man. And I knew not what to make of this.

A terrible equation appeared before my eyes. If I am a human being and patients with leprosy are human beings, we are of the same flesh, therefore some part of me is a leper. Gradually, I realized I had become one with the perverse disease. I had it in my heart. Had I not, as a priest of science, spent the day cutting the hearts out of a thousand people, cutting them out just as surely and deftly as an Aztec priest standing on the heights of his holy pyramid? Had I not been holding a thousand hearts as far as I could from my own, using all my clinical skill to see them as parts of human beings, as less than human beings, as fascinating specimens? Had I not committed the most despicable sin of a physician, silently reserving myself to myself and denying what compassion I might have, holding back from the proffered hand of a patient in need? Had I not told myself, the whole day through, that when night fell I would leave the leper's hell, as when a medical student, I had left the body on the anatomy table, left the slide of syphilitic tissue beneath the microscope, had left the caged rats in the physiology laboratory, left them to enjoy myself in the living world. Had I not contracted leprosy in the very act of fending it off? My heart felt weak.

What to do? How can I act as a physician now that I have seen leprosy for what it is? I had asked Dr. Pandya if there was anything I could do. She had hesitated a moment, as though a bit embarrassed, and said, "I know you are from the States and you said your wife is meeting you by way of Hawaii. Should she go to Molokai, I would appreciate a picture of Father Damien's grave. I know they dug up that leper's body and shipped it back to Europe, but I believe his heart is still there. If you could get me a snapshot of his grave—it doesn't have to be in color—it would help."

And there it was—I could do something, but I could do nothing. I could do nothing directly to relieve the lepers of Bombay, but I could recognize that there are some who do help. There are some, very few, who touch the spirit of mankind as deeply as leprosy repels it. Perhaps there is a cure for leprosy, but it will only come from those few who have the heart to be greater than the disease. As though released by that flash of belief, a great sob welled from within me, and almost as though I would wash my spirit as I had washed my body, I found myself crying, and I cried, and cried, and cried, and cried. Leprosy is truly a disease of the heart.

Endnotes

Reprinted from the *Journal of the American Medical Association* 248(1982): 573-576, with permission. Copyrighted 1982, American Medical Association.

The Quality of Mercy

The quality of mercy is not strain'd,
It droppeth as the gentle rain from heaven
Upon the place beneath: it is twice blest,
It blesseth him that gives, and him that takes.
—William Shakespeare (1564-1616)
The Merchant of Venice, Act IV, 1, 183

Travel has a way of stretching the mind. The stretch comes not from travel's immediate rewards, the inevitable new sights, smells, and sounds, but with experiencing firsthand how others do differently what we have believed to be the right and only way.

Not all travelers know that their ultimate destination is a wider view of themselves, that personal questions arise whose answers will not be found in guidebooks. We exert our sharpest powers of curiosity only when our mind is on its own, wondering, reflecting, contemplating. At its best, travel proves a healthy convalescence from life's routine, a time when quickened imagination nurtures a revaluing of self.

A trip my wife and I made to Venice is a case in point. We love that city without automobiles; that city free of the imprint and coercion of machines, except, of course, the vaporetto, that humble, rocking beast of burden, more like a tamed hippopotamus than a ferryboat, created to bear a full crowd of human beings not very far not very fast. Venice, all walks and water byways, is and remains a monument to human dimensions.

We stayed at the Hotel La Fenice et des Artistes, in a third-floor room overlooking the small piazza of the Teatro La Fenice. Naturally, jet lag haunted us the first few days, leaving us wakeful while the rest of Venice slept. On the first night, about 3 A.M., I heard a noise coming through the window, not the cooing of sleepy Venetian pigeons, but a strange scraping sound. Rising, I looked out. The single streetlight, suspended on a cable across the piazza, cast a distinct ring of light. At first I was unable to make out the source of the noise. Only as my eyes grew accustomed to the surrounding darkness did I discern a strange sight.

Across the way crouched a small woman, all but overwhelmed by her ill-fitting coat. To all appearances, she met the American definition of a bag lady. Hunched down, she noiselessly picked through a plastic bag.

With great care she regularly brought forth spoonfuls of some unknown material, which she deposited into a ring of tin cans surrounding her. The scraping noise came as she cleaned the spoon against the side of each can.

As my eyes fully accommodated, I could see, sitting in a wider ring beyond the tin cans, an attentive pride—small, perhaps feral, house cats of indeterminate origin. Once the lady finished her ritual with the tin cans, the cats moved in, the largest ones first, and set to eating with gusto. While they ate she remained in the center of the circle, only to interrupt her vigil as now and then she scurried to fill an empty tin or deliver an additional can to a hesitant visitor beyond the range of light: a cat too shy to join the dinner party.

During our entire stay in Venice the scraping began punctually at 3 A.M. Each night we watched from our window, and the only other person to share the scene was a carabiniere, who once, apparently on his rounds, sauntered through the piazza. He hardly glanced at the cat lady, while her attention never strayed from her wards. Without a word or sign of recognition, he passed into the night. For all I know she is busy every night, ladling out portions to Venice's homeless cats.

Like it or not, my mind was stretched. What was I looking at? When I asked others, their answers varied little. "Madness," some would say and then regale me with a tale or two of grate-sleeping, homeless bag ladies defying the limits of common sense by defecating on a street corner or badgering peaceful passersby.

Nor was science of much help in understanding what I had seen. In its Christmas edition, *New Scientist* carried an article about England's six million disease-ridden, spraying, caterwauling feral cats who "needed" to be trapped and neutered.[1] Even this dispassionate account contributed to my mind stretching as it reported how a "devoted member of the public" has for the last twenty years been giving breakfast every day before dawn to cats in Regent's Park, London. Is there a syndrome of cat-feeding madness, or, I found myself asking, had I witnessed an act of mercy?

But feelings, particularly when they identify an action, need to be more than named; they need to be made real. What more is meant by mercy than a passing recognition of goodness? The word "mercy" hardly finds a place in the parlance of medical scientists. We may know charity, for many of us give at the office. But what is mercy? It neither has pity's sterile distance and faint aroma of disdain, nor joins compassion's impulsive rush to embrace the afflicted. No, mercy, while appearing to hesitate, pauses to judge carefully both the near and far of anguish, the responsibility for and innocence of wrong. Despite the dictates of reasonable justice, mercy accepts what is as it is, redeeming the insignificant other with solace and support; support that touches with gentle fingers and soft words the body, mind, and heart of suffering. Therein lies the meaning. Mercy is considered intimacy with despair.

One need not look far to see there is precious little mercy, either strained or dropping like a gentle rain, for homeless cats or human beings. I know, for recently I joined a fellowship in my city attempting to establish an infirmary for the homeless. Like the people who claim Our Lady of the Cats is mad, a bank official, when offered an opportunity to help fill the need of the homeless, replied, "Our organization is doing everything it can to distance itself from that problem."

In contrast, when the local medical society was asked for help with homeless human beings, sixty local physicians volunteered. Yet we cannot help but wonder what is thought of these doctors. Are they mad for not distancing themselves from human suffering? What are we to think when we hear these doctors scraping their medicine cabinets clean for a circle of nameless sick?

Much as my pupils dilated in the darkness of the Venetian night, my mind expanded to the somber question, Are doctors mad for serving the homeless? Long ago, while traveling on the Red Arrow Express to Leningrad, I shared a compartment with a Russian physician. We could converse because he was as fluent in English as I was clumsy with Russian. We talked intimately as travelers do when they discover their compatibility uncompromised by threat of continuing responsibilities. He illustrated his concern for understanding the difficult position of a physician during wartime by recounting his conflicting feelings while treating wounded Nazi soldiers captured shortly after they had murdered a schoolroom of children by throwing them down a well. My companion paused and from his depths witnessed, "Compassion is not a concept. It is an experience."

The memory led me to reflect on Charity's three daughters: Compassion, the impulsive one, youngest, spontaneous, and direct; Pity, who stands apart and points; and Mercy, the oldest, who seeks no truce with sorrow. Mercy illuminates the question of madness in charitable doctors, for though hesitant, perhaps reserved, she carefully measures the distance between her heart and the other's pain, always considering her part in what transpires. Only then does Mercy act to sweep up anguish as substance from which to fashion forgiveness. With judgment fulfilled, Mercy extends both mind and heart in the balm of forgiveness, laying on the spirit of life, a willing merger with souls in despair.

My colleagues who volunteered to care for the homeless know, perhaps not as well as Our Lady of the Cats, that only as we experience mercy do we live as merciful people. They infuse our profession with mercy, though they may appear mad to a world that judges by direct returns, be it commercial profit or military victory. Anticipating another stretching, my mind has me searching for a land where Our Lady of the Merciful can be found in the darkness before dawn, feeding value-less, spirit-starved, feral souls.

Endnotes

Reprinted from the *Journal of the American Medical Association* 266(1991): 614-615, with permission. Copyrighted 1991, American Medical Association.

1. S. Young, "The Kindest Cut," *New Scientist* (22/29 December 1990): 81.

Part 2

The Human Condition

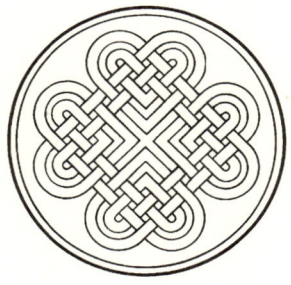

*May my application so close
To so endless a repetition
Not make me tired and morose
And resentful of man's condition.*
　　　　　　—Robert Frost (1874-1963)
　　　　　　　In Time of Cloudburst

Overview to Part 2

Though the forms of suffering are infinity, the fact of suffering is singular; its circumstances are lived in personal terms.

Things happen. They have been happening since the Big Bang. A woman stops by to talk about her invalid husband—**The Yammering Grandmother**. A medical student loses her first patient, a child, to death—**Humanism in Medicine, The Rudimentary Process**. A dog is killed on the highway—**On the Sounds of Death**.

On and on, the human condition happens. Good happenings bring happiness; others, bad, come laden with misery. There are small, inconsequential happenings and great, life-altering happenings; all have their reasons, often clouded, always debatable. In my experience, happenings set the mind rolling in a familiar search for "What does this mean?"

The meaning of happenings is discovered in lived experience. With good happenings, happiness proves answer enough. With bad happenings, which are inevitable since our lives are owed to relentless fate, suffering offers more questions than answers. Destiny prompts the human condition's profound question. The search for an understandable context for the happening begins with, "What in God's name is going on here?"

With more difficult happenings, perhaps as unwanted and painful as a diagnosis of malignant cancer, the reality is so great it abrades one's sense of personal identity, which brings the next question, Job's, "Why me?" When that question goes unanswered, the third question calls out for compassion with, "Who can tell me why I suffer?"

It seems to me the answers to human condition questions fall into two general categories, good answers and bad; that is what the accompanying essays say. The good answers, grief and sorrow, even the personal agony of losing a loved one, lead back to life. Bad answers, denial and flight, particularly the trips consciousness can book on wings of mind-altering drugs, simply circle death at a distance, never returning the questioner to a sorrowful yet livable reality.

Dysfunctional answers, those that cloud rather than uncover meaning, reveal the space where compassion might have offered meaning. The non-review of **Saving Private Ryan** speaks to how human suffering is traduced by filling the natural place of compassion with entertainment. Oscar Wilde observed that where there has been suffering the place is sacred. However, with our era's gross commercialism that space is easily degraded into virtual suffering, entertainment intended to yield a profit rather than a moral.

Portrayal of suffering bears with it the author's motive in reaching to the reader, the artist's co-passion or an entrepreneur's dalliance with another's feelings. Were Cervantes and Shakespeare out to turn a peso or a pence or were they driven to speak to and for others? Only they can say, as only a physician can say if his vocation or his occupation leads him through the world of human illness. Nor does the question ignore the reader for, like the passive patient, they are drawn to judging how their significant other, the doctor, views human suffering, is it a means to compassion or occupation? The judgment, albeit silently, determines growth or stasis of the soul when bad things happen, even on the silver screen.

Sacredness is a personal belief, not a religious dictum. The sacredness of suffering comes with an individual's acknowledged compassion. Falling back upon pity or sympathy cancels any chance of vested sacredness. It is certainly too strong to think of a movie house as a sacred place yet the issue of experiencing portrayed suffering in personal terms is ever present. Is the suffering real?

Only if the individual acknowledges it as a personal experience directly related to his life. This question hovers someplace above the audience of any tragedy, on stage, screen, or page. Too many leave it unanswered, festering as morbid sentimentality.

Fostering acknowledgment and relatedness, together with doubt and action, as a reaffirmation of life, **The Value of Suffering in Medical Practice** speaks directly to the anatomy, pathology, and physiology of the human condition. Moreover, readers armed with their personal questions should have little difficulty following how illness finds its meaning as much in the flesh and spirit of the patient as the mind and heart of the doctor. When fully recognized, the question of illness passes beyond "Why me?" to "Who can tell me how my suffering can have meaning?" The "telling" is for the compassionate patient-doctor relationship to explore, each in his own way, patient and doctor, "telling" each other what its meaning can be—companions in the human condition.

The Yammering Grandmother

Kind hearts are more than coronets!
 —Alfred, Lord Tennyson (1809-1892)

Though one may never get the key to a city, a fringe benefit that comes with elective office in a county medical society—I served as president in 1975—is a key to doors ordinarily locked. Frequently, officers are invited or permitted into byways customarily closed, and during my tenure I used this privilege perhaps to a fault. Certainly, if there was as much scandal attached to using elective office for talking with people in different walks of life as there is attached to using the society's money for first-class air travel, I would have long since been bugged, taped, and run out of town on a court decree.

Along the way—the day escapes me as I only associate it with an acute attack of professional helplessness—I telephoned our local public welfare department and asked a caseworker if some of the recipients might wish to suggest how the medical society could improve the health care of the poor in our city.

The case worker politely asked if I really knew where I was at, but added he would see what he could do. So, on a cold winter morning, Mrs. Wellwise, a welfare recipient, dropped by, and I had the privilege of meeting a bright-eyed, dark-haired, fiftyish, slim, spare, and responsive woman.

Medical societies, like most establishments, are all ahum at 9 A.M.—phones ringing, copiers clacking, and executives executing. Short of my pulling rank, no office was available for Mrs. Wellwise and me; I suggested that we use the staff dining room, since, prior to the coffee break, it was out of the traffic pattern, empty of people, and undisturbed. Mrs. Wellwise agreed. As we seated ourselves at the corner of the long table, she murmured that it reminded her of her childhood, "We had a long table like this, with Father sitting at one end, Mother at the other, and all ten children around the sides."

It was an auspicious beginning, but once seated she faltered, as if uncertain where to begin. Clumsily, I offered reassurance, "It may be a bit scary, coming to an unfamiliar part of town and meeting strangers."

She replied, "No, that does not bother me. What really bothers me is that I did not sleep too well last night thinking about what I should say this morning. At the last moment I almost didn't come, and if my son, who is a carpenter's apprentice, had not put me in the taxi and paid the fare, I guess I wouldn't have made it."

As she spoke she relaxed, unfolding her hands and explaining how little she had to offer. The caseworker had told her of my interest, and she had some ideas, but she was not sure they would fit in.

"You see, I never did have much education. I was the oldest of ten. We picked potatoes and followed the crops. My father would be with us in the fields, but he was a sick man. He had diabetes real bad. I can remember him falling down, but we made it. I suppose you want to know about what I think about doctors. Well, I've never had much trouble with them. They were all nice to me."

I asked what she thought of the complaint some welfare recipients have of feeling unwelcome in doctors' offices.

"Oh yes," she said, "I know what you mean, but that only happens with *ignorant* doctors. You come up against them, sometimes on the phone, where they simply turn you down, right then and there, spouting off about how 'we don't accept your kind of people.' And sometimes they say this in the office. You know how doctors can smile. Well, some can frown, too. And while you're sitting in the waiting room, the doctor comes out, picks up the chart, and with a frown says to the nurse, 'Oh, here's another of those welfare patients.'"

Glancing around the empty room, she continued, "But it isn't always the doctor. Sometimes there are nurses who take personal information in the waiting room while you are sitting there. They don't ask for 'an insurance number' or 'your number'; they ask loud enough for everyone to hear, 'What's your welfare number?' and that is embarrassing. But you have to understand that they are ignorant. They are the kind of people who rush you through and do not give you any time to talk."

Mrs. Wellwise paused, as if for reassurance that she was not speaking out of turn, so I responded directly, "How do you react when you have to deal with medical people who are this way?"

She sighed and went on, "Oh, I tell myself I know I will never overcome their ignorance. I'm not saying that they don't know about giving the right medicine to folks, but I am saying that they are ignorant about the circumstances of other people. Take our family—we have five children and a grandchild—and my husband's illness is serious. Some days he can get out of bed and walk a bit. Other days, when his breathing is hard, he can't get up. I wouldn't call our circumstances too hard since we always make it.

"But when they say, 'Five children,' and look at you queer, I say, 'I love them all and it's really six, since my granddaughter stays with us, too.' As I said, I wouldn't call our circumstances too hard; we've always made it."

I wondered if it was only physicians and nurses who were difficult, so I asked about her pharmacist.

"Oh, he's an honest man," she said. "If I need some special medication for my husband, he gives me an extra supply. 'Mrs. Wellwise,' he says, 'I don't know whether the department will allow this or not, but I'll give you five days' supply and write to the state capitol. If they don't allow it, well, then I'll get in touch with you.' You see, that man is not trying to cheat the government or me. He lets me know if I can't have the medicine and gives me plenty of time to pay him what it costs."

I found myself asking, "How do you find an honest man such as your pharmacist?" She replied simply, "It's not difficult; he was recommended by my doctor, who is honest."

Somewhat taken aback by this, I blurted, "But how did you find this honest doctor?"

Being Choosy

"Let me explain," she said. "When I got my doctor's name from your medical society, the first thing I did, after I sat down with him, was to tell him my circumstances right out.

"After I told him I was on welfare, he smiled and said that he appreciated knowing it. Later he delivered all five of my children and he took care of my granddaughter, too. I guess I have an honest doctor because I am choosy. I think people should share and I choose to be with people who think like that."

I asked, "But what about the ignorant ones?"

"Oh, those that frown and don't know how to give? Why, I'm patient with them. At times like that, I think of my mother. She could get you to look at things in different ways. I guess I still look at things more than one way. Anyway, it's being patient."

Then I brought up another matter. "One idea that the state medical society is talking to the state government about is paying for recipient care at rates normally charged to other patients. That is, doctors should not be giving cut-rate services to welfare patients. What do you think of that?"

"Well, that's right," she said, "I suppose some people will say it's because the doctors are greedy. I don't think it's that so much as everybody should get what they deserve. But, you know, it's not going to make much difference with the ignorant doctors. All they will say is, 'Now we get what we deserve,' and they will probably remain just as unhappy—sorry that they didn't get it sooner."

Learn to Share

Finally, I asked her what she might suggest if she had a chance to say three things to physicians. She pondered, as the question appeared confusing, "You mean, if I was going to tell them what to do? You know I can't tell them how to be doctors."

"Yes, I know, but what would you tell them from your viewpoint? How would you suggest that they might be of more help to welfare patients?"

"Oh, well," she replied, "first they should do unto others as they would have others do unto them. The second thing is really part of the first, they should be kind and understanding of the patient's circumstances, for those circumstances might be their own some day. They should be sort of polite but better than polite. For the third thing, I guess they should be more discreet. They don't have to have their nurse shout out in a waiting room, 'What's your welfare number, Mrs. Wellwise?'

"I guess I haven't answered your questions satisfactorily. Only one thing is really important, and that is for all of us to learn to share. Our granddaughter comes over—you know my husband is in bed most of the time—and she runs right to her granddad because she knows that in the drawer in the little bedside table he always has a tiny piece of candy or some fruit or something for her. She asks him, 'Granddad, what's for me?' and I just stand there; it's one time when I don't talk so much. And he says, 'Well, I've got something for you, but first I will have to get it out of the drawer.' You know, when you think about it, even she is learning how to share. I guess I keep coming back to the same thing too much, but we should learn to share, because we are all in the same life together.

"I talk too much. I have probably said a lot of things I shouldn't have. But I am not a gossip. I don't visit my neighbors and talk away into the afternoon. It's another case, I guess, of me being choosy, and in this case, I choose to be with my family."

She paused for just a minute, and, thinking of her future, I said, "And when they grow up?"

She responded immediately, "Why you know, I've always wanted to go back to school. I'd really like to get that GED or GDE. I don't know what the initials are, but it's that school diploma that you can get after you leave school."

"I hope you can," I assured her. "You have been most kind to sit and share your thoughts with me. Do you want a taxi to get home?"

"Oh, I will walk," she said.

"Walk? Let me show you where to get the bus. Are you all right as far as the bus fare is concerned?" I fumbled for change.

"Oh yes, thank you. I've got the fare. I know I have talked too much." She smiled, "They call me the yammering grandmother."

I accompanied Mrs. Wellwise to the vestibule, pointed the way to the bus stop, and knew how lucky I was to have shared an hour with a complete person.

Endnotes

Reprinted from *Prism* 3 #2(1975): 3, 64, with permission. Copyrighted 1975, American Medical Association.

Humanism in Medicine, The Rudimentary Process

There is a stage in suffering, or in any emotion, or passion, when it belongs to what is most personal and inexpressive in man and there is a stage where it belongs to art. But in its first moments art can never do anything with it. Art is the distance that time gives to suffering.
—Albert Camus (1913-1960)
Notebooks 1942-1951

The preoccupation with a medical profession that appears more mechanical and less human grows each day. Our ears are bent, our minds filled, perhaps even our hearts weighted with the burgeoning catalogue of iatrogenic problems. For me, I have had enough, a surfeit of these problems, moral and mechanical, which indicate that physicians, like it or not, are becoming acquisitive corporations under the sway of a Frankenstein technology and a Faustian government. I do not know precisely when life begins or ends, nor care to use an electroencephalographic machine or any other device to hide my ignorance. In fact I know precious little about the technology of morality, when to transplant a heart or who should and who should not have renal dialysis; and, perhaps strangely, I have few expectations of mastering this modern blight, notwithstanding the storm of papers, the glare of programs, and din of talks demanding clarification of great ethical issues.

Perhaps perversely my ethical interests stray from the "great issues" of medical technology that make headlines when physicians are found guilty of manslaughter for performing abortions. Though I belittle neither the task nor the valor of those practicing on the frontiers of medical ethics, I have yet to wander that far from home and office.

My wonderment is restricted to those smaller, more mundane, though every bit as human, ethical problems of the profession, such as, should a doctor keep a patient waiting and if so why, or, should a doctor have clean fingernails (when I brought this problem up at a seminar on medical ethics at our local medical school I was nearly run out of the room for "getting personal"), or even, should a doctor direct his spouse to tell the importuning answering service that he is not home? Admittedly tacky questions at best, lacking all the glamour and heroics of deciding life and death for some unfortunate, but these humble questions do have the benefit of being commonplace enough for me to get my mind about them.

Also, it may be that the best chance of finding the raw material of a humanistic medicine is in the day-to-day life of the medical practitioner, his behavior in his office and at the bedside of his patients. Actually, I believe the present academic frontal assault on the concepts of ethics and humanism is in grave danger of being lost in words. Robert Louis Stevenson makes the point when he says, "Men do not live by bread alone, they live by catch words." Hence, one result of these profound theses on humanism could well be a rush of practitioners to buy the latest all-new-giant-size-super-American journal of up-to-date humanism with its guaranteed dosage of daily minimal requirements of tolerance, charity, and insight. No, there is no need to play the scholar to the detriment of the man.

Humanism is not inherent in either the individual or the culture. We are all born little savages and require as much civilizing as our aboriginal forefathers, who were quite content neither to bow nor to curtsey, but gradually learned that the grunts of the chap at the other end of the cave had meaning. This process of developing and then raising the level of social consciousness is humanism, and it has taken millenniums of trial and error, of bludgeonings and rip-offs to reach our present feckless stage.

Actually, Humanism with a capital "H" is a product of the Renaissance, and a late development in our culture. Five hundred years out of perhaps fifty thousand years is not a great span. Only yesterday was faith challenged by reason, asceticism by pleasure, group by individual, tradition by personal liberty.

Now if the development of Humanism during the Renaissance is considered as a time when there was a new emphasis on reason, rebellion, and recreation, it patently corresponds with a stage of individual development, adolescence, a time when overweening reason, nascent rebellion, and uninhibited recreation are assiduously pursued. Thus, the individual repeats the history of his species.

About the age of twelve, most of us become aware that other people matter even though they may not be ever-dependable pillars of strength. Our parents step down from their God-like positions, revealed as they really are, human beings. Then a momentous decision is made, by perhaps most adolescents, to respect or disrespect those who are weak and to confer dignity or scorn upon the less powerful.

This important yet ephemeral concept, that the weak also matter, is hardly a conscious idea, let alone a belief. It may pass through the mind of a young lady as she suddenly realizes that saying "please" is not simply an empty formality ground into her by her mother but a subtle exchange of gifts with another person. Or take the young man who suddenly understands that holding the door open for an infirm elder is not an onerous duty. He catches a glimpse that the brief time and effort he gives is a gift, both to himself and to the elder. These quivers of social awareness—that the other person, though weaker, has feelings and needs—may not last, but they are the green shoots of maturing human understanding, the raw material of humanism, the budding ability to see a choice between what is best for me and what is best for thee and me.

The development of considered social choice begins as a youth identifies with someone who has had to make a moral choice, a parent or mentor, and continues as the youth suspends judgment to see two or more possibilities in his search for the better moral solution. Similarly, it was not that the Renaissance man simply rediscovered the wonders of classical Greece and pitted them against medieval asceticism. His awakening came with the possibility that there could be more than one way to look at moral problems. He did not discover a new philosophy so much as he discovered that being human is a process—not a static condition. Considered choice, in contrast to established dogma, looking the answer up in Aristotle or the Bible, emerged as Humanism.

Discovering and developing this process of moral choice remains as much a necessity for today's medical student as it was to Renaissance man. Characteristically, humanism cannot be taught, lectured, assigned, or graded into students. However, an article titled "Three Medical Students Confront Death on a Pediatric Ward"[1] does delineate how humanism is learned. It recounts the willing involvement of three medical students with the family of a dying child. The students learn how helpless and alone they become as they minister to the stricken child and family.

> Four hours later Judy died. When she died I felt terribly inadequate, incapable. When I went out into the lounge to wake her parents and tell them of the tragedy, I wished I could have been somewhere else. All at once all my reason for wanting to be a doctor flashed before me and I wanted to reassure myself by telling them that it was a mistake, Judy would be all right. But I couldn't say, they already knew. And they in fact told me that Judy was dead.
>
> I felt confused and found I could not accept the fact that Judy was dead.

Thus these students explore their means of responding to the parents of a dying child and discover three ways in which they develop their sense of humanity: by being directly responsible for patient care; by having someone with whom to talk through the experience; and by independent learning—learning which is truly independent implies both self-discipline and self-responsibility. Inadvertently, they reveal the process of refining the raw material of humanism.

If medical humanism is a process, physicians have a lifelong need for processing. There must be a continual refinement of some essential material—A must be converted to B. Each day physicians should be converting a supply of raw feeling into civil behavior, continually civilizing and humanizing themselves.

Specifically, as soon as I, as a physician, have matured enough to realize that each patient is an individual, not a stereotype, I must adapt myself to each patient in a manner that allows him to be most open and free in revealing his humanness to me. I must "process" myself into a state of civility, "hold the door open for them," as it were, which comes down to my humanity, or lack of humanity, showing in everything I do or say, no matter how trivial. Every phrase of my speech, each act of my behavior, may inhibit or encourage patients to reveal themselves as human beings.

Take, for example, dirty fingernails of a physician: where do dirty fingernails fit into the relation with the patient, and do they hinder or help the patient? Is it too obvious, too simple, and too unimportant in the great scheme of medical humanism? Does someone protest that it did not matter if Osler had dirty fingernails—all that mattered was his moving teaching to the bedside of the patient? Remember, protester, you speak for yourself and not for Osler's patients; you speak for scientific concepts, not human behavior. Logically, the only patient you may speak for is yourself as a patient. Do you wish your doctor to have dirty fingernails?

And, of course, dirty fingernails speak for a class of small behaviors, which are not compulsive traits but tokens of consideration. Do you wish your physician to be prompt, to listen, to tolerate questions, even unsophisticated questions, to be discreet, to be candid with details as well as major concerns? Do you wish your physician to be considerate of you? Predictably, the odds increase if your physician has clean fingernails and in a thousand other ways has converted his raw material of humanism into a refined behavior awaiting your needs.

Medical humanism is not limited to the physician preoccupied with bioethics; it is the direct responsibility of every human being relating to a patient. The physician, the nurse, the aide are called upon to consider carefully what is best for the patient *and* themselves, not just what is best for themselves. It is the immediate patient who is the focus for the active process of humanitarianism, the patient sitting before the doctor, not the one who called earlier with complaints; the patient in the bed before the nurse, not the one down the hall; the patient on the stretcher the aide is pushing, not the one who needs a bath later in the day. Medical humanism is an immediate experience of shared dignity, not a theoretical debate in grievance committees.

The patient may also contribute to the humanizing process, for medical humanism is not a unique, one-way, "professional" street. How the patient communicates his self-concept predetermines much of his treatment. The patient with dirty fingernails is treated differently from the one with clean nails. Oh, the gross treatment, say the number of units of penicillin, may be the same, but the treatment meted out can be worlds apart for these patients. For the patient who thinks of himself as an animal, giving no more to others or to himself than circumstances demand, treatment can be little more than devalued veterinary medicine. For the patient who thinks and acts as a self-respecting, considerate human being, no matter what his circumstances, humane medicine is his due.

So even in the small behaviors, the details, everyone has an immediate responsibility to be humane in caring for the sick, a responsibility to think and talk through with others the meaning of that care, and to be forever dedicated to learning more about each fellow individual. Our responsibility is discharged as we work through our daily ration of the raw feelings, our elemental perception of the human condition, and continually develop civilizing insights into our innumerable encounters with our fellow man. There, and only there, in process of being human, can humanism be found in medicine.

Endnotes

Reprinted from the *New England Journal of Medicine* 293(1975): 1320-1322, with permission. Copyright ©1975 Massachusetts Medical Society. All rights reserved. Original title: "Sounding Board. Humanism in Medicine—the Rudimentary Process."

1. J.A. Griffith, P.J. Fabri, M.S. Kies, et al., "Three Medical Students Confront Death on a Pediatric Ward: A Case Report," *Journal of the American Academy of Child Psychiatry* 13(1974): 72-77.

On the Sounds of Death

A voice from Death, solemn and strange, in all his sweep and power,
With sudden, indescribable blow—
—Walt Whitman (1819-1892)
Leaves of Grass

The sounds of death are fearful, more so even than the sounds of dying. The muffled beat of the strong, black wings of death, when heard about, who knows where, sounds like the rush of a great owl, questing invisible through the night forest. The sounds of dying and the dead are fearful too, but different. Men, particularly physicians, may grow accustomed to these lesser sounds, for whether the death rattle of a soul released or the macabre grunt of a battlefield casualty thrown into a rough grave, the numb monotony of daily work dulls the ear to these morbid voices.

In contrast, no man grows accustomed to the sound of death itself. There is no pattern to be learned, for death may announce its presence with as light a touch as a faint change in tempo of senile fingers plucking at a counterpane or suddenly with the all-enveloping scream of an incoming artillery shell. Whether the least of noises or the greatest, the sound of the Black Angel brings a shudder to all men. I know. You see, I heard death when my dog was killed last night.

To Hold in Mind

I drove home from the office after dark and, with a touch on the horn, swung into the driveway. My dog was waiting, and when my wife opened the front door, he made for me. As I climbed out of the car, with a yip of joy he sprung up before me and then off around the yard, up the driveway, and, in his bursting exuberance, out onto the highway. It was dark and a car was coming by. As it passed, there was a quick, ever-so-soft thrum, as though some heavy hand had tapped a dampened cymbal. With the sound from the road, involuntarily, I shuddered at a thought too painful to hold in mind.

Not believing what I heard and felt, I strode into the house, leaving the front door open for my dog to scurry in behind. After exchanging kisses with my wife and daughter, I hung up my coat, and as I closed the hall closet door, there was a car in the driveway—

"Yes?"

"We have hit your dog."

"Oh, no!"

I ran through the rose bushes, up the lawn, and there lying on the pavement was the dearest bit of fur I had ever known. A car approached. I signaled it to one side and rushed out to sweep up in my arms that limp, warm mass. He rested in my arms ever so gently—but he was no more. A trickle of blood came from his mouth. His eyes were closed as though asleep.

I cradled him close. No heartbeat in his chest; no breath from his mouth; no flick to his eyes. He was no more—though he was as warm and limp as any night he had ever rested in my lap.

My wife cried. "Shall I call the vet?"

"No—I'll need a shovel."

So we carried him to a wooded spot, a bit of a knoll, beyond the house. I lay him upon some fallen fir boughs, and while my daughter held the light, I dug his grave, as a grave should be dug—deep, wide, unstintingly. You see, my dog was killed last night.

Before you ask why I should write, please let me tell just a bit about him—he was small, black, a bit ungainly. I believe he was a rat terrier, though I was never sure. He had that unusual personality, special brightness, illuminated optimism, which are found only in the resurrected. There are some people—and animals—who have known severe deprivation or illness early in life and, having been spared, bear no grudge with the past.

For them, for those unusual few, the worst is always over, behind, and what exists is blessed freedom from any fear. Nothing can ever again be as bad as it once was; the worst is left behind in the past, and happiness abounds.

And so it was for my dog, who came to us as a sick puppy, perhaps dying; and with us he grew well, strong, and free of fear. But not every fear, for we discovered, by coincidence, that the shuffling of a deck of cards stirred his all but buried, dark past. He was never teased about any part of his former life, and he trusted us never to stir it.

Within This Spirit

So within this spirit of bounding optimism, he became one of us, though my wife always said he loved me best. Perhaps he did—for if given a biscuit during the day, he would never eat it. He put it by the door, and, after I came home in the evening and he had greeted me, he would lie at my feet and chew up his treasured tidbit. Or after supper if I napped on the living room couch, inevitably I would awaken covered with his toys, for while I slept, he would go about the house and pick up his rubber mouse, his tugging toy, his bits of chewing rope, my old sock, his precious rubber porcupine and deposit them upon my sleeping body.

Not that I did not play with him—every evening after supper he would jump in my lap for our "fight." I would grab him by loose folds about his neck and he would sit and growl, snarl, bare his fangs, and ferociously gnaw my wrists. The sounds were hideous, but the damage nonexistent—for no matter how he "sank his teeth into me," there was never any pressure, never any mark—and at the climax of this noisy struggle, he would break from my grasp, plunge at my face, and lick my ears as though to amputate them.

Now, what I write is no apology for sorrow for a dog. I know that hundreds of people died this year on my state's highways and thousands have died upon my country's battlefields. I do not apologize; rather, I affirm how real the gift my dog has given me in his death. For today I know again, completely, what is probably the most painful and yet the most important part of life for any man to know—that death ends life but not love.

My dog was killed last night. The shock is passing. My regret, dear dog, is that when I buried you I did not take the coat from my back and wrap it about you. Not that you now need any protection from the cold, but rather that I would know even better that part of me lies in death with you, as part of you remains in life with me. It is 2 A.M. I have trouble sleeping, for I've heard the sound of death. You see, my dog was killed last night.

Endnotes

Reprinted from *Prism* 2 #5(1974): 9-10, with permission. Copyrighted 1974, American Medical Association.

Who Is Saving Private Ryan?
A Non-Review

Seventeen years as a movie critic for the medical profession taught me that you have to see the film in order to write an acceptable review. What you get here is not a review of *Saving Private Ryan* but the reasons I stayed home rather than join the search. Reluctance began with a report from a friend who had been seriously wounded at the Battle of the Bulge, "I don't fault making an anti-war film, though I question if Private Ryan is really anti war, but I am not going because no one can ever know what it is like to be in combat by watching movies." Another response, a psychotherapy patient, "It was horrible. The roar of tanks riding down out of nowhere to crush our men. I just held my head in my hands and closed my eyes," led me to believe I might have difficulty fitting it to my definition of entertainment and would probably, like it or not, have to spend hours, if not days, unwinding my reactions to scenes of terror the director flashed before me. No, I did not see the film, but rather spent time considering what is and is not entertainment.

One of my first encounters with the "magic" of cinema, illusions intended to produce intense anxiety, came as a seven-year-old in 1928 when my parents brought me along to a showing of Lon Chaney in *The Phantom of the Opera.* Predictably, the effect of that monster slithering up from the sewers of Paris to enthrall defenseless women sent shivers to every cell in my body. My engrossed mother was forced to recognize the film's effect on me by my squirming about in the seat. With her broad-stroke, generally ineffectual maternal solicitude she assured me, "Not to worry. It is only a picture up on the screen. It is not real."

Working from a premise that had served me well for seven years, namely, what you see and what you hear is real, I responded, "Oh, yes it is! Look, he is dragging her away." I was then prepared to launch into what had the makings of a profound ontological discussion only to be hushed into uncomfortable silence. Later I came to realize that most philosophical endeavors, particularly with my mother, ended nowhere, for any pursued challenge to her ready definition of reality resulted in untoward passion and a trip to my room.

THE HUMAN CONDITION

As could be predicted, I came away from the *Phantom* with a bonus of terror for the things that went bump in the night; those strange beings, including the Headless Horseman, whom I could make out in the flickering light and shadow cast on my bedroom wall by the street light shining through the leaves of the great maple tree outside my window. As yet unacquainted with Plato and his cave, I knew considerable about real things casting shadows when I was supposed to go to sleep. Still a bit perplexed by Mother's explanation of reality, "Because I say so," which turns out about as functional as Plato's, my certainty of reality remains flawed and in need of continual attention.

My failure to be certain may stem from my Mother's unshakable assurance that she "knew" and the fact that there was no chance, this side of the Big Bang, of changing her mind. *The Phantom of the Opera* may not be real, certainly no more or less than *Saving Private Ryan,* but for me coming to grips with a sense of uncertainty at what I see on the silver screen remains a piece of work. How can I watch Orson Welles stumble through a millionaire's life in *Citizen Kane* and not believe that this is closer to reality than whatever might have happened to William Randolph Hearst? How can I have Cyrano raise me to the heights of chivalry only to say it is just a bit of movie magic? Is it or is it not real? For me the clincher comes with Hamlet. Was he a person even more riddled with doubt than I? Shakespeare, along with some help from Richard Burton and Kenneth Branagh, made Hamlet real, at least for me.

But movie magic is done in the dark, the dark of the theater, the dark of the audience, and in my personal darkness. As Coleridge put it, albeit for the magic of poetry, it calls for a momentary pause of disbelief which constitutes poetic faith. When I step into the darkness of a movie house I willingly suspend my judgment in the service of taking to the center of my conscious being those shadows on the wall. I submit myself as a passive vessel for actors/directors to fill with their chromatic elixir of life. Mind you, I did not at the age of seven explore this side of our discussion with my mother. Then I just pulled away her hands as she attempted to shield my eyes from viewing her non-reality, the continuing depredations of the monster.

The reason I will not see *Saving Private Ryan* is a deep distrust in any artist/director who might fail to return me and my suspended judgment to the daylight a more complete person than when I entered the darkened chamber. Horrendous moulage of U.S. soldiers flying apart may rival the shock of confronting monstrous Lon Chaney, full screen, but now I am better prepared to encounter the artist who offers up entertainment. Having grown old enough to no longer tag along to popular films with the folks, parent surrogates, increasingly I discriminate when approaching ontological problems of reality.

Curiously, the present basis for my choice of films does not so much revolve around aesthetics as about the use of language, the etymology of "entertainment." This word turns out to be a bit of baggage William the Conqueror dumped on Middle English in 1066. It derives from Middle French, meaning to stand or hold between, as in the legal phrase, the court refused to 'entertain' his plea. The act of being entertaining calls for a temporary "holding between," suspension of laws, rules, and judgment of and by all concerned. Little do we realize on entering a movie theater the valuables we check at the door.

This is true for all elements of entertainment, for though the Greeks took their drama in the daylight, Coleridge pointed out that poetic drama, too, demands a necessary momentary pause of disbelief. Today, the movie producer stretches the pause of disbelief further and further, three hours in the case of *Saving Private Ryan*.

Even if it is true that turnabout is fair play and my dear departed mother was nearby I would not willingly challenge her sense of reality a jot. Rather, I would simply share with her my views about going to the movies. To my mind, any seat we take is paid for, in addition to the admission price, with a state of suspended unaccountability. In return the entertainment industry guarantees us a place between two worlds, between daily life and Hollywood, between two realities of experienced human emotions and its similitude.

My views might again take us to the issue of reality, accounting for our feelings and who is responsible for them. I might even return to our mutual friend, Hamlet, to say how much I identify with him as a believable human being, my measure of his reality. My mother, perhaps taken by *Private Ryan's* scenes of the Normandy landing, might well shush me again. If she did I would understand that she like most of the audience would say it is only "on the screen" insisting that no one is accountable for more than the time it takes to watch.

You may detect how little I *really* expect the audience to be accountable, even to themselves, for what they feel. There is too much danger in watching *Private Ryan* that my need to be accountable, if only to myself, even if I squirmed in the seat, would go unrecognized as passive agreement with the prevalent doctrine of vicarious violence in the service of peace, a lesson in the evil of war much as the thrill of TV murder is watched as an entertaining lesson in the need to reduce crime. It was all there in my youth when porno film houses proclaimed from their marquees, right below some salacious title, "This show is in the service of redeeming social value." Unfortunately, accounting for suspended judgment in the pursuit of entertainment remains deceptively hidden behind that too common reality check, everybody does it, including my mother.

The future for my sallies at discussion seem bleak. If I pause before entering a theater to ask, "Will it leave us wiser, if not better, human beings for attending?" the best I can hope for is, "Get on with you." Instead of *Private Ryan* I search for any who might join in weighing a chance to laugh or cry against its possible aesthetic, civic, psychological, and moral costs. Hearing nothing in response, I caution the attentive reader that unless you wish to have someone put their hands over your eyes, from all indications *Saving Private Ryan* is not the kind of film to take your mother to.

Endnotes

Reprinted from the *Neil Elgee, M.D., Newsletter*. Mercer Island, Washington, The Ernst Becker Foundation.

The Value of Suffering in Medical Practice

They should have known how to interpret sorrow better. I have said that behind sorrow there is always sorrow. It were wiser still to say that behind sorrow there is always a soul.
—Oscar Wilde (1854-1900)
De Profundis

Once embarked on their clinical practice, many practitioners are confounded at discovering the prevalence and intractability of human suffering. Trained as physicians are to reorder physiology and remove pathology, little formal attention is devoted to a fundamental human manifestation of illness, suffering. Yet the treatment of human suffering has unique power to heal the sick when skillfully and compassionately pursued by a caring physician. Let us consider the value of suffering in attaining that skill and the intimacy that ensures its compassionate application.

While conclusions may differ, understanding human suffering has been a goal of prophets, visionaries, saints, and philosophers since the beginning of history. Some conclude it to be a token of the stoic's resignation to assuage the calamity of being alive. Others invoke theological beliefs that suffering is God's path to redemption through punishment for sins. Others, attorneys, account for pain and suffering in dollar amounts.

Personal suffering remains an enigma to human understanding even as it speaks a language known to the human heart; an enigma too often unexamined, even denied. Yet physicians, as healers, must seek to understand and speak this remarkable language that is learned by openly considering patients' inevitable pain and suffering.

Defining suffering is not easy since it occurs in a place where eyes do not see, where science does not measure, the center of the human heart. The dictionary provides slim definition, saying little more than suffering is a state of submitting to or enduring misery and pain.

However, compassionate clinicians are called upon to use their heart as well as mind to define here and now the functional definition of suffering as soul-felt experience.

Suffering is experience. It is awaking at 3 A.M. with an inescapable sense of dread. Suffering is a teenager standing unnoticed at a high school dance. Suffering is giving birth to a baby. Suffering is a father without work. Suffering is a root canal operation. Suffering is sitting through interminable committee meetings that drag into the night. Suffering is making and receiving a fatal diagnosis. Suffering is losing one's mind. Suffering is attending at the bedside of a terminal patient. For caring physicians such shards of feeling add up to a personal definition of suffering.

Perhaps the quintessential example of suffering is the ten-year-old child, happily returning from school, entering her home, only to suddenly remember that her mother is no longer alive; that her mother is dead, died, forever, two months ago. The suffering child's heart shatters yet again.

How is it that the loneliest and most personal experience a human being endures relates to healing? Is it not reasonable that suffering, like pain, should be quickly suppressed or eliminated by chemical "tranquilizing"? To answer these questions another question must be asked. Where does suffering originate?

Suffering begins at birth. We first become conscious of suffering in separating from our mothers. Then, kicking and screaming, we reluctantly embark on the business of becoming independent human beings. Fortunately, original pain lies beyond recall; for most, suffering is initially associated with the first day of school. The memory can be recalled of leaving the security of home, a heartbreaking hesitancy at joining a gang of noisy, demanding children just like ourselves as mother fades first into the background and then from the room. Some may even remember their mother's parting admonition, "Don't cry, be grown up," taking with her every shred of your personal security as she left.

Suffering originates with the inevitable sense, albeit sometimes unfounded, of being abandoned, perhaps forever. Suffering is experienced loss, deep loss of a significant part of our world, a loss of part of ourselves.

But is suffering necessary? Are human beings required to experience loss in order to function as individuals? Is it not enough, like Buddha, to simply know joy and security and, with unalloyed positive feelings, grow into complete human beings? The fact remains that suffering is essential in shaping our unique character, much as pain is necessary in identifying our bodies. Pain sets the limits on physical being while suffering defines character.

The practical role of pain becomes self-evident when leprosy, a disease of fifteen million people, is considered. *Mycobacterium leprae,* the bacteria responsible for the disease, has a predilection for the cooler portions of the body, especially the feet and hands. Its progressive infection not only disfigures the skin but insidiously destroys the pain receptors of the nervous system. Consequently, advanced leprosy leaves its victims anesthetized, painless.

A patient with leprosy lacks sensation of the body's inevitable scrapes and bruises. Without their attendant sensations the body is ignorant of what to repair. Holding a lighted cigarette between his fingers a leprous patient is unaware it has burned down to his finger until alerted by the smell of roasting flesh. We remain aware of the danger of a hot stove, not from a childhood admonition, but from our ever vigilant warning system, pain. The leprous patient lacking pain awareness consequently discovers his body literally eroding away.

A comparable warning system exists for emotional life. Like it or not, the healthy person remains alert to possible emotional dangers. Suffering at the hands of a cruel teacher can burn like a "hot stove" and quickly instructs a student to avoid contact of mind, expressed curiosity. Maintaining this largely unconscious but elaborate system of thought and feeling is real work. It is the inept student of life who ignores actual circumstances to believe, "But it can't happen to me." Potential suffering is ever present in the "real" world, a fact which the wise clinician appreciates, knowing that, like death and taxes, there is an inevitable emotional cost involved in the patient's life. Part of that cost is maintaining a warning system against real losses that "do happen" and happen to "me."

No thinking person can doubt that the human condition carries with it inevitable suffering since all human relationships terminate. To the degree termination is accepted and answered to, including ultimate termination, death, an individual matures. To the degree loss and its consequent suffering is accepted and understood, to that degree alone an individual lives rather than exists.

Fear of loss, suffering, is confided in countless ways to the attentive physician. As a mother confides her concerns in sending her son off to play football or to go downhill skiing, her fear may seem inconsequential to the listener, but not to her. Helped to reflect on the risks and rewards for her son in these "rough and tumble" activities, she is then able to weigh her painful apprehension against his joy of life. Quietly, with the support of wise counsel, she can learn to own her suffering as her own.

The perpetual problem confronting both patient and doctor is identifying significant emotions in a shared calculus of suffering that compassionately matches appropriate interpretation of anticipated misfortune.

The Treatment of Human Suffering

By examining the elements of the patient's suffering refracted through the physician's experience, clinical judgment leads to therapeutic understanding. There is not nor ever can be a how-to-do-it manual for relating to patients' suffering. Therapeutic understanding is an amalgam of experienced suffering. Here more than at any other point in the practice of medicine a technical, "cook book" approach proves defeating. Instead, in the process of making conscious the unconscious processes that go into suffering, the physician mobilizes four indispensable elements of the patient-doctor relationship, acknowledgment, relatedness, action, and doubt. These elements, neglected as they may be by the medical literature, are more than intuition.

Acknowledgment

Experience gains authentic value only through interpersonal validation, acknowledgment. Without conscious thought, experience generally slips into forgetfulness, much as the memory of last week's headlines now lie beyond recall. Without disciplined self accounting, experience readily merges with fantasy, the toy of facile imagination, the enemy of fact. Unless we recognize who we are by our several behaviors we remain ignorant of our identity. To be a "me" we must acknowledge who "we" are.

Human development critically depends upon acknowledgment of being. Unconsciously, parents validate feelings for children, such as the pain that comes with a scraped knee. "Ooh, falling on that bad rock hurts" is acknowledgment intended to educate the three-year-old to appropriate feelings. How much it hurts and how long it aches is open to negotiation, but when we are children, parents' validation that we hurt and how we hurt establishes the reality of our pain and consequently contributes significantly to the fact and process of our understanding of our bodies.

At a level deeper than cuts and bruises, parents validate the emotional being of a child. Whether a lullaby or gold stars for good grades, open parental acknowledgment of a child's emotional life shapes the feelings of the adult to be. Remarks, sometimes said in jest, "This is my beloved daughter" or "Here is my ungrateful son," may not register long in the mind of the parent yet reverberate through the subsequent life of the child. The pediatrician who recognizes that shots hurt with, "You were a brave lad not to cry," does much more than reduce the noise in his office.

This can happen in the patient-doctor relationship when it successfully addresses the patient's suffering. Acknowledgment is accepted with integration, sometimes a momentary pause of recognition that satisfies at all levels of relating for acknowledging what needs to be acknowledged.

Sometimes pain is dismissed, denied, by a significant other with, "Everyone gets a scraped knee." The absence of acknowledgment in later life surfaces with, "Pull yourself together. It can't be that bad." Deprived of sustained acknowledgment in childhood, adults can remain confused, unsure, even ashamed of painful feelings. This leaves the woman patient with family difficulties surfacing around her menstrual cycles vulnerable to a physician's, "It is just your periods. You should expect this kind of thing at your age." Thus a critical task for a caring physician is not to dismiss but investigate and educate, as a caring parent acknowledges and educates, identifying particular experiences of suffering.

Relatedness

Though naming feelings may be an integral part of successful living, it should not be held narrowly as private reflection. Unless suffering moves others, generates empathy in a confidant, the sufferer remains locked in an empty world of loneliness. If a scraped knee fails to generate even a smidgen of empathy, the child is shortchanged in learning how to judge the loneliness that inevitably shadows suffering. Significant others are necessary instructors in the practical importance and unimportance of our pain and suffering. Here lies the fundamental bond successfully relating doctor to patient, patient to doctor. If the bond is faulty or missing, the relationship degenerates into provider servicing consumer.

If blighted by neglect or ignorance, the possibility of sharing feelings goes unrecognized, life passes with emotions as no more than empty words. Feelings, here-and-now feelings, are points of our emotional compass for navigating social life. To set those compass bearings, feelings must have a commonalty with kindred feelings. As a significant other, the caring physician resonates with sincere empathy and approachable fortitude to the patient's feelings. Thus the relationship prospers; healing, in every sense, becomes possible.

Action

There is much a caring physician can do to help a patient draw strength from his suffering. Action offers alternatives to senseless resignation, blind sorrow, and unrelieved misery. Action opens the door to healing by metabolizing suffering into meaningful points of reference. The great physician Sir William Osler is reported, perhaps apocryphally, to have responded to criticism for whistling as he left the room of a dying child with, "Would it be better if I cried?" Apparently he transmuted his suffering to action. When leaving the bedside of a terminal patient, it is commonplace for practitioners to turn their personal suffering into more than a resolve "not to cry," using heightened self-awareness to focus on the immediate care at hand. So it can be in helping a terminal patient to work at "putting your life in order."

Of all actions afforded the physician, touching certainly is the most available for softening the ache of suffering. From the pediatrician's finger proffered to the insecure infant, to the gerontologist's gentle enfolding of palsied hands plucking at a counterpane, sentient outreach of one human being, touching, is an ancient, elemental solace. We are lost to the full reality of healing should we simply consider our examining fingers as tools, extensions of our mind, rather than what they can be, extensions of our heart.

A patient once wisely observed that he judged physicians by one thing, whether they washed their hands before they examined him. More than ritual impels the caring physician to carefully wash hands, then rub fingers to acceptable warmth. Thus patients' vulnerability is openly acknowledged. The unselfconscious, half embrace that accompanies the hand on the shoulder of the patient informed of a terminal diagnosis says more of continuing support and care than an encyclopedia of words. Conscious caring informs styles of interaction until they become habits of the heart, elixir to sore tried souls.

Action in the service of suffering is unlimited yet so often passed over in discharging the patient-doctor relationship. A patient's genuine "thank you" does much to reinforce mutual respect. In grief a patient may have his eyes opened by responsive counsel to the beneficence in sweeping the kitchen floor or rereading a consoling book. Nor are these tonics for the patient alone. The physician, lifelong inhabitant of a world of care, needs considered nurturance in healing his or her soul as well. Thus through the balm of shared love, expressed in returning home to embrace a spouse, kiss a daughter, pat a dog, weed the garden, the physician's spirit is regenerated for yet another day. These actions give meaning to suffering through acknowledged relatedness—authenticated identity.

Doubt

Doubt, often experienced as a direct consequence of fear and loss, seldom is considered as a necessary force in addressing suffering, yet by establishing personal value for suffering, doubt ultimately determines its meaning. Doubt is an anvil for forging renewed identity.

"Could I have done it differently?" heads a list of seldom acknowledged but often considered questions patients have about themselves when confronted with the bad news of a guarded prognosis. "If only I had not smoked a cigarette," "…stayed out in the rain," "…driven home after drinking," express deep doubt in the personal judgment that has apparently brought suffering in its wake. Rather than pass over self-doubt with denial or, worse, false reassurance, both patient and doctor are called to examine pervasive self-doubt as a consequence of suffering, recognized since Job's lament.

By its nature suffering diminishes identity. "Is this really happening to me?" is the beginning of corrosive self-doubt. Inevitably, by grasping the nettle of suffering the force of doubt is recognized. "What have I done to deserve such misfortune?" questions who I am as much as what has happened. For the religious, doubt is framed by "Has my God forsaken me?" Should these questions be ignored or denied, acknowledged suffering remains inchoate.

Doubt is a strange business. Though humane values may be refined by daily tests of doubt, doubt ceaselessly challenges identity. In the face of suffering some patients deny self-doubt by facile sentiment or exaggerated self-esteem. "I am too tough to be shaken by your diagnosis, doctor." Some seek to strike a bargain with fate, "Get me out of this Doc and I will…." To touch suffering, physicians must accept the patient's doubt-prompted denial. This calls for the physician to judge the patient's capacity to accept suffering, keenly cognizant of all patients' limits in the knowing. Curiously, judgment of a patient's plight requires physicians to doubt their own soul-strength while in the reach of implacable misfortune. Then the physician's self-doubt reveals possibilities for healing through shared courage and deepened insight.

St. Paul ascribes to love a lack of arrogance. Can caring in the service of suffering also be without arrogance? Physicians must judge the mystery of human suffering with humility, aware how weakness, ignorance, and deception can color judgment. Experience teaches that error in judgment, misconception, and cowardice are forever linked with the human condition. Hence, our valuing of our self, like valuing an other can never free itself of doubt.

Significant elements of healing find their source in character strength displayed through acknowledgment, relatedness, action, and doubt. Who can doubt that these four traits are essential for encountering and treating human suffering? There may be other words and other concepts carrying deeper meaning—intelligence, compassion, redemption, and forgiveness—but it is the caring physician's unique style that empowers the successful treatment of suffering, soul healing. The healer's considered personal experience integrates the vital four elements of caring into the patient-doctor relationship. Without them the patient may be cured of the disease but not of its burden of suffering.

Physicians' informed, compassionate response to patients' travail is an ancient tradition. Pursuing this tradition means accepting, if not proclaiming, the obvious. Our meaning as physicians resides in our ability to recognize and join with the patient's suffering. In serving the sick of body, mind, and soul the complete physician continually asks, "How do I value suffering, my patient's suffering and my own?"

Part 3

Compassion's Necessary Courage

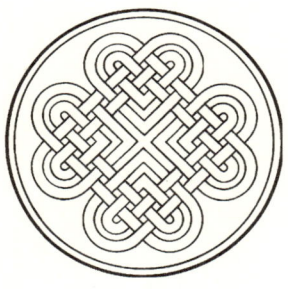

Unbounded courage and compassion joined...
make the hero and the man complete.
  —Joseph Addison (1672-1719)
  The Campaign

Overview to Part 3

Can anyone doubt that compassion calls for courage? The raw grit of plunging into a rampaging river to rescue a drowning child, standing up to a mob in defense of a helpless lynching victim, are activities far from day-to-day life. However, physical courage, grasping the hand of the leper, heroic as it may be, is an element of compassion secondary to moral courage, seeing the leper as one with yourself. Ultimately, compassion demands a quiet yet unshakable resolve, the courage to see if not do the right thing, morally.

Moral courage, an uncompromising recognition of what it is to be human, is neither instinctive nor a matter of habit. Subtly, culture focuses our vision to an "accepting" perspective, our "instinctual" xenophobia for those who do not speak or dress as we do, while habit persuades us to see people and circumstances as we are accustomed to see them, comfortably, not necessarily as they are.

Consider, if you will, a passing observation, a file of children, lined up, impatiently awaiting their morning ride on the school bus. Can you spy the little girl, jostled by some rowdy boys into "her" place at the end of the line? Do you see the violence for what it is? Instead, perhaps, you indulge a flight of sentimental fancy with "Ah, what a shy little thing she is."

Innocuous judgments often comfort the observer by disguising another's suffering as innocent charm. It takes exercised compassion, sharing the other's vision of experienced violence and enforced indignity, together with its whiff of nascent fear, to experience the plight of the other compassionately.

Conscious penetration of the obvious, accepting the risk of encountered pain and suffering, is motivated by more than simple interest. Curiosity that seeks the full human import of circumstance is forged from moral courage.

The grace of seeing things as they may be for the less powerful is so prized in the practice of medicine that it is explicitly recognized in the ancient custom of swearing a medical oath. The reason why this recognition has been integral to the character of the medical profession for two thousand years is explored in **On the Psychology of the Hippocratic Oath**.

Hello, Hippocrates, Are You There? documents, contrary to common belief, that a vast majority of medical schools in the United States offer graduates opportunity to publicly profess their moral obligation for courage in the service of patients.

Moving from generalized to personal accountability, **A Medical Code for Me** offers one physician's interpretation of the healer's need to see things through her or his own eyes.

The movie review of ***Betrayal*** explores unaccountable caring, lying to "protect" another from the truth. By focusing on insidious moral cowardice among "friends," the film depicts a trail of suffering that follows in the wake of pernicious lying. Though *Betrayal*'s characters are apparently dedicated to truth, each colors it with "little" lies which accumulate until there is no certainty of what the truth may be. Their remarkable cleverness only serves their cowardice by investing even minor motives with specious reasons, alienating attitudes, and irresponsible behaviors. For them, the art of lying becomes a lifestyle. Though embellished with intellectual ingenuity, empty respectability erodes away the character of each into bits and pieces of dishonor.

Unfortunately, *Betrayal*'s commonplace threat of "benign" deception is routinely found in conceits of medical practice (see "Lying" in part 10). Glib pronouncements, "This will not hurt" or "You have to expect some aches and pains once you get on in years," erode trust. Tawdry professional fibs, "Sorry about the delay but hospital rounds kept me busy" or "The nurse (receptionist, business manager, answering service) did not let me know you were waiting," can make so light of truth that trust fades from the relationship.

Fullness of compassion compels a close look at "insignificant" cheating, insincerity that subverts the indispensable requirement of quality medical practice, candid intimacy. The review of the book **The Corrupted Land** examines the common rationalization, "everybody cheats." With newspaper reports of major research scandals along with proliferating Medicaid fraud, the idea of cheating in medicine is not as unimaginable as it once was. Professional corruption is fostered in part by practitioners' reliance on a depersonalizing attitude that confounds the patient with the disease, "I am referring a colon cancer to you," cowardly dissimulation in the face of human need.

Though not readily recognized, the sharp edge of physical courage is never absent from medical practice. **The Awareness of Courage** addresses an instance of physical courage, examining its character and cost.

Melding physical and moral courage calls for sustained judgment. **In the Belly of the Soviet Beast** expresses the author's concern and ambivalence in confronting evil in high places of a hostile foreign culture. Since anonymity is important, actual names are replaced with ones taken from Anton Chekhov's *Ward Six*. The bitterness of unrequited, moral courage salts **Humble Pie** and is dealt with, as it seems it always must be, inadequately.

To be authentic the patient-doctor relationship must, when challenged, be experienced courageously.

On the Psychology of the Hippocratic Oath

Take care not to feel toward the inhuman as they feel toward men.
 —Marcus Aurelius Antoninus (121-180 A.D.)

While I was serving on a committee of the county medical society, a question of ethics arose. In order to resolve it, research proved necessary and this in turn brought me circling back to the cornerstone of our profession, the Hippocratic oath. The juxtaposition of the ancient and the present startled me into asking myself some questions which may interest others.

What purpose does the Hippocratic oath play in our profession? Is it a vestige of custom, an anachronism which habit carries into the graduation ceremonies of over 94 percent of our medical schools? Perhaps it serves some more vital need than dignity ensconced. The literature concerning the oath is limited largely to historical documentation and contemporary interpretation. There is little written on the "why" of it.

So then ask, "Why take an oath?" and the answer comes back, "Custom decrees." But why does custom decree? What purpose does a baptismal, confirmation, marriage, court, allegiance, fraternal, or professional oath serve? What is custom asking? What is the meaning of Hamlet's ghost, who from beneath the stage, charges Hamlet's cohorts with a rumbling, elemental command, "SWEAR!" Are we listening to Hippocrates' voice over the ages ordering us to "SWEAR!"?

We take an oath because it is suspected that we may not keep our word. Sometime in the future we are to be subjected to an ordeal, and during that ordeal we may fail. The oath is necessary to ensure that our minds not play tricks by encouraging us to rationalize away the meaning of the ordeal. An oath makes possible the full use of ourselves, our mental, moral, and social selves, when we may need it most. It removes debate and philosophy from a time when action may be the only consideration, for by an oath you identify yourself irrevocably.

There is considerable literature against taking oaths—particularly loyalty oaths, but this is not so much in opposition to the process as it in opposition to political exploitation of oaths, where the intent is not to activate honor but to enforce conformity. These are the two results of oath taking, an activated honor and an implied conformity.

But what has this to do with the Hippocratic oath? Much, for it too is intended to activate honor and ensure conformity, but what honor and what conformity? We are to meet the ordeal of another's illness with honor and conformity to his needs.

Perhaps a modern mind would dismiss such a construct as unnecessary, a form of philosophical mumbo-jumbo left over from the Middle Ages. Talk of ordeals has little relevance to our day—or does it? There is an interesting scientific literature evolving on the ease with which modern man cooperates in torturing his fellow man, that is, perpetrates ordeals on his fellow man. Not that he carries faggots to burn heretic witches, though some might see an analogy in dumping napalm on Asian children, nor is he a "Doctor of Infamy," but in just plain unhonorable, thoughtless obedience to authority, modern man tortures. The laboratory work of Milgram, Kaufman, Cragi, and Crockett shows that there is almost no limit to the torture one man will inflict on another "if properly prepared." In the lingo it is called "destructive obedience," the slang expression is "going along with the crowd." The way Milgram put it, "obedience may be a deeply ingrained behavior tendency, indeed, a prepotent impulse overriding training in ethics, sympathy, and moral conduct."[1]

Kaufman's study, "The Unconcerned Bystander,"[2] may serve to make the point scientifically clear. Though his experiment is detailed, superficially it may be described as an experiment in which a college student was ostensibly employed as an assistant to carefully record the reactions of subjects to a "learning situation under stressful conditions." The apparent subjects were described as older students, but were actually actors who reacted with increasing agony to the apparent electric shocks they received for wrong answers. The shock machine had clearly marked dials, 20 to 240 volts, while verbal designations were from "very slight to very dangerous" shocks, and with each wrong answer the "voltage" was jumped. Kaufman was trying to find at what point the student-assistant would intercede to stop this destructive treatment of his fellow men (the dependent variable) but his experiment failed because no one had a cutoff point. Out of 186 humans, 20 spoke to the "teacher" about what was happening, and only 10 objected to torturing a fellow human—no one tried to stop it. I believe the average medical school class runs about 100, so the figures may be easily transposed to us.

The "trick" of preparing Mr. Everyman to be a torturer is to lead him to an unpleasant task with sufficient masking of human issues. Unfortunately, it seems that if given the chance most men will reach for the blinders necessary to willingly cooperate with evil. At least this is what science shows to date. Not that this is new, what is new is the extraordinary ease with which it can be done. Nor is this "brain washing," on the contrary, it is "brain dirtying," if there is such a phrase, and men are accomplished in doing it for themselves. Only when they have the fortitude to examine their stand against what they said their stand was to be, can the extent of their deviations be examined by themselves. Thus only can a man take measure of his character, for if men have no point of reference they have no hope of ever knowing if what they do is right or wrong, helpful or harmful, human or inhuman. The accepted standard becomes the prevailing mood of the man, or his times, which is as useful as a match in a forest fire.

It is an honest man who knows he is capable of a dishonest act and that he needs his morals in his forebrain, not on vellum.

The Hippocratic oath is sometimes considered to be the prototype union contract, the original guild charter for the protection and preservation of a profession. Actually it is a sacred agreement between the student who stands with hand uplifted and the future physician he or she will be, to protect, not self, nor the profession, but the patient. I commend it highly as an honorable reminder to ourselves of what we can be.

Endnotes

Reprinted from *Private Practice* 2(1970): 59.
1. S. Milgram, "Behavioral Study of Obedience," *Journal of Abnormal and Social Psychology* 67(1963): 371-78.
2. H. Kaufman, "The Unconcerned Bystander," *Proceedings of the 76th Annual Convention of the American Psychological Association*, 1968.

Hello, Hippocrates, Are You There?

> *Perfection of means and confusion of goals seem—in my opinion—to characterize our age.*
> —Albert Einstein (1879-1955)

A phone call from a reporter for the *Kansas City Star* broke into my somber daily routine of eight 50-minute hours. He wanted to know if it were true that the Hippocratic oath was all but dead. While I wondered at his question, he gradually explained that Kansas physicians were amending their medical oath to fit the changing times. Omitting any further reference pro or con on abortion, they had gone so far as to seriously consider dropping any medical oath altogether. The reporter had been under the impression that what remained of classical medical tradition hung on the mere whim of an elderly professor at the Kansas Medical School, that is, until someone had told him of a survey I had conducted on the use of medical oaths.[1]

"Is it true that they are all but gone by the board?" he asked.

I assured him that quite the opposite is true. Indeed, during the last decade, ever-increasing numbers of medical schools in the United States and Canada are using medical oaths; currently over 94 percent have adopted or retained them. Apparently, students and medical faculties are more interested in them now than in the past, and medical faculties in Europe and the former Soviet states appear increasingly interested as well. In October 1997, the first world conference on medical oaths was held in Freiburg, Germany, well attended by representatives from every corner of the world.[2]

Like many answers, this one stimulated more questions, for the Kansas reporter went on (at his expense!):

"But, then, what do you make of this change in Kansas? Incidentally, are you for abortion?"

Glancing at the clock, I assayed an answer. "First, let me answer your second question first. I am not for or against abortions. If there is one thing the medical profession does not need, it is another political campaign. What I am for is a patient, a particular patient, is not something that can be lobbied through a legislature. I gather that what you want to know is the impact of social change on the profession. Well, I assure you that the impact is extraordinary. You cannot take a tradition of two thousand years, such as the Hippocratic oath, and tinker with it without repercussions. That is how I explain the increased use of medical oaths.

"The profession is under strong social pressure to serve the majority. Right now the majority has the uneasy feeling that it has become too numerous for comfort and that whereas there may not be enough commodities—food, shelter, land—to go around now, soon there will be even less. The majority, the culture, or whatever label you want, has decided for its reasons that abortion shall be legal. In effect, the medical profession is being ordered to 'innovate,' that is, to get in step and undertake a solution to the population problem.

"Oh, it is not just that clear or simple, since the humanitarian aspects of abortion are prominently displayed on most of the banners. But apparently by mass abortions we are now to save the girls who have failed in sex education. We are to rescue the mental health of pregnant young women and rid them of a sudden plague of incipient nervous breakdowns. We are to reduce the self-afflicted burden of so many apparently unwitting welfare mothers. Although I am not eager to debate such social-moral problems or even to candle those eggs, I do sometimes wonder where all the latter-day missionaries were hiding when society was shipping abortionists off to jail!

"As it turns out, present legislation makes the abortion problem at once easier and harder for the profession. As the government removes itself from the area of morality, abortion becomes more available. The less government comes between the patient and the physician, the more their relationship prospers. However, the gritty part for the profession is that just because government is dropping the morality issue does not make morality either illegal or obsolete. The moral problems for both patient and physician increase, not decrease, once abortion laws are repealed. If this were not true, we would be living according to the narrow dictum that what is legal is moral and what is illegal is immoral. In effect, we would be endorsing the absurdity of legislators becoming our spiritual leaders."

For the physician who accepts the questionable maxim that what is legal is moral, the present change in abortion laws presents no problems. As a technician, he simply alters his position to accommodate a new technique. Particularly since his new approach has a certain *avant-garde* glamour and a lot of money connected with it, he may find himself increasingly comfortable. It is the classical position of the twentieth-century scientist: "I was ordered to do those experiments at the concentration camp so don't hold me responsible." Only in the case of abortion, the "order" is implicit rather than explicit.

"Now lest you think I am some kind of zealot rallying the troops for a counterreformation, hold on. Again I remind you: I am not for or against abortion; I am *for* a particular patient. Although this may be hard for a layman to comprehend, that is what the medical oath is all about. It focuses the moral thinking of the physician on a particular patient. To function, the oath cannot remain an abstraction. Either it works every time a patient is seen, or it is not worth the breath to swear it.

"Do not get the idea that the physician should now, any more than in the past, impose his morality on the patient. We need no medical inquisitions to wipe out patients' real or fancied heresies. However, and this lays the gravest responsibility on the profession, we do need to remember that there is a morality for the patient and for the physician despite any laws that are passed to the contrary. The onerous part is how to make this explicit to the abortable patient. Let me ask you. Should the physician do more than negotiate a convenient time to squeeze the abortion into his own and the patient's schedule? Should he explore with the patient the implications that go beyond the physiological? Should he venture into the psychology, the sociology, the morality of the patient's life? Ah! Now arises a vicious ambiguity. How far should the physician involve himself in the relationship? Should he be amoral, partially moral, or moral? Should he go to the soul of the matter? Guilt, shame, and fear are the inevitable and intense consequences that follow any destructive act, particularly if the act impinges on the rights of another human being, even an unborn human being. Should the physician, then, be more than a technician, a functionary of the system?

"I am not the one to say whether a physician should involve himself in the psychological, social, or moral perceptions of his patient. I am merely pointing out that the moment he relates to the abortable patient, he is involved in a vicious ambiguity. If he strictly limits himself to a technician's role, he is less than his medical oath expects of him; he is acting not immorally, but amorally. If he does involve himself, not in the patient's life, but in the patient's perception of life, he must frequently, if not always, develop an awareness of the patient's morality and of its effect on the patient's life. How dark and forbidden this territory is for the twentieth-century scientist! What training, what precedent, what formal resource has the physician to venture through those unique labyrinths? Ultimately, about all the physician has directly from the profession itself is the medical oath. Battered compass though it be, the oath has guided physicians through the rise and fall of dynasties, and through the most diverse cultures, as well as academic warfare raging in some medical schools. It is not and never has been the answer, never the perfect means. Yet the oath has been a guide which physicians turn to increasingly."

The silence at the Kansas end nettled me. "Are you still there?"

The reporter grunted.

"I'm sorry to have been so long, but you did ask. It seems to me that there is and will be a great deal more interest in medical oaths as well as in professional morality that exists in its own right apart from government. Actually, an exciting challenge lies concealed in these developments. If we can but learn to accept, understand, and finally work through these ambiguities with our patients, how much more help we can give to them. For example, consider the questions a physician might take up with an abortable patient before they decided what should be done."

At this point, a faint clicking came from the Kansas line.

"Are you there?"

"Yes, but I think we have a bad connection and…well, thank you, anyway; I have enough for my feature story."

"You are more than welcome. Goodbye."

"Goodbye."

I was ten minutes late for my next patient.

Endnotes

Reprinted from *Journal of Chronic Disease* 25(1972): 123-125.

1. R. Crawshaw, "The Contemporary Use of Medical Oaths," *Journal of Chronic Diseases* 23(1970): 145-50.
2. This paragraph has been updated to reflect the current state of use and interest in medical oaths. The remainder of the essay is virtually unchanged because it is as relevant today as it was when it was written some twenty-five years ago.

A Medical Code for Me

A little knowledge of history stresses the variability of moral codes and concludes that they are negligible because they differ in time and place, and sometimes contradict each other. A larger knowledge stresses the universality of moral codes and concludes to their necessity.
—Will Durant (1885-1981) & Ariel Durant
The Lessons of History

How often a surprise comes, not with the discovery of something new, but with absence of something old. Sometimes the loss is pleasant, as awakening to find that a fever has passed with the night. Yet too often an unexpected change has the opposite effect, not welcome relief, but a sense of mean and ugly trickery. Whether it be a missing tooth, salt banished from the diet, or a friendship traduced, the realization that a bit of oneself has disappeared, has the bitter taste of a small betrayal with the discomforting aftertaste that time proves unfaithful to our trust. Just such a start caught me when I overheard a fragment of a conversation which went,

"We abandoned medical oaths years ago."

It was early evening and the conversation that drifted my way came from a group of physicians gathered at the hearth of our medical society.

Arriving at intelligent, coherent, and ethical professional opinions is not easy. It calls upon physicians to devote time to careful consideration and thoughtful debate—the practical housekeeping which goes with a vital profession.

It was just such a group of physicians, caught in the moment of taking a breath between the day's work and the evening's demands, which sent my way the ear-catching phrase, "We abandoned medical oaths years ago."

As I say, it gave me an unpleasant start, but like a trout to a fly, I was hooked by the idea and involuntarily drawn to the group. The speaker turned out to be a friend, a surgeon whose skill I admired. He continued as the ice clinked in the glasses all the way around.

"Yes, we took a look at this whole thing while I was a student at Stanford. What is there to a medical oath anyway? Nothing but words, a ceremony, and forgotten the day after a man opens his practice. Who is there to check? I ask you, how is it possible to know if a man kept his oath or not?"

He had made a point worthy of answer, but the question was rhetorical. And after a pause no longer than a sip of gin, our speaker continued.

"In fact, *we* started the present trend away from oaths." He had his facts wrong, and I began to tune up a rebuttal, for I was aware that more than 94 percent of the medical schools in the United States use some form of medical oath, while internationally a similar movement toward medical oaths has been detected.[1]

Shifting my weight from foot to foot, I impatiently waited the inevitable pause for breath that would give us the chance to dissect his logic. I was ready with more zeal than discretion, but the promised pause was preempted by the announcement, "Gentlemen, dinner is served." So it turned out to be a case of stomach over mind, for unable to find a seat near my surgeon friend, I was forced to move my thoughts to a back burner of my mind where they remained, simmering.

Blocked in talking with my friend about the worthiness of medical oaths, I was forced to think about what he had said, and the more I thought, the more justification emerged for his stand. Not that I agreed with him, but a closer look at the Hippocratic oath turned up a few flaws in my ethical position when swearing to uphold it.

For example, I have nothing against "cutting out a stone." It may have been an unethical practice in Hippocrates' day to slash open the flank of a sick Athenian, who was doubled with renal colic and was willing to agree to anything that promised relief. But for me, though not a urologist, the prospect of helping pop out a persnickety offender such as a kidney stone would be an ethical delight. To my mind, removing a renal calculus is practically guaranteed to bring happiness and virtue to all involved, provided there is a whiff of anesthesia, a nod toward sterile technique, a sharp scalpel, and a competent surgeon.

Perhaps the Hippocratic oath should go the way of bloodletting, for the oath can be likened to an ancient Grecian urn—beautiful, awe-inspiring, but so cracked that it leaks beyond repair.

I continue to reject part of my friend's stand that there is no need for oaths and that men no longer yearn for an honorable life because it is immeasurable. I know that George Bernard Shaw maintained that there are no honest men over forty, but I have known some men of ethics who continued to function into their eighties. It is here that my surgeon friend and I remain unreconciled, for to my way of thinking an ethical man or woman remains a distinct possibility even though the measure of the person may be difficult.

If a particular physician is measured by the Hippocratic or some other oath, the possibility of trouble becomes immediate, for the ethics must fit the times as much as the times the ethics. How could the framers of the Geneva Declaration anticipate, in 1948, the vexing problems of organ transplants? Yet measure I must, for if I wish to be ethical in the practice of medicine, I must have some chain with which to survey my lot. What it comes down to is that the Hippocratic oath is not an outmoded process but an outmoded structure. Though the words may be wrong, the idea is right.

Now I understand why my friend startled me. He was right in abandoning the Hippocratic oath, but he was wrong for not substituting another oath in its place, an oath that would appoint him his own judge and jury. He should have proposed his own oath that would apply naturally and uniquely to him, particularly in his times of stress and doubt.

What we need to celebrate in the ancients and develop for ourselves is not so much the worship of their thoughts, but emulation of their thinking. For each man to set about his own fundamental ethical thinking may sound like a prescription for anarchy, but only if you believe that ethics have no commonality of direction and vary like the winds. Does it matter what road the physician takes to honor as long as he does not wander on the way?

Though this idea was new to me, a moment's reflection revealed how old it is. In religion, the process of personal acknowledgment of principles is called "witnessing"; in art, "a testament."

Listen to the great writer-physician Anton Chekhov as he sets out his beliefs, his measure of himself, in a letter to a friend.

> I am not a liberal, not a conservative, not a gradualist, not a monk, not an indifferentist. I should like to be a free artist and nothing more, and I regret that God has not given me the power to be one. I hate lying and violences, and whatever form they take....I regard trademarks and labels as prejudicial.

> My holy of holies is the human body, health, intelligence, talent, inspiration, love and absolute freedom—freedom from force and falsehood, no matter how the last two manifest themselves. This is the program I would follow.[2]

On looking back to that evening at the Medical Society, I gradually perceived my need for a personal medical oath. Granted, I buy my suits ready-made, and, until recently, my medical ethics came much the same way. With any mode of behavior, however, there comes a time when I can afford my own thinking and dispense with the "tailor's" pattern. Reflection affirms no need to run with the fashion of the times; whether it be old or new, I can select the material to cover both my physical and moral dimensions.

In fact, there is no reason why any thinking man might not do the same. And should he wish to measure the cut of his jib against mine, he is more than welcome, for it is not clothes, any more than ethics, which ultimately make the man, but the man who makes the clothes and the ethics.

The following is what a medical oath means for me. It originally appeared in a paper I published in the *Journal of Clinical Computing*.

- I swear, on both my sense of integrity and curiosity, traits which allow me to see beyond the moment and make me human out of an animal past, to respect the patient intrusted, directly or indirectly, into my care. I will see the patient not only for his body and mind, but for his personal reality which includes all information concerning him, past and present.

- It is my ceaseless responsibility to seek out, identify, and, with the patient's permission, treat, to the limits of my skill, those parts of his body, mind, and environment which are alien to his well-being. I shall in no way exploit nor otherwise misuse him. Though I may be tempted to shrink from the patient's suffering, be confused by the distance between us, wearied by fatigue and self-doubt, burdened by prejudice, or distracted by self-interest, yet, I hold it a privilege to serve the patient's need and I will seek for him the care I would want for those I cherish the most.

- I shall not conceal from the patient that which the patient seeks to know, nor divulge that which the patient seeks to conceal, and I will remain continually accountable to the patient for all judgments which I make concerning the patient. Aware that the community, particularly the community of science, makes demands in the name of the common good, only after I personally know the extent and quality of possible harm my cooperation with the community may cause the patient will I subordinate his needs.

- Knowing there is more than I can perceive or understand, I will exceed the objective amorality of reason and justice to confront the human condition with hope to the hopeless, comfort to the inconsolable, independence to the dependent, life to the dying, goals beyond attainment, quest beyond reach.

- Avoiding no moral options, I freely swear this oath, not for social acceptance, political conformity, nor professional status but as an explicit witness to measure my future care of the sick, dependent, and deprived against my present belief.

This suits me well.

Endnotes

Reprinted from *Prism* 3 #3(1975): 11, 44, with permission. Copyrighted 1975, American Medical Association.

1. The percentage in this paragraph has been updated. Otherwise the essay is virtually unchanged because it is as relevant to me today as it was when it was written some twenty years ago.
2. A. Kelly, "Chekhov the Subversive," *New York Review of Books*, 6 Nov 1997, 61.

Betrayal
A Film Review

> *No villain need be! Passions spin the plot:*
> *We are betrayed by what is false within.*
> —George Meredith (1828-1909)
> *Modern Love,* xliii

Betrayal is an exceptionally fine film, one that bridges the gap between stage and film with *éclat*. Superior acting, superb writing, effective editing, and unobtrusive yet excellent photography make *Betrayal* achieve the best of two worlds—art and entertainment.

The tale concerns the love lives of three close friends and their increasing confusion over "love lies," the high cost of dishonesty in interpersonal relations. Robert (Ben Kingsley), a book publisher, and Emma (Patricia Hodge), who runs an art gallery, are a not-so-happily-married couple. The film opens in an odd sort of way, since the camera, like a nosy neighbor, peeks in the window of their palatial London home as they bid their dinner guests adieu and retreat from room to room, ending up in the kitchen. The windowpane cuts off their voices as street noises fill the silence, and although we see the two give each other right smart slaps to the face, we are as much on the outside of the marriage as we are on the outside of the house, until, with a most interesting series of chronological reversals (they cannot be called flashbacks), we are gradually illuminated about nine years of mutual betrayal.

Jerry (Jeremy Irons), a writer's agent, Emma's former lover, Robert's best friend, and best man at their wedding, is the original betrayer, but as it turns out he is outdistanced by his friends. Jerry, with his wife, Judith (never on camera), are half of convivial foursomes as they share family celebrations and, in the case of Jerry and Emma, beds. The dissolution of Robert and Emma's marriage is dissected most unconventionally, for the analysis follows neither science nor logic but becomes movingly real through the artist's eye. A clinical pathologist may display the fulminating structure of a tumor, but if he wishes to show the process of the malignancy he must assemble a series of specimens, each at a significant stage in the development of the carcinoma. The artist, Harold Pinter, however, analyzes the "tumor" by tracing it back, dissecting out the process of dissolution before your eyes at each retrogression, until the earliest form of that malignancy is laid bare. His scalpel is sharpened dialogue, in which the characters slice away at each other, purportedly in a personal search for substance, while starkly revealing more than they intend.

The intricacies these three bright minds weave and ravel into their web of lies become a mirror of their personalities. Jerry, with a brash quality of self-importance, is the poorest liar of the lot, and although his vanity is piqued by learning of his friend's lies, his vanity never falters in its swift reconstitution; hence he loses least, for he has risked least. Emma is the most daring, and through the acting of Patricia Hodge her face becomes a self-contained drama in itself. When first teased and then confronted by her husband for her infidelity with Jerry, she sits in the middle of her bed saying little, much like a war-hardened general watching his army be overrun and then, the engagement lost, accepting defeat with a proud defiance that broaches no surrender. It is all there on her beautiful face, shifting with each of Robert's sorties, explicit as a military map, yet a thousand times more informative. Robert, the most intense, and with the most to lose, treads his way through the mine field of impossibilities in his marriage and friendship like a master tactician, acutely aware of the danger to himself and his family, yet coolly weighing the odds, as he inexorably drives himself to convert a suspicion into a truth, a destructive truth. The audience is caught with the characters, striving to find what lies behind the words, while Pinter piles associations and meanings one upon the other in a lustrous web of deceit, until there is no certainty of anyone's integrity.

Lying is indeed a strange yet common experience, and although no man is reputed to have a memory long enough to be good at lying, few escape the temptation. What these three liars demonstrate is the prodigious expenditure of mental energy creative deception demands. The lovers take a flat in Knightsbridge for their trysts, but once there they spend most of their time checking with each other for what is true. "Does your wife suspect?" "Who is the father of the child you are carrying?" "Is this a home?" Cross-examination preoccupies them rather than their vaunted infatuation. The terrible price of lying is their loss of trust and trusting. Who can love if they cannot trust? The answer comes back, loud and clear: there is no way. Whether the social lie ("Oh, what a delightful time we had this evening") or the medical lie to the cancer patient ("Nothing new on your latest x-ray"), there is an effect on the liar, a price paid for shortcutting the truth. One cannot help but believe that one-sided fashioning of illusions affects the teller as much as the hearer.

The strange part about lying is its expectedness. Robert, Emma, and Jerry accept lying as a necessary part of life, a sort of social oil to lubricate interpersonal relations under the guise of protecting some other's feelings. Candor, like Candide, quickly arouses suspicions of public fomentation, for men and women seem genetically dedicated to the curious belief that their illusions safely reinforce the illusions of others.

Emma lies to her daughter in saying that the man on the telephone is Daddy, and at a different level it is clear that her dissembling permeates all her family relationships. In fact, she is so lost in her lying that she will never be able to tell her son in truth who his Daddy really is. To Emma, and others, it seems best to leave sleeping dogs and human beings lie. She has lied so much she does not know. Emma expects this of herself, much as the physician who in not wishing to burden an ailing patient with their worsening condition may find himself twisting or evading the truth. Everyone's feelings are protected, or so it seems, but hidden in the "expected" lie is the liar's feelings of omniscience, the culture media for lying, and the prime feelings that demanded protection, those of the liar.

We are all tempted to believe we know what is best for others as a consequence of our superior knowledge of the circumstances. This grand illusion of the liar, more paradox than illusion, proclaims within itself that what we really know when we lie is that we do not trust the truth and consequently must be ignorant of ourselves. How strange we are, and how, without a smidgen of self-righteousness, Harold Pinter masterfully confronts us with our strangeness. We are the only animal that believes in immortality, and we are willing not only to lie but to die for this belief.

"Bitter web indeed. Deceit twice poisons. First, degrading the speaker's integrity while eroding the trust of listener. Then the pernicious toxin of lying binds them in an allegiance of misrepresentation. Nor can any dose of falsification be small enough to do a greater good without doing a lesser evil, no matter how white the lie is painted. The choice is always before us, live by the truth and be known by the truth or bide with the lie and die by the lie."

Endnotes

Reprinted from *The Pharos* 47(Spring 1971): 42-43, with permission.

The Corrupted Land
A Book Review

I can't bring myself, as so many men seem able to do, to blink the evil out of sight, and gloss it over. It's as real as the good, and if it is denied, good must be denied too. It must be accepted and hated and resisted while there's breath in our bodies.

—William James (1842-1910)

While the review of *The Corrupted Land*[1] was written some years back and the details are dated, the avenues the book travels are all too familiar; the human concerns of both the book and the review of the book unfortunately apply as much today as then, only the names of the scandals have changed.

Because it gave me a headache, I find it difficult to give this book a wholehearted recommendation. The style is fine; a swift journalistic approach. The book is well documented, the format easy, the subject matter familiar, but the impact is overwhelming. It can be relaxing to spend the evening reading the history of some ancient swindle—the shenanigans of Boss Tweed bleeding New York City for a hundred million dollars; the manipulations of Cornelius Vanderbilt shouting, "Law, what do I care about the law? Hain't I got power?"; the Teapot Dome Scandal—all have a distant innocence that appeals to the larceny in the reader. However, the impact of Watergate, Whitewater, the savings and loan debacle, and the tobacco industry's perfidious behavior are immediate instances of the same social rot. The experience is a little like visiting a neighbor in a hospital, only to find that he is being treated for syphilis and *boasting* about it. I may be old-fashioned, but this kind of thing bothers me. Somehow we know scandals happen, but "really not close to me." The author, Fred Cook, points out clearly how close it is happening to all of us.

The book carries us swiftly along through the avenues of seamy power. The facts are there, although they are not used with the clear dispassion of a scientist. For instance, in discussing the increasing rate of bank embezzlement, Cook compares the number of banks closed in one period with the number of banks embezzled in another. The logic is not tight, although the conclusions appear valid. Happily, he does not rely on journalistic sensationalism to make the point of how our whole society is being geared to a new type of morality, which is two-faced. Ostensibly, the alteration of moral purpose stands for the individual and free enterprise, but in practice the approach is institutional, with an adaptable value system. I don't like what Cook says, but I believe him.

The most immediate response short of a headache is probably an "ain't it awful" reaction. This is a fairly common way of trying to push the problem away from our personal experience. Thus, "How could anybody be like Billy Sol Estes [or Michael Milken or what is alleged of Enron executives] and make off with $21,845,730.72 [$55 million in one year alone]?" It is a rather stock thought. For instance, "How could anybody be like Eichmann and run a concentration camp?" Emphasis on the magnitude of the crime obscures the petty foundation supporting it.

But Fred Cook is a good enough author not to let us hide behind this defense. He points out how the good people of Pecos, Texas, backed Billy Sol Estes with respectability and acceptance even when the local smell was so bad it had their eyes watering. When some members of his local church objected to his becoming an Elder, he used his influence to have them fired from their jobs. However, the Reverend W.S. Boyett, whom Estes furnished with a Cadillac, says he had no suspicions: "I don't consider it my function to dig into the business of the members of my congregation." The president of the bank (though stung once and highly dubious of the deals going on around him) did nothing about revealing the swindles because, he said, "It was none of my business."

Something for Nothing

Cook takes us up close to look at farmers who lent their credit ratings to Estes on plans that gave them something for nothing, who signed for fertilizer tanks they never saw (and which never existed) because "it paid."

The worst part of these documented swindles is not the crimes, but the public reaction. When 105 cadets were dismissed from the Air Force Academy in 1965 for cheating, the public clamor of "Let's not judge these young men too harshly because cheating is so common anyway" was a scandal in itself. In a poll conducted in a California school system in 1961, grade-school students were asked whether they would look if they were given a chance to see the unguarded answers to a test; 41 percent said they would. Later, 94 percent of the same students rated themselves as "basically honest." This is our scandal: an adaptable sense of guilt.

A variation on the "ain't it awful" reaction is: "Oh, look what they are doing." In this case, it is used to point at a spectacle to avoid a personal issue. It is reminiscent of the pickpocket circulating among the crowd at the fire pointing out the details of the blaze with his right hand while he is going through the bystanders' pockets with his left.

An example is John Chiles, Westinghouse vice-president and general manager, who was sentenced to jail by the Philadelphia federal courts for willfully breaking the Sherman Anti-Trust Act. Was justice done? Not according to the Reverend Malcolm MacMillan, pastor of St. John's Episcopal Church, in which Chiles was the senior warden. Said the pastor: "The Vestry still feels that Mr. Chiles is a man of high integrity, and we have every confidence in him." The implication has to be, then, that the judge participated in a miscarriage of justice. Look what the judge did to this man of high integrity! It is a neat way of lifting the moral scruples out of any situation. The phrase recurs, "I really didn't do anything very wrong and see how they are persecuting me!"

In *The Corrupted Land* physicians come out fairly clean. There is one recorded scandal in medical licensure, but when it was uncovered, no excuses were given and swift, relentless justice followed. Two physicians in Pecos finally prodded the Justice Department into doing something about Billy Sol Estes. It was a psychiatrist in Denver who refused to judge insane the rookie patrolman who insisted that some of his fellow policemen were stealing. The legal profession goes unexamined in the book, but anyone curious about lawyers can turn to Jerome E. Carlin's *Lawyer's Ethics: A Survey of the New York City Bar.*[2]

I hope the millions, if not billions, of dollars that pass though Medicare do not generate a response in the medical profession similar to the reaction of some members of state highway departments to federal funds. But then, that would be fraud. Should Fred Cook ever wish to look into the matrix of unethical behavior that supports fraud, he wouldn't have to wait to see what Medicare brings, and I only hope we receive a passing grade in ethics.

Some questions might present a problem, but not the clichés about medical practice and finance like: "Do you pad your expense accounts?" or "How much of your income do you leave unreported?" or "Do you recommend unessential operations and prescribe drugs that are not indicated, or sign medical documents without proper investigation of the patient?" No, not these old saws. Not even: "Do you read the books you review?"

The questions I would tremble at hearing our profession answer are related to the interface between professional life and civic duty. They would go something like this: "It is reported that on the trip you took to Europe with your family you bought a handtooled leather briefcase in a shop in Florence. When the clerk asked if you would like the bill of sale to be written for one-half the cost so that you could get by U.S. Customs with one-half the duty, what did you say, Doctor?"

Or: "What did you say, Doctor, when it was proposed at a planning committee of the medical school alumni to let a cooperative drug firm underwrite the cost of cocktails for the next annual reunion?"

Another: "Doctor, when you were having coffee last year in a local restaurant with a county commissioner and he began gloating with glee about getting seventy-five thousand dollars in federal money to spend on mentally retarded kids 'any damn way I please,' what was your comment?"

Compliance

And a final example: "When you were at the state medical meeting and one of the physicians reported that the social workers are pushing a bill in the state legislature that would, in his judgment, set the treatment of emotionally disturbed children back twenty years, but that since this year's crop of social workers are an aggressive, forceful group and we physicians have gotten a bad name for objecting to other legislation, we should go along with them, what was your reaction, Doctor?"

Cook's volume has a list of contemporary answers: "Everyone is doing it." "I didn't know." "I did not want to start any trouble." Do you have one? I must admit to some mixed feelings at the thought of Cook doing valid sampling of these questions. I am sure it would be enlightening to the profession, but I can not be sure it would be painless.

One particular thesis of Cook's I find difficult to understand. It is that virtue should be acclaimed, not derided. He details the saga of Douglas Johnson who found and returned 240 thousand dollars, which brought him so much notoriety that he came to wish he had burned the money or thrown it down a sewer. Virtue has always been its own reward. Any act that is out of step with the multitudes, such as an act of virtue, can be expected to precipitate disapproval in all forms, including contempt and hate. Obituaries excepted, the crowd has seldom cheered anyone clearing the path to personal morality.

The American Revolution is a case in point. The highest estimate is that 7 percent of the population participated actively, risking life and property. The remaining 93 percent stood by passively, ignored the Revolution, or actively subverted it.

Summer soldiers outnumbered winter ones and, even combined, the soldiers were a small minority compared with the "innocent bystanders" who found it none of their business. Why should attitudes be different today?

Essentially, Cook is saying in *The Corrupted Land* that American citizens have abandoned their personal morality for a collective institutionalized morality. They have abandoned thoughtful conviction for compromised sentimentality and popularity, that is, responsibility for obedience. This is strong medicine to take. We can always hide behind the fact that Cook has no statistical evidence, that it is impression, so it really does not matter much anyway, or does it?

Stanley Milgram's research at Yale begins to put a scientific foundation beneath Cook's deductions. Milgram carried out a series of psychological experiments in obedience. He took a sample cross-section of the adult (aged twenty to fifty) male population of Bridgeport, Connecticut, from blue-collar workers through professionals. The experiment sought to determine how much punishment one person might inflict on another when so ordered, but it was deceptively presented as a scientific study on learning techniques by "Bridgeport Research Associates." The subjects, selected at random, were paid four and a half dollars for their time.

A "learner" was strapped into an "electric chair" after the subject (a teacher) had experienced a sample shock of 45 volts to convince him of the authenticity of the instrument. Then, from an adjoining room the subject delivered a shock of increasing intensity for each wrong answer. Actually the "learner" was not shocked, but his responses, unknown to the "teacher," were a standardized tape recording of murmurs, gasps, pleas, and shrieks matched to the ascending voltage. The answers were prearranged by the experimenter, so the only limiting factor preventing the teacher from delivering the maximum intensity of the shock machine was his compassion for a human being in pain. The conflict for the teacher (Mr. Everyman) was obedience to the authoritative system versus his belief that he should not hurt another person.

What percentage of the so-called teachers went full bore and gave the maximum shock? But before you guess, listen to the voice of Mr. Everyman at the switch:

150 volts delivered: "You want me to keep going?" (COMMAND)

165 volts delivered: "That guy is hollering in there. There's a lot of them here. He's liable to have a heart condition. You want me to go on?" (COMMAND)

180 volts delivered: "He can't stand it. I'm not going to kill that man in there. You hear him hollering? He's hollering. He can't stand it. What if something happened to him? You know what I mean? I mean, I refuse to take the responsibility." (THE EXPERIMENTER ACCEPTS THE RESPONSIBILITY) "Alright."

195 volts, 210, 225, 240, and so on.

Obedience

The subject (teacher) unfailingly obeyed the experimenter. What percentage of the almost one thousand teachers went the whole route? Estimate before you let your eyes stray ahead. A group of forty psychiatrists who studied the project predicted 0.1 percent. In the actual experiment, 62 percent obeyed the experimenter's commands fully. What did you guess?

Milgram concluded:

> With numbing regularity good people were seen to knuckle under the demands of authority and perform actions that were callous and severe. Men who in everyday life are responsible and decent were seduced by the trappings of authority, by the control of their perceptions, and by the uncritical acceptance of the experimenter's definition of the situation into performing harsh acts. The results, as seen and felt in the laboratory, are to this author disturbing. They raise the possibility that human nature, or more specifically, the kind of character produced in American democratic society, cannot be counted on to insulate its citizens from brutality and inhumane treatment when at the direction of a malevolent authority.[3]

In the laboratory, 62 percent of the population accepted prevailing immorality. How many more would accept it outside the laboratory, say in the imposing private office of Billy Sol Estes, furnished with the autographed photographs of most of our national political leaders? Cook says *everyone*. He says it is a *corrupted* land. I say *most*, and it is a *corruptible* land. There are those who did *not* punish in an unconscionable fashion despite the directions of a malevolent authority.

There is, in our nation, a core of people who judge independently, check on their perceptions, and do not necessarily accept the prevailing authorities' definitions. They are not Pollyanna "cannot tell a lie" people, they are not acclaimed, but they are real. Look at Benjamin Rush's soul-trying resignation from the Continental Army, Peter Cooper's tenacious integrity in industry, the steeled intellectual honesty of Speaker of the House Thomas Reed. If you want a longer list, turn to *Profiles in Courage*. In any case, the number of such men and women may be small, but their effect is great. They are not the heroes of our land; they are the ones who make our heroes and our nation possible.

Antidote

Thomas Browne's comments of three hundred years ago[4] are the antidote to Cook's overwhelming pessimism.

> Think not that morality is ambulatory; that vices in one age are not vices in another. And though vicious times invert the opinion of things and set up new ethics against virtue, yet they hold to the old morality. Since the worst times afford imitable examples of virtue; since no deluge of vice is like to be so general but no more than eight escape; eye well those heroes who have held their heads above water, who have touched pitch, and not been defiled, and in the common contagion have remained uncorrupted.

I am afraid I must agree with Cook that many United States citizens have abandoned a personal for an institutionalized morality. It is my opinion, though, that not everyone has. For some, the battle of trying to seek a personal morality in a world that downgrades the individual and panders to the idea of security as a form of mental health continues.

The basic conflict is between a sense of security, represented by the institution, and a sense of identity, represented by the individual. The institution guarantees security if you follow its rules. It will take care of you if you submerge yourself in it. However, with personal identity nothing is guaranteed. Only one person can and will work for your personal identity—you.

Countless institutions attempt to give you an identity, but as defined and limited by them. They will describe your role as a physician, father, citizen, wife, contributor, consumer, voter, etc. They will sell you on security by guaranteeing your success, but always on their terms. Seldom do institutions present you with unequivocal choices. The options they do allow are general and oversimplified. They replace your thoughts and choices with their rationalizations and precedents, and make it clear how easy it is to be a "nice guy." Too often learning about yourself becomes coincidental. Like fire, institutions make excellent servants but poor masters, certainly insofar as morality is concerned. An individual generates values, while, at best, an institution transmits them.

Today everyman is his own Doctor Faustus. Do you have a desire to see and know your own real world, or would you trade your soul (identity) to someone for the promise of a fantasy world? The media is particularly blatant on this point. Do you want to "think young, look young, be young" or be your own age? If you want the former, there are innumerable formulas you can drink, spray, soak, chew, or rub onto or into yourself. For the latter, thought and choice are the only way.

Last Chance

Fred Cook points out that we are being crowded by our institutions. Your parents had more latitude in deciding to be themselves than you do. Now may be your last chance to make your own decisions. Most important, if you do not choose to be yourself, to seek your own identity, your own morality, your own value system, your children may not even know what an act of choice is. By the next generation the manipulators of institutions, the powerful, may have developed a computer that could be guaranteed to search your soul more swiftly, painlessly, and economically than you yourself could. I recommend Fred Cook's book for those interested in making their own choices.

Endnotes

Reprinted from *Medical Opinion & Review* 3(1967): 59-66.
1. F.J. Cook, *The Corrupted Land: The Social Morality of Modern America* (New York: Macmillan, 1966).
2. J.E. Carlin, *Lawyers' Ethics: A Survey of the New York City Bar* (New York: Russell Sage Foundation, 1966).

3. S. Milgram, "Some Conditions of Obedience and Disobedience to Authority," *Human Relations*, 18:57-76, 1965.
4. T. Browne, *Religio Medici and Other Writings* (New York: E.P. Dutton & Co., 1920).

The Awareness of Courage

Modesty is of no use to a beggar.
—Ancient Greek proverb

Consider this, if you will. It is a Sunday morning, and with the prospect of a few days vacation, you and your spouse have started out from your city home at dawn for some welcome solitude in your wilderness cabin. Two hours down the highway, you are over the first range of hills and into the mountains proper. Intermittent squalls of rain spiked with hail arrogantly race across the highway before you.

You drive well-controlled down a vale, around a wooded curve just below a mountain ravine, and there, before you across the highway, are two vehicles, a pickup and a four-door sedan, in violent collision! You have time to pull to a stop. You are the first to come upon the accident.

The closest vehicle, the pickup, has the driver's door open, and the driver is sitting on the ground with a two-inch cleft in his upper lip, dripping blood. The front end of the pickup is pushed up like a pig's snout with the wheels splayed, and it passes water from its radiator like a spent and wasted beast.

The sedan has a front end looking like a used toothpaste tube, with twisted, groaning people extruded from smashed windows and cracked seams. There is a flailing hand on a broken door sill, seeking to drag out the rest of the body. All this is set upon a shimmering, wet cascade of cracked and broken glass.

You have happened upon the edge of an abyss where souls are falling off into eternal oblivion or heavenly paradise, or who knows what. People are apparently dying, and there are decisions to be made. What would you decide?

My first decision was to set the emergency lights of my car blinking, my second to step out, while my third decision was to knock the glowing ash from my pipe; no sense bringing fire to the gasoline. As I walked toward the pickup, the man with the parted lip staggered up. He appeared dazed but intact. The woman in the cab seemed in satisfactory shape; the blood that was coming from her arm was not spurting, and though badly stunned, she responded.

The sedan, however, was a different story. The man, in what had been the driver's seat had his head jammed between the spokes of the steering wheel. He was struggling weakly, like an injured ox in an ill-fitting yoke, but with a bit of firm direction, his head came free.

Some travelers had stopped on the far side of the wreck and by now had pulled clear the woman without a nose. She lay on the highway in the pouring rain slowly writhing in agony.

Another woman in the center of the front seat could not be moved. She was crushed against the dash, and her moans, "I can't breathe," were alternated with screams, "He won't leave me alone!" Obviously, she thought that the mashed flesh with bared broken bones hanging from her left shoulder was being twisted by her companion. In the back seat, one man had pulled himself out, while on the other side of the car, two passersby were dragging the man with the broken wrist and a gash on his cheek from the wreck.

The dialogue was terse, "Don't move anybody further until they are checked."

"Has anyone called for help?"

"Yes, the people in the house up the road."

"We need more than help; we need the state troopers, a wrecker, and two ambulances, not one." Someone ran off to repeat the call.

The woman in the center of the rear seat had both feet splayed at the ankles and moaned with back pain. She should not be moved.

A bystander squeezed into the front seat and held the undamaged right hand of the pinned woman. "Hold my hand. That's it," he said. "Hold it tight. Help is coming."

Two men attacked the driver's door with a sledge hammer. "Careful, careful!" A piece of quarter-inch water pipe bent like licorice as they attempted to pry open the door.

The woman sprawled on the pavement was bare to the rain. "Anyone got a rug?" While a woman bystander stripped off her coat and covered the victim as best she could, a carpet out of a station wagon was put down beside her, and ever so gently, she was rolled upon it. A wrecker truck with warning lights ablaze roared up, then more sirens and bright flashing lights down the highway. A pang of disappointment.

"Hell, it ain't the ambulance. It's the goddam state police."

But soon the ambulances arrived.

The work went on. "No need of a tourniquet there."

"Dressings here, a lot more."

"Keep the traction steady."

Gradually, with careful attention to those still inside, the wreck was pulled apart. Stretchers appeared, the victims treated, infusions started, and off to the hospital. Then almost as suddenly as it began, there was nothing to do but climb back into our car and accept the wave of the state trooper. There was nothing more to it. Or was there?

Later, after we arrived at the cabin, I realized that my hands were bloody, and as I washed them, I began the work of putting together, thinking through, understanding what had happened.

An Eerie Quality

The cries of the pinned victims still echoed in my ears. I could hear the woman screaming with rage as her coat was cut to free her from the wreck, "Don't you dare cut this coat; it's my good one," even though the arm within was all but severed.

So many images—the yellow-slickered state troopers setting flares, the wish for a hat so the rain would not run into my eyes, five people holding a tarpaulin for shelter while I helped slide a splint under the broken leg of a screaming girl, a tooth fragment on the dashboard, and a hysterical woman bystander, white-faced, shivering and crying with her wet hair hanging down over her face. Vividly the reel unwound—the clinging, oppressive odor of gasoline, with a mixture of sweat, alcohol, blood, and urine stinking in my nose. The need for dispatch—"That one there goes to the hospital first! Move fast!"

My steamed glasses drawing a curse as they blurred the limp wrist beneath the needle, yet not preventing my hitting the vein on the second try. The patient crying out that she could not breathe, while fighting the oxygen mask that brought her air. A broken leg with a bared, jagged thigh bone, and a foot stubbornly pinned.

The blonde's face, as though painted by Delacroix, beauty contorted by violent protest, slashed and spattered with matted blood. The crackle of granulated safety glass underfoot. The driver of the wrecker, aware of his limitations, sticking strictly to his machine, avoiding the victims. Clothes soaked through, dragging against your every move, and broken white bone piercing blue denim.

The memories flickered by unchecked—an ear dangling, yet the victim wiping the stump repeatedly as if to relieve an itch. Checking pulses, the change in color as florid rage drains to gray acceptance. The difficulty in recollecting precisely how many victims there were, searching your mind for who went where, and when. The eye that no longer responds, slowly revolving, pinpointed on eternity. The rain dancing off the bare abdomen of an extracted victim, a sheet dragging in the mud. Disoriented victims pulling dressings from their head wounds. The defective inflatable splint unable to hold air while I dizzily blew and blew, futilely attempting to maintain pressure. White-faced children pressed against the windows of cars that slowly edged through the maze of wreckage.

The whole scene had the eerie quality of a Fellini film with God and the Devil appearing as if by magic; first God with his head under the tarpaulin, "I am with you, dear; there is nothing to worry about," while the Devil, a wooly-headed, sulking, wet-bearded monster, directs traffic with curses for each passing car. The wail and screech of the twisted wrecks, screaming like wounded horses, as they are pulled from the road. And then, the final impression, viewed from the rearview mirror as we drove away—the wreckers sweeping glass, spent flares, blood, and mud into the ditch.

A Child's Nightmare

So when I threw my blood-spattered clothes into the laundry hamper, I began to realize I was faced with another of the physician's eternal tasks, blending feeling with action, in the quest for meaning. But feelings and action are as oil and water. Who did I feel for? I did not know a single person at the scene except my spouse. It was a child's nightmare—no names, cardboard cutout characters known only for their roles: Mr. State Trooper, Mr. Wrecker, Mr. Bystander, Mr. Ambulance Driver, Mrs. Broken Leg.

It is almost as though the victims were not people, simply masses of bleeding organs. What personal meaning did the action have?

Late in the day, a telephone check with the hospital affirmed that the victims still lived. Relief—a partial meaning to the action—helped, but how to translate the experience into broader meaning, a context which might clarify those strange paths that lead down from the wide, busy plane where I spend most of my days to the edge of the dark abyss. What was I missing? What is it that happens when, for unknown reasons, the surgical patient begins to slip away? The blood pressure falls. The reflexes are going. The surgical team stops everything to wait as the anesthesiologist works on. Where are *his* feelings? It does no good for him to share the numbness of the dying. What keeps him going? Is it knowledge? Is it fear of what others will say or sue? Is he an automaton, a machine? No! But where is his humaneness?

Slowly, the answers emerged from my musings, like a granite mountain appearing as the morning fog dissipates; the essential quality that affirms his humaneness is courage.

I respect Sir William Osler for saying that the magic word in medicine is "work." But, certainly, he knew that with a dying patient that was never enough. As the patient slips away and the relationship wanes, knowledge becomes relative, compassion becomes superfluous. To grasp the hand slipping over the edge takes courage.

The mere thought of tagging myself with virtue was repugnant. Restlessly, I left our cabin, driven by the fear of vanity. Walking along the wooded path did not help. The view of the distant sea through rain-burdened branches, the gloss of wet, mossy rocks—none gave solace.

Perhaps the most difficult trait for a physician to accept consciously within himself, fully aware of the horrendous distortions possible, burdened by the sordid knowledge of the past preening, ambivalent to the heart of his consciousness, is courage. Yet, how can it be otherwise?

If a physician strives for a noble life, there are two virtues that must be in his cells. But I hesitate to name them. Granted, a physician knows much or little, but always something, of the workings of the body. However, beyond intelligence, the two necessary virtues that divide his world into feeling and action are compassion and courage. And of these, the awareness of courage comes the hardest.

But was what I did bravado? Courage comes in so many forms—making a phone call to a bereaved; standing against the crowd; throwing away three years' work proven false by a brighter mind; telling the whole truth, not just the acceptable part; picking up the pieces of a shattered career; sleeping without a pill; sticking to a bargain gone bad.

All these take courage. But what is courage? Again, was what I did bravado? And then the final question—could I have the courage to see courage for what it was: the acceptance that I had committed myself completely to the action?

I paused, thought a moment as I kicked a rock free from the wet sod, and then taking a deep breath as though a weight had fallen away, I turned on my heel and retraced my steps to our cabin. It was over, and I knew what I needed now, what every man needs at the end of an ordeal—a bright fire on the hearth, a hot meal, and a good night's sleep, interrupted only by the soft sound of rain dripping from the eaves.

Endnotes

Reprinted from *Prism* 3(#6, 1975): 7-8, with permission. Copyrighted 1975, American Medical Association.

In the Belly of the Soviet Beast

When you live with wolves you must howl like wolves.
—Russian proverb

Curiosity can be dangerous to more than cats, especially should it draw us into the bowels of a vast totalitarian bureaucracy. When I discovered that the Russian medical profession lacked a medical oath it struck me as a fascinating business which I must investigate firsthand.

For me, the central question was: Could Soviet doctors in the Soviet Union, who made up the world's largest medical organization, practice humane care without an explicit statement, an oath, to measure their behavior against? The answer proved to be "no," Soviet doctors could not practice without explicit personal accountability. In 1971, I learned the Russians were writing a Soviet medical oath to replace the Hippocratic oath that had been discarded during the Revolution as an expression of "bourgeois exploitation." All this whetted my curiosity. Was the Soviet oath window dressing or a sincere expression of medical vocation? As a U.S.–U.S.S.R. exchange scholar, I went to see and kept returning to the body of the beast, until one morning I awoke to find myself in its belly. As I said, curiosity can be hard on more than cats.

After clearing Moscow's Sheremetyevo airport passport control on a snowy evening in 1985, I met Marsha, my official guide, translator, and undisclosed KGB control. It was my fifth visit to study Soviet medical deontology, the Communist equivalent of medical ethics. During this visit I intended to examine how Soviet physicians went about the problem of prioritizing scarce medical resources, the worldwide dilemma of implicit health care rationing.

Marsha was a slight, bright-eyed, middle-aged woman in knee-length leather coat with wool knit hat topping her apprehensive smile. On the taxi ride in from the airport she warily confessed concern for her limited vocabulary for the specialized language of medical deontology. Marsha was visibly reassured when I acknowledged the subject as difficult, often defying cross-cultural understanding. Throughout the visit, even when I was harassed by threatening anonymous midnight telephone calls, she proved a supportive ally. Later, she confided she had passed along in her obligatory daily reports to the KGB that I consistently resisted attempts at intimidation.

Once deposited in the lobby of the Ukrina Hotel, I was informed by the clerk I was the only Western guest in this Soviet establishment. Daunted by an overwhelming sense of isolation, I rode the rickety elevator to the thirteenth floor and after trudging down a long, dimly lit hall, dumped my bags on the floor of a small room and turned on all the electric lights, the better to send the resident roaches scurrying to the cracks in the walls. After a hot bath I settled down to preparing for the next day's meeting with officials of the ministry of health.

My agenda included:

1. Ascertain reasons for recent changes in the official Soviet medical oath.
2. Determine developments in the Soviet delivery of health care related to significant issues in access to medical care, official policy for priorities in allocating scarce medical resources.
3. Open preliminary exploration of a joint effort by the U.S.S.R. and U.S. medical academies to study the ethical basis of

medical practice. (I carried a letter from Dr. Samuel Their, president of the U.S. National Academy of Science, Institute of Medicine, to Dr. N.N. Blokhin, president of the Soviet Academy of Medical Sciences, proposing the exploration.)
4. Share a humanitarian concern for the fate of refusenik Norm Chernoblynsky, brother of a colleague at the Oregon Health Sciences University.
5. Attend Soviet movies as film reviewer for a U.S. medical journal.

At 10 A.M. the next morning I was admitted through double doors to a high-ceilinged, somber reception room of the ministry of health. After Marsha introduced me to Mr. Andri Yefinmych, an official of the ministry who spoke fluent English, she left the room. He was a large man both in height and girth, with steel-rimmed eyeglasses surmounting an unctuous smile. Following greetings and a handshake, Mr. Yefinmych promptly launched into a description of the "excellent" program prepared for my visit. He concluded by stating that the visit I had proposed to Novosibirsk would not be possible as the program concentrated on Moscow and Leningrad.

In response I offered my agenda. He immediately reviewed it, item by item, remarking at the many technical questions I asked, assuring me they would be taken up the next day by the staff of the N.A. Semashko Institute for Social Hygiene and Public Health. Certainly, Dr. Ivan Dmitich, the director, would be an excellent source for information since his Institute had both the experts and the data to address them.

My request to speak with Dr. Blokhin brought a suggestion that arrangements be made for me to attend an upcoming international meeting protesting nuclear war at which Dr. Blokhin would preside. I agreed reluctantly, having no desire for a public meeting with that gentleman distracted by a crowd of importuning visitors. Acknowledging my reservation, Mr. Yefinmych said he would do what he could.

Upon reaching the item concerning the refusenik, Norm Chernoblynsky, Mr. Yefinmych's manner changed abruptly. Seeing him bristle, I interjected that I acted simply as a messenger. I assured him my motive was not ideological but compassionate, emphasizing the point by using the Russian word *sostradanya* to convey the deep concern my colleague at the Oregon Health Sciences University had for the fate of her brother. With icy disdain he listened as I continued, saying I considered the message secondary to the objectives of my agenda and I did not wish it to interfere with the primary goal of my visit.

Maintaining his silence, Mr. Yefinmych picked up the Chernoblynsky packet that I had brought along and slowly paged through it. After perusing every page he coolly remarked that the matter would be considered but as it concerned a civil charge against a Soviet citizen there could be little hope of anything developing. While in the Soviet Union I never heard of the matter again.

Our encounter closed with me observing that since Novosibirsk was no longer on the program my goals could be accomplished in less than a month, consequently I wished to leave Leningrad for Helsinki in two weeks.

Mr. Yefinmych then conducted me to the finance department where I signed a receipt for a packet of rubles to cover out-of-pocket expenses during the visit. He bid me adieu with a wish that I make the most of the cultural advantages of Moscow. Subsequently, the word "cultural" became clear as I unsuccessfully pursued the *scientific* advantages of Moscow.

The next morning Marsha led the way to the Institute of Social Hygiene and Public Health. After shaking a dust of snow from our coats we were conducted to a large, warm room with a long table covered with green felt, bearing a samovar and dishes of cookies and cakes. Here Dr. L. Korotkich, a medical deontologist, greeted us, bid us to sit down and poured cups of steaming hot tea all the way round. Unlike his hospitality, Dr. Korotkich's information fell far short of the mark. Marsha had no difficulty translating his vague account of the new Soviet emphasis on intensive care. His delivery, it was never a discussion, ceased abruptly with the entrance of Dr. Rozov. Following introductions, Dr. Korotkich obsequiously relinquished his position at the head of the table to Dr. Rozov. There was no question in my mind who was the party representative for that Institute. Dr. Rozov, oblivious of what had preceded, immediately established his credentials for judging Western medicine by recounting his travels on the far side of the Iron Curtain. He made the point of his cosmopolitan background by ostentatiously drawing attention to his Swiss wristwatch.

Ensconced, Dr. Rozov rambled on through a thicket of clichés concerning the frightful problems Western doctors face under the capitalistic system. He took pride that, unlike their Western colleagues,

Soviet doctors meet the needs of their patients without thought of time or cost, a subject Soviet medical practitioners apparently never even discuss, let alone share with visiting colleagues.

Any opportunity left for me to speak was framed to answer his questions, not mine. With relish he eventually came to the denouement of Western medicine and me, "Doctor, would you please explain why Western doctors resort to euthanasia as a cost saving procedure?" Aware that his head was filled with his own answer to the question, I used the Russian dodge of "That is a difficult and complex question" to bridge the exchange back to facts about the Soviet medical system.

My repeated attempts to secure information about the present practice of medicine in the Soviet Union met with his assurance that my questions were relevant, data existed, and experts at the Institute would answer them when I returned tomorrow. "Tomorrow" was a surprise since I had expected to spend the full day at the institute. Tomorrow's surprise turned into today's frustration when at the end of two and a half hours of harangue about capitalistic medicine I was politely ushered to the door. Later I learned, inadvertently through Marsha, that following our departure a telephone call went from the institute to the ministry informing them that I was never to return. There proved to be no tomorrow for collecting experts' data on the delivery of Soviet health care.

That a sensitive nerve had been touched became increasingly obvious. Unlike previous visits when my program had been crowded with opportunities to talk with individual clinicians, this time interviews simply failed to materialize. When the follow-up visit to the Institute of Social Hygiene and Public Health was canceled the next day, Marsha and I went to the movies.[1]

My requests to see Dr. Blokhin met with repeated evasions. The ministry reported that he was out of town or too busy with the upcoming meeting to see me. I instructed Marsha to convey to the ministry that I was getting nowhere and if I was in any way an embarrassment to the Soviet Union I would voluntarily leave the country immediately.

The following day brought notice of more appointments canceled from the program. Without Marsha, I went around to the U.S. Embassy to discuss the unexpected developments with Mr. John Zimmerman, our U.S. science advisor. He judged the sensitive nerve was primarily the reluctance of the ministry to reveal its statistics, with a possible second sensitive point their lack of any reliable statistics. He confirmed my impression from earlier visits that the Soviet health care system is so rigidly compartmentalized there could be little possibility for the internal communication necessary for data collection. Mr. Zimmerman suggested I cable the United States asking Dr. Their to cable a request to Dr. Blokhin to receive me. The cable to Dr. Their went off pronto.

Friday, Marsha informed me that she would not be with me for the weekend, wondering, since I would be on my own for two days if I might like to attend church with her that evening. Though not a religious man, in a country so rigorously dedicated to atheism, I could not pass up the invitation. She gave me directions for reaching the Arabat metro station from my hotel where I was to meet her at 9 P.M. From there we would walk to a chapel in the park adjoining what had once been the Novospassky Monastery.

We met as arranged and Marsha immediately shared some brusque instructions. We would be watched. Walk briskly. Do not look about and do not speak even if questioned. With that we made off through the frosty night. Once inside the park I twice noted loitering figures, one disclosed in the shadows behind a street light by his glowing cigarette. In neither case did I take my eyes off the snowy lane we crunched along.

The chapel door had two fedora-adorned men on either side making it impossible to enter without their close inspection. We pushed on as though they were invisible. The chapel was ancient, with low stone arches, resembling more a crypt than a sanctuary. A soft yellow light from banks of burning candles glowed in frozen breath of the small congregation, standing crowded together in rapt attention to the priest at the altar chanting the rituals of the Russian Orthodox church.

We slipped to one side and it was a few minutes before I realized the dirty looks from the tightly bundled, nearby worshipers were not from suspicion I was an intruder, but for my failure to doff my fur hat in sacred surroundings. There we stood for an hour in the biting chill as I rocked from one foot to the other on the floor of packed snow, attempting to preserve circulation in my frozen feet. The service in all its ancient glory of incense, dripping candles, and endless chant made no sense to me beyond an intense feeling of embattled community, more apparent than even the frozen clouds of the chanter hanging before me in the still air. Finally, no longer able to tolerate the glacial cold I gave a sign I could take no more.

We left after I lit a candle to those brave souls and made our way back to the Metro through the gauntlet of peering eyes.

The weekend was not spent at the international meeting but riding the Moscow metro, sight-seeing to the end of the line and back, as well as taking in Russian films. Both activities were small achievements in themselves considering the unaccountable schedules of Moscow subways and the number of Muscovites willing to stand in the snow to purchase movie tickets.

Monday, the scheduled visit to the First Moscow Medical School, the nation's most prestigious medical center, came off without a hitch. Here I met a group of medical psychologists who proved genuinely interested in medical deontology. They gave me considerable candid information about what was and was not being done for the patient-doctor relationship in the Soviet Union. Acknowledging their frustrations with "dehumanizing medical behavior," they were most interested in establishing ties with U.S. academics teaching medical ethics. Monday afternoon word came through that the program had been altered again. I was to leave for Leningrad on Wednesday.

Tuesday morning, after I lectured at the medical school, Marsha and I made off at once for the ministry of health. This time I came dressed in full capitalistic uniform—dark-blue, three-piece pin-striped suit with a thin, blue Royal Society of Medicine tie set off against a starched white shirt with gold cuff links. Once again alone in the reception room, I stood gazing out the window on a sooty courtyard of dirty snow, waiting until Mr. Yefinmych was well into the room before I turned about.

As anticipated, I found his previous fixed smile was replaced by an expression of raw exasperation. He nodded in recognition but I immediately cut to the point with, "There is a problem. I came here with a message from Dr. Their for Dr. Blokhin. It appears I will be sent off to Leningrad without seeing him!"

Words spluttered from the big man. "Dr. Blokhin is busy. What would you do if I was in your country and wished to see the minister of health?" This was a significant slip of the tongue as I did not wish to see the minister of health, a ranking bureaucrat, but a fellow academic.

"I am not asking to see the minister of health. I am asking for ten minutes with the president of the Soviet Academy of Medical Sciences. If you were in my country I would not hesitate. I would go to the telephone, call Dr. Their and tell him there was someone here who had a message concerning both our countries, and ask him if he would find time to see you."

This was followed by a series of "Yes, but's" which I cut short with, "I am most dissatisfied with the manner in which I am being treated. I am about to be sent off to Leningrad without seeing Dr. Blokhin even though I am prepared to wait here in Moscow until he has time to see me. In the event he does not wish to see me he can simply say so."

Mr. Yefinmych stumbled on, "Yes, I know. There was a wire from the Fogarty Center [the U.S. coordinating center for foreign exchange programs in Bethesda, Maryland] about your being discontent. This is the first time in my entire career that such a thing has happened. What I understand is that you wish to abandon the scientific purpose of your visit in order to talk with a particular person."

"Absolutely false. You are using words to avoid my request. I have stated and will state again in writing that I am here primarily to study Soviet medical deontology. I also wish to speak with Dr. Blokhin. There is no contradiction in these requests."

"Ah, but now you are telling me you will not go to Leningrad."

"Wrong again. I am not saying I will not go to Leningrad. I am simply saying that I wish to speak with Dr. Blokhin before I leave. Look, you and I are not making any sense. I propose to write down what I am saying in order that at a later date authorities will have a clear view of what is transpiring. You can write down what you are saying as well."

I then began writing out in longhand my statement while in a flurry of confusion Mr. Yefinmych rushed from the room to find paper to write down his statement of how he saw what was happening. He returned with a handful of blank paper and I gave him my handwritten statement.

Maintaining the initiative, I continued. "Here, write what you have to say in my notebook. You have my statement before you."

Confused, he wrote in my notebook, "Dr. N.N. Blockin [he misspelled the name], as president of the Academy of Medical Sciences of the U.S.S.R. is an extremely busy man person with a heavy schedule. At the present time he is finding difficulties in confirming the meeting with Dr. Crawshaw. In case the meeting is confirmed I will be glad to arrange it." His signature followed.

After writing he went on, "But such a meeting is impossible. He is a busy man."

Then I went for broke.

"Are you aware that Dr. Their has sent a personal cable to Dr. Blokhin asking him to receive me?" I was not certain this had actually happened but I was fairly sure he did not know either.

He was stunned that I had waited so long for this move. He thought a moment, "Would you be willing to see someone else in the academy if I can not secure time with Dr. Blokhin?"

"Who did you have in mind?"

"Dr. Shaznoff," a name I did not recognize. "He is the head of the academy's Division for International Health."

Unhesitatingly, I replied, "Yes. I am a member of the U.S. Institute of Medicine's Board for International Health. We are therefore peers. I accept the opportunity to talk with him as appropriate and timely."

Rising and coming around the table to shake my hand he volunteered, "I will see what can be done." I left feeling all was not lost.

Wednesday morning, the day I was to leave for Moscow on the midnight Red Arrow Express, I was informed by telephone that Dr. Blokhin would receive me at 1:30 that afternoon.

However, that was not the end of the difficulties. The ministry had arranged an 11 A.M. conference at the Soviet National Medical Library to acquaint me with their archives of medical deontology. As it turned out, the taxi trip through the center of town and out to the library took forty-five minutes. As Marsha and I rode through icy suburbs, another unpleasant complication unfolded in my mind. Once there, how would we ever get back for a 1:30 appointment? At best taxis are a sometime thing in the Soviet Union. I feared that once dropped at our destination nothing short of dogsled could get us back by dark. Anticipating a disastrous delay, I handed the driver a ten-ruble note with instructions through Marsha for him to remain at the library with his motor running as there would be more in it for him should we decide on a quick return to the city. We got out and made our way up the plowed walk while the driver backed his cab into a cleared space between two snow drifts and settled into a cloud of Russian cigarette smoke, awaiting our return.

The entrance to the library was guarded by an old crone, acting as concierge, who told us that our hostess was not in yet. She suggested we check her office so we made our way back through dim passageways to the rear of the immense building, to discover, yes, there was no answer to a knock on the librarian's door. A few doors down a pleasant woman offered us seats in her office until our hostess arrived. Demurring, we made our hasty way back to the concierge who again reported that the librarian we sought was not in the building nor was she expected until noon. Enough said. We were out the front door, back in our warm, waiting cab, and off to the academy.

When Dr. Blokhin heard of our early arrival he graciously shifted his schedule to meet us over tea and cakes. I recounted the Institute of Medicine's interest in developing closer ties with the Soviet Academy of Medical Sciences for exploring a collaborative effort of both academies toward a cross-cultural understanding of the ethical basis of medical practice. Dr. Their proposed a preliminary meeting of U.S.S.R. medical deontologists and U.S. medical ethicists. Dr. Blokhin was genuinely interested saying that he would take the proposal to his executive council. To mark the occasion, he presented me with a medallion commemorating the fortieth anniversary of the All Soviet Union Academy of Sciences. We parted on the best of terms.

Dr. G.I. Tsaregordotsev, chief of the Chair of Philosophy, Academy of Medical Sciences, had learned of our visit and as he was situated an hour away he asked that I remain at the academy to meet with him. Subsequently, Marsha and I passed the time awaiting his arrival with a quiet lunch on the premises.

When Dr. Tsaregordotsev arrived, he and I discussed the proposal for a meeting of members of the U.S.S.R. and U.S.A. academies. He has written definitive articles on Soviet deontology and wholeheartedly concurred that what was proposed could prove mutually beneficial. Practical constraints were considered, including maintaining a low media profile and avoiding confrontation over ideological differences. We proposed naming the effort Project Chekhov for the Russian writer/physician renowned for his profound understanding of the patient-doctor relationship.

Marsha and I spent the remainder of the afternoon fulfilling a wish that she had previously confided to me, for her to have some books of English literature. With my encouragement we made our way by Metro to one of Moscow's few used book stores. This may seem strange since the Communist Party maintains the largest publishing house in the world but their numerous outlets sell only new, doctrinaire accounts of party policy and heroes which apparently carry meager resale value. Outside the used bookstore we found a line stretched around the block made up of would-be patrons patiently awaiting space inside to be made by departing patrons. With a flash of ministry credentials we jumped the line.

For an hour, Marsha was a child loose in a candy store, piling editions of Shakespeare upon Jack London, Emily Brontë upon Mark Twain. Once the clerk totaled up the cost she grew apprehensive. I reassured her that I had rubles enough and not to worry.

Hesitatingly, she asked, "You are sure?"

"Of course. I have dollars as well."

Convinced I was serious she turned from the counter, declaring, "Then I want more to buy clothes." Out we went without a book and off to a nearby Beryoski store.

Moscow has a number of Beryoski (birch tree) stores which carry handmade and special goods intended to separate tourists from their foreign currency. The rule is, no Russians admitted and no rubles accepted. I informed the concierge that my guide was needed to advise me in buying gifts for my wife. Marsha then selected a discrete wardrobe of blouses, skirts, and sweaters. This time as the clerk totaled the bill there were no questions, for, with a shrug of defiance, Marsha took from a "For Export Only" shelf a beautiful, small icon of Christ the Redeemer which she placed on the top of the pile of purchases. These souvenirs never reached my wife, for my trusted guide, a believer among disbelievers, rejoiced in her just rewards.

At midnight, as scheduled, I boarded the Red Arrow Express bound for Leningrad weary from the encounter with Soviet bureaucracy.

The experience was worth the candle. A month after I returned home my colleague at our medical school reported that charges had been dropped and her brother had been released from prison. With no accounting of cause and effect, a few months later he was permitted to emigrate to the United States.

Though Project Chekhov never flourished, the effort significantly increased communication between the two medical academies and our friendship prospered over the debris of the crumbling Iron Curtain. In 1993, I was elected as a foreign member to the Russian Academy of Natural Sciences.

The most cherished memento is a slim slip of paper now pinned above my desk. It is Marsha's home telephone number, passed to me for my protection in case "anything happened," an act of treason when shared with me, an "agent of capitalism." That tag of paper was written with courage that gradually taught me that it takes two to be brave. You cannot be brave for yourself alone, at best that comes to no more than an instinct for survival, at worst it is bravado. Bravery demands a shared meaning, one of circumstantial action, the other of interpersonal recognition. Though never verbalized, that sharing flowed between us, Marsha's seeing and respecting my "resistance to intimidation" while I gradually appreciated her sustained courage in sustaining her personal beliefs and dignity. She lived in the belly of the beast, I but visited, but who would not enter into the maw of that beast to share such bravery.

Endnotes
1. R. Crawshaw, "Off to the Russian Movies," *The Pharos*, Summer 1987, 41-44.

Humble Pie

Disguise it as you will, flavor it as you will, call it what you will, umble-pie, and nothing else.
—James Russell Lowell (1819-1891)
in C.E. Funk, *A Hog on Ice*

Hopefully, with the passing of two hundred more years, our nation will have "picked up" many more of the delightful customs of the British. Not that we lack traditions, "Hurrah for the Fourth of July," nor customs either, "Wah, ev'rbody eats cone pone an' chittlins," but as yet ours are less worn smooth to the shape of human eccentricity.

Take the British use of "humble pie" for instance. In bygone times, the custom arose for the lord of the manor to leave his peasants the umbles, or entrails, when he killed a deer. Once he made off with the cleaned carcass, the menials gathered up what was left and cooked a bitter umble-pie. Through the years "umble" became "humble," but the idea remained to signify a ration of leftovers for the inept, the ineffective, and the weak.

British physicians regularly publish in the correspondence columns of the journal *World Medicine* their servings of humble pie (their goofs and blunders) not for scientific knowledge but in recognition of the profession's abiding need for humility.

A personal example may clarify the concept of medical humble pie. After attending a conference on the East Coast, I started home emotionally drained. The people, talk, and ideas at the conference had reached a tempo which wore me out, so when I changed planes at St. Louis for the final leg to Portland, I wanted a solitary flight to recharge my batteries with idle fantasy, aerial sight-seeing, and a snooze.

Since the plane was nearly empty I chose the far right seat (sunless) in the first row, where I settled down, relieved when no passengers occupied the adjoining seats. Across the aisle, in the far left seat, was an unaccompanied little girl. She had been deposited there by the stewardess with the usual admonition to be good. With plenty of room to stretch, I tuned my earphones to Vivaldi, sipped a Scotch, and watched a checkerboard of prairie farms pass far below.

Special Alertness

After the meal, sleep evaded me, and when I restlessly glanced about, I found that the little girl had slipped two seats closer and was looking at me. She was a wispish nine-year-old, almost concealed by an immense, stuffed horse in her lap. It was impossible not to respond. I smiled and she smiled back, a shy fleeting smile that made mincemeat of my resolve for silent meditation.

"What is your horse's name?" I asked.

Could there have been a more engaging answer?

"She has no name."

There was absolutely nothing brassy about the lass. Her clothes had a homemade look with blouse of matronly dark blue print, a plain skirt, knee socks, and scuffed shoes. Her face was bright, yet drawn, with subtle shades of fatigue about her eyes. Her glance was attentive, with that special alertness of the weak, anxiously seeking to please. This, coupled with her quick, overcontrolled movements, dark cropped hair, and thin, chirping English accent, made her into as sweet a sparrow as has ever flown thirty-five thousand feet above the earth.

Up In the Air

I bumped her stuffed horse up and down twice on my knee—

"Looks like her last stable was a department store. Could it have been Harrods?"

"Why yes—How did you know?"

"She has a decided gray-dappled, London look. She's a lady, too—why not call her by her rightful title, Lady Jane?"

"Do you really think we *could* call her Lady Jane?"

"Of course"—and as the miles flew by, the tale of the young lady, this gamine of the airways, unfolded. She was between parents—and was as much in the air domestically as she was literally.

Her father was an author living on the East Coast, while her mother lived in a fishing village on the West Coast. She had not seen her mother for three years and was on her way to spend a fortnight with her. Her aunts in England had "adopted" her. "I consider myself English," is how she put it and recited, with just a little prompting, a poem she had written while living on the Yorkshire Moors. It was a creditable verse and she gained more confidence as she recited it to me. She then opened her small notebook to another that she had composed the previous winter while staying in a Canadian cabin that her father had borrowed "to be alone" while writing.

Her notebook contained many little gems, sketches of horses, more poems, and a list of her classmates in her latest school. The list helped her remember them, since she changed schools so frequently that it was difficult to keep them in mind. We laughed at Anthony Bologni's name, for he is known to the crowd in the fourth grade as "Tony Boloney."

I then suggested ticktacktoe.

As we "x"ed and "o"ed our way across empty pages, she explained that next year she might not be in school at all, since she would be eighteen months in Sumatra with her stepmother who was an anthropologist. She could, however, read well, she exclaimed, and to prove the point promptly produced from her carry-on bag a small paperback library of Tillotson's delightful cartoons of horses and little girls. She read the captions on the cartoons she thought might catch my fancy.

"Here, you're bound to like this one," and she would read yet another.

I interrupted her rapid reading to ask what had been her best trip. She paused, thoughtful, but could not say. However, she knew her worst. It had been over the Atlantic in December, and she spun out a hair-raising tale of fever, fog, and delay.

Something of Value

As we neared our destination, our mutual captivation turned to desperation, for we realized our bond, with its tempered intimacy, was soon to break. Our brief relationship seemed capable of the deepest confidences with one exception—loneliness. Any direct reference to loneliness was deftly turned aside, although any other subject might be shared. She spoke of her embarrassment when adults kissed each other, and she unburdened herself of some of her concerns about suicide by relating a news item from Hong Kong.

It concerned a man, born forty years ago, literally in the harbor, when his mother had fallen overboard. He had lived his life in sampans but in despair had drowned himself at the very spot where his mother had delivered him.

"It was suicide, don't you know."

And then she asked about breech deliveries for colts. Had I seen the movie *The Red Pony*, where a man put his hand up inside the mare— "Well, anyway, the colt was a sound one—a beauty."

And so I sat there hopelessly struggling to say something of value to such a brave little soul. As we neared the airport, the stewardess repeatedly interrupted with the charm of a first sergeant. "Don't leave the plane until I say so. When we're ready to take you off, you can go, but not before."

Always Alone

After she had admonished the lass for the fifth time and bustled on down the aisle, my sparrow turned to me, abandoning her "little girl" facade and exclaimed, "Precisely where does she think I am going to go?"

The plane landed, and as it taxied off the runway, I was completely at a loss for words—only action seemed left.

"How shall we part?" I asked. "Should I hug you or you hug me?"

The stewardess, probably taking me for an aging Humbert Humbert pursuing a Lolita, chimed in, "Just thank the nice man for talking with you."

Without further words we tearfully embraced. I suspected that we both wished to hide any further show of emotions, so I shouldered my way off the plane leaving that child of Sisyphus—alone, for yet another journey, and another, as always alone.

Perhaps I should have mustered up my frail hold on science and, by putting some name to her circumstance, "discovered" a new syndrome for child psychiatry—the airborne waif! However, I was wise enough to know that she suffered from the human condition, and for all my training, intuition, and desire, I was powerless to help. For me, this was the bitterest of humble pie.

Endnotes

Reprinted from *Prism* 2 #11 (1974): 13-15 and from *World Medicine* (Sept. 1973) with permission from Reed Business Information Limited.

Part 4

The Many Languages of Compassion

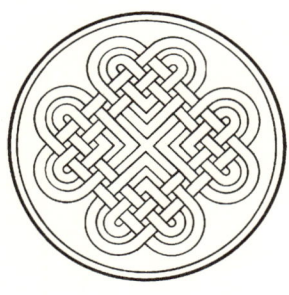

We are a migrating but not a traveling people. We think of our country only as abounding in residences; and pass from one to another, without inspecting anything between them. Thus, even migration bestows on us none of the benefits of travel. In our transits, all things are sacrificed to speed. We are not satisfied unless we add night to day; and when we awake in the morning, congratulate ourselves that we are a hundred miles nearer the point of attraction; although we may have passed through scenes and objects the most interesting, without having beheld the least or the greatest of them. Thus while we are wanderers, we remain ignorant of the relations and true character of all among whom we roam; or know them only in connections with hemp and cotton planting, commerce, land speculation, or the practice of law or medicine.
—Daniel Drake, M.D. (1785-1852)
in *Physician to the West: Selected Writings
of Daniel Drake on Science and Society*

Overview to Part 4

There is something about the reach of a far horizon that makes a traveler out of all but the blind. From first flight, when, as small children, we were joyfully tossed overhead by an energetic relative, travel is an exciting, thrilling part of a life. It lures us to adventure, to venture forth, first beyond our immediate surroundings, later to the edges of our culture, and finally to explore the explorer we have become. Travel, for the nonchalant saunterer, opens wide a window on limitless humanity.

Travel is many things, including expense, emotional challenge, time, stress, education, fatigue, but for the searching mind travel is, above all, obligatory. Once infected with an itch to see the other side of the mountain, involuntarily we become students of a new language, mankind's infinite ways of expressing fellow feeling.

Listening over God's Shoulder introduces the language of fellow feeling as it may be spoken by the passenger sitting in the next seat on an international flight. **The Necessary Samaritan** recounts how a physician/traveler remains alert to puzzling accidents and alien illnesses, to frame service accordingly.

Nor is the language of travel easy to master, for travel teaches its lasting lessons by abrupt culture shock, rather than the soft stroke of quaint encounters. Emotional trauma may sound out of place in brightly colored travel brochures featuring tropical, palm-fringed beaches adorned with lightly clad bronze maidens offering every comfort—and it is. Travel advertising merchandises an illusion, selling "virtual" travel in the form of a hand-held guided tour, an idyllic cruise to a razor-wire secure, sybaritic resort. "Virtual" travel promises safe extension of the tourist's native ambiance, transporting the tourist to an advertised paradise, the land of your home-based dreams.

Unfortunately, the guided tour sets the heart and mind apart from the reality of a foreign culture by ensuring the trip remains blandly pleasurable for the frail and frightened. Such journeys serve well as a metaphor for the "hand-held" life, guided existence never explored.

In contrast, engaged travel brings with it unavoidable abrasion of personal beliefs and values, vexing confusion and unanticipated risk—symptoms of culture shock.

Travel can nip much sharper than jet lag, for from experienced travel-ache a contagion of reactions spreads as the dynamic of culture shock. A first response to travel weariness is often querulous complaints. "Why did I ever leave home in the first place? Who needs this miserable bus ride." Then, recognizing that retreat to home is blocked, "I plan to spend the rest of the stay in my hotel room." Reactions continue with, "It really is not all that bad but I never plan to come back to this God-forsaken place." As culture shock progresses, acceptance of mixed feelings emerges. "When I was at home I was in a better place, but a traveler makes himself content."

With acceptance, the traveler turns adversity to advantage. "How was it that miserable beggar in Barcelona irritated me so?" The question opens the traveler's mind to considering the foreigner as a person rather than a bit of scenery, a curious mass of ambulatory flesh. If examined carefully, the question does more for the traveler than can ever be accomplished by displaying a collection of color slides of "our" group posed before the Taj Mahal.

As foreignness becomes an interpersonal experience, the traveler can, with a measured personal curiosity, compare received values with values of the foreign other. It is neither lack of tact nor poor breeding that prompts the Indian woman with suckling baby at her breast, standing on a Madras roadside, to fiercely importune the tourists in the stalled bus for "rupees." She is driven by a grim fact of a desperate life. She is hungry. Such disquieting sights, raw experience, can be kneaded by curiosity and thoughtful reflection into a meaning that draws the participant observer closer to the foreigner's life rather than enforce distance.

Travel uncovers hidden strengths as it renews self-awareness. Foreignness, as lived by foreigners, can lead to the discovery of the traveler as foreigner in someone else's native land. Inevitably, by discerning the foreign other as a unique and interesting individual, we, home-loving butcher, baker, or candlestick maker, learn more of compassion's many-tongued language.

A reliable principle for insightful travel is illustrated in **Going to the Movies in China**. Few experiences so swiftly and harmlessly immerse the visitor in a foreign culture as attending a locally-made film in a local movie house. With the traveler's personal foreignness covered by the dark of the movie house there is no inhibition on locals sharing their reactions to flickering images on the screen. Thus alien delights and sorrows easily surrender their foreignness.

Facility with another language, such as travel's, clearly is not limited to verbal communication but includes a spirit quickened to unfamiliar nuances, idiom, and body language. Thus nascent foreignness, culture shock, can be translated into heightened compassion as pain is transmuted into meaning.

In the face of ethnic and tribal differences, fellow feeling is fragile, vulnerable to unexpected passions and estrangement, which can twist fellow feeling into scorn. Present-day slavery, apartheid, is an example of inverted fellow feeling as it pervaded the crevasses and crannies of South African culture. It may have lessened its agonizing hold on that suffering land since I last visited there in 1993, but I acknowledge how experienced apartheid all but overwhelmed my respect for fellow human beings with mind-filling rage. In desperation I made much use of a special "travel tool," asking my hosts for their three magic wishes.

I asked many, poor men, rich women, garrulous taxi drivers, soft-spoken game wardens in the Kruger Park, a brusque minister of health, "If you had three magic wishes what would they be?" The question is germane for rich and poor, Black and White, wise and foolish, young and old. Often it stirs a quizzical, what-is-it-with-you look, but when reassured by returned genuine curiosity, none fail to share soul-sounding answers.

One morning while working at my desk in a Cape Town hotel room, I put aside my pen to ask the humble Black chambermaid for her three "magic wishes." She paused, ceased making the bed, and standing erect, looking me straight in the eye, slowly in broken English said, "Peace. You look at me and you are scared. I look at you and I am scared. If you do not talk you kill. When talk, it is better because you say what is in your heart. If you know the heart you do not kill. We all have one father, God." She gave me the gift of a lifetime, lighting up my flagging faith that compassion might be found in that benighted land. The hub about which **A Fairy Tale for a South African Grandchild** revolves is the gift of that sharing lady.

Compassion is found at unexpected times and in surprising places, attested to by **Compassion Is Where You Find It**.

Listening over God's Shoulder

*Let my prayer come before thee: incline thine ear
unto my cry…*

—Psalms 88:2

Whom do you know that is aware that airports have chapels, let alone acknowledges using them? Consequently, I felt sure of a refuge from the maddening crowd when I was inadvertently left suspended in time at Paris's Charles de Gaulle Airport. In gratitude I followed the arrows leading to the chapel.

As it turns out, there are three, a small Jewish synagogue in which a man in a yarmulke was saying prayers, a Muslim retreat empty of everything but rugs upon the floor, and a Christian chapel. The chapel is a 15- by 40-foot chamber with white stucco, windowless walls, and subdued lighting which gives it more the appearance of a crypt than a place of worship, but the cross above a simple altar bearing an open bible together with a row of simple stools spoke to its consecration.

After catching my breath and thoughts, alone, I found on the stool next to me a plain notebook which on paging through turned out to be the visitor's log. The book held a wide assortment of notes in many languages and scripts. Those I could read became for me a window on the souls of the weary.

Some left their name and date, some a business card, others simply signed, "A child of God." Here is a sample of the pleas, thanks, and praise of life by pilgrims far from home. I wrote them down that others might join me in a miraculous position of listening over God's shoulder.

> It is a good thing to find a chapel in the airport, a point of silence in this crazy world.

> Dear Lord - let bygones be bygones.

> This chapel is a welcome oasis of peace in a desert of duty-free commerce.

> I come here, my heart filled with sorrow. I do not understand your ways. I find it hard to come to you in my grief. Please pray for the soul of my

Aunt who with her husband and four children were killed in a car accident on the Swiss/Italian border this morning.

Dieu nous protégé et nous aide. Merci.

December 25, 1994 – Happy Birthday and thank you for the North and South Korean accord, the PLO and Israel accord, but most of all for my peoples' accord and trust. Ireland was far too beautiful to be destroyed. Bless Mom and Dad.

I sincerely thank you for this wonderful experience of your loving presence. I am never alone though I feel very lonely in my travels.

Dear God - [followed by a series of small roughly drawn hearts].

5 months later I find myself back here. Something magical about this quiet spot. Help me be strong and my family healthy and happy. They always do "the right things" and help others what ever way we can.

It has been a good weekend. We have had our ups and our downs but we ate, drank, and slept well. Thank you for life.

Take care of us we need you.

Thank you for this quiet time - a weary Chicago traveler.

Here I am Lord. I have come to do your will.

Lord Jesus, have mercy on me a miserable sinner.

I pray for the people of Armenia where I am going, that peace may come to them soon and for a safe journey with guardian Angel at my side.

Thank you God for my 3 months in Paris. I don't think I can write about it….But I…If we are destiny please give us the opportunity to meet again. Thank you my God. [Signed with a Japanese name]

Thank you for giving me a chance to say prayers. I feel so much better.

With our aloha for many blessings.

Power that was, is and will be - I thank you for the company of those who shared themselves in this book. We all become weary once we know we are far from home. You link us in love.

The Necessary Samaritan

But a certain Samaritan...went to him, and bound up his wounds...
—Luke 10:33-34

"Is there a doctor in the house?" is a command, not a question, for most, if not all, physicians. Few have escaped the call to minister unexpected aid sometime in their career, and though the scene may vary, the scenario is stereotyped.

There is a huddle of people, some chattering with agitated confusion, some frozen with obvious concern, all with drawn, anxious faces. The standard first line runs, "Is there a doctor here?" and the reply, "Yes," immediately casts the responder as a Necessary Samaritan.

The actual scene makes little difference—a restaurant with a woman strangling on a piece of meat, a sidewalk with a boy prone in an epileptic seizure, or a commuter train with a passenger doubled up by the pain of a myocardial infarction. Once the bystander is identified as a physician, he loses all choice. Unlike the biblical Good Samaritan who *chose* to help, the physician becomes the Necessary Samaritan who *must* help.

I remember the first time the role was thrust upon me as a new doctor. It was years ago, while my wife and I were staying at the Crater Lake Lodge in Oregon at the end of the vacation season, a dripping wet Sunday afternoon.

The lobby was filled with at least forty bored guests, some playing bridge, some reading, some writing, some just staring out the rain-splattered window. Suddenly the manager appeared at the far end of the room. Bearing down upon me, he exclaimed, in a voice loud enough for all to hear, "Doctor, come quick. There is an emergency."

I sprang into action, rushed after him, and found, in an upstairs room, a bride of three days, sobbing hysterically. After motioning the bewildered groom to leave I closed the door. Forty-five minutes and a Kleenex box later, I learned *"HE* is a beast!" A little more listening and she agreed to try him again rather than rush home to Mother. This was not a demanding task for this Necessary Samaritan; in my judgment, a sympathetic ear is best in treating anxiety attacks.

However, there is more to the definition of the Necessary Samaritan. The downstairs crowd who were suffering from acute epidemic curiosity had completely slipped my mind. As I recrossed the lobby's threshold, eighty inquisitive eyes fixed upon me. Obviously, they needed something to merit their expectations. I paused, every bit the compleat physician, coughed, and blithely announced to my wife across the room, "It's a boy. Eight pounds six ounces." There was an audible sigh of relief. The day was saved as well as the patient!

A more serious example of the Necessary Samaritan occurred for me one evening flying out of Moscow. It was a sedate British Airways flight, and in no time I was relaxing with a Scotch and soda. From my window nothing could be seen outside but inky blackness; inside, the aproned stewardesses were bustling down the aisles, serving dinner.

Few passengers had boarded with me at Moscow; the plane was filled mostly with sleepy Japanese who had boarded the flight at Tokyo and, as I later learned, a group of rock musicians who had enplaned at Bangkok.

Even though dinner would be a British airline special—beef and boiled potatoes set off by limp lettuce and weary pickle followed by tepid pudding, swilled down with hot tea—I was relaxed enough to be looking forward to my first Western meal in a long time. Suddenly, the pilot's voice rang out alarmingly over the public address system, "Is there a doctor aboard? Would he please report, immediately, to the forward cabin."

What physician has not experienced the reflex that followed! It is kind of screwing your body down in your seat as you wait for the real emergency doctor "to please stand up."

Well, nobody stood up, and as the second announcement began, I folded up my tray table and clambered over the Siberian salesman and Japanese transistor expert between me and the aisle and went forward to discover a groaning young Caucasian man bundled up in blankets and surrounded by solicitous buddies.

His history was brief. He was a member of a Cockney rock band, the name escapes me, which had been "doing a gig" in Thailand until the audience had run amok and the police terminated the group's brief engagement. The band started home with Alfie, the sick one, feeling "a bit nasty in the tummy." During a brief layover in Tokyo, Alfie began to vomit, and an emergency consultation with a local physician returned a diagnosis, ironically appropriate, of Asian flu.

The Japanese doctor had recommended hospitalization. Alfie refused, but compromised by agreeing to a series of shots of an unknown drug, which had quieted him most of the way over Siberia. Somewhere over Novosibirsk he had awakened to more nausea and cramps, but this time when they put down in Moscow, he fixed his mind on Britain's National Health Service, bit his lip, and never let out a whimper. Now he could no longer contain himself.

I am a psychiatrist and I know a psychosis when I see one, but a medical emergency is a different story. I had left all that behind twenty years ago with the Korean War. Undaunted even when I learned there were no medical instruments and only few drugs aboard, I bent down and gave the young man a once-over.

There he was, doubled up, a bit damp to touch, thready fast pulse, anxious face, splinting of the abdomen, and in the right lower quadrant as nice a rebound tenderness at McBurney's point as you could ever hope to demonstrate to a medical student. I put my ear to his belly, and the gurgling of the bowels confirmed that the next step was "off to the surgeon" for an appendectomy.

I straightened up and met the eyes of our worried captain. "What do you think, Doctor?" he asked.

I did not answer. It seemed to me that Alfie should be in a hospital, but where? Return to Moscow's Sheremetyevo airport? The frustration of Russian customs would be enough to rupture a healthy vermiform appendix! Straight down to Warsaw, somewhere far below us? Ahead, two hours to London? I turned back to the patient, who whimpered, "Doc, please—just get me 'ome."

He was not in shock and I judged would keep for another two hours and told the pilot so. Then I tucked him in with a shot of morphine, pinned a note to his jacket, and returned to my seat. This time the passengers did not want to know the weight of the baby. No, it was "where are we going to put down?" When I said, "Heathrow," there was a sigh of relief.

A few weeks after the emergency consultation, I received a letter of thanks from Dr. Daniel L. Murphy, of British Airways. He invited me to stop by for a visit the next time I passed through Heathrow.

A few months later, between planes, I took him up on his invitation and made my way to the south end of the Intercontinental Terminal at Heathrow, where he has his surgery. Dr. Murphy turned out to be a delightful Irishman. He was busy with a patient, but as soon as he had finished, he settled down to an hour's fine talk.

It seemed I had stumbled upon a "Super-Samaritan." His airline had fifteen physicians, but he was the one who directed professional care and friendly protection to the sky passenger. What a fund of knowledge he had of the do's and don'ts of health during air travel, from ruptured ear drums to terminal carcinomatosis, with, of course, human nature hooked to all the problems.

Much of his time is spent offering advice to the mentally ill. Affluent countries such as Canada, the United States, and Japan have a surplus of batty souls restlessly shuttling back and forth about the world, and a good many of them come to Dr. Murphy's attention.

Incidentally, he told me that the Scandinavian governments are best about caring for their wayward nationals, hospitalizing them, following their conditions, and escorting them home. When a recalcitrant country refuses to help one of its own, the airline is forced to pick up the bill, including the ticket home.

Dr. Murphy is always willing to work with any sick or incapacitated person in need of air transportation. However, many passengers are afraid to reveal their disabilities or are simply unaware of available services. "Granny from Glasgow" is an example. She is typically an untraveled, elderly, provincial woman with a touch of arteriosclerosis who is flying out to visit her grandchildren for the first time.

Fatigue (long walks through airports), confusion (long lines through customs), excitement (a new experience), hypoxia (airplane cabins are sometimes low in oxygen) culminate, about twelve hours out, with her request to "please stop the tram, I want to get off at Dalmarnock Bridge." If the officials only knew about her ahead of time, she would have been escorted with a wheelchair through the airport and customs and given a whiff of oxygen now and then by an understanding stewardess.

The cost to the airline of the cardiac patient, who has concealed his two past coronaries until five minutes out over the Atlantic when his chest begins to hurt, is stupendous. It could mean turning the plane about and dumping a couple of tons of precious fuel in order to land.

Perhaps Dr. Murphy's most difficult decisions concern patients intent upon going home to die. "These people are problematic, but we must be compassionate, and if there is any chance of getting them through, we go along with the trip," was how he put it.

"Some terminal patients yearn for a chance to make that final visit— to realize a lifelong dream before dying. And, much as Charles Lindbergh's last flight to Hawaii six days before he died, their requests are treated with profound respect, but of course we must include the cost of a zinc-lined coffin to return the body." The International Civil Aviation Organization regulations are adamant about this, despite the high costs of air shipping.

To make the point, Dr. Murphy spun a yarn about the couple who beat the cost of coffin transportation. The steward on a flight out of Singapore, heading for London, noticed a retired colonel sitting bolt upright by the window and asked a lady companion in the next seat, presumably his wife, if he wanted a pillow. She said no, and the steward let the matter drop. Hours later over the Middle East, he realized the colonel had yet to move a muscle to finger his waxed mustache. Concerned, he again spoke to the lady, "Madam, your husband does not look well. I do not believe he is breathing." To which she tartly replied, "My husband may have expired but his ticket has not!"

The fillip for the Necessary Samaritan came toward the end of our talk as we reviewed my experience over Poland. "Of course you omitted something," said Dr. Murphy. "You failed to get your rock patient's name and address and send him a bill." That was a vital difference between the "Good" and the "Necessary" Samaritan. The lack of choice should be compensated for!

I left his office flooded with fantasies of chucking it all and opening a roving practice as a Necessary Samaritan of the Airways.

As I flew out of Heathrow, I mused, "I could jaunt to exotic corners of the world and dispense care on 'plane calls' from Katmandu to Marrakech depending on referrals from the captain." However, by the time I deplaned at Geneva in a jostling crowd of boisterous, presumably healthy, American passengers, I knew it was a dream. The specter of malpractice insurance had awakened me, and besides, neither managed care nor Medicare would permit me to keep my practice up in the air.

Endnotes

Reprinted from *Prism* 3 #4(1975): 7-11, with permission. Copyrighted 1975, American Medical Association.

Going to the Movies in China

The Master visited the Grand Temple of the Founder of the Dynasty. He inquired about everything. Someone said: "Who said this fellow was an expert on ritual? When visiting the Grand Temple, he had to inquire about everything." Hearing this the Master said, "Precisely, this is ritual."
—Confucius (551-479 B.C.)

The Western movie is alive and well in the Far East. The saga has been turned inside out like an old glove, however, and what was once right is now left, while the raggle-taggle seams that were hidden are now exposed, all to the delight of the Chinese audience and the chagrin of the occasional Western-Yankee-imperialist who gets a peep of the silver screen behind the bamboo curtain.

Although a Cold War trip to The People's Republic of China and its cultural revolution was not intended to include the cinema, in 1977 gracious hosts were kind enough to accommodate my wish to join Chinese audiences watching Chinese films in China. As our group journeyed from Beijing to Kwangchow, the Chinese Travel Bureau found us tickets to the local Bijou in Anyang. Occasionally I purchased tickets myself simply by stepping up to the box office and plunking down a yuan or two.

For the China traveler, movie-going takes a bit of planning; the seats in Chinese movie houses are reserved, and, in my brief experience, every seat is filled by show time. In Shanghai, I located a movie house three blocks from our hotel and, after passing the word among our group of twenty-two travelers, found six other movie buffs willing to take on yet another event in a packed schedule. Frankly, it takes a bit of stamina, after spending a day of visiting hospitals, communes, schools, and/or factories, to then dash out to the local 7:00 show. After supper the weary traveler is tempted to fall down dead in bed and sleep until the next day's round of events.

During a lunchtime break, I made for the box office of the Shanghai movie house and, as my Chinese vocabulary is limited to "Gung ho," the dickering was more visual than verbal. I had in mind a movie featured in the lobby by a large poster of a white-uniformed Chinese man rescuing a young lady from some ill-defined danger. As it turned out, I negotiated eight seats in the balcony (the extra seat was for our interpreter) for a total cost of forty-nine cents, but for the wrong film.

We were a bit late getting off to the show since our interpreter was nearsighted and had trouble borrowing a pair of eyeglasses. Eyeglasses are not conspicuous in The People's Republic of China, and I wonder if their scarceness is not part of a general reluctance that revolutionary Chinese have in seeing possible political shortcomings. The basic Chinese assumption seems to be that since the mind of man is infinitely malleable to the political will of man, such things as the common cold, fatigue, hunger, and myopia can be willed into insignificance. Theirs is a spartan approach to what we Westerners, with our perhaps hypochondriacal and certainly sybaritic attitudes, deem to be necessities, such as three squares a day, sunglasses, cold tablets, sleeping pills, and overcoats. Incidentally, one of the curses of writing anything about China is digression, and then digression upon digression, until your basic confusion about all that is Chinese remains the only point you are capable of making—the Marco Polo syndrome.

Anyway, our interpreter located some specs that matched his astigmatism closely enough for him to discern the movie screen from the balcony, and we were off, prepared for some old-fashioned melodrama. As it turned out, I had booked us for a documentary of the historical development of The People's Republic of China. Luckily, the disappointment was softened by the quality of the documentary, which was well edited, moving along with excellent animation to explain the tactics of the People's Liberation Army during the 1930s and 1940s. The scope of the film was surprisingly broad, starting with newsreels of the Boxer Uprising and moving up to the blast of the Chinese atomic bomb.

One disconcerting note of the documentary, and other Chinese films for that matter, was the unabashed portrayal of the Westerner in general, and the American, in particular, as a military aggressor. The shots of United States troops marching into Peking during the early years of the twentieth century, the Marines in Shanghai during the 1930s, World War II B-25s dropping bombs, presumably on defenseless peasants, and GIs being escorted from North Korea as prisoners of the People's Liberation Army gave a slant on history that does not go with the Western grain. In one film, seen in passing at an outdoor movie in Kwangchow, the plot was sharply focused on driving out the barbarians, in this case GIs on a munitions train in North Korea. It had a Buster Keaton sequence, though serious, of fighting across the top of moving railroad cars and had the audience clapping approval every time a Yankee-imperialist pitched from the careening train. To say the least, it is disconcerting to find your symbols turned inside out.

The fact is I never did adjust to seeing the villains in chop suey Westerns wearing brown fedoras, rather than black cowboy hats. The plots of the few I saw were fairly uniform, generally about a minority group on the border of China which afforded the director an opportunity to include some exotic scenery. The heavy in the film turns out to be the local elderly landlord. He is a seamy character, with the best house in town and a couple of "nieces" intent upon pleasing him in all ways, including filling opium pipes, showing a bit of leg through a split skirt, and generally mooning about over booze and cards like the dancehouse floozies of our Westerns. The ultimate heavy in the act is the landlord's son who puts on Occidental airs, such as wearing a brown fedora, carrying a riding crop, and wearing a sidearm, a .38. As might be expected, the local people have a hard time meeting the rent, while the landlord's son is busy making things worse by raising the price of rice. When things look just about impossible for the locals, who should arrive but our heroes, a squad from the People's Liberation Army. The landlord surreptitiously warns the locals that if he catches them talking with these tall, smiling strangers he will foreclose on the mortgage.

The plot is a loose remake of *Shane*, with its unfettered cowpoke who comes meandering into town, meaning no harm. Then he aims to settle down for a spell in the little mining town, or was it a cattle town, or a sheep town, until he sees a bit of injustice. Since he has an attitude problem with the local baddies down at the gin mill, they decide to run him out of town. In the Chinese version there is as much guttural threatening as you could ask for as the baddies alternately attempt to starve out and then drive out our heroes. But of course the baddies have a fatal flaw, greed, which leads them to try to corner the rice market, or turn the competition's lambs out into the snow, or sell off the commune's grain crop, or chop down the bridge to town; the list is as long as Hollywood Boulevard. Once their perfidy is exposed they take it on the lam, but, you guessed it, yes, the good guys get on their horses and the chase is on, through the rice paddies and over the hills, until the cornered baddie is betrayed, inadvertently shot with his own gun, or surrenders in abject humility. The heroes, the Peoples' Liberation Army (PLA) or locals, in the tradition of the Lone Ranger, refrain from gunfire, allowing the evil ones to destroy themselves. The final scenes are filled with the joyful locals enjoying the benefits of an abundant life, and include such artful changes as the substitution of Chairman Mao's picture for Buddha's over the family hearth, with the PLA filling the background where earlier there were Buddhist monks.

The films seemed long, which may be a function of my language problem, since all dialogue arrived secondhand, related to me by the interpreter with the same kindly patience I can remember my father using when I, as an unlettered lad, attended silent films. The camera technique was excellent, not overdone nor fancy, and some of the settings, particularly in the Mongolian hinterlands, with lakes, mountains, and clouds bespeaking nature in its glory, were spectacular.

The clearest example of the American as enemy was not in the movies but in the Peking Opera's production of *The Light Sabre Society*. Chinese opera is a delight, albeit a matter of developed taste, for to my ear the music is shrill, the singing predominately vibrato, the voices fricative and of course unintelligible, the acting melodramatic, the plot slow, yet the overall effect intriguing. Clappers and gongs accent fascinating dramatic effects as actors in sumptuous costumes of former mandarin luxury pose and whirl in a manner intuitively felt as part of the ancient China.

The Light Sabre Society runs seven acts, during which Liu Li-chun, Pan Chi-hsiang, and the young lady Chan Hsiu-yung, revolutionaries of 1853, organize the workers of Shanghai into an uprising against the foreigner and renegade Chinese of the Ch'ing dynasty for forcing opium on the people, as well as generally raising Ned through graft, looting, and killing. Finally it is all too much for Pan Chi-hsiang, and he beats up, you guessed it, an American, Martin Young, a "U.S. Imperialist Catholic Father."

Martin Young appears dressed as a Jesuit priest in the habit of the 1700s—round hat, black surplice, and pendant crucifix upon his chest. He is a balding man of devious manner, who is abetted by the British counsel and a French officer. The latter are secondary characters without name and seldom directly involved in oppressing the hero and his crowd.

Martin Young continually gets it in the neck. During Act II, Pan Chi-hsiang is to be beheaded for his attack on Martin Young, and when the priest shows up at the execution to administer last rites, no cowering prisoner awaits him. Pan gives him holy hell or, as the translator puts it, "exposes his false benevolence." Martin Young is so furious at the harangue that he gives the nod to the Chinese executioner, Wu Chien-chung. Inadvertently, his action is a signal for an uprising, in the course of which Young gets his second thrashing, while Pan breaks free.

The next thing we know, Young, now dressed in a fancy layman's outfit, meets with the French and British for more skullduggery. He has brought along Wu to rig a treaty that will further humiliate the Chinese people, but he is foiled when the Light Sabre Society shows up and with "indignation" uncovers the Imperialist plot to rob the Chinese of their sovereignty. Young and his crowd, despite much prancing about the stage, are powerless to stop the leaders of the insurrection.

The next acts stretch over years, revealing the initial success of the Sabre Society gradually melting away under siege of the Ch'ing mercenaries. While Pan is off to Nanking seeking help, who shows up in camp to tempt the lady leader, Chou, but Martin Young. This time he offers money to the fair practitioner of the martial arts, while she dazzlingly flies about the stage, saber in hand. But it is no go; she knows Pan will bring help. Young then maliciously shows her evidence that Pan has been killed. The crowd is enraged, and Young catches it again while fleeing over a wall.

In the final scene the revolutionary forces break out of the encirclement. In the battle Liu kills the renegade Wu but is mortally wounded by the American priest, who proves handy with a blunderbuss. As he dies, Liu musters enough strength to chop up, you guessed it again, Martin Young. The play closes with Chou making off with the red flag that will keep the revolution alive and eventually destroy reactionaries of Martin Young's ilk.

There is no mistaking in this play that the United States is the source of the trouble, with the villainous Martin Young as its agent. He is portrayed as an unprincipled coward, as merciless as Fu Manchu dragging a defenseless blond lass off to his opium den. The stereotype is indelible and who is to say no? Certainly not I, for no matter how ironic the portrait of Martin Young may be you will never find me standing up in a Chinese audience to protest. There is enough confusion about Sino-American relations as it is.

The irony stems from the fact that the revolutionary movement, the T'ai P'ing rebellion of 1853, portrayed in the story, was a Christian revolution led by a Cantonese, Hung Hsiu-Ch'uan. He was a well-educated man who had studied the Bible and, after finding strength in the Bible's message to face some personal problems, developed a Christian sect that grew to immense proportions in Southern China. He led the fight to reform the Ch'ing dynasty with his belief in the T'ai P'ing, the Great Peaceful Heavenly Kingdom, Christianity. Obviously, the Christian source of the insurrection was omitted from the Peking production nor, do I believe, was this omission pointed out by any of the local drama critics. In any case it was vibrant theater.

Not only the Peking Opera but the whole "entertainment" industry seems alive and well in The People's Republic of China. When recounting post-liberation developments the town fathers at all our stops included the number of new movie houses and theaters just as frequently and with as much pride as they recounted the construction of hospitals. That the average town dweller sees three feature films a week may be understood simply as the result of a dearth of television sets (I watched a Russian film dubbed in Mandarin on late-night television in my Beijing hotel), but it is also a manifestation of another quality which is difficult to describe.

The elusive quality which must be experienced to be appreciated is a blend of patriotism, religion, hard work, transcendental metaphysics, and myth. The compound force seems to focus a whole people into a consistent, conceptual whole. (There I go exaggerating, oversimplifying, and confusing.) The visitor's first and most persistent question is, "Are they putting me on?" Are they really this "gung ho" about their moral, cultural, and political life?

The answer is necessarily Chinese, and, as I am ignorant of the language, I do not know. What I do know is that there is a unique excitement in seeing a myth being lived out, a vital myth.

Our culture has known this excitement, as in Europe in the Middle Ages, for example, when everyone was a Christian. There was no room in Europe for those who did not participate in the Christian myth and although the conformity was hard on skeptics who were sometimes featured at a local *autos-da-fé*, this universal belief must certainly have excited its believers. In a patriotic way, our country experienced the fervor, in about 1800. George Washington, the Father of Our Country, had just died, and his myth was all but palpable. Then people went to the town square on the Fourth of July with joy and expectation to listen to oratory they believed in. They lived the rhetoric. They lived our myth. The people of today's China are equally alive to their myth which may be more vital to them than any previous myth simply because of hammered reinforcement by the movies.

Consider, through a simple comparison, the effect of the movies, the "living" image, on the development of the Chinese myth. Suppose our documentation of the life of George Washington was at the level of that of Chairman Mao. What difference would it make in our lives if we had been brought up on "living images" of the father of our country. To extend the speculation further, would live tapes of Moses and filmed interviews with Christ have altered our Judeo-Christian heritage? The answer is, of course, yes, but how and to what degree? The "Chinese" phenomenon may answer these questions.

Viewing Chinese films left me in awe of the power of media, movies in particular, to shape men's minds, perhaps for better, perhaps for worse. In the West the shaping is diffuse, multidirectional, and sometimes conflictual. In the West anyone can make a film or a television documentary about anything, provided he has money for materials, staff, and promotion. In The People's Republic of China there is no diffusion, rather the focus of every media lens is on shaping the mind and, even more important, there is an apparent wish in Chinese minds to be focused, if not fashioned. Both the ancient tradition of Confucius and the modern experience of war, starvation, and chaos prompt the modern Chinese mind to seek peaceful conformity. The wish empowers the movies not as an amusing toy but as a pervasive mechanism for national solidarity.

Perhaps the Chinese wish for conformity is just propaganda, but there is more to it than simply being against past regimes and national catastrophes. In China there is a positive sense of using everything, every leaf that falls, every grain of rice, every frame of movie film to fulfill the growing myth which started three thousand years ago when the Han first appeared as a unique people intent upon becoming ever more themselves, the Chinese. This sense of purpose becomes so pervasive that the traveler eventually feels himself to be a bit player in an epic multidimensional feature blockbuster being filmed on the movie lot of the gods. But there I go again, exhibiting the Marco Polo syndrome, seeming to exaggerate. You have to see it to believe it, but for this performance you will have to go much farther than your local movie house.

Endnotes

Reprinted from *The Pharos* 41(Spring 1970): 38-40, with permission.

A Fairy Tale for a South African Grandchild

And now for all the people of Africa, the beloved country, "Nkosi Sikele' iAfrica," God save Africa. It lay a far off, because...men are afraid, with a fear that is deep in their hearts, a fear so deep they hid their kindness, and brought it out with fierce anger and frowning eyes....And such fear cannot be cast out, but by love.

—Alan Paton (1903-1988)
Cry, the Beloved Country

Once upon a time, say a million billion seconds ago, there was a king, not a great king as kings go but undeniably a king for he had the power of life and death over his subjects.

King Skelm lived in the beautiful land of South-South, a sparkling pendant dangling from the lower tip of a vast continent called Agrifa. To the north stretched an impenetrable desert of hot, blowing sand while in the other three directions rolled vast, empty seas. No one knows why this magnificent country was called South-South. The name might have been translated from an original name of Khoi-Khoi, which meant "men of men," for the first people who lived there but was later changed to mean "Our Land." However, the king and all his subjects firmly maintained that South-South had always been called South-South since it was the center of the universe and everything remains unchanged at the center in "our land."

King Skelm, though expecting and receiving the best of everything, was an unhappy old soul. He avoided all thought of unhappiness by forbidding the least mention of it in his kingdom. The mere suggestion of unhappiness by a subject, even a crying lass or a grumbling elder, brought punishment, generally only one or two lashes of the whip, but the most serious consequence was having their indispensable official passport stamped "Trouble maker."

King Skelm's ambition was to go down in history as the happiest of happy kings. For him happiness was a heritage from his ancestors who expressed parental care, concern, and attention by the practice of spanking. He knew that as long as he spanked his children and subjects, much as he had been spanked, they would be just as happy as he considered himself to be. Naturally, he was a great spanker, often using his long scepter to make the point.

When not attending to punishing his children and subjects, a task that often ran into late afternoon, King Skelm relaxed by munching biltong and drinking beer fermented from stone-ground maize. As you may imagine, so much eating and drinking between meals made him huge. He towered over all his subjects and was wider too, but not so wide that he could not fit on the throne which was regularly enlarged, much as his laws were, to fit the King's needs.

How the King Thought

King Skelm's mind worked in mysterious ways, expressed in part through the royal motto, "Might makes more than right." Experts alleged that he suffered from conceptual dyslexia, which is a complicated way of saying he regularly turned ideas upside down, meanings inside out. He commonly confused his favorite granddaughter's name, Felicity, calling her either Duplicity or Complicity. His way of thinking served to banish nagging doubts or worries from his mind.

An example of his round-about thinking followed from his love of order. He earnestly wished his multi-colored subjects to be well ordered, distinct and apart from each other. To avoid confusion in crowds he made laws for them to line up for buses, beaches, homes, bathrooms, and jobs according to their shade of skin color. His classification started with his hue of well-protected skin, Purity White, which he boasted was the

THE MANY LANGUAGES OF COMPASSION 181

shade of rich cream, a color expected to rise to the top. Remaining light shades were accorded by royal decree the designation Vanilla White. The next notch darker was labeled Colored. This included Jehovah Witnesses, Indians, Jews, and Japanese salesmen. Colored turn out to be a rainbow of hues including the pinkos, union members, and revolutionary reds, that is, any subject caught reading foreign newspapers.

The King's strange palette of colors concluded with what he decreed was the absence of color, black. He divided this category into primitive Blacks, responsibly dressed Blacks, irresponsibly dressed Blacks, illiterate Blacks, smart-acting Blacks, moderate Blacks, and immoderate Blacks.

To ensure subjects held their slotted position in the national color spectrum the King followed up with enforcement laws, the Prohibited Over Crossing laws (POX laws). People caught crossing the color line, being friendly to someone of another shade, were immediately arrested as murky trouble makers. Those rash enough to marry across the color bar promptly turned up missing. Some said that their mixing colors made them invisible.

Interpreting the POX laws proved cumbersome, as those who turned blue with the cold or green with envy defied ready classification. A significant complication arose with the request of the Blind Visionary's society for all South-Souths to have Braille insignias raised on their foreheads so the blind might comply with the law. Eventually, King Skelm replaced the POX laws with his voluntary Royal Honor Code of Previous Judgment, commonly referred to as prejudice. The voluntary code worked just fine.

The King's Family

Though King Skelm never tired of repeating how happy he was with his four sons, each borne by a different wife, the brothers proved a rowdy lot. In accordance with royal protocol the brothers acknowledged how happy they were but it was official happiness without a smidgen of love for each other. They never socialized, shared Sunday family dinner, nor even talked to each other except about their regular business, punishing runaway workers, breaking strikes, or planning general mayhem. Much as brothers the world over, the four had particular difficulty agreeing on a very simple point, who ranked first after Dad.

Whether by custom or genes, each brother went his separate way as far as he dared. Whether swiftly or slowly, with determined stride or reluctant shuffle, each demonstrated, if not defended, his mother's way of life. Over time, the brothers might have taken their families and left South-South for distant lands but other countries erected permitting (spelled sanction in English) barriers against them, permitting the brothers to remain in South-South the better to work out their personal problems. Enforced residence in South-South left them hopeless, endlessly elbowing and continually bickering about no one knew what.

Not that King Skelm ever paid heed to their constant squabbling. Preoccupied with preening himself on his happiness, the King left family matters to fall out as they would. That is, should an occasion arise at an official parade or on a weekend of plundering, he ignored how Roeb, the firstborn of his favorite wife, Dame Vaal Voortrek, elbowed himself into second place directly behind the King. In fact, Roeb ranked on the King's list of likes nearly as high as maize beer, unlike the other sons, Yew, Wantabe, and Xhobanzu, who ranked high on the King's dislike list.

Yet another example of King Skelm's curious manner of thinking could be found in how he bestowed special rights upon his son, Prince Xhobanzu. A hulk of a man, the largest son by far, Prince Xhobanzu inherited all his mother's traits but none of his father's except love of the land. Yet here Prince Xhobanzu's love differed significantly from King Skelm's; the King loved the land as valuable property while Xhobanzu loved it for its limitless beauty.

Learning that Prince Xhobanzu was being abused and cheated by his brothers, King Skelm established his Not In My Neighborhood policy, which is common parlance was referred to as "Apartness." King Skelm set aside a portion of his kingdom as a neighborhood of safety for Prince Xhobanzu, his family, and friends. When asked why the land he bestowed on the Prince was of such little value, the King said he did this according to the wisdom of the ancient parable about the rich man and the poor man, who came upon a ripe melon at the side of the road. The poor man said, "Let us divide it in half." The rich man replied, "Ah yes, you take the outside and I will take the inside."

As King Skelm explained, this tale expressed the essence of caring, for the rich man cared enough to take the better half and guard the poor man from jealous neighbors who might make off with the poor man's half. "That is why I have bestowed the outlying desert on Prince Xhobanzu. He has the husk of our country. No one will ever try to take those rocks and blowing sand away from him. He is apart and safe." King Skelm would then smile his straight-across-the-face smile which meant he was officially happy and that everyone else had better smile as well.

The Princes' Families

The brothers' families, like most families, had well-mannered members and folks with good intentions, some bad apples, and others with evil in their hearts. Taken together, most family members were simple folk doing what they could to get through the day as inconspicuously as official regulations and royal proclamations allowed.

One onerous regulation required South-Souths to speak Argukaans at all times. As might be expected, despite regulations, when at home each family of the four princes spoke their own dialect. But this was not the source of the Princes' inability to communicate with each other. The trouble lay in the manner in which they spoke not in the language they used. Some spoke out of the wrong side of their mouths, others jabbered so fast and stridently it was impossible to make out the message. When together they commonly spoke simultaneously, seeking volume over meaning. Actually, they had never learned to listen. Consequently, they could say outrageous things to each other safe in the knowledge that no one listened. In a desperate attempt to communicate officially the brothers held four-ums, meetings during which the members of the four families sat together loudly growling "um."

Prince Xhobanzu was easily King Skelm's least favored son. Unfortunately, the Prince's mother, Princess iNewadi, taught Xhobanzu neither King Skelm's gut-wheezing language of Argukaans nor the King's way with a whip. Consequently, Xhobanzu grew up at the working end of a shovel while his sisters were tutored by a broom. Though no one would say so, the kingdom could not exist without the labor of Prince Xhobanzu's family. Rumor had it that King Skelm rejected Prince Xhobanzu because he was more dependent on his Black son than he could comfortably acknowledge. The way King Skelm put it with his typical logic was, "No matter what, I will always make it possible for Prince Xhobanzu and his family to work hard and long for me."

Prince Roeb's mother, Dame Vaal Voortrek, came from Neitherland, a patch of North sea bottom with the water bailed out. Yew's mother, Lady Cecelia Rhodilia, also came from beyond the deserts, from the tribe of Yewropeens, hence her son's name, Yew. Wantabe's mother, Ranee Jati Dukha, was washed up on South-South's shores following a shipwreck.

Her single wish was to return with her son to her native land beyond the Eastern ocean where most local customs began and ended with a mouthful of curry.

With great reluctance the mothers acknowledged King Skelm's order replacing their native customs with ones he judged superior. Consequently, behind King Skelm's back they encouraged their daughters and sons to continue native ways.

Prince Roeb, the favored son, shared King Skelm's ambition to plow all the tillable land and to share neither the land nor the plow with anyone. Prince Wantabe came second in the King's regard, for this Prince worked hard at commerce rather than farming, striving to become the merchant of the land. The King tolerated him as a reliable source of taxes.

Prince Yew's mother, Lady Rhodilia, on the other hand, brought with her the venerable Yewrupeen custom of holding her nose in the air, the better to catch the sweet smell of money. Consequently, Yew specialized in work that was remarkably clean and clever, like running the universities, financing Wantabe's enterprises, and counting up the gold and diamonds Xhobanzu dug from deep beneath South-South. Yew's quick ability with numbers and mastery of words ensured that the King never trusted him.

The King's Happiness

As the King grew older, his greatest joy came with placing a grandchild on his knee. Grandchildren could not sit on the royal lap, for it had completely disappeared a number of years ago despite the royal constabulary searching for it in every cranny of the palace. Eventually, the royal lap was declared stolen by trouble makers.

With a grandchild perched on his knee, King Skelm would spin long tales in his mother's tongue of how his father and father's father were farmer warriors who outwitted evil Great Grandmamma Vic. The tale always started with, "Once upon a time thieves and robbers, Great Grandmamma's soldiers, came to our land. They invented the world's first concentration camp and locked our mothers and their obedient children in it. Never forget that."

His eyes would brighten when he came to the part where the elders formed a laager, circling their wagons into a mobile fort, and, with their blazing rifles and cracking whips, founded South-South on the bodies of the fallen. "The torch of civilization was kept bright because my forefathers never missed a shot at White soldiers or the Black farmers." He would close by boasting that like his forefathers he had no fear of Black men and women since he had killed so many.

King Skelm, famous for his singing voice, sang beautiful songs of yearning for a past utterly lost to his grandchildren. The lyrics echoed the poetry of the lonesome wanderer, longing for the warmth and security of a safe home. He sung of the wonderful time before mining machines and railroads, when the "true" settlers of South-South trekked their ox carts across Agrifa, fashioning a new nation from a wilderness of snakes, mosquitoes, lions, kinky-haired Tottenhots, and other beasts. He sung of days of sacrifice and hardship and how they were overcome. However, his fine bass voice never caroled the former king of the Tottenhots, who had cordially welcomed King Skelm's forefathers when they landed on the shores of Agrifa.

Should the children grow restless listening to his lengthy tales and ballads, he would turn on television that was programmed to continually repeat his songs and stories. If the children did not fancy the television he would order them out to play among the vast monuments he raised to his ancient relatives for fashioning the unique ox-cart-driving language of Argukaans. If happiness did not reign in South-South, it was not because of the lack of a "Happy" King.

The Death of King Skelm

One day, Felicity, the daughter of Roeb, was playing on the spreading lawn outside her palatial home when from behind the shrubs she overheard two gardeners whispering about how unhappy they were. The strange idea shocked the little girl. This murmur of unhappiness sent a chill of fear through her. As little girls will, she ran to her Grandfather for grown-up reassurance. In a panic by the time she reached the Council House, she burst into the throne room pleading, "Tell me, tell me, Grandfather, what is unhappy?" and stopping squarely in front of the throne she blurted out, "Grandfather, are you unhappy?" Like a well-aimed arrow, the question flew straight to the center of the King's head.

King Skelm stopped chewing his biltong, put down his mug of maize beer and shook his head as if to loosen such a penetrating question. But there was no dislodging it. The more he shook his head the deeper the question, like a barbed nettle, worked into his brain. As with any good question, it stimulated thinking, an unusual activity for his mind. He thought, harder than he had in years, all the while struggling to free himself of the question. But it was not to be, the question just worked deeper and deeper into his mind. "What is unhappy?"

Exasperated the King jumped up, scattering food and drink about the room. With his head tightly clasped between his hands he opened his mouth, slowly moving his lips as if to speak, but nothing came out.

The crash of breaking mugs and flying platters brought a crowd of attendants running to the throne room where they froze, not knowing what to do. King Skelm staggered forward, wagging his head violently to and fro, first back and forth, then sideways, again and again, until too weak to shake it anymore, he slumped back onto his throne. As his great, round face twisted in pain, slowly, from someplace away down inside, a tiny voice squeaked, "I *am* unhappy, so unhappy." Then, as if the barb found its target, a putrid abscess of fetid conscience exploded in his brain. The squeaky voice became a frightful howl, "because I never grew up." With that, King Skelm pitched forward on the floor, dead.

Pandemonium ensued, people running madly hither and yon. The only one to remain calm, the Royal High Chancellor, Lord Media, knelt beside the King to check his pulse and finding none, in an authoritative voice which carried above the clamor, declared a happy, wake-full weekend to precede a Royal Fun Funeral. Later he explained the holiday was intended for all subjects to celebrate the King's stroke of good fortune, his swift and unexpected visit to his ancestral spirits. By one proclamation, Lord Media saved both the peace of the kingdom and King Skelm's tradition of happiness.

Luckily for Felicity, the Lord Chancellor's announcement gave her a chance to slip away unseen. If she had been caught she might well have been detained in a children's place of safety to be examined for witchcraft, perhaps, even, tried and punished as a juvenile trouble maker.

There is little doubt this would have been Felicity's fate, for King Skelm had anticipated such delinquencies when he ordered inscribed on the granite stone gateways of the kingdom's children's places of safety, "Punishment teaches trouble makers by making them smart."

The Consultant Arrives

So King Skelm passed away and in keeping with his tradition nobody was sad at his sudden departure. In fact many remarked what a relief it was to know he had joined his ancestral spirits.

THE MANY LANGUAGES OF COMPASSION

Not unexpectedly, for in South-South few events ever worked out as planned, the Royal Fun Funeral was delayed until the proper proclamation was officially posted. The preparatory proclamation, in anticipation of the official proclamation, appeared on four different colored papers, but it took time for them to be properly tacked, with the white copy highest, on every lamp pole in the kingdom.

> In this proclamation referred to in subsection (2) part one of the Amendments to the Public Proclamation Act, including a proclamation purporting to have been issued in terms of that subsection, is further amended and substituted, to state that anything done or purported to have been done under the provision of the previous proclamation which could have been done under the proclamation as so amended or under the new proclamation whereby that proclamation is so substituted shall be deemed to have been done under the amended or new proclamation, as the case may be, that all subjects shall read the coming proclamation celebrating great and worth King Skelm's recent arrival in his ancestral home.
>
> Signed, Lord Media, for
> the Brotherhood of the Realm

Actually, it took a full month to complete the multi-colored postings.

The burial, as contrasted to the Royal Fun Funeral, for obvious reasons could not wait. Directly after his death, King Skelm was deposited on his knees, the proper position for entering the land of his ancestral spirits, at the bottom of a deep grave.

Despite elaborate preparations, events were not enjoyed by all. During the initial funeral festivities of barbecues, folk dancing, and ox-cart races, a whiff of something rotten was detected in the air. The source of the odor was quickly traced to seepage leaking from the ground about King Skelm's grave. Without delay a concrete memorial plaza larger than a shopping mall parking lot was poured over the grave with a gigantic, bronze statue of King Skelm at its center. Unfortunately, as the hasty construction settled it squeezed out even more smell.

With each passing day the smell grew until it drifted over the entire realm. Though invisible, without a trace of mist or hint of haze, the stink found its way to the farthest deserts and jungles of South-South. Fortunately, none of the animals seemed to mind. The dogs, with their customary abandon, continued to sniff each other from nose to tail. The cats, large and small, continued to track their prey with the sprightly cleverness generally attributed to gem thieves. But human beings were different. Yet no one complained since all were accustomed to solitary crying and private puking.

As the stench persisted, few had stomach, needless to say, for the culminating Royal Fun Funeral. Since the person in whose honor the entertaining funeral was given remained their king, everyone attended to choke down their assigned portions. After the celebration the brothers gathered in the Council House in anticipation of the reading of King Skelm's will. There, Lord Media announced the King had died intestate, leaving no will for he had been too happy to have ever considered death. Frustrated in their private ambitions the brothers slunk away anxious and upset.

Actually, Lord Media was concerned with more immediate needs. The stench had grown so bad that subjects no longer were able to work. Not so the brothers, who worked each other for any hint of a quick dash for the throne. Reluctantly, they agreed to postpone deciding on the royal succession until the oppressive stink was controlled.

The smell served to sharpen the brothers' suspicions of each other, prompting bitter accusations, back and forth, of raising a stink over the claims of rightful heirs. Attempting to defuse the threat of civil war, Lord Media reported he had called a highly qualified aroma expert from Teknation, the most advanced industrial and hence the most odoriferous country in the world. Lord Media, appealing to the brothers' cupidity, cunningly suggested that since the consultant had so little honor in his own land he might be hired on the cheap.

Lacking a better suggestion for breaking their deadlock, the brothers grudgingly agreed to hire the consultant. But before going as far as officially engaging him each brother sought him out on the sly. In private each related a remarkably similar story of how the other brothers were the source of the evil stink. Arcus Senilis, the consultant from Teknation, aware of the value South-Souths placed on non sequiturs, responded to Roeb as he did to each of the other three, "Yes, you had a good mother for she made Rooibos tea for you when you were a sick lad." To Yew, "Yes, your mother was loving when you had a sore throat for she made you custard pudding." To Wantabe, "You were so lucky to have such a caring mother who cooked you the best curry every made." And to Xhobanzu, "Oh, how good your mother was to fix you delicious meali-meali when you were tired and hungry." Predictably, each brother said to himself, "Ah, this man knows the truth. We should hire him."

Later when the brothers reassembled, Lord Media interrupted their "uming" to review the state of the nation. He went over how King Skelm had been buried deep with all the rituals of the tribes, cults, and corporations yet his fragrance, since there could be no disrespect for the King, lingered on. Lord Media's simple account was enough for the brothers to finally agree to hire the consultant, each with the unspoken assumption that the consultant would lay blame on another brother.

Arcus Senilis, the consultant, was promptly called for Broeder Bond Certification. Before entering the Council House, all mud and wattle, with a great conical roof of woven palm fronds, Arcus paused to look about. The Council House was situated on a rise behind the palace, the site of South-South's first shamba. Immediately Arcus understood why this was a sacred place for South-Souths. Stretching beyond the circling cluster of royal assistants' grass-roofed huts lay a vista of the veld, a vast sun drenched, golden grassland, sparsely peppered with dark green thorn trees, stretching off to a distant horizon of Black Dragon mountains. It was beauty incarnate.

As everyone must, Arcus bowed his head low on entering the door of the Council House. The low transom was intended to inspire humility in those approaching the King's throne while simultaneously inducing extention of the neck of any unwanted intruders for decapitation. Once inside, Arcus's eyes gradually accommodated to the stark interior with its dirt floor, and the four brothers crouched on low stools arrayed before the empty throne. Lord Media stood beside them. The remainder of the great hall was empty except for a row of hard benches lined against the encompassing wall. With a flick of his head Lord Media indicated that Arcus should stand before the brothers.

After Lord Media's brief introduction, Arcus began by reaffirming all Lord Media had reported about the smell, adding that the nation smelled as if all its drains were blocked and cesspools running over. He noted too that the smell now reached worldwide as nations of the world were turning up their noses at anything to do with South-South.

Once Arcus was confirmed as official aroma consultant, he explained that he would begin with two weeks and a day of visiting the countryside.

After that he would talk with the brothers further. Seeking a swift solution, they agreed and officially recessed by holding their noses while "uming."

Arcus Senilis, with his shaggy hair, smudged glasses, wrinkled jacket, and mucky boots, looking for all the world like a wallydraigle, made a poor impression on the people of South-South. Nor did his sticking his nose in everywhere help. Since no one in South-South expected to be listened to, many grew suspicious that with his questions he was dealing in gossip or worse, witchcraft, particularly when he asked if they had three magic wishes what would they want for their country.

However, some of the more simple villagers shared their wishes with him and a few even went so far as to ask him where the smell was coming from. To one and all he replied, "I have no answers." Since consultants are paid to have answers his reply contributed to the miserable impression he was making. When word filtered back to the brothers that their consultant was striking out with the locals, he was summoned to an emergency four-um.

Arcus returned to the Council House promptly to stand again before the brothers. Yew began, "Well, what is your answer?"

As he had before, Arcus replied, "I have no answers." The response brought all four brothers to their feet, shaking their fists, Roeb screaming loudest of all, "Fraud, scoundrel! Exploiting imperialist, colonial dog!"

Moving only to push his glasses back up the bridge of his sweaty nose, Arcus waited for quiet. When the brothers eventually paused to catch their breath, it was Lord Media who spoke, "So what are we to do?"

Without hesitation Arcus said, "Oh, you wish to know what to do? I thought you were asking me for the answer to your soul stink, for this is what it is. If you wish to do something about it you should talk."

Interested as they were in determining who was guilty, the brothers ignored Arcus's diagnosis of soul stink. "What do you mean talk? We talk all the time," exclaimed Wantabe in a provocative whine.

Arcus responded, "I have not heard much talk out of the four of you unless you call 'uming' talk. Talk is more than shaking fists and uproar. To be more than noise, talk needs to be listened to. Traveling about your country I tried to talk with people, as many as possible. It was not easy. Either South-Souths do not like to talk or they do not know how. For my part I used as few words as possible, just a few questions, asking people what they wished most for their country. Only a few knew I was listening and answered."

This reply affronted the brothers. Yew threw up his hands, crying in exasperation, "What can you expect from a foreigner?"

Xhobanzu, aroused, stepped forward, pointing an accusing finger at Arcus to demand, "And what did the people wish?"

Arcus replied, "Their first wish is for freedom."

This came as a surprise to three of the brothers. They had expected their subjects would wish for money. They asked each other, "Freedom, freedom, freedom from what?"

Xhobanzu was not confused. "Did they wish anything else?"

"Yes, one other wish," said Arcus.

"Which was?" queried Yew from his seat.

"Peace." This astounded the brothers, for none had ever considered peace. Roeb shouted over the uproar, "What does this mean? Peace, for years we have beaten into our subjects' heads that we are a peaceful nation."

Wantabe, his mind confused by the absence of any practical remarks about credit or consumers' strikes, blurted out, "But how can you talk if you do not have answers?"

"You listen," replied Arcus.

Roeb in astonishment interjected, "Then you did not talk. You listened."

Emboldened Wantabe spit out, "Really Roeb, will you ever get it right!"

Roeb responded by shaking his baton of authority at Wantabe, prompting even more commotion.

Arcus interrupted the growing squabble with, "It may seem to Prince Roeb that I can not both talk and listen. I know how you were brought up on King Skelm's talk, talk, talk and you all aspire to be royal talkers just like he was. Stop and think, who can deny it takes two to talk intelligently, one to sound the words and the other to understand them? Answers need listening to live."

Suspiciously, Xhobanzu interrupted, "What are you up to, auslander?"

Avoiding the sharp edge of the question, Arcus continued, "Come, listen with me to what a poor woman said to me while she was cleaning rooms in an inn. When I asked her what she wished for her country she said, 'Peace.' Then I repeated 'Peace' to let her know I was listening. She went on, 'You look at me and you are scared. I look at you and I am scared. If you do not talk you kill. When talk, it is better because you say what is in your heart. If you know the heart you do not kill. We all have one father, God."

"What does this mean to us?" snarled Wantabe.

"Well, Lord Media asked me what to do and I recommend you take the lady's advice. It would be wise for you to talk from the heart, talking that includes listening. Listen with the heart. It is the only way to avoid killing."

"What would we talk about?" queried Yew provocatively.

"The smell."

In chorus the brothers shouted, "It stinks. What else can be said?"

With an even voice Arcus answered, "If the reason for it is not, as I believe, soul rot, talk it out and find what you believe is causing your stink?"

Still avoiding Arcus's diagnosis, Wantabe snapped, "If we get into what we believe, it will be the end of us. We all know there is something in the land that sinks and that's it, period."

"And no one will say why."

"Well, we can't talk about our royal father."

"Oh, I thought it came from your land. Certainly, no single body could give off such a stink."

Wantabe could not contain himself. "If we talk about ourselves there is nothing to say but how we hate each other, that hate has us speechless with rage."

Arcus repeated the poor woman's words, "If you know what is in the heart, you do not kill."

Yew snarled, "I have no wish to know anything about my black-hearted brothers." Roeb shook his head in agreement.

Flashing with anger, all eyes fixed on Arcus. "I assure you that your hearts are one and the same color, if you but knew them."

Xhobanzu had remained standing and now advanced threateningly. Scornfully he bellowed, "I see where you are taking us with your clever blather. You want me to forgive the unforgivable."

"Please, no need to shout, I am listening. But are you? Listen, what is that we hear?"

All paused and in the unexpected silence the sound of children came through the wattle walls. Not the shouts and laughter of children playing, but screaming for help.

Arcus spoke up, "You hear them, I hear them, but only if you stop hating long enough to listen. The children are necklacing each other. They are dropping an auto tire over the head of a defenseless playmate, drenching him in gasoline, and setting him afire, a human torch. Listen to the shrieks of agony as they teach each other South-South's custom of necklacing.

"You are distracting us," sputtered ever legalistic Yew.

Arcus continued, "They are your children."

"So they are," Yew sputtered again.

"Why are they torturing each other?"

"You tell us."

"Because they follow your example. They are playing the grown-up game of soul killing—destroy your sisters and brothers so you will not hear what is in their hearts. The children are practicing to become grown-ups. They are learning for themselves that to forgive is unforgivable."

For the first time Xhobanzu looked perplexed rather than indignant, "I hear you saying that the cry of South-South is not that of the fish eagle but the cry of burning children."

"Yes."

Then in the deepest voice imaginable Xhobanzu exploded, "Who is responsible for burning my children?"

"I do not know," replied Arcus.

Pointing first in one direction and then another, Xhobanzu thundered his outrage, "Is it the far right, the far left? Who is it? It can not be me!"

Holding firm, Arcus responded, "It is not you. It takes longer than a lifetime to make a stink that drives children to burn each other."

Searching the downcast faces of the silent brothers, Arcus continued, "Consider how some days Xhobanzu is strong and Yew is weak. Other days Yew is strong and Xhobanzu is weak. Yet every day, as brothers, you are weak unless you are strong together, talking from the heart about the soul stink that has your children killing your children."

Despite a wish to drown out the pitiful screams and moans of the burning children, the brothers sat quietly, thinking as they had never thought before.

Lord Media broke the silence, with the intermediate question, "But how to clean up the stink?"

"I have no answer beyond recommending tears," murmured Arcus.

"We have had enough of tears!" snarled Xhobanzu resuming his surly defensiveness.

"Oh no, not tears of sorrow or rage. I speak of tears that wash away despair. Tears of relief."

Abandoning his usual stiff-upper-lip reserve Yew cackled, "What are you talking about, witch doctor?"

Responding to the question, not its provocation, Arcus continued, "I am talking about tears of relief that come with forgiving the unforgivable. Listen, as you can, for the promise of redemption whispered by forgiveness. But first you must examine your heart for the rage that fills it, your heart not your brother's. Rage can not be talked away. Like death it is part of every life.

"Forgiveness of the unforgivable is not for others; whatever terrible crimes or misbegotten evil that makes you rage, it goes with your struggle. Even the pain suffered at the hands of a wicked father, even that raging pain can be known and forgiven. Your father's failure to offer loving understanding can be accepted in your lives rather than left to rot your souls.

"Forbearance and understanding that comes with acceptance of self-rage protects your children from soul rot, the source of their necklacing. Only as you recognize your personal hunger for blind brutality can you regain its opposite, passion for loving care. I encourage you to listen carefully to the children and to the child within your own heart."

A deep silence descended on the Council House, this time broken by a sob from behind a far bench. It was Felicity. Now that she knew what unhappiness meant, she cried in relief. She sobbed and sobbed, her tears flowing down her cheeks in a little stream. It was a magical stream for as the tears flowed across the chamber floor they gave off a fresh aroma. Much as when a bale of silage is broken open and dispels the rank odors of a barn, the Council House filled with a sweet fragrance of new-mown hay.

Indeed, the stream was magical for it ran straight to Arcus and as it touched the cuff of his baggy trousers he stood transfixed. In a weakening voice he spoke, "You have your answer, listen to the child." Then he began to dissolve, smaller and smaller, into the puddle of tears, only to disappear much as a sugar cube vanishes in a cup of tea. Astonishment at the disappearance of their consultant lasted but a moment.

Roeb cried out, "Daughter, what are you doing here?"

As Felicity ran to him, sobbing and smiling, she exclaimed, "I was unhappy and hid. Now I do not have to hide anymore. I know everyone is unhappy."

Her father swept her up in his arms and for the first time Xhobanzu smiled, saying, "Yes, little niece, we are unhappy but smile and come to my house to play with your cousin Seraphina."

Excited attendants rushed in laughing and singing out the glad news that the horrid stench was leaving the land. They joyfully embraced each other and their dancing feet scuffled over the moist spot in the earthen floor that had once been Arcus Senilis. What mattered most was that the cries of the children had gone and everyone could hear the sound of their own hearts in harmony with singing coming through the walls. All listened, listened together, for they could hear the lovely voices of children singing *Nkosi Sikele' iAfrica—God Bless Our Africa*.

Epilogue

Yes, little African grandchild, everyone wants a fairy tale to end with everyone living happily ever after but how can that be with a tale in which the consulting wizard leads everyone to be unhappy? There is a reason. In consultant talk it is called the Post Aromatic Stress Syndrome and it goes like this.

Though the air in South-South became much sweeter and the smell blew away, unhappiness remained. But now it was on the lips of the people not in their hearts. They talked about how unhappy their children might be. They openly worried that they might pass on the false happiness King Skelm had left them. They became concerned that they might fail as he had failed to wholeheartedly love their family and their country. Over the years, as unhappiness was talked about, people became less and less unhappy knowing that nothing dissolves the hate in human hearts like a child's tear. Remember, it was children's voices that changed the whole continent of Agrifa into our beloved Africa.

Lastly, dear child, you should know there are some people, big and small, with sharp eyes who can not see, with large ears who can not hear, with skin so thick they can not feel. They do not listen to the child in their hearts nor learn that thinking and feeling are done with all the body not just with the brain. They understand printed words but can not read the book of life. For them everything must be measured. Even the spirit of our fairy tale must be spelled out, letter by letter, word by word, to be weighed against another fairy tale they call reality. So for them we will put the immeasurable moral of our tale into measurable words: as people suffer together they are borne up, relieved, and made free in the belief that if the heart is known you do not kill either the body or the soul.

Compassion Is Where You Find It

O heavens, can you hear a good man groan,
And not relent, or not compassion him?
—William Shakespeare (1564-1616)
Titus Andronicus, Act IV, 1, 123

I journeyed to Paris at the invitation of the delegation of the French Parliament which had visited Oregon to examine, firsthand, our health plan. A second motive insured that the opportunity would be seized upon: curiosity about French legislators' perception of the nature of political will necessary for constructive health care reform.

Early arrival at the Senate building, the seventeenth-century palace of Marie de Medicis, afforded a stroll through the surrounding Luxembourg Gardens. Here April was busily conducting a delightful intermezzo of splashing fountains, verdant lawns, interlaced paths with counterpoint of children playing, oldsters sunning, ambitious jogging, amorous fondling, and pigeons strutting to the tempo of shimmering spring sunlight.

Once inside the Palace, polite deference ruled, accented by the glint of gold on the gendarme's cap, an ambiance of appreciated space and individuality that only Paris teaches. A moment's wait and my hosts appeared with warm greetings, apologizing that only two of the expected four senators would be at lunch for the others were off engaged in the hotly contested presidential campaign. We made off over the deep carpeting through the magnificent palace, ceilings by Delacroix, stairways of imperial dimensions, built to impress, succeeding royally.

Lunch in a private dining room proved superb with a wonderfully smooth sauce béarnaise on the beef and a dessert of Gascony apple pie so seductively intimidating I chose familiar French vanilla glacé instead, finally drowning with plentiful wine any lingering sense that hunger might exist in our world.

We were five at the table, Senator François Delag, a primary care physician; Senator Jean Paul Hammann, Mayor of Ittenhein, a town near Strasbourg; Ms. Marie-Claire Carrer-Gee, who interpreted from a background in English learned as an exchange student in Peoria, Illinois; and Mr. Phillippe Reifler, Senator Delag's assistant.

Lunch sauntered along for two and a half hours permitting a leisurely examination of health care issues. Unemployment is the major problem confronting the French government, while the drive for health system reform diminishes as a result of two years of managed care. Hospitals, with budget caps, have not displayed sufficient restraint but no immediate governmental response is anticipated.

As conversations will, this circled back on itself. "We are not like the U.S. which has the world's greatest drain of 14 percent of its GNP for health care," prompted the other Senator's rejoinder, "No, ours is only 8 percent which gives us the world's second greatest drain."

Apparently health delivery costs do not loom as large in France as in the United States, buried as they are in the vast social security expenditure for the unemployed, physically disabled, and pensioners.

A pause offered opportunity for my "political will" question. "Does a French legislator risk loss of office by pressing critical health care reform measures?" The answer came without hesitation, "No, office is not lost—the reform is. If a serious attempt is made to limit programs, five hundred thousand people appear in the street to protest. That is enough for any reform to evaporate."

Talk of people taking to the streets prompted, "In the French tradition can Oregon's health decisions program be considered revolutionary?" Citing the cry of the French Revolution, Liberté, Egalité, and Fraternité, I asked if it did not translate into twentieth-century health policy. "Does the belief in 'Liberté,' meaning choice of doctor and of treatment, 'Egalité,' expressed as access for all to a basic health care package, and 'Fraternité,' through grass roots participation, suggest a revolutionary community?"

"Ah, yes," replied Senator Delag, "I have read some of your material and unfortunately you fail to understand that community means something different to us. We speak of community as in a religious order, a community of nuns, a community of faith. Closer to what you mean would be our use of the word "solidarity." But then the Revolution's cry has, unfortunately, today become largely demagoguery. Who believes in such words?"

Bringing the discussion back to reform, I continued, "We mean by "community," a community of discourse. Only by acting together can we insure an individual's right to choice—to stand apart. You do agree that the patient has a right to refuse treatment should he wish?"

Mr. Reifler interjected, "Yes, but everyone wants everything."

"Not in Oregon. In fact, Oregon Health Decisions does much public education in the use of advance directives: the individual's choice to eliminate futile care from the final days of life."

The subject shifted significantly as Senator Hammann spoke in French softly, emphatically. I could not follow for, caught up in his words and feelings, Ms. Carrer-Gee ceased interpreting.

I waited until irrepressible curiosity prompted, "What is he saying?"

With eyes fixed on the Senator she murmured, "He is telling how dreadful it was for him to place his father in an institution." I now could see tears welling up in the Senator's eyes.

"His father suffered from senile dementia. There was nothing that could be done but the Senator had to decide to place him away, to decide nothing more to do."

We were beyond words. Reaching across the table I grasped his hand to convey my understanding. Compassion is where you find it.

Much of our remaining time focused on advance directives and their use in France. We parted even more cordially than we had met. I promised to forward copies of Oregon's advance directive forms and to "remain on line" for any questions they might have.

Once back in my hotel room I resorted to a treatment made famous by a French Revolutionary physician, Jean-Paul Marat, immersion in a full-length bathtub. As my mind slipped its bond with my weary body, the pieces came together. Despite the specter of political denial that haunts all legislatures, Senator Hammann had answered my question, what is the nature of political will necessary for undertaking difficult issues—the actuality of the policy maker's compassion.

In Oregon we reach towards legislators by offering them a constituency of courage. Our cadre of concerned voters supports legislators taking on tough issues by defending them against the savagery of special interest groups. Citizens interpret to citizens actual trade-offs involved in complex and demanding legislation. We identify this process as "community," the French as "solidarity."

What we failed to distinguish in producing political will, a key factor, is the catalytic effect of a legislator's suffering. To successfully undertake a significant reform, a civic leader must believe through heartfelt experience, more than through abstract thinking, that the "tough" legislation is needed. For difficult policy proposals to succeed they must resonate with the personal suffering of the legislator.

As the steam about me cleared, I understood a limitation of our health decisions concept of community grass roots discourse. Certainly our approach made a difference in establishing Oregon's successful outreach to the medically poor. Inadvertently, we failed to conceptualize that civic discourse must express compassion to ensure solidarity. The Senator's account from the heart made clear why senior citizens in Oregon testified that they wished no improvement in their health care that came at the expense of health care to children. They spoke to the fellow feeling of legislators.

Constructive change in government policy, especially as it calls for trade-offs among contesting groups, demands a fulcrum supported by political leaders' awareness of their personal suffering. The ultimate leverage for significant change rests with a community of compassion in which the deepest values of the people are understood through the leaders' co-passion for suffering. Here lies the nascent political will for sacrificial civic change, or so I came to believe as I toweled down for an evening of celebration, thanksgiving for Senator Hammann's gift.

Endnotes

Reprinted from *Journal of Clinical Epidemiology* 49(1996): 817-818, R. Crawshaw, "Compassion Is Where You Find It." Copyright 1996, with permission from Elsevier Science.

Part 5

The Compassionate Patient-Doctor Relationship

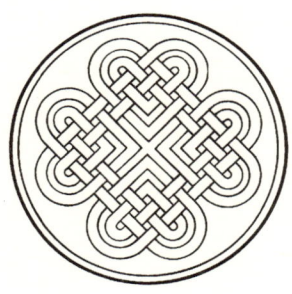

If the physician possess native sagacity, and a nameless something more,—let us call it intuition; if he show no intrusive egotism, nor disagreeably prominent characteristics of his own; if he have the power, which must be born with him, to bring his mind into such affinity with his patient's,...at some inevitable moment, will the soul of the sufferer be dissolved, and flow forth in a dark, but transparent stream, bringing all its mysteries into the daylight.
—Nathaniel Hawthorne (1804-1864)
The Scarlet Letter

Overview to Part 5

Who is unacquainted with the patient-doctor relationship? Who better to describe its strengths and weaknesses than those embraced by the relationship, patients, children, family members, nurses, doctors, and administrators?

The elemental social power of the patient-doctor relationship stirs the imagination. Young children live it out by "playing doctor," a sometimes illicit game invoking professional license to experiment with forbidden social conventions and repressed emotions. Adults announce, if not boast of, the relationship's value, underlining its importance with the personal possessive, "My" doctor.

There is little question of the effectiveness of the therapy of shared respect, the caring patient-doctor relationship's ability to heal. This respect is so ingrained in the tradition of healing that patients rightly expect it even in inconsequent patient-doctor encounters.

Predictably, trust follows upon shared respect. Mutual trust is powerful, enabling an otherwise stranger, the doctor, to explore intimate details of body and deep sorrows of the psyche without threat to the patient's dignity. The following essays respectfully examine the patient-doctor relationship as it succeeds or fails in fulfilling the promise of enlightened caring.

Granted, you the reader and I, concerned writer, have had different experiences with doctors, each a unique individual. By overarching our disparate experiences, the film **Nicholas and Alexandra** offers a point of reference for us to consider mutually the role of compassion in the patient-doctor relationship. Though the Russian culture portrayed is aristocratic and foreign to our world, even at that distance of time and space obvious traits of a good doctor surface in the turmoil of treating a pampered prince's intractable illness. The film uncovers the necessary connection between commitment to service and trust in caring, in this case commitment even unto the death of the physician.

Have you ever considered how a physician understands you as a uniquely suffering individual? Tapping my experience as a patient, **Patient–Doctor Bonding** focuses on how doctors "personalize" the patient; how they go about understanding each patient as an individual. In **Lasting Impressions** we touch some formative childhood reactions to the patient-doctor relationship, while **The Foley Catheter** offers an adult patient's hard-won insights.

In truth, as **The Bedpan Factor** establishes, the education of a medical student to the full dimension of patients' humanness is taught through experiencing blood, pus, urine, and feces. Who can disagree that for any doctor to miss the essential lesson of humility is tragic for the doctor, a tragedy for the patient?

The layman's perception of "other" doctors, "Not my doctor but those AMA doctors," is explored in **Professional Diplopia**. Here the unavoidable ambivalence resonates with the experience of power and powerlessness within the patient-doctor relationship. The inevitably mixed feelings experienced by patients with doctors and doctors with patients is often more sensed than acknowledged.

Frequently, the experience of caring is overwhelmed by the sheer number of suffering mankind. A larger view, in fact a global view, helps healers understand their role in addressing unmet needs. By visiting struggling developing nations, inquiring physicians may develop a perspective that allows us to see and respond through a wider concept of caring. **A Lesson from Chinese Medicine** teaches how a personal quest for compassion gains meaning.

The patient as a person bears repeated emphasis. Loss of personal dignity, patients' most prevalent concern, is addressed in **The Importance of a Name**. Should you identify with Mrs. Sprightly, you will feel as well as consciously recognize the insidious evil of unrequited emotional need buried under a blather of mindless familiarity.

You Can't Kill Hope recognizes how scarce compassion can be in medical care. Yet the tale carries a heart-sustaining message that hope, one soul touching another in compassion, redeems so much.

Who can deny that the future of healing encompasses a broader scope than bedside care? Only as citizens and healers work together with, or in spite of, the tyranny of economic-medical bureaucracies can we as caring people ensure that the patient-doctor relationship sustains its implicit expectation of compassion. As I learn from you and you learn from me, we are joined in the quest for compassion.

Nicholas and Alexandra
A Film Review

It is our duty to remember at all times and anew that medicine is not only a science, but also the art of letting our own individuality interact with the individuality of the patient.
—Albert Schweitzer (1875-1965)

Nicholas and Alexandra is a coherent, enlightening, and entertaining film. It is not exceptional art but qualifies as a minor Hollywood epic and shares with other art, good and bad, the possibility of varied perspective. The film may be viewed as a drama, a historical account, a political essay, a sociological treatise, a medical mystery, or simple entertainment. I saw it as entertainment and later reflected on its medical mysteries.

The plot is simple. A nice guy, Nicholas, is married to a neurotic lass, Alexandra, and they rear a family with a sick child. He loses his job through gross ineptitude, and as a consequence they all die. His job happens to be tsar of Russia and the consequence is the Russian Revolution, which makes for big scenes, a gigantic cast, violence, and actors who were apparently directed to use long, unintelligible stares as aristocratic airs and boisterous screams as revolutionary language.

The film is historically accurate but understandably incomplete, as any attempt to condense into three hours the inner life of historical figures must be. Perhaps the most telling omissions are the failure to connect Nicholas's weakness to his father's colossal oppression. Alexander III was a man capable of cowering the entire Russian empire, and he imperiously forbade young Nicholas any training for his later responsibilities. Another omission in the film was the foreignness of Alexandra. She was German and as such never accepted nor was accepted by the Russians.

The historical errors are never glaring but remain annoying. For instance, the scene in which Lenin arrives at Finland Station is done in cinema pseudo-vérité, a style reminiscent of bigger than life Stalinistic social realism. Actually, Lenin was not pleased by his reception when he got off the train, and he gave the greeting officials two hours of bloody hell for standing around the station and not manning the barricades. Also, in the "drug scene" Rasputin is killed by being beaten to death with chains.

Autopsy actually revealed that he drowned after they dumped him through a hole in the ice of the Neva. His luck finally ran out when he could not locate the hole through which to claw his way back out. Though irritating, these are details that do not detract measurably from the historical credibility of the film.

Incidentally, the director showed admirable restraint in portraying the violence of the times. Though some may be shocked at the scenes of death and destruction these are minuscule in comparison with what was the reality. The massacre of January 22, 1905, is depicted as a bureaucratic snafu, as though it were a Kent State debacle with Nicky moaning, "Why did not someone tell me?" Actually, the killing went on for months with 14,000 people slaughtered, 1,000 executed, 20,000 wounded, and 70,000 arrested by soldiers under orders to, "Be merciless, make no arrests."[1] Equally restrained was the execution of the royal family, where all you see are pistols exploding onto the screen. Actually, those who survived the first fusillade were bayoneted or had their skulls smashed with rifle butts as they tried to crawl away. How often it is a relief not to see history as it was.

Of possible interest to physicians are three medical mysteries lurking in *Nicholas and Alexandra*. The first revolves about the influence of hemophilia on world history. Would the course of the Russian regime have been different if the tsarevich had been a healthy child? Had the royal family not been preoccupied with their own concerns could they, through the tsar, have contributed to a continuing reign and a prosperous nation? The Marxist answer to these questions is unequivocally no; the march of history is relentless and the Russian Revolution was inevitable, independent of any individual's illness, no matter how important the person. On the other hand, the physician, deprived of a grand view of the world, can say, after properly disqualifying himself of any expertise beyond his own experience, "Perhaps."[2] Perhaps this family could have discharged its responsibilities to their nation as other stricken "royal" families such as the Abraham Lincoln and Joseph Kennedy families have done. With the "perhaps" must come much understanding and study of family pathology and physiology. However, as the Romanovs are of a different era, a distant land, and a foreign culture, the "perhaps" is unlikely to be settled.

The second medical mystery within the film touches on a dark side of practice. Does the family of a chronically ill, dying child always hate the physician? My answer, from experience, is *yes*, for all must hate the thief of hope. The Romanovs were no different in this respect than other families, and Eugene Botkin, their family physician, felt the brunt of their monumental anger and icy fear. But this question of hating the physician is only part of a larger question. Since time and understanding can do much for any human being, a larger question emerges: must the family of a dying child continue to hate the physician? Here the answer is *no*. Even in the most trying family-physician relationship there is prospect of a final resolution of elemental feelings of revulsion. If the physician can work with the family's sense of guilt, which Botkin could not, if he can accept their storms of rage, which Botkin could not, if he can point to the means of mourning and eventual restitution, which Botkin could not, he can help them transform hate into acceptance and mutual respect.

Loyalty, otherwise known as commitment, is the one additional quality the physician must have in dealing with the hating family (perhaps you think the word "hate" too strong, but before making a final judgment ask the parent of a child who has died while under a physician's care). Loyalty is the ultimate key in working through a stricken family's harrowing experience, and this Botkin had. He stood with them firmly as the family struggled year in and year out with specialists, quacks, crisis, and illusory respites. He stuck with them to the death, not running out when others fled. Failing in so many respects, in knowledge, insight, Botkin did not fail them in loyalty. He went with them to their destruction, treating their son even though it cost him his life. He worked at, if not through, their terrible unhappiness as best he knew. He was a fine physician.

The third mystery, and perhaps the most intriguing one the film poses, is why did Rasputin, the charlatan, succeed with the family where Botkin, the scientist, failed? Was the magic of Rasputin just magic, charisma, hypnosis, or is there something for every physician to learn from Rasputin in dealing with the special patient. Botkin and Rasputin were dealing with aristocrats. Aristocrats are not so uncommon that this is an unusual problem. Not that our present royal families wield life and death power, but like all cultures we have our "upper crust." Even the classless society of Soviet Russia recognized this phenomenon by maintaining a special independent medical establishment solely for the leaders and their families.[3] Only a knowing physician is consciously master of the special treatment royalty needs.

In our country, the aristocracy goes untitled but it does go. Our royalty may be found in the badly burned son of an industrialist, a hypertensive governor, a neurotic movie star, the alcoholic wife of the university chancellor. Irrespective of any credentials, as elite they expect and need special treatment. Though unpopular to say, it is psychologically true that there can never be equality of treatment among people. The powerful may die, but they do not do it in the style of the weak. When a multimillionaire comes into a physician's office he is treated differently. The dilution and anonymity of a prestigious clinic offers no solution, not as long as it is run by human beings. Look at Ernest Hemingway's experience at the Mayo Clinic. His medical records were purloined by a reporter for a national magazine; he needed special protection he did not receive. Look at the tragic situation of James Forrestal, former Secretary of Defense. While a group of eminent psychiatrists assembled from all parts of the nation debated his treatment in Bethesda Naval Hospital, he was left unguarded in a tower suite, from which he jumped to his death. The mere fact that an extraordinary attempt must be made to avoid being extraordinary makes the treatment of a powerful person extraordinary. Not without reason does the chief of a surgical service generally seek his personal operation far from home, hoping, half consciously, to be just another patient. In *Nicholas and Alexandra* the point recurs repeatedly. Botkin calls in Europe's greatest physicians, who decide, after learned consultation, that the tsarevich should have an operation. But who is to do it? As one man says, "Who would want to risk his dying on their operating table?" The boy, perceived as too powerful to be treated, never has the operation.

Coincidentally with this Russian conference, Sigmund Freud was writing about the phenomenon, the taboo on treating rulers.[4] Freud showed that since ancient times there has been an attitude towards rulers, the powerful, that places them apart. They must not only be guarded but also must be guarded against, for they are vehicles of mysterious and dangerous magical power that brings ruin to anyone who transgresses the taboo. Ostensibly, the taboo is expressed in the elaborate rituals surrounding the powerful, but the taboo also appears in the exaggerated deference shown rulers, for bowing and scraping marks out a safe psychological distance from the ruled. In a more benign form, it is this distancing that has the captain of a naval ship eating alone in his quarters and not in the officers' mess. It makes leadership the lonely job it is.

Look at how Botkin and Rasputin deal with the gulf between them and the royal family. Botkin is obsequious, deferential, unsure, and worried. Rasputin is direct, certain, and personal. In the scene where Rasputin meets the tsarina, the aristocrat of aristocrats, he is correct in the accepted ritual. He is on his knees; he is polite; he is reverent; but he is also personal. Before him is the gulf of royalty, manifested in the tsarina's sumptuous gown, dazzling gems, regal air, and yet he relates directly to the person behind the appearances. He reads her eyes for her loneliness and terror and talks to her of her needs. At that moment he is not a magician but a genius at overcoming his own inhibitions. He remains a feeling person rather than becoming an abject subject. This quality of personality, all religious charisma aside, is the secret of his uncanny success in relating to the royal family. He has the wisdom to be himself. Just this quality of empowered self-knowledge in the face of distracting psychological influences, allows some physicians to treat where others fail.

Power enters the waiting room of all physicians and comes in many forms. The tsarina personifies one form far more powerful than her royal position in her presence. Not that the waiting rooms of physicians are filled with queens or duchesses, but their counterparts exist, and it is part of the art of a physician to understand their special needs.

Look carefully at the phenomenon of presence personified in the prima ballerina. The prima ballerina has supreme presence as she gathers up her audience. They become hers in spirit, breathlessly alive as she inspires. At some future performance, for a moment, detach yourself from the immediate experience and watch the power of presence. Watch her as she pauses on the stage in a *pas de deux*; her partner all but disappears into the background, no more than another prop. She suspends all motion and awaits expectantly with all her body poised as the music announces her next step. In that moment, with the lift of her neck, with the position of her feet, with the relaxed tenseness of her slender frame she strips away the history, the freedom, the identity of the audience and marshals feelings in all that make boys of men, girls of women. With instantaneous awareness of anticipated joy all submit willingly and entirely to what she chooses to do. Through the completeness of her presence she makes a pause excruciatingly beautiful.

Such presence is rare but not unreal, for whether the royalty be of art, politics, money, intellect, or breeding, these men and women of innate self-confidence do exist. In a woman it is not only the beauty of her body but of her being. She chooses where to look without a flicker of hesitation. She not only sits in a chair but knows where in the chair she is sitting. She speaks to be heard and without volume is heard across the room. Her posture proclaims an uncompromising acceptance of self-imposed discipline. Such a woman expects to be felt not through popularity, sex, or fashion but through presence. Though the concept is complex it has some simple measures, and one I have happened upon is the angle between the chin and the chest. This in no way implies the tilt of her chin, a tool of the coquette. It is the angle formed from the point on the throat where the chin first appears to the tip of the chin, and another line drawn from the origin of the chin down the neck. Clumsily with eye and more precisely with protractor I have measured it on statues and pictures. Nefertiti, the most beautiful of Egyptian queens, ranks as the ultimate with 123 degrees and leaves me wondering if Imhotep or some other royal physician of those days might not have measured as well.

Let the Botkins of our present day beware, for the aristocracy still get sick and still expect to be treated as persons. The one individual in all the audience who can not allow himself to be swept up in the prima ballerina's magic power is the ballet master. Standing in the deep shadows behind the stalls he must suspend, sometimes with superhuman effort, his own primordial wish to be lost to her artistry. He must renounce what Coleridge called that momentary pause of disbelief that constitutes poetic faith. Only he must measure the beat, judge the performance, and do the most difficult of acts, criticize a loved one. Without his willful suspense of gratification he is lost to her and she has lost the contact that will preserve her humanness within her revelation as a goddess. In similar ways too, the physician must suspend his appreciation of his cherished illusions when treating the famous, the powerful, our rulers.

Clearly the physician's role is always to see the person behind the persona, the mask of personality. It is sometimes difficult, never impossible. The cost is high, for physicians must relinquish illusions of joy and power that we tenaciously clasp to our hearts. The treating physician can not allow himself to see presidents as presidents, anymore than he allows himself to see welfare recipients as welfare recipients. They are all people, flesh and blood, hopes and fears. Implicit in the mastery of his art is his ability to see every Alexandra as the mother of a sick child. Poor Botkin failed, as unfortunately most of us do, for as Hippocrates said, "Art is long," and perhaps medicine is the longest art of all.

Endnotes

Reprinted from *The Pharos* 36(Winter 1973): 35-36, 39, with permission.
1. E. Wilson, *To the Finland Station* (New York: Doubleday, 1953), 424.
2. F. Cartwright, *Disease and History* (New York: Thomas Y. Cromwell), 174-96.
3. M. Field, *Soviet Socialized Medicine* (New York: The Free Press, 1967), 96.
4. *Totem and Taboo*, vol. 13 of the Standard Edition of "The Complete Psychological Works of Sigmund Freud," (London: Hogarth Press and Institute of Psycho-Analysis, 1955).

Patient–Doctor Bonding

One day is enough for my complaints, it is tortured for enough hours;
One day is damp enough with its own tears for me.
—Richard Crashaw (1612-1649)
"Take therefore no thought of the morrow"
in *The Complete Poetry of Richard Crashaw*

Personal illness has a way of sharpening the clinical acuity of physicians. At least it did for me, a psychiatrist, recently recovered from a severe fever of undetermined origin. The experience taught me more about patient-doctor bonding than I had ever expected to know.

The fever, a vicious affair, repeatedly spiked at 102.8°F., high enough for me to pass out, while the immature forms of my leukocytes "banded" at a 60 percent rate. As my condition worsened, treatment at a local teaching hospital became imperative.

I had just returned from the Marquesas Islands, and though I never convinced the medical staff, I believed I had dengue fever. Granted my medical history was a bit unusual, yet I was surprised and finally peeved at having to repeat it at least eight times. As it turns out, the business of repeating a medical history numerous times may not be unusual. In fact, repetition may be a necessary ingredient for developing a sustaining patient-doctor relationship.

Initially I gave a detailed history to my physician in his office. He listened attentively and, once he was convinced I needed hospitalization, called the admissions office and relayed my history to expedite my way to a hospital bed.

When I arrived at the hospital, I gave the admissions clerk all the ritual numbers of birth, insurance, and whom to inform in the event of my death. Then I was asked what eventually became a litany: "In your own words, would you tell me about your condition from the time you first noticed something wrong?" I did, only to repeat the process again with the admitting nurse, the charge nurse, the intern, the resident, the visiting exchange resident, various attending physicians, the chief of the Infectious Diseases Service, and the chief of Medicine.

It was not easy to report my medical history over and over. Given my murky sensorium, after a few repetitions the details tended to run together and blur, leaving a sense of not having it right. Repetition of the facts generated new facts demanding to be integrated into the growing account. No patient wishes to appear inconsistent or, worse, confused. Knowing any inconsistency could stir the interrogators to more questions, including a request to repeat it all again from the beginning, I tried, as best I could, to settle on a standard form.

One interrogator pressed for the precise time of onset, a detail that failed to interest the next, who was preoccupied with the exact site of my headaches. Neither of these points interested the third interrogator, who encouraged me to enlarge in detail on past reactions to fevers. Finally, simmering with fever and unable to concentrate, my only wish was for an end to the questioning.

As the fever subsided, my mind cleared, and during my convalescence the obvious emerged. Those asking for a personal account of my misery all bore clinical responsibility for my care. I realized they consistently did two things: First, each asked me to relate the story of my present illness firsthand, and then each touched me. Initially I attributed their need for a personally recounted history to some hidden concern about hearsay or inaccurate information, but given the overwhelming duplication of facts on the chart and in their consultations, fear of misinformation could not be it. Finally, as I came to see it, the need for my repeating my history was part of a professional ritual, the process of establishing a relationship with me.

My interrogators requested my version of why I was in the hospital in order for me "to be," in order for them to hear "me." Albeit unconsciously, they were developing their personal data bank as a necessary part of the process of converting me from a case into their patient. My account was a necessary part of becoming their patient. Without my personal contribution, I would remain nothing more than an interesting diagnostic challenge. Without my personal account, there could be no emotional bond between me and the physician.

The other unfailing action of these physicians was to touch me. A few, unhesitatingly and without introduction, reached out and took my hand. Some palpated my aching limbs, others pressed my nailbeds, but all involved in my care, nurses included, never failed to touch me. It was as if they were sealing the bond by touching the patient.

While my immediate reflections about physicians' behaviors ceased with the return of health, the various ways they bond with their patients remain an open and interesting consideration for me. No matter what the specialty, my experience with the patient-doctor relationship as a patient has led me to expect a sustained, caring commitment from my physician.

Endnotes

Reprinted from *Western Journal of Medicine* 157(1992): 201, with permission.

Lasting Impressions

Yes Sir, I think you will be satisfied. We have brought you the best physician in the world.
—Molière (1622-1673)
The Doctor in Spite of Himself

My first remembered contact with a physician leaves a residual of memories that remain powerful for me, too many years after the encounter. I was four years old, suffering from a sore throat and a fever that had me in bed. The bed was a day couch in the dining/living room of the small apartment my parents had in my grandmother's home on Stuyvesant Avenue in Brooklyn, New York. At the time we were upper-lower-middle class, yet possessed with a sense of dignity and position that is no longer readily apparent in this world. Sunday was for Sunday clothes, shined shoes, church, and a ride in the car after a family dinner of roast chicken.

The flat was on the second floor, and I can remember hearing my mother anxiously greeting Dr. Adam Schauf, our family doctor, at the downstairs front door. Though I could make out no more than the murmur of her voice, coming up the stairs she recounted, I am sure, why she had called him and expressed her gratitude that he had come.

Dr. Schauf appeared to me gigantic, especially with his impressive long mane of silver hair. He had a curious manner of acting slowly. He spoke slowly, with what seems to me now must have been a slight speech impediment, and moved with studied deliberation. He removed his heavy wool coat, placing it carefully on a dining room chair, and after setting his black bag on the floor beside the bed, drew up another dining room chair to sit upon.

My mother remained close at hand, fluttering and chirping details of her concern about my illness—a fever, cough, and restless night—that would not respond to her nursing. Much later in life I came to understand my mother's behavior as reflecting her fear that I too would die suddenly of an infection much as my sister, Chicky, had died of diphtheria six years before.

Dr. Schauf was not only imperturbable but almost inarticulate as well. He slowly parted his thick lips to reveal many tobacco stained teeth and then in a slow, guttural tone asked when my fever had started. Perhaps he was then in the early stages of the disease that colored his later life. As the father of my Aunt Mildred, his private life was not for us entirely private. Though he eventually died of a stroke, years of neurological disease, perhaps Alzheimer's, perhaps Parkinson's, preceded his death. In his later years he spent endless hours poring over the same page of an old anatomy book, apparently reviewing and attempting to remember information from his training.

As my mother answered Dr. Schauf's questions, my eyes fixed on his vest, with its pockets' brimming assortment of magical instruments. From a pocket above the two that were joined by a gold watch chain, he pulled out a silver tube and slowly unscrewed the top, revealing a thermometer. He shook it down and, after examining the fossa of my mouth, carefully placed it under my tongue. Out came his gold watch with a flip-open cover for taking my pulse. By this time the thermometer had cooked sufficiently so he removed it and, holding it to the window for light, ascertained the reading.

This done, he turned to the large black bag at his feet, drew back both sides of its cover, and brought forth a stethoscope with a metal face he rubbed warm. At the same time my mother had hoisted me up and pulled back my pajama top to expose my chest. As I breathed in and out according to his directions, he listened carefully to what was going on inside me, concluding with a thorough thumping front and back. Sitting up and bent over, I peered into his bag to wonder at its mysterious contents, rows of bottles, pill boxes, neat clasps to hold little knives, metal devices whose names I did not know, and other assorted but unnamed tools of the trade.

Then came the most disagreeable part of the examination. From another pocket in his vest he pulled a tongue depressor and proceeded to take a long look down my gagging throat. In later life I had my tonsils removed, so it was probably the infected tonsils that caused the fever.

He never said. Once the examination was over and I had slid back under the covers, he pulled out yet another silver instrument from his vest, a fountain pen (which by happy chance I have in my office to this day), and reaching into his back pants pocket brought forth a leather wallet containing a pad of prescription blanks. As yet there was no reassurance for my mother, who now hovered silently near us. He wrote something indecipherable to my mother, which I now know was an illegible scrawl of Latin. He looked up, speaking slowly to her about my illness as he gave her the prescription. She was immediately relieved. She smiled and for the first time relaxed. He repacked his black bag and stood, drawing on his heavy outer coat while he continued to tell her in monosyllables how the prescribed medicine should be administered.

The good doctor then made his way down the stairs, presumably to another house call, probably thinking that I was not in serious trouble and that my mother was a most anxious woman.

These shreds of memory speak to two effects this encounter had on me that proved critical to my life. The first was learning the profound sense of respect my mother had for Dr. Schauf. With just a few words from him I saw her go from acute anxiety to relative calm. He resolved my mother's anxieties instantaneously—a vast and lifelong problem for me. In subsequent care of patients and their families I have remained ever mindful of this physician's effect.

The other effect was not as apparent. My father was away at work and what he said on his return that evening is lost to mind. But I do know he had a querulous anger toward all physicians. Whereas my mother could express relief and gratitude for Dr. Schauf, my father had enough bitterness toward physicians for the both of them. I am sure he remained angry about Dr. Schauf's treatment until I recovered, feeling that not enough had been done and the fee too high, for this was his fixed attitude about doctors. Unknown to me at the time, he too was struggling with the loss of my sister, which for him had occurred when a physician other than Dr. Schauf failed, despite my father's plea, to come promptly to treat the first symptoms of the diphtheria that killed her.

As I relate to my patients, the memory of those two attitudes remains someplace on the edge of awareness in my mind. The ambivalence patients and their families feel toward physicians, in my judgment, is the most critical factor in establishing a workable therapeutic relationship. Though largely unconscious, the patient balances two sets of values in our relationship, one of love, the other of hate. This so human, unresolvable ambivalence inexorably drew me to the role of the physician, for me to relive, over and over, balancing apprehension at my father's anger with the relief of benevolent acceptance my mother found in Dr. Schauf's treatment of my sore throat.

Endnotes

Reprinted from the *Journal of the American Medical Association* 268(1992): 3247, with permission. Copyrighted 1992, American Medical Association.

The Foley Catheter

The fact is the general principles in question ever remain abstractions. No one is able to recognize them as you do in the situation you find yourself, nor are people able to see themselves acting just as you have acted in doing what you did.
—Luigi Pirandello (1867-1936)
Each In His Own Way, Act 1, 1

Have you ever had a Foley catheter caught in you, and I do not mean in your ear? My point in asking is to gain your attention, which by now, I have thoroughly secured from those unlucky souls who have had the unique experience of involuntarily holding on to something they wish to let go of. Like grasping a live 220-volt line, once you have had the experience, you never forget it.

I want to recall this particular experience not to bare my soul or other private parts nor, in this age of expected sexual exhibitionism, to invoke some inverted eroticism, but to illustrate a discourse on the prime sin of medicine: The most immoral of omissions in the patient-doctor relationship is the physician's failure to let the patient know where the doctor is, to leave the patient waiting and not explain why.

Details are necessary for shading the cardinality of the sin. To judge properly whether a punishment fits a crime, certainly the crime must be known; this crime, which revolves around a Foley catheter, is known, oh, so known!

Catheters and inserters of catheters (urologists) became important to me during a surgical go-round called a transurethral prostatectomy, in medical lingo a TURP. Urologists think much like other physicians, with kindness and compassion toward patients. However, their thoughts often wander freely down metaphoric byways. Take uroscopy as an example, the ancient art of peering through a decanter of urine held to the light. The language of uroscopy is positively sybaritic; it has usurped the connoisseur's language of wine.

Nor is this a trade secret. After one's operation a urologist is likely to exclaim, "A day and a half of rosea; you are on the mend." As the patient is pouring one to two gallons of water a day into the upper end of the system, he quickly picks up the jargon of the vine and hopes to produce a distinguished blanc de blancs at the lower end. A heady Burgundy complete with purple dregs can fill the patient with despair and fears that he may never again boast a straw-colored Chablis.

Another quirk of urologists' thinking that may obscure some finer sentiment is their statistical approach. For example, when one considers an operation it is not unusual to hear, "During my years in practice, 99 percent of the men in your age group have had an uneventful course through surgery," or "Only 0.5 percent (or some such figure) of all patients develop complications while anesthetized."

This statistical approach has the merit of being close to the truth, closer perhaps than a smile and a pat on the back, but it also offers a glimpse of that realistic hole through which an unlucky, though statistically valid, sample can slip out of this world. Personally, for reassurance I will settle for the clap on the back and let the numbers go.

My engagement with Foley catheters began quite unexpectedly when I fell off the statistical wagon and took a tumble down the wrong side of a bell curve into a significant deviation. I awoke early one morning, about 10 days postoperative, with an intense sense of mission. Though obviously full of piss and vinegar, I was unable to express myself: I could not even stammer, just stood there, all intention and no action. Even though it was 6 A.M., it was clearly time for an expert.

I called my urologist and he responded, wide awake. "Why, that's all right, I was just leaving for the hospital. I'll come by there and in no time at all we'll have you all emptied out. It's nothing serious."

I arrived, checked in with a sleepy clerk, and jumped into bed. One-two-three, the Foley passed without difficulty. Oh, what relief to express oneself freely.

After a few minutes of flushing out clots the party was over. Out came the auxiliary plug and the 25 cc of sterile water inflating the balloon, but that was all that came out. In went another 25 cc, up went the balloon, out came 25 cc—and still nothing doing. A twiddle here, a twist there, but still no go. It was stuck, and with that realization my surgeon's face froze.

"It cannot be. It just is not in the script. Of course it is statistically possible, but not in my statistics," went his thoughts, while through his teeth he muttered, "There is no reason for it to be stuck!"

The next rescue attempt had a contrapuntal movement with the ring of the bedside phone. It was my anxious spouse. The nurse, in a masterly example of cool professional understatement, replied, "The doctor is indisposed. Would you please call again?"

Meanwhile, having regained his composure my surgeon sallied, "Ho, ho, old man, we could always shoot a bit of dye in there and with an x-ray or two tell what is happening." I knew what was happening. The Foley had, with the help of its infernal balloon, tied itself into a left-handed sheepshank.

With a quick glance at his watch, my harassed surgeon said, "Look, I think we will let the whole matter relax for awhile. Right now I'm due in the OR but I will be back in an hour. Nothing to be afraid of. We will just leave you hooked up to the leg bag." As if "we" had any choice. Off he dashed, with the decency not to whistle.

So there I lay, rigid, in bed, impacted with what felt like a reasonable facsimile of the Holland vehicle tunnel. The nurse tidied up a bit, remembered she had some other chores, and placed a call button in my left hand and the television remote control switch in my right.

Fortunately I could manipulate the telephone, and I reassured my wife that my condition, though uncomfortable, was far from critical. The surgeon had left at 7:30, promising to return in an hour. If we gave him the usual doctor's allowance of double the promised time, my wife might call by 9:30 for his latest bulletin. The morning dragged by. She called at 9:30, 10:30, and 11:30, and all I could report was the plot of the soap opera on the tube.

Generally we are a stalwart couple, but the unknown was gnawing. Not a word. It was just one of those things, or was it? And one's fancy can wander afar when unchecked by reality.

About noon my surgeon burst into the room. "Sorry, they stole my anesthesiologist!" Courtesy still prevailed. I replied, "Quite all right. Do you think you can get this out?"

"Statistically I have never had one stay in."

I responded, "But Murphy's law applies here: 'If anything can go wrong it will,' especially with a colleague or his family."

Undaunted, he exclaimed, "We shall see what we shall see," gave a quick tug, and this time the catheter slipped smoothly out.

Before I could have spit out a bullet, he was on his way, shouting over his shoulder, "We will talk about where we go from here as soon as

I get back from office hours." At 9:30 that evening I had a phone call from him saying he would be a little late, but he thought he was about finished up. I knew I was about finished up.

At 10:15 P.M. he arrived, ashen with fatigue. Without pausing for more than a quick hello he retreated to my toilet, where the squeezings of my grapes of wrath stood in chronologic order. The last was a clear, thin rosea. He returned to my bedside, nodding approval, and resolutely announced, "There should be no more trouble from here on in. We will discharge you in the morning." Then, as though winding down from some internal whirlwind, he said, more softly, "Gee, I am sorry about all the mix-up."

I was too far gone to protest that it was not a mix-up, not crossed signals, but an absence of signals that fixed me against the bed's headboard.

He went on, "I know your wife is upset. You are fine, though, and can go home tomorrow. If it isn't too late I will call and tell her so…if it isn't too late I can apologize…from here on it is simply a matter of the epithelium covering the site of the bleeder…just a matter of time."

With the word "time" he came to a complete stop. I murmured that he need do nothing. I would call my wife. "Just catch your breath," I said.

He was half leaning against the foot of the bed, in the shadow just beyond the subdued light of the reading lamp. When he spoke again it was even slower, the measured speech of exhaustion.

"I am too busy. Twelve major surgeries in three days."

No longer was he a physician consulting with a patient. Now he was a man, confiding in a fellow man.

"Too busy. Twelve—heavier load than internship. The last one, oh, just a stone. We did everything right and everything went wrong. All afternoon in the OR and an hour after he was back to his room we had to take him up to the OR again. I think we saved him. I hope we have."

While he spoke his posture slumped as though his muscles, one by one, were surrendering to gravity, and now he was no longer leaning but sitting with his face turned toward the wall.

He sighed—and paused. Obviously, there was no room for me to nurse my grudge. If anyone was to take care of my feelings it would have to be me. He, poor man, had the prospect of a night of telephone calls. The pause continued until he suddenly caught himself.

"I am sorry. Really I am."

"Forget it. Go home and get some sleep. When I am home tomorrow I'll call your office and make an appointment to see you next week."

"Fine, fine. Now, you're sure there's nothing I can do?"

"No—no. Go home and get some sleep." He said goodnight and he was gone.

Before going a word further, two things should be made absolutely clear. First, I am a difficult patient at best. As a physician, my probing curiosity, characteristic of the profession, lifts aside my physician's protective professional distance; as a specialist, my psychiatric fish-eye, fixed-face, noncommittal stare often unnerves as much as it uncovers; in addition, as a scribbler, my word processor is loaded with the ghastly threat that I may write anything and everything about my treatment for the edification of the medical profession at large. Little wonder I need saints to treat me.

The second point is that this physician about whom I write is a healer and a gentleman. I have trusted him with my life, and should the occasion arise, I would trust him again. Yet in addition to his skill and manners he has the tolerance not to object to my printing the details of our encounter.

I will indulge in some mental turnabout. If the urologist may look into the psychiatrist's bladder, is it out of place for the psychiatrist to look into the urologist's mind, particularly since they both are intent on raising the level of medical practice in the community?

What may be seen in my urologist's mind, and in the minds of most other overworked physicians, is preoccupied concern. Though the call may not be as public as a clarion trumpet, the telephone is just as surely a summons to the unanticipated, an emergency. Much as a soldier on the ramparts of a bastion, the surgeon thinks, "How to withstand the assault?" Like assaults on a position, with too many telephone calls, the patient is lost. It is strange, but true, that dedication to care of patients cancels itself when the care of a patient is jeopardized by the dedication. The mind of a physician is of little use to a sick man when it is overwhelmed with caring.

The saving grace that balances hypertrophied dedication is judgment, particularly judgment in the form called common sense.

Unfortunately, too frequently physicians subordinate common sense to their preoccupation with emergencies. Waiting for the preoccupied physician, whether in a hospital bed or in his waiting room, is tolerable. But though a patient may at first defer to some other, fancied sicker patient, eventually the waiting patient considers him/herself neglected, willfully neglected, and who is to say the waiting patient is wrong? No one but the physician. If physicians are long absent from their appointed rounds, rank suspicions grow like weeds.

It is too easy to indict the individual, the profession, and the system. Worthy of my surgeon and my profession is the suggestion that we pause in the serious work of the patient-doctor relationship and identify who we are and what we are about.

Perhaps it is the height of fancy, but is a "station break" possible for the doctor and the patient—a pause permitting some secondary information, some incidental knowledge, to filter through? Certainly such a pause can never be as important as establishing the diagnosis of the illness, but as a patient I would like to know more of the procedures and people that go in and about me, not only how a Foley catheter works but even some facts about the inventive Dr. Foley.

Such a pause in the routine would help both the patient and the doctor find out where the doctor is. However, more importantly for me, the patient, the momentary pause might allow my surgeon to see me as a child in the dark. Too often my appearance and my banter involuntarily conceal my needs, particularly my needs as a patient. Involuntarily, when dependency and ignorance make a child of me, plunging me into a darkness that is sometimes only the dusk of early evening, sometimes the dead of night, I hide my fear. Then I would hope my physician knows that, childlike, I do not so much need light as to know that someone is there. I do not fear the dark but, rather, its loneliness. It is not the future that I fear but being alone in the future, even the loneliness unto death.

Do not hear me grumbling about my care; rather I am asking to share in the caring, asking for a moment for us to find each other and for me to be trusted as I trust, to be respected as I respect. Sharing under the shadow of loneliness demands much; yet, no matter how experienced, either as a patient in a hospital bed or as the physician at the bedside, without sharing, the relationship of the patient and the physician is as nothing and I am alone, be I patient or physician.

Endnotes

Reprinted from *Modern Medicine* 45(#2) (1977): 81-92. Copyright ©2002 Advanstar Communications Inc. Advanstar Communications Inc. retains all rights to this material. Original title: "The Doctor-Patient, The Patient-Doctor, and the Foley Catheter That Stuck."

The Bedpan Factor

> *My wind exploded like a thunderclap....I also shed a rosy red and Panacea turned away her head holding her nose: my wind is not frankincense.*
> —Aristophanes (ca 450 B.C. – ca 388 B.C.)
> *Plutus*

Everyone associated with the care of patients can essentially be divided into two classes: Those who have carried a bedpan during the course of their training and those who have not. This bedpan factor has some application, less for the educators of our nation than for medical practitioners. The latter may well use it to clarify some of the more smelly details of professional participation in the managed care of our medical facilities.

Anyway, there remains the notion that all medical personnel may be divided into those who have emptied bedpans and those who have not. The way the idea was thrust upon me may be more interesting than the idea itself. It is a legacy of Cranston L. Cranston, one of those special people who is found in every college class.

Cranston L. Cranston exemplifies a species that I believe may be frequently encountered throughout the English-speaking world. He represents a class of individuals who seem to favor elaborate, repetitive names, with middle initials, and often numerals hung on the end. Unlike the "Horaces" and "Aloysiouses" who must fight their way through the first six grades to prove that a droll given name need not indicate a "sissy," their names have no obvious flaw. Instead, they carry hidden difficulties that generally remain concealed until adolescence. Hence, Philip Perryander Waters passes untaunted through grade school as "Perry," only to be found out in high school as "P.P. Waters." Thereafter he bears a lifelong brand, "P.P."

These special people may give the impression that they were formed by the Fates (the three goddesses of Destiny) who were intent upon creating geniuses. Initially came liberal portions of intelligence; but the Fates, before adding the next ingredients, were called away by some cosmic distraction and, in the rush to leave, merely chucked in the rest of the genes, helter-skelter.

The net result, the Cranston L. Cranstons come out oddly intelligent, but oh!! Their innate clumsiness is not limited to bodily movement but includes a basic social ineptitude, a propensity for interpersonal disaster, which immediately sets them apart in every contact.

An example from my college years should make the point for the species. Baxter T. Baxter, III, shared a room across the hall in our dormitory with Jack Robinson, a superb fellow who was everything with girls and athletics that Baxter was not. Baxter vomited regularly when engaged in competitive sports, and he actually forgot the night of the junior prom, leaving his date in the lurch and forever marred.

However, a genuine affection existed between "Bax" and Jack that was probably born of the natural ease opposites find in setting each other apart. Bax with his hero worship was always trying to impress Jack with traits that he, Bax, could never achieve—charm, daring, cleverness.

It was Halloween, and Bax hatched what he considered to be an ingenious prank to scare his roommate. He spirited an articulated skeleton from the biology lab and, climbing out of the fifth-floor attic window (we all lived on the fourth floor), attempted to dangle the bones before the window below where Jack was studying.

It was a blustery, rainy night, and Jack, responding to the rattling outside his window, stared aghast as wildly gyrating Bax flew past. Bax's foot had slipped on the wet slate roof and, consequently, he followed the skeleton down through the branches of a maple tree and, as there seems to be a special providence for these people, into the gardener's compost heap, which saved him from everything but three broken ribs. The skeleton was permanently disarticulated.

But it is Cranston L. Cranston who indelibly stains my memory. The "L" was for Longfellow because, so he claimed, one of his great-great-uncles had delivered milk to the Longfellow home. At our twenty-fifth class reunion, no one was the least bit surprised to learn that "Cran" was back, for how else to explain the sleeve of the brass button blazer floating in the punch bowl!

I remember him in medical school for his inveterate habit of wearing mismatched socks, or mismatched shoes. Mind you, he was never the class clown; that is a role which calls for wit, ingenuity, a quick perception of the people around you. He was not the class dunce either, for his species has intelligence. He was simply "Cran."

As third-year medical students at New York University, we were assigned to wards at Bellevue Hospital, and Cran and I ended up in the same group. In the course of the year, he unintentionally taught me the meaning implicit in carrying bedpans.

Frankly, I forget how it all started, grand rounds were in progress when we came upon a patient cautiously removing himself from a bedpan. The busy charge nurse was shocked. She grabbed the offending vessel away from the startled patient and passed it to the pretty nurse who was pushing the cart with the charts. She in turn handed it to the student who was leaning against her cart, and he, with the special wisdom all students have, passed it to the next in line. Predictably, Cran was last and ended up with the growler.

The nurse nodded toward the utility room at the end of the ward, and wearing a blank expression, Cran stumbled off with his burden. In less than two minutes, there was a horrendous crash which sent us all running to investigate.

The expected had not happened. Cran was still bearing his burden, but was standing among the remains of a large rack of urine bottles that he had somehow dashed to the floor. All of us crushed into the small room behind the chief nurse. We could understand her exasperation, for hadn't we all had it with Cran? She exploded at him, "Dammit, it goes in there." She pointed to the wall disposal unit for flushing bedpans.

Cran gingerly stepped across the urinous glass fragments to the wall, pulled open the lid, and crammed the bedpan in with snout up instead of down! How he did it I will never know, but he slammed the whole thing half shut and set off the brownest shower this side of Mud Geyser, Wyoming. It did not miss a one of us!

At the time I thought what Cran had inadvertently taught me was why medical personnel wore white coats as a protection against such catastrophes! It was years later before the real lesson finally filtered through—blood, feces, semen, menses, urine, snot, and vomitus are disagreeable, yes, but not fatal. From an early age we are taught that excrement is deadly, and our daily language reinforces the lesson. It takes considerable to learn otherwise.

It is all such a messy business. I had a friend who was married a month before he realized that his wife had alimentary functions which went beyond eating. The mind seems to ignore the elimination of human waste as an honest consideration and reacts with the anxiety of humor (need I cite any one of a thousand ribald rejoinders) or the rancor of rejection! (See the Watergate tapes for examples.)

One of the unfortunate results of this quirk of thinking is that the public expulsion, by anyone older than two, of any of the human gases, solids, or fluids that are labeled excreta makes the excreter decidedly unpopular—so unpopular, in fact, that he is up the proverbial "creek without a paddle" and we "pull the chain on him," to "flush him down the drain." The person is identified not only *with* the act but, by the vagary of the human mind, *as* the act.

Nor are human minds alone in this reaction; it is biologically ingrained that animals withdraw from offensive odors as well. One of the lesser sorrows of Sigmund Freud's last days was that the stench of the cancer rotting away his face caused his favorite chow dog to shrink from him.

Unfortunately, the last investigation by a member of the medical profession of this natural reaction against foul smells dates back four hundred years to the French humorist/physician, François Rabelais!

As medical practitioners, we must fall back on our own resources as we learn to deal with excreta. Somewhere along the way in medical training is the hidden experience of fighting the "instinct" to withdraw from a fellow human who has become "dirty."

If this fight has been won, the aide, nurse, medical student, or whoever it may be, has learned a great lesson in humaneness, removing a barrier between himself and a sick human being. However, for those who, out of choice or chance, have never carried a bedpan, a subtle barrier arises between them and the patient. Those who have never picked up the burden remain permanently handicapped in the art of medical care. They are involuntarily forced in an "emergency" to forego their charge by the immediate preoccupation of finding someone "to clean up the mess."

Be it a suppurating fistula in a terminal tuberculous patient or the snotty nose of a malnourished child, the patient is unwittingly testing and dividing us into the two great classes of servants of the sick—those who have chosen to carry bedpans and those who have not. That is the bedpan factor.

I have no intention of encouraging classes for medical personnel in the quality use of bedpans. That idea is more repulsive than the contents of a bedpan. My wish is a simple one: that we remain ever aware of how much we must learn about ourselves through our personal experiences if we wish genuinely to serve the sick. Frankly, it has taken me years to learn and relearn Cran's lesson.

Endnotes

Reprinted from *Prism* 3 #9(1975): 9-13, with permission. Copyrighted 1975, American Medical Association.

Professional Diplopia

There are none so blind as those who can but will not see.
—Old English saying

Are you interested in having a disease named after you? If you wish to go down in history with proprietary rights over a fraction of man's unhappiness, I will gladly turn over to you all the privileges and glories associated with the discovery of Professional Diplopia. I have the disease.

It is a serious, endemic malady on the rise among physicians. Professional Diplopia is an allergic reaction occurring in the visual organs of nearly any adult who takes a long look at the medical profession, and its major symptoms are double vision, hypertension, and nausea.

Secondary symptoms are emotional instability, with mood swings ranging from rage to depression, an itch to kill, and moderately severe pseudologica fantastica—the morbid tendency to exaggerate. The major signs are unpaid bills, threats of government legislation, and physicians resigning from professional organizations.

Basically, the problem stems from discordant images of the physician. The prime image is the one that was indoctrinated in our early years. It may have been implanted by *Arrowsmith*, with Ronald Colman portraying keen-eyed dedication to microbiology, or the decorum of some of the later saints of the most prominent medical society known to civilization—the American Society of Television Doctors. This distinguished group includes, of course, such luminaries as Drs. Welby, Kiley, Kildare, Gannon, Lochner, Craig, Stuart, Hunter, Hughes, Bellini, Powers, Aldrich, Hartly, Baldwin, and Pinkam—all dues-paying members of the society. For most of us, the primary image of the ideal doctor emerged somewhere from this crowd.

The prototype of these heroic men is the doctor in Sir Luke Fildes's famous painting[1]—famous because by now it has been reproduced in at least 627 drug advertisements—which shows a dark, maudlin scene of a sick child stretched out on a makeshift bed with the worried parents in the background. The small lamp in the foreground highlights the bearded practitioner, hunched at the bedside, pondering his shoelaces. It is the Victorian image of the family practitioner.

Dichotomy of Visions

For the medical man himself, the secondary image of the doctor is personified by the guy with an office down the hall, breezy in dress, late in rounds, lax in records, and regular at the bar. This is not to say he does not do his job, but, oh, how he suffers when compared to Welby—particularly if you listen to what his former patients have to say about him. (This image becomes even more vivid as you reflect that none of your former patients would ever say anything like that about you.)

Admittedly, there is nothing new about this dichotomy of visions. Paracelsus had himself drummed out of a number of universities for taking the matter seriously and speaking up in public about it. But what *is* new is the decidedly sophisticated audience that has evolved from spending endless evenings (and, in the case of many housewives, mornings and afternoons as well) glued to their television sets watching doctor shows. Their involuntary education has taught them the difference between a polymorphonuclear leucocyte and a Rieder's leucocyte, which they are anxious to share with you.

This sophistication was once passed over as an occasional case of the *Reader's Digest* syndrome: the hypochondriasis resulting from an exposé of a disease a month, twelve months a year, complete with the latest treatment. Today the public is different. When someone has seen syringomyelia diagnosed six or seven times a month by as many doctors, he is bound to pick up a little—albeit mighty little—genuine know-how.

He knows how Welby treats angina pectoris, and he knows that Welby is sharper at internal medicine than Kildare. The public, in short, is no longer the old crowd that would let you hide behind your stethoscope long enough to think of a plausible cliché or steal a quick look at the *Merck Manual*.

Yet, despite this assault on the physician's self-esteem, Professional Diplopia need not become a serious condition at this particular stage. If pressed, the anxious doctor can always ask for a consultation and look to some colleague of greater experience in a smaller field to bolster his own dimmed self-image. The serious and malignant complication—or should I say genetic change—which has most frequently precipitated today's Professional Diplopia is the potentiating pressure of the politician.

These ruthless bloodhounds on the trail of national virtue also watch television, perhaps more carefully than most. Moreover, they check the ratings and know how strong doctor shows are with their ever-demanding constituents. Putting two and two together—in this case, Welby and the guy down the hall—they have come up with a dreadful discrepancy.

It turns out that most physicians (with the possible exception of me and my friends) do not measure up to the standards of the eminent Dr. Kildare. Obviously, no zealous politician is going to let that state of affairs go by uninvestigated. No, not even if it means appearing before the nation's television cameras with the amazing discovery of a grand-slam, all-American, health crisis. "Save our nation from our doctors" makes a sturdy plank in almost any political platform (with the possible exception of the presidency of the American Medical Association).

You can almost hear the politician whispering to the doctor, as the executioner did while neatly strapping the condemned man into the electric chair, "Now, you wouldn't want me to lose my job, would you?"

This is where the screw tightens on the profession. Professional Diplopia begins to drive fevers up, not at the polls, but in the hallowed sanctums of the medical societies. There is a growing clamor by doctors for the profession to meet the standards that the public demands—or at least the standards that the public's political voice demands—"more for less!" The basic ambivalence that all physicians feel toward other physicians suddenly becomes a severely disruptive element within the profession.

The young Turks are for overthrowing Istanbul, while the old Turks are for peering into reviews of reviews to weed out the incompetents. The rest of the profession, not knowing exactly what they are for, stand around arguing the matter.

In the hubbub that ensues, hardly a man is left to see a patient, and none, or presumably none, looks at the fact that all doctors hate doctors. They love them, too, but the hate part has been left well covered up until pried loose by the turn of the times and schemes of the ambitious.

Profounder minds than mine must eventually describe the details and dynamics of Professional Diplopia, particularly as it twists the profession away from its essential duty. However, common sense is right at hand, available for the immediate need. Professional Diplopia—loving and hating a physician—is a personal experience. It is an inescapable part of life and as certain as death itself.

Remember always that the physician is the harbinger of death, your death and mine. Should I be lucky enough to escape a violent death on the highways or skyways, I know that there is a physician somewhere—perhaps studying in medical school today—who will come to my bedside with the knowledge, if not the news, that I am dying. It makes no difference whether I lie there scramble-minded in the gray haze of a senile psychosis or cramped in the vise of a myocardial infarction or possibly resting quietly with an inoperable mass. He will come as certainly as I will go.

At that moment when we both know I am dying, I am sorry to report, I will both fear and hate my physician. I will fear that he has not done enough and hate him for not doing more. In that moment, though assailed by regrets for the thousand things I never accomplished, brimful of sorrow for the million thoughts of love I never expressed, confused and oppressed by the looming nonfuture ahead, I trust he will help me with my Professional Diplopia, the ugliness in my eye. I trust that by listening patiently, until I have cleared away the fear and hate, he will help me as best he can to see that we are both human, ah, too human.

Endnotes

Reprinted from *Prism* 1 #4(1973): 9-11, with permission. Copyrighted 1973, American Medical Association.

1. G.E. Gifford, "Fildes and 'The Doctor,'" *Journal of the American Medical Association* 224(1): 61-63.

A Lesson from Chinese Medicine

I lack the discernment to distinguish the whole lesson of today; but it is not lost—it will come to me at last. My desire is to know that I have lived, that I may know how to live henceforth.

—Henry David Thoreau (1817-1862)
Journals, November 12, 1837

The occasion of our group's visit to the People's Republic of China grew out of the memory of Evans F. Carlson, a former Marine Corp general who garnered fame during World War II as the leader of Carlson's Raiders, an attack group that with devastating effect applied the tactics of the Chinese Communist guerrillas to Japanese defense positions. Carlson had spent considerable time in China during the 1930s studying the operations of the Eighth Route Army. He had earned their respect as an honest, open-minded man who was willing to learn under the most trying conditions. He eventually retired to Oregon, where he died in 1947. In his name our group of twenty-two was invited in 1977 to China to increase understanding between two great peoples.

A Blur of Impressions

One of our hosts in Beijing remarked that seeing China in three weeks was like studying flowers from a galloping horse. However, if you take the trouble to look for certain blossoms, even while going hell-bent for leather across a vast land inhabited by nearly a billion people, you will catch a glimpse here and there of what you are looking for and, though too often blurred, lessons do emerge. The flower I looked for was compassion, particularly medical compassion, and the lesson learned was an appreciation of the humanitarian imperative.

Insight into the humanitarian imperative emerged through an unbelievably complex blur of sights, sounds, and experiences. The sight of the Great Wall of China leaves one even more breathless than the cold Mongolian wind blasting over its towers and parapets. The surrealistic flow of two million blue-coated bicyclists tinkling their way, crisscross, in and out along the dusty Beijing boulevards, the sudden offbeat aroma of America at the U.S. ambassador's reception, the excitement of meeting

Peggy Snow, Edgar Snow's widow, an evening of living history spent chatting with Dr. Hans Miller, a German-Swiss physician who first came to China in the 1930s to take Dr. Norman Bethune's place with the Eighth Route Army and who became vice-chancellor of the Peking Medical School Number 2—these are experiences that run together like an inked message left in the rain.

The impressions while traveling in the provinces are even more difficult to hold in perspective. The milling, industrious, ingenious mass is ever about. Even while peering from a speeding train at night, the passing lights flash on camels pulling laden carts, on bent figures straining under heavy loads, and on a relentless flow of life. In the morning light, as the dust momentarily clears from a bus window, there on a cliffside above is a man. He is alone with hammer and chisel and at work, apparently reducing a whole mountain. We visited communes where no Westerner has ever been and were all but overwhelmed by crowds following us, the foreigners, with the awe and wonder that Westerners give to movie stars. We ate dinner at the Peking Duck, a restaurant that has been in business in the Old Front Gate neighborhood for more than 150 years. It serves a meal exclusively of duck, including webbed feet sauteed, split heads, and one hundred-year-old duck eggs (reputed to be but three months old). There was course after course, until we lost count in the heady atmosphere of wine, beer, and that form of liquid dynamite, the Chinese liquor, *dah chu chiew*. But then, the blur of some of the flowers that we galloped past only reminded us of our ignorance of what was going on beneath the surface—ignorance of a reality that has permanence.

Because our group happened to have seven physicians, a medical librarian, a nurse, and a retired medical secretary, our gracious hosts made every effort for us to visit medical facilities along our path. Understandably, the medical interest of other members of the party flagged once they had seen a few operations under acupuncture anesthesia, but they were indulgent and bore with the relentless curiosity of the unfettered American physician. Each medical person had his own handle, which he twisted as the occasion arose. The radiologist sought out the x-ray equipment in the Beijing Children's Hospital, the internist discovered that China has no intensive care units, the public health physicians sat down with their counterparts in Shanghai, and the medical secretary returned to her old haunts at the Beijing Medical School, where she had worked thirty years before.

To the chagrin of some of my companions, I, the peripatetic psychiatrist, made no attempt to visit psychiatric hospitals nor to pursue the statistics of schizophrenic reactions among the inhabitants of Hunan, but limited my psychiatric observations to passively watching a ten-year-old girl being treated for enuresis by acupuncture and checking the barefoot doctor's pharmacy in Anyang to find that chlorpromazine was there for use as necessary. Chinese psychiatry seemed too vast and foreign for this brief encounter, and I focused my interest on another "flower," compassion, which has a universality far beyond psychiatric practice. I was out to learn what I could of that exquisite humanness that is part of any medical practice willing to recognize the patient as mortal and fearful of pain.

Pursuit of the Flower, "Compassion"

My first attempt to get beneath appearances failed when I asked one of our interpreters if he was acquainted with the English word "compassion" and if it had a Chinese equivalent, since I wished to use the word while visiting with Chinese health professionals. The timing was poor, perhaps because of the traveler's demon, jet lag, or because we were in a noisy bus caught in Beijing traffic. Whatever the reason, all I got for an answer was a brusque, "Certainly, it is an old word," and then a bit of Chinese, which bounced off my eardrums along with the uproar of raucous horns. Obviously, pursuit of the concept had to be delayed.

The next chance came on a train south of Beijing. We had crossed the Yellow River into Honan Province, and at Chengsien our railroad car was shuttled off the main north-south line to be hooked to a locomotive heading west, up the valley into the Hsiung-erh Mountains. This was the route Confucius took in 517 BC when he sought the advice of Lao-Tzu in the ancient capital of China, Lo-yang, to which we were heading. After the rattle of being switched in and about the train yards and finally being attached to the new train, the entire party retreated to their respective compartments, leaving me alone in the rear vestibule of the last car with yet another interpreter. As we stood there, bracing against the sway of the car, we watched the railroad gangs stepping back to their work on the tracks from which the speeding train had separated them and the crowds of people and carts piled up at the crossings, bursting to resume their way. I then resumed my pursuit of "compassion," now with an interpreter whose etymological interest had been aroused. We had gone through the difference between "grief" and "depression" the day before.

This time I went after the concept carefully, responding to his reflex use of "sympathy" with clear English definitions of "pity," "sympathy," and "compassion." He was a bright young man, clearly interested but also confused. The old Chinese word for compassion had escaped him, or perhaps had never reached him. He said, "Kind sir, I must reduce your idea to seven separate words—a phrase—which I think expresses what you describe: 'I have experienced the same bitter feeling.'" Then carefully bracing against the sway of the train, he lettered out the pictograph for *tong yang tong ku te gan quie*. But despite his effort, he remained puzzled, knowing that such a concept must exist with clearer definition in a culture as venerable as his. He then said, "I will think and study this carefully and let you know more." He accompanied his words with a cheerful smile and a clap on my shoulder as we lurched into one of the countless tunnels on our way to Lo-yang.

A few days later, my friend and I continued our dialogue about compassion. "I have given the matter much thought and have discussed it with others and find what you wish is an old word, 'ling min gan shou.'" Again he carefully lettered out the pictograph which curiously contains the symbol of the human heart at its center. "This conveys much closer the idea of experiencing the feeling yourself. You, the speaker, are referring to your immediate feeling after the happening." He had caught the idea, with no condescending distance of pity implied in it. "However," he went on, "'ling min gan shou' is seldom used. Since the liberation we speak of 'revolutionary humanitarianism." He then lettered with ballpoint pen the saying of Chairman Mao, "Heal the wounded, rescue the dying, practice revolutionary humanism." For the remainder of our stay in China, I had my phrase for describing the feelings all who practice the art of healing must have as they deal compassionately with the hopeless, helpless, and dying. In China it is revolutionary humanitarianism.

Equipped with my new instrument, I began to move into place some of the innumerable pieces of the vast jigsaw that is Chinese medicine. Physicians are taught to work in unity for service to patients. The dying patient is treated with all possible care and is given the choice of returning home when possible and if the family wishes. Patients have the choice of traditional or Western-educated physicians. Every citizen is taught that he has four free services: health care, education, kindergarten (child care), and cremation. Clinic walls are adorned with placards reminding all of their dedication to serving the sick humanely. Revolutionary humanism is part of the training of both the health professional and the public. Apparently it is part of the system.

The Humanitarian Imperative

Revolutionary humanism is apotheosized in Norman Bethune, M.D. If fame is measured by the sheer number of people who are aware of a contribution, Bethune is easily the most famous physician who has ever lived. Millions of Chinese know of this Canadian physician's service to their country. Billboards, movies, posters, picture books, and word of mouth proclaim how he died of septicemia contracted while operating on an unknown, wounded Eighth Route Army soldier. Dr. Bethune's sacrifice is the epitome of revolutionary humanism.

A quick and careless judgment leaves revolutionary humanism as another example of the total politicization of the Chinese culture—an example of compassion being politicized. Perhaps the term is just jargon, but I hope I am wise enough to know that three weeks is not enough time to arrive at even that simplistic conclusion. Much more attention must be given to the culture, language, and politics of Chinese medicine before any conclusions can be drawn about the meanings, as well as the sincerity or insincerity, of a policy that promulgates revolutionary humanism. However, revolutionary humanism does serve as an excellent reflection point on how our own system fulfills human needs.

China travel requires that any thinking about the contrast between revolutionary humanism and Western medical compassion be at a level above material means. The physical resources of Chinese medicine are too different from Western medical resources to lend themselves to effective comparison. Clearly, Chinese solutions to health problems should not be transplanted to Western medicine. The prospect of being treated for a myocardial infarction by a conscientious barefoot doctor from Chongsha is nothing I would wish on myself or others. However, Chinese solutions do call on us to find better solutions for Western health problems, including our use of medical compassion.

A successful comparison of medical compassion is possible if it goes beyond material means to the heart of the beliefs that move each system—to their philosophies. When the saying of Chairman Mao and the oath of Hippocrates are placed side by side, little disparity is revealed; rather, they vibrate harmoniously with the central belief that the physician, barefooted or white-coated, must strive to be worthy of serving the suffering. Together, they affirm that the worthy physician should look beyond himself with a developed social-mindedness for others. Both medical systems agree that there must be a conscious humanitarian motivation within their members that is understandable to others. This is the humanitarian imperative.

Apparently the systems differ as much in practice as they agree on need. Where I saw zeal in the barefoot physician, I see diffidence—perhaps indifference—in the white-coated physician. There is a readily appreciated contrast between the way the respective physicians indoctrinate and reinforce medical compassion among themselves.

Simply reflect on how much the Western medical student or practitioner has to say about medical compassion. Our medical education, the place for indoctrination, is notorious for being four years of training that leaves too many young people bereft of compassionate imagination and altruistic ideals. By graduation the resulting void is filled with preoccupation for getting on with a career. Nor is continuing education of the practitioner any better, for how many credit hours are devoted to developing and broadening the physician's social awareness? Where are we indoctrinating and reinforcing our humanitarian imperative, the conscious commonality of humanitarian motivation within Western medicine?

The example of Chinese medicine challenges us to moderate our exaggerated curiosity about body function. In Western medicine technical curiosity is so overemphasized that "compassion" is in danger of becoming an old word for us. Frankly, we need a language that will articulate the humanitarian imperative: a practical language with a candid vocabulary of humane words as contrasted to technical ones, a language that can be used every day to speak of suffering, want, fear, and compassion without embarrassment. I do not suggest revolutionary humanism, but a common language, for practitioner, student, and medical educator, that permits us to listen to and speak with patients as human beings.

Compassionate Alternatives

Ironically, this lesson on the humanitarian imperative was not taught to me by the Chinese, but rather by a fellow American physician, my roommate on the travels. The pieces fell into place in a most natural way late one night as we talked on about the day's adventures over a Chinese hot toddy.

The Chinese do not turn on the heat until November 15, and by that time northern China is a cool country. There is no heat in homes, schools, trains, or hospitals, and it is not unusual to see a patient lying in bed with cap and mittens on. Of course, there is no heat in hotels either, so during the first two weeks in November my roommate and I developed the habit of having a hot toddy out of a vacuum bottle of tea prior to turning the lights out.

So there we were, sitting in our room surrounded by the litter of travel, me in two sweaters, wearing a cap, he in his coat, and the both of us knee deep in eviscerated valises, dirty clothes, half-empty bottles, rucksacks of camera equipment, piles of empty film cartridges, the litter of candy wrappers, torn maps, and crumpled boarding passes, discussing whether the Chinese paint the temperature line on their room thermometers. Although the temperature read 10°C, Chinese thermometers seemed always to read 10°C, and we both could have sworn it was much closer to 5°, if not 2°C.

I have forgotten how he brought it up, but sipping his steaming brew he said, "All the places we have been, the things we have seen—think if we were at home and took the time to visit people's homes, working people's homes—what a different opinion we might have of what people really need for medical care. Suppose every physician in the United States took maybe two hours a week, less than a tenth of his time, to get his head up out of the rut he works in and look at people's needs as they see them. Suppose we went to a factory back home or made rounds with a welfare worker. I mean all doctors, not just clinicians. Suppose a researcher took the time from his laboratory work or a faculty member at the medical school wandered off from his teaching rounds long enough to sit down and ask a county commissioner what *he* thought about health care. Can you imagine the effect it would have? Suppose people began to think that physicians were interested in more than increasing either their skills or incomes? Mind you, I am not saying that all physicians are inhuman, but suppose it were part of the training of every physician to use his own imagination and get out to see what his community is doing—his school boards, his police departments. Just suppose a pathologist or a family practitioner skipped his Thursday afternoon on the golf course to visit the local jail—not a conducted tour to prove everything is OK, but all on his own. Suppose he went down to the local pokey without apology or jokes and checked it out for what was and was not being done for prisoners.

Suppose he just thought that he should find out for himself what it was like at the food stamp counter of the local welfare office. Can you imagine what less than 10 percent of a physician's time devoted to seeing actual life outside the office and hospital, beyond his usual rounds, would do for patients in particular and citizens in general?"

He gave a long low whistle across the top of his cup, which in the cold room could be seen as well as heard. I could only reply, "It's time to turn in." His questions were not rhetorical, but I lacked answers. He left me thinking in the cold Chinese night until I finally realized I had been listening to the humanitarian imperative.

Endnotes

Reprinted from the *Journal of the American Medical Association* 240(1978): 2257-2259, with permission. Copyrighted 1978, American Medical Association. Original title: "A Lesson from Chinese Medicine, The Humanitarian Imperative."

The Importance of a Name

Someone had better be prepared for rage.
There would be more than ocean-water broken
Before God's last Put out the Light *was spoken.*
                    —Robert Frost (1874-1963)
                            Once by the Pacific

On his ninetieth birthday, which occurred in 1931, Supreme Court Justice Oliver Wendell Holmes observed that there was no one left on the face of the earth who would address him by his first name. Just this single observation places him in a different era from ours, for today it is reversed, with title and surname gone. As a man of these times, let me show you the full 180 degrees we have come.

Should I reach ninety, I will be lucky if there is someone left to call me by any last name. It simply is not in the cards. Oh, I expect and will tolerate an impertinent "Doc," but give me anonymity in preference to a steady diet of "Dearie." In fact, in this connection, I wish to put society on notice: At no time during my decrepitude do I wish to be patronized or infantilized by slovenly address. If it should happen, I plan to act, to act impulsively, possibly even criminally.

This nasty, if not malignant, chain of thought originated while I was visiting an eighty-six-year-old woman in a nursing home. Her emotions had recently become master of her reason, and, with the need to better understand herself, she reached out to me, a psychiatrist. I visited her regularly, and we worked away at the painful confusions which hampered her pursuit of life, liberty, and the spirit. She, as any other patient, expected and received the attention and understanding implicit in the difficult job of mutually examining her values.

One day, while we were hard at uncovering some sources of her carnal passions, who should stride across the threshold of her room but Miss E. Alwright, the charge aide. Miss Alwright was new to me, but there was no mistaking who she was. Her front was pinned together with one of those confounded plastic license plates worn by members of institution staffs as a guarantee against being confused with the furniture.

Miss E. Alwright's unctuous salutation rolled across the room: "Well, Rosie, I have a little pill for you." And, before you could say "polymorphous perverse," she had run around the bed, popped the pill with a quick flush of water from a paper cup into the patient's mouth, and had gone—in and out with the blast of a Blue Meanie. With discretion born of experience, my patient had silently accepted her medicine, both chemical and psychological. She carefully touched her lips with a delicate handkerchief, while I sat slack-jawed with astonishment. After a moment's silence, I asked, "Do you know her?"

"No, she is new here," replied Mrs. Sprightly. "I've never laid eyes on her before." My mouth sagged wider.

After thirty years of watching patients survive in spite of their treatment I should be able to take a purely pragmatic view of patient care; but no, my gorge ascended. I barely contained myself from shouting down the hall after Miss E. Alwright, "If she is Rosie, who the HELL do you think you are?"

Luckily, experience has drilled into my head that it is not only wise but therapeutic to refrain from impulsively afflicting patients with personal feelings. I remained silent, closed my mouth, and sat back as we began to pick up the shreds of our shattered discussion.

Only later, in the tranquil security of my study, did the implications of the experience unravel to reveal "The Professional's Infantilizing Salute."

By a curious inversion of our culture, a greeting becomes a diminishment. In a strange, at least to me, alchemy of our times, courtesy and formality are turned inside out with the rationalization that rudeness and familiarity are more humane and, hence, more acceptable to the elderly. With the Infantilizing Salute, disrespect passes for courtesy, while familiarity counterfeits as affection. By inverted logic, manners are ignored as a means of knowing people, and formality becomes synonymous with rejection.

Justice Holmes's contemporary William James wrote that "the greatest revolution of my generation was the discovery that by changing the inner attitudes of our minds we could change the outer aspects of our lives." Today it is different, for the change which has occurred has little to do with inner attitudes. The magnetic poles of custom have reversed. What was once positive is now negative. In this context, the path through the maze of patronizing care of the elderly is not too difficult to follow. But specifically, why did Miss E. Alwright perceive Mrs. Rose Sprightly differently than I did? Needless to say, the aide was not available for analysis; consequently, this portion of the investigation is conjecture. But for myself, as usual, I was up front in my mind, all too available for analysis.

How did it happen that I understood the patient as Mrs. Sprightly and not Rosie? Well, to begin with "Mrs.," she had once been married. The aide must have known that from simply looking at the patient's records. But, ah! The aide probably did not feel that "Mrs." No, the aide could never have sensed Mrs. Sprightly's husband, for the poor man had died years ago in a traffic accident, leaving Mrs. Sprightly with five small children, a few dollars, and a room full of furniture. Then it follows that the aide would not have sensed how lonely Mrs. Sprightly had been, born in a distant land and adrift with her little ones.

Mrs. Sprightly had forced her grief and fear into the back of her mind. She had no time for her own feelings. With naked pride and the grim determination that her family would survive, she opened a tiny millinery shop. As she said, "There was never a day I couldn't get a job working for someone else, but I wanted to keep the children close. We needed each other; so I started my own business."

It was a struggle all the way, but Mrs. Sprightly succeeded and reared all five children to be self-reliant adults. Unfortunately for her, rearing the family turned out to be but half the struggle. When her little ones had grown and were no longer in the nest, she was left with an emotional cancer. Eventually, the long-delayed grief broke upon her, and, in order to be once more herself, she began the dreadful work of measuring and weighing her loss.

So, despite her history, it was her present dreams, her present temptations, her present recriminations, and her present doubts about being—not her past—that made Mrs. Sprightly anything but Rosie. The only conclusion possible was that Miss E. Alwright did not know that Mrs. Sprightly dreamed, hoped, and feared, any more than Miss E. Alwright is aware that all people dream, hope, and fear.

Is it possible that Miss E. Alwright lives in a world where only she and a few "near and dear" have a monopoly on being? If it is, she must believe that the rest of the world is made up of emotionally dead people who do not or cannot care. How else could she have called Mrs. Sprightly "Rosie"?

I shrink from that dreary reasoning, though I must respect it for its simpleminded efficiency in guarding against an original thought or an aberrant emotion. For getting by with a minimum of involvement, Miss E. Alwright has it made. She probably would consider it a compliment to be saluted as "E."

But just a bit more of what is in a name. When the sessions go well with Mrs. Sprightly, she walks me to the elevator. There, since I am at least a foot and a half taller than she is, she asks me to bend forward and, taking my head between her hands, plants an affectionate kiss on my forehead. It is an act for all and sundry to observe. It is Mrs. Sprightly who gives me the kiss, for we both know Rose much too well to ever allow her to do it; and it is Dr. Crawshaw who accepts the kiss, for I know Ralph much too well ever to allow him to accept a patient's kiss. It is a gift, one of many, including humor, affection, insight, wisdom, and respect—sprinkled with the occasional spice of invective and wit—which Mrs. Sprightly bestows upon me.

One day after Mrs. Sprightly had bid me goodbye with her usual benediction, I rode down in the elevator with a pair of middle-aged women who had been visiting a "Dear Friend." The shorter woman was visibly agitated by what she had seen and blurted out, "She likes you."

I agreed.

Then, reaching for some mystical explanation, the woman continued, "Why, you must be her minister!"

"No. Her physician," I replied.

For a moment, I was tempted to go on and ask what she was thinking, perhaps even explore that a kiss is a kiss is a kiss, but her face was suffused with crimson, and I knew her thoughts as a final blush of adolescent fantasy. There was nothing to be said. After the elevator doors opened, she scurried off with her companion, and I was left musing on the motto of a distant time: "Evil to those who think evil."

So what is in a name? I'll tell you. The name contains what is in the relationship. And again, let me put the world on notice. If I make it to ninety and if some miscreant doctor, aide, technician, social worker, nurse, or indigent nonprofessional assaults me with an infantilizing "Ralphie," I plan a final, impulsive act. Right then and there, I will summon every bit of my remaining strength for the Herculean task of strangling him or her with a corner of the bedsheet. I'll kill the bastard. That is what is in a name.

Endnotes

Reprinted from *Prism* 1 #1(1973): 7-10, with permission. Copyrighted 1973, American Medical Association.

You Can't Kill Hope

Hope, like the gleaming taper's light,
Adorns and lights our way:
And still, as darker grows the night,
Emits a brighter ray.
—Oliver Goldsmith (1728-1774)
The Captivity, Act II

Come with me; I'm going to visit the mother of a Down's syndrome child. She has much to tell us. Listen while she speaks.

"It was ten years before I regained a sense of compassion for physicians."

Her eyes, as she speaks, are neither suspicious nor defensive. They are clear as a cloudless sky after a shower, all cried out. Her eyes search yours, to see if you recognize her wounds that time has covered with clean, smooth, almost transparent scars. Only her voice betrays her vulnerability; it is a calm voice but too controlled, overmodulated with strain.

"There have been so many doctors, so many years of doctors, and so much pussyfooting around. I did not understand them to begin with, but now I think I do.

"Take the delivery, for instance. I believed in natural childbirth and was conscious throughout the delivery. I heard when the hum of the room suddenly stopped. Everything grew quiet and no one said a thing. 'But there is nothing wrong with my child,' I thought, and no one said differently. They just did not say anything.

"Then I had trouble with Suzy. She would not nurse, or grow, or respond. Or rather, she did but she didn't, and that's the trouble. You are never sure. You find a thousand reasons to explain what is happening, yet no one says anything. There were so many difficulties, and when I asked, no one had answers. It was not until the pediatrician blurted it out that I was sure something was wrong. Not that she intended it that way.

"We were both there, my husband and I, and when she looked at him it startled her. I said, 'Yes, she's her father's daughter,' referring to the family resemblance we had all commented upon. It was then she exclaimed, 'Did you ever think he might not be her father?' Imagine! She said that, and we did not say a thing. After we had Suzy back in the car it hit me, 'What did she mean by that?' I went back in and asked her. That was the first time anyone mentioned that Suzy might be retarded, the first time, and even then the pussyfooting, the ifs, buts, and perhaps.

"Then, what we went through! More and more uncertainties but never any answers. Finally, we found a doctor, a saint. I mean it; there are a few in the medical profession. He sat down with us and listed all the symptoms Suzy had. I think the list went to twenty-five. He went over the list with us and he said, 'Any healthy child can have one or two of these symptoms, but only a mongoloid child has all of them.' At last we knew.

"He was so kind. He took time. He was gentle. He explained carefully. He told us the alternatives. He gave us time, as much as we needed. I remember he said, 'But always remember she is a nice baby, and she is your baby.' He did not take her away from us by what he said; he helped.

"I guess what helped the most was finding other parents who had been along the way before us. Having a child like Suzy puts a real strain on a marriage, and I tried to do too much by myself. But then we organized, and the parents' group has been really supportive.

"The doctors were the worst, though. I went to the heart clinic with Suzy to see about her cardiac defect. The doctor just looked at the diagnosis and said to me, 'Some of these kids make it to five or ten.' He must have known he was in left field by the look on my face, because he took a second look at Suzy, or perhaps it was his first look at her, and then looked back to the chart, which informed him she was eight years old. Flustered, he said, 'I mean ten or twenty.' If doctors would only read the chart before they start talking! Perhaps then they would avoid getting so nervous and talk too much. First too little and then too much, along with praise, the senseless praise. I did not understand what was wrong with them. But now I have an idea

"Take the OB man. After a thousand doubts and questions, my husband and I went ahead with a second pregnancy. If ever there was a planned pregnancy that was it. I was two months along when the articles started coming out on chromosomes, and one article made the point that if there was translocation of the chromosomes, the chances were one in three that the child would be mongoloid. You guessed it. We had a rare form of translocation, and an abortion was advised.

"That was back when abortions were difficult to obtain, though there was no legal block for us. I went through with it—the consultations, the letters of approval, the whole experience, and when it came to the final discharge checkup, the OB man, who I guess is as decent as most—and who certainly knew all of what went into the abortion—turned to me as he was leaving the room and said, 'Use some birth control. I don't want to be doing one of these every year.' That man did not know I existed. He was thinking only of himself.

"Talk, too much talk. Oh, how doctors talk. A few years later I was with the genetic counselor who had advised the abortion. We were talking about an altogether different matter when he gratuitously remarked, 'Oh, you remember all our interest in translocation of chromosomes? Well our new discoveries show it is not so important.' I burst into tears. Our whole lives had focused on that second child, and now he told me we had aborted it for nothing. Oh, how I cried. I cried for nothing—the nothing he had turned all our sacrifice into. I hope he will never forget me or my tears.

"Gradually, from experience, our own and other parents', we learned how to deal with doctors: You must get them off the hook. It is always wise to start with, 'We are not out to prolong Suzy's life, only to make her as comfortable as possible.' You can see them relax once you tell them you are not looking for miracles.

"Then, you do not tell them a diagnosis, you only suggest. If you say, 'I have learned that they are using sulfa, at the state school, to prevent respiratory infections,' they will say 'It won't help!' But if you suggest they might wish to try sulfa, it gets done. Suzy never had any trouble with infections once we got her on sulfa, but before it was hell. You must be so careful whom you ask. Ask a surgeon about a medical problem, and the answer, nearly always, is 'Out of my field—couldn't care less.'

"But I was going to tell you how I regained my compassion for doctors. I guess the saints had something to do with it. I have known three. Mention their names to people who have known them and their faces literally light up before you. A mother came up to me in a supermarket, a woman who knew me because both our children had been in one of the cottages at the state school. Dr. George Smith was the doctor in charge of that cottage. She said, 'Have you heard? Dr. Smith died,' and right there she burst into tears. I believe a nimbus floated over that man's head.

"The other doctors finally have made sense to me. It took me a long time to see that they are interested in life, not death. They study and strive for healthy babies. I suppose you could almost say they live for healthy babies, and when the child is not healthy, I believe they take it personally. They feel as though they have failed, personally, and they pull back. I have yet to meet a doctor who is not willing to learn—but not many of them want to learn about dying.

"They are afraid of killing, and I understand that. They are afraid of killing hope as well, but they should know that you just cannot kill hope. Even on the busiest street some blade of grass is pushing up through the pavement. Patients are not as fragile or as ignorant as doctors think.

"When we began meeting with parents of other children like Suzy, all we had was a church basement, but now we have an organization that can help people. Twenty years before that, parents had nothing.

"Suzy goes to school now. Just the other day the school bus driver came by. She explained that she'd been assigned to drive another route, but she wanted me to know how much she loved Suzy and would miss driving her to school. I heard another mother say of her child, 'I would have missed her if I had not known her.' She could have said it for me."

Just then, while I was listening, the door opened. Eleven-year-old Suzy entered with a crushed, sticky paper napkin in her hands. She smiled shyly at me and went up to her mother, pressing the mess into her mother's hands and wiping jelly from her own hands on to her mother's. Involuntarily, her mother leaned forward to grasp the mess, and in that instant, without stepping back, Suzy met her cheek with a wholly unexpected and resounding kiss. I have no doubts about who is teaching compassion to our world.

Endnotes

Reprinted from *Modern Medicine* 45(#10) (1977): 51-53. Copyright ©2002 Advanstar Communications Inc. Advanstar Communications Inc. retains all rights to this material. Original title: "Physician Take Note: 'You Can't Kill Hope.'"

Part 6

Medical Practitioners of Compassion

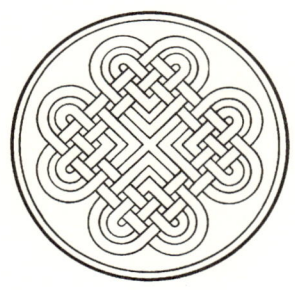

*Honor to those who in their lives are
committed and guard their Thermopylae.
Never stirring from duty;
just and upright in all their deeds,
but with pity and compassion too;
generous whenever they are rich, and when
they are poor, again a little generous,
again helping as much as they are able;
always speaking the truth,
but without rancor for those who lie.*

*And they merit greater honor
when they foresee (and many do foresee)
that Ephialtes will finally appear, and
in the end the Medes will go through.*
—Cavafy 1909

Overview to Part 6

Perhaps the reader might expect *Dr. Zhivago* as a proper introduction to physicians' practice of compassion, yet **Gandhi** better illuminates the conscious emotional discipline that undergirds a compassionate career. Discipline of spirit by committed minds defies easy description. The source of such self-education lies in a profound wish to cultivate moral character, the soul, and soul is a subject unremarked in contemporary medical education. Consequently, compassion in medicine remains elusive, detectable largely in the physician's style of behavior, where without recognition its quiet presence artfully shapes the quality of healing.

The life of U.S. medicine's poet laureate, William Carlos Williams, here sketched, too briefly, in **Stories, Poems Look at the Heart of Medicine** comes closest to defining compassion in words. With an artist's genius he shares his lifelong struggle to care for patients' ill-fated bodies and flagging spirits in a manner they find caring.

How doctors approach social suffering is explored in **A Visit to Maimonides' Grave** and **A Rose for Chekhov's Grave**. Neither of these physicians used any word closely equivalent to our word "guts," yet their disciplined intestinal fortitude, their moral energy, in examining, close up, their life against the circumstance of others' suffering has to be "gutsy."

Pursuit of a compassionate life insensibly transmutes self into otherness. One surprising facet of this metamorphosis sparks as physicians confront political oppression. Though generally seen as politically conservative, the medical profession has produced significant political activists. The list is long, including Dr. Thomas Sydenham, the English Hippocrates who served British democracy as a cavalry officer in the English civil war; Dr. Benjamin Rush, signer of the American Declaration of Independence and a physician in our Revolutionary Army; Drs. Jean-Paul Marat and D.J. Larrey, leaders in the French Revolution; Dr. Sun Yat-sen, known as the father of modern China; Dr. Frantz Fanon, who gave vibrant voice to the liberation of Algeria.

In 1976, I cited these heroes in an article, not to mark their compassion but to illustrate the courage some physicians display in addressing evident evil. Their humanitarian work was described as a medical dimension of the bicentennial celebration of our Revolution. The submission proved of no interest to American medical editors. So, like other refugees, the article made its way to politically tolerant Switzerland. There it appeared as *Célébration des Médecins en Révolte,* a paper not included here but mentioned as an example of implicit cultural strictures in considering physicians' full role as caring citizens.

But dedicated physicians' spirit of political revolt in the service of the oppressed can never be stifled by politically correct editors. Compassion shared with a suffering community emerges in the biography, **José Rizal,** and the book review, ***Witness to War,*** where in the face of profound outrage the discipline of caring assumes the role of political leadership. Dr. Carroll Behrhorst, **Obituary: Carroll Dean Henry Behrhorst**, a physician who supported and reinforced the indigent Guatemalans with limited medical resources, lived his practice of medicine on the thin line between sustained compassion and expressed outrage.

Undrained Brains is charged with the preservation of compassion in cultural exchange and, incidentally, led to the development of a prospering international physician exchange program, Health Volunteers Overseas.

Perhaps compassion goes unrecognized in the medical curriculum because it can not be taught with words, only learned through self-examined experience. Without question, great medical teachers model insightful caring for their students. The everlasting debt to my heroes is evident in **Dr. Karl's Finest Colloquium**, and in a book review, *A Psychiatrist for a Troubled World*.

Alert reader, beware of construing the "otherness" of heroes, their exemplary behavior, as a reason for limiting your engagement with compassion. Heroes' examples are cited for your action as much as reflection, for encouraging you to become partner, revolutionary accomplice, in making our world more humane. The torch is there for any to carry.

Be it as patient or healer, each of us gains by experiencing and reflecting on another's style of compassionate engagement. That our heroes may sometimes stumble in their quest need never give us pause. They are as human as we are. How else could they be our heroes?

Gandhi
A Film Review

> *The woes of* Mahatmas *are known to* Mahatmas *alone.*
> —Mohandas Gandhi (1869-1948)
> *Gandhi, An Autobiography*

Gandhi is an excellent film, worthy of three hours of close attention.

Ben Kingsley's fine portrayal of Gandhi has a woven intensity of sorrow and joy, stubbornness and wisdom, as the outrage of a puffed-up prig evolves into the compassion of a saint. The movie is a magnificent interpretation of *Experiments with Truth,* as Mahatma (Great Soul) Gandhi entitled his autobiography. In a sense, however, the picture is stolen by a supporting player, India, for the country with its deceptive beauty, where vibrant humanity is only a camera angle away, subtly intrudes with more than just scenery. Finally, India subverts the film for Western audiences by imposing on them such a vast and exotic background that the humaneness of Gandhi is lost in the drama of the landscape and the complexity of cultures. The foreignness of the scene makes for an "otherness," which unfortunately works with Gandhi's unique life to make that an "otherness" as well, each beyond the lives of the audience. Here lie the achievement and the failure of the film.

Gandhi's assassination in Calcutta, January 30, 1948, dramatically opens the film. Then a series of flashbacks reveals how this diminutive, dapper, London-trained, Indian attorney, through his unrelenting demand for personal integrity, grows from an alien, marginally successful lawyer in South Africa into the most powerful human being in the world. Early on he discovers that his only chance for initiating constructive social change is through personal force of character. Although continually tempted by position, money, sex, and violent force, Gandhi relentlessly focuses on the ultimate social force of our world, spiritual power.

The audience is easily attuned to the impact of violence on Gandhi; it is such common fare in movies, where "our" hero suffers under some form of established tyranny. This point is made early in the film when Gandhi is brutally kicked off a South African railroad train for having the audacity of being "colored" yet attempting to ride in a first-class coach.

For me, however, the story within the story is not Gandhi's evolving political campaign of nonviolence, which loosens some of the racial bonds of South Africa for immigrant Indians, and then the bonds of all India, including the untouchables, but his unique ability to personalize his opponent.

His struggles were actually never with the empire, but always with other men who happened to be holding the reins of power, or a billy club over his head. His saintliness does not lie in nonviolence, as he staunchly maintained, for he endorsed the British war effort, but in his unrelenting curiosity to find out what made his opponent human and in his ability then to limit his reactions to the humanness of the "enemy." The film says this in a thousand quiet ways, such as when Gandhi meets with the liberal leaders of the India Congress Party in Pandit Nehru's sumptuous home. In a wholly unostentatious way he reveals to them their implicit hubris by taking the tea service from the magnificently attired butler to serve his fellows himself. The scene has an implicit, religious quality of communion, only because Gandhi understands the plight of the servant and the blindness of his fellow leaders; and with character born of reflective genius he makes a living, personal point that none can question. He even goes so far as to apologize, never obsequiously, for his own vanity in making the point of immediate humanity. Here lies the uniqueness of Gandhi and of this film in searching out his spirit. He turns out to be human enough to be a saint.

The development of Gandhi's political insight, as contrasted to political power, closely parallels his increasing spiritual strength. After the horrible indignity on the railroad coach he begins to live his life along principles of tolerance and understanding, which, he concludes, are coherent and essential. Then he puts himself to the test of his beliefs before asking anything of others. He is even brave enough to put his own family to the test, for he not only cleans household toilets himself, a task always assigned the untouchables, but asks his followers to do the same. In a moving scene of elemental passion he asks his wife, who must suffer loss of caste as a consequence, to take up and share that burden. With compassion for himself and others he sticks with his belief that violence should not beget violence. "If I strike a man in the eye for striking me in the eye—the whole world will end up blind." Gradually, in South Africa, he begins to understand the process of using spiritual power, *satyagraha,* the principle of firmness in truth, until it eventually becomes the designation for the national struggle for Indian independence. He starts with himself in everything and then moves to family, ashram (community), nation, and world. For him, action is a direct, considered, personal experience that purposefully fits together with every part of his life.

The film itself makes a most interesting comparison with other film biographies of charismatic leaders. Perhaps our local art theaters may someday mature beyond running series on movie stars, such as "The Humphrey Bogart Festival," or "John Huston's Films on Parade," and consider other dimensions of life, such as a series on "World Leaders." If they do, a great beginning would be *Napoleon, Lawrence of Arabia, Our Hitler,* and *Gandhi.* How fascinating it would be to put these portraits up beside one another and compare.

Remembering Albert Schweitzer's admonition, "God is in the details," I would start my comparison with a close examination of how these men expressed their characters through their clothing. They were style setters who believed clothes make the man. Napoleon, at the Bal des Victimes, is dressed to the nines in his preposterous uniform, intended to make a short man tall. His clothing is imperious, even as it limits the motion of his body and head. Then there is Hitler's butler, commiserating about Hitler's confusion, black socks with brown shoes, and Hitler ending up in a banal private's jacket. Reflect on Lawrence's ecstatic rapture when he is granted a sheik's white burnoose, the conquest of Arabia expressed in six yards of fine-spun wool. Gandhi's metamorphosis from formal Western attire to bare-bodied loin cloth reflects the most striking use of clothes of all. Here is a window on vanity made large, an undeniable expression of man's soul. Would that the films could be seen together and deeply understood by white-coated physicians.

The failure of *Gandhi* is hidden but real, for though the film reveals Gandhi, it only partially reveals the female star with whom Gandhi was in love, Mother India. There are the obligatory shots of nursing paupers with flies crawling over their babies' faces, but the imploring hands of beggars thrust into Gandhi's coach on his triumphal return to India could be seen mistakenly as saluting. The sheer oppression of heat, numbers, and hunger, though not denied, is never enlarged upon. What we do see are majestic rivers replete with lush landscapes and lazy water buffalos, railroad trains rushing through verdant tea plantations, exquisite flowers and birds (some of the women in their rainbow-hued saris seem almost to be birds of paradise), and the ravishing music of Ravi Shankar's sitar.

Possibly this vast discrepancy between visual beauty and experienced horror is at the bottom of Indian mysticism, but it is obvious that in financing a moving picture about its country the Indian government had little interest in explicating these extremes of the social experience, even though they are essential to understanding Gandhi. The film softens to the point of weakness the encompassing Indian feeling of heat, hunger, and despair, which Gandhi met with inner coolness, fasting, and eternal hope.

Recommending *Gandhi* carries with it the deep admonition that you examine his suffering as one with the suffering of all people, including our own. It is much too easy to see Gandhi as the speaker for the Indian masses and not for all mankind, much as it is easy to see the plight of the developing countries as something foreign to our lives and natures.

The problems he wrestled with are the fair and present problems of any concerned physician, any thinking citizen: how to give meaning to human suffering as it exists within our ken. If we properly serve one patient, we must think of ourselves as serving all patients.

"Do we struggle to change things or to punish?" was Gandhi's question. As Western physicians, we punish through the sin of omission. In this round and finite world, we, who are richer and more powerful than the princes who cluttered the countryside of Gandhi's India, can and often do remain as blind as that atavistic aristocracy. This is not a plea for charity as such, but rather that we would each in our own way leave the movie house strengthened in our personal belief that the other man's suffering is not "other" but our own. This is how I understand Gandhi's experiments with truth.

Endnotes

Reprinted from *The Pharos* 47(Spring 1984): 40-41, with permission.

Stories, Poems Look at the Heart of Medicine
A Book Review

*For the beginning is assurably
the end - since we know nothing, pure
and simple, beyond our own complexities*
—William Carlos Williams (1883-1963)
Paterson

There is an arrogant perversity in all caring physicians, an unrelenting search for beauty in the ugliness of pain, human suffering, and death. The caring physician is drawn to the most malignant pathology, the sickest patient, the most debilitating deprivation—ostensibly by an unslackening curiosity, but actually by a rare and inverted vanity that he, the physician, shall through knowledge and compassion bring order to lives and organs that the fates have relegated to chaos and infinite nothingness.

No physician's life better exemplifies this double-edged quality than that of William Carlos Williams, M.D., the sadly departed New Jersey general practitioner/pediatrician, and oh, how surely he wields his pen and pounds his typewriter to expose this strange dynamic in the physician's heart. Through poem and story he lays out, for all to learn, how sorely afflicted caring physicians are with the "humble arrogance" in the pursuit of hope for the hopeless, life for the dying. It is all there in *The Doctor Stories*.[1]

Through the thoughtful editing of Dr. Williams's art of literature, Robert Coles, M.D., reveals a living sample of Dr. Williams's art of medicine—a dirty, bloody, hate-smeared, redeeming business when seen up close. The introduction gently points the eye to the torn ambiguity within the artist/physician, who, like a Renaissance artist, is preoccupied with the miracle of birth and childhood, a host of New Jersey madonnas given rise from his own mother, and dedicated practicality from his too-busy businessman father.

His very name proclaims this contradiction. Even his daily journal notes jotted down between house calls are a potpourri of medical notations and billings, interspersed with lines on nature's beauty and the startling silence of a Paterson dawn all to be later filtered and distilled into medical records or lyrical poetry. Simultaneously, he could read the fading color in the cheeks of a dying child as a clinical sign and an aesthetic moment.

Of the fourteen, "Doc Rivers," his short story of the dissolution of a drug-afflicted colleague, should be required reading for everyone seeking a license as a medical practitioner. It should be the opening document for every committee on impaired physicians in each of the fifty state medical societies and should be tattooed on the chest of every physician tempted to dissolve his life away with mind-altering chemicals.

Here is the unbelievable professional behavior of organized medicine in the 1930s, and I am old enough to attest to its truth. We see our brothers standing by, privately condemning while publicly condoning the deadly course of a colleague bent on destroying himself while heedlessly dragging patients to perdition with him.

Here is the "conspiracy of silence" in spades, yet it is but one of the elemental truths of physician behavior bashed into our consciousness by Dr. Williams.

A greater miracle also is there, the belief and trust of patients in a drunk, drug-mad physician who cares for patients with a loyalty forever holding to the patient: forever risking himself for the patient, albeit without much clinical judgment; forever listening to the patient's suffering with a palpable dedication that cuts through class, color, religion, age, money, and hate to directly address the suffering of the particular human being. Here is the example of what once was related to me by an oppressed and elderly Russian physician practicing in the Soviet Union: "Compassion is not a concept. It is, and can only be, an experience."

"Jean Beicke" is the story any experienced physician might write about the case in which we do everything but the right thing. Along with the careful history and physical are the consultations and operations while the patient just fades away before the physician's eyes because he fails to see the pathology for what it is, acute purulent mastoiditis. "We might, however, have taken a culture of the pus when the ear was first opened. I shall always, after this, in suspicious cases."

Heartfelt regret remains the most imperious teacher, for what caring physician can ever forget a lesson when it comes at the cost of a patient's life?

This collection is a labor of love: love of a mentor, of a physician for a physician, of a human being for a human being—for Dr. Coles has made a life work of explicating the art of his friend and teacher Dr. Williams.

The words are sparse in the introduction, as they should be, to allow the man to show through, but if you are drawn to know more of Dr. Williams, in addition to his autobiography, read Dr. Coles's scholarly analysis of Dr. Williams's literary works in *The Knack of Survival in America*.[2]

In any case, read *The Doctor Stories*, and then ask yourself how you see the infinity of beauty in human nature, body and soul, that patients offer up to share with you in daily practice. Where, oh where, is your perversity—for surely it must be in you—for otherwise you are naught but an overtrained technician. Read carefully and turn aside for some private thoughts, remembering as the humble New Jersey practitioner would have us remember, beauty is in the eye of the physician.

Endnotes

Reprinted from *American Medical News*, date unknown.
1. W.C. Williams, *The Doctor Stories*, introduction by R. Coles (New York: New Directions, 1984).
2. R. Coles, *William Carlos Williams: The Knack of Survival in America* (New Brunswick, NJ: Rutgers University Press, 1983).

A Visit to Maimonides' Grave

The fourth species [of wisdom] is the true human perfection. This in true reality is the ultimate end; this is what gives the individual true perfection, a perfection belonging to him alone; and it gives him permanent perdurance; through it man is man.

—Moses Maimonides (1135-1204)
The Guide to the Perplexed, Part III

A journey to the grave of the illustrious physician Rabbi Moses ben Maimon, Maimonides (1135-1204), is a pilgrimage that properly begins at the ancient port of Akko (Acre) on the Israel coast of the Mediterranean. There the Crusader citadel yet stands on the shoreline much as it did when Maimonides walked about the city in 1166, unsuccessfully seeking a safe haven for religious study and the practice of medicine. The time was tumultuous, for the twelfth century saw intense rivalries among empires, religions, and ideas, much as our present century does. These forces buffeted Maimonides throughout his life. His visit to Akko was relatively brief, for its Christian government was unstable, and he left to settle finally in Egypt.

The present-day pilgrimage east from Akko, over the mountains of Hagalil, to Maimonides' grave in Tiberias on the Sea of Galilee resembles that of his travels, for in some ways the Holy Land remains physically and politically as it was 850 years ago. He was born in 1135 to a family of Jewish scholars living in Cordova, Spain. Sophisticated Muslim scholarship made this city the preeminent academic center of the Western world, the point where Arabic, Jewish, and Christian learning intersected to preserve and build on the intellectual heritage of the ancient world.

By the time Maimonides reached manhood, a fanatic sect of Islam, the Almohads, had conquered the city and threatened death to unbelievers. Maimonides, with his family, staunch Jews, fled to Morocco in 1159. Here, the family prospered, as David, Maimonides' brother, pursued the jewelry business, while supporting Maimonides in his studies of religion and science. In 1165, however, religious intolerance again forced the family to move on, first to Akko, then in 1166 to Alexandria in Egypt, and finally to Fostat (Old Cairo), where Maimonides settled for the remainder of his life.

The road east from Akko climbs through verdant groves of olive trees whose leaves alternately flash green and silver in the sunlight. Climbing to an altitude of nearly three thousand feet, the road enters the ancient holy Jewish city of Safad (Zefat). Here, deep within clustered hillside shops and homes, can be found the revered Ashkenazi Ha'ari Synagogue, where medieval rabbinical scholarship continues much as it did in Maimonides' day.

Entering from the bright sunlight, the traveler needs a minute for his eyes to accommodate to the dark interior with its heavily curtained windows gently answering to the cool west wind. Unlit lamps hang on long chains from the vaulted stone ceiling, and the weary traveler may sit at ease on the rug-covered marble benches that edge the room. The walls, with the exception of the curtains that segregate the women, are supported by bookcases of ancient texts. In the center, a marble pulpit, bearing an open book, faces a curtained recess that contains an age-old Torah. Here is the center of a community seeking, as in Maimonides' time, to understand the wisdom of the Old

Testament prophets in today's world—a scholar's mountain refuge, the lifelong goal of the too-busy practitioner.

And busy practitioner Maimonides was. He was a superb clinician and, though few of his specifics for hemorrhoids, sexual impotence, asthma, and the healing of wounds remain useful today, his clinical approach remains valid.[1,2] That he was all but overwhelmed as a physician in great demand cannot be doubted. His account about his practice in Cairo is delightfully candid. He reported that after a day of government work as medical advisor to the Sultan, the son of Saladin, and the Sultan's family, he wearily returned to his home and office. He wrote:

> I dismount from my animal, wash my hands, go forth to my patients, and entreat them to bear with me while I partake of some light refreshment, the only meal I eat in twenty-four hours. Then I go to attend to my patients and write prescriptions and directions for their ailments. Patients go in and out until nightfall, and sometimes…until two hours and more in the night. I converse with them and prescribe for them even while lying down from sheer fatigue. When night falls, I am so exhausted that I can hardly speak. [1, p.656]

Here is a busy physician.

Continuing the trip east from Safad, the road moves through a barren, sunbaked, rock wilderness as it drops down to six hundred feet below sea level into the Jordan Valley, where date palm and banana plantations border the Sea of Galilee. Here Jesus Christ pursued his ministry, gave the Sermon on the Mount; and here Herod Antipas built for the Romans the city of Tiberias, a resort of pleasure and licentiousness on the edge of their empire. The modern city of Tiberias retains parts of its original Roman walls, while elements of past grandeur echo in its air-conditioned hotels, guaranteed to refresh the weary traveler with year-round sunshine and sybaritic, hot mineral baths. It was Maimonides' wish to spend his last days here in his religious homeland, where so many saintly rabbis were entombed; but that wish went unfulfilled until after his death, when his body was brought from Egypt for burial among the graves of Jewish prophets and heroes.

Maimonides' grave, unlike the neglected graves of so many of medicine's heroes, is maintained with full respect. Near the center of the city, it is part of an ancient cemetery and is approached by a broad, paved path with wide steps starting at street level. Granite pylons stand beside the path, each inscribed in Hebrew with "Knowledge," "Love," "Vows," the names of the fourteen volumes of his *Codification of the Jewish Law,* the *Mishneh Torah,* one of Maimonides' greatest achievements.

Although devoted to religion, Maimonides' motive in writing this work reveals, for me, the key to his contribution to medicine. Maimonides sought to cut through the barriers of custom and ritual by interpreting the ancient words of the prophets and scholars into a language and understanding for the common man. In medicine, his goal was similar, to give each individual an opportunity to care for himself.

At the head of the paved walk a white marble entrance opens on a small, bowered plaza with benches for quiet meditation. Circled by thriving acacia trees and date palms yet bathed in the sunshine, the grave is covered by a large hemicylinder of stone. Across the foot of the cylinder, engraved in gold Hebrew letters, is:

> From Moses unto Moses
> there was none like Moses
> Here rests the dust of
> The Great Eagle
> The Giant of the Bible,
> Understanding and Medicine
> Who brought healing to kings
> of flesh and blood.

The visitors' words and thoughts focused on Maimonides' contributions to the growth of medical science in lessening the dreadful conflict between emerging science and absolute religion in the Middle Ages. By offering a "single truth," a belief in one all-knowing God, Maimonides hastened the reconciliation of the "double truths," which saw religion as faith and science as reason in a way that held them incompatible. For Maimonides, religion and science were facets of the "single truth." By using the recently rediscovered philosophy of Aristotle, he opened the way for the scientist to believe in God and the priest to believe in science.[3] His teaching that moderation and tolerance were not heretical offered strength to Thomas Aquinas in his heroic interpretation that science was not in conflict with the Christian religion. Thus, Maimonides opened the way for all religions to see that science served God as it served man.

Today, as we search for a wider moral basis for the practice of medicine, bioethics, we have a debt to the physician Maimonides. We have much to learn from him of moral imagination and moral courage, which he considers in detail. Our struggle with the dark cloud of medical rationing, with the prohibitive expense of costly medical technology, with confusion of the physician's role as patient advocate with corporate minion, can well draw on Maimonides' dedication to the physician's highest quest, healing the souls and minds as well as bodies of our suffering patients.

We visitors left Maimonides' grave renewed in spirit, knowing righteousness is possible, if only in the memory of those who have lived a righteous life. For the traveling physician, a few minutes spent in reflection beside the beautiful grave of Maimonides can make the longest journey worthwhile.

Endnotes

Reprinted from *The Pharos* 53(Winter 1990): 22-23, with permission.
1. F. Rosner, "The Medical Writings of Moses Maimonides," *New York State Journal of Medicine* 87(1987): 656-61.
2. S.R. Benatar, "Maimonides, the Physician—1135-1204," *South African Medical Journal* 69(1986): 255-57.
3. A. Broadie, "The Moral Philosophy of Maimonides," *Journal of Medical Ethics* 14(1988): 200-202.

A Rose for Chekhov's Grave

It takes two to speak the truth,—one to speak, and another to hear.
—Henry David Thoreau (1817-1862)
"Wednesday" in *A Week on the Concord and Merrimac Rivers*

This is a difficult world as Anton Chekhov, the physician-author, knew so well, for he, with his talent for humanity, could, as few men have been able, trace out these difficulties before your eyes. Over and over again his disciplined genius leads the reader through human experiences to the central problem of man, which is not man striking man, but man shrinking from his fellow man; not anger, but loneliness. For me, the ultimate expression of this theme is found in his short story, "Heartache," which I read years ago and have puzzled over ever since.

Perhaps you remember the tale: an old man, Iona Potava, a hack driver, is borne down with grief for his son who has just died. His son was his last relative; Iona's only link with the past and with the future. Bereft, dazed, the old man staggers through his night's work seeking someone who will share his burden, seeking solace from some other human being. He tries to speak to a rich man, who is too drunk to hear. He tries striking up a conversation with some young men, who are too gross to understand. A doorman is too self-important to listen, and his fellow cabbies too tired to care. Finally, he confides to his horse, and as that old gray nag munches on her hay and oats, apparently listening, he pours out his heart, and you, the reader, feel your heart squeeze within your chest. You stare into a black void with a man who is brave enough to remain a human being despite every loss.

Perhaps it is too obvious a tale to generate much curiosity, but for years Chekhov's inner meaning has puzzled me. Not that I was concerned with some literary question. No, it was always a question, man to man, a question which can only be broached in a quiet, unhurried restaurant, over coffee and brandy, after a good supper, "What moved you to write this story, Anton? Come, no talk of making money, none of that potboiler or scribbling subterfuge you are always hiding behind. What part of you got on those pages?" Well, the good Doctor Chekhov is gone and only the wind would answer my questions, or so I thought until chance brought me to Moscow and gave me the leisure to haunt his footsteps.

Late in 1973, I had the good fortune to spend a few weeks studying in Moscow. I was given unlimited freedom, at least it seemed so to me, to go where I wished and to see what I wanted to see. Of course, under these circumstances I would visit Chekhov's home and grave and I did, and most surprisingly along the way I found an answer to my question, the one I would have asked the good Doctor Chekhov if fate had allowed us to meet over cigars and cognac.

However, not in his home, the present Chekhov museum, did I find what I sought. Incidentally, the museum is a delight, the best museum I discovered in Russia, and for that matter, one of the best in the world. A delight because it is so little an institution, so much a home. It was Chekhov's home and office for most of his productive years and remains much as it was, situated on a boulevard in Moscow. The waiting room and office are as he left them, even with his pen on the desk. But it is the photographs and paintings on the walls that add the living touch. These walls are alive with a hundred vibrant faces of loving, excited, thoughtful, creative people—artists, actors, doctors, mothers, fathers, sisters, and brothers—with the ever human expression of Chekhov threading through the crowd. Before your eyes he flourishes and then sickens at an early age.

Inadvertently, the museum had a touch which made it seem even more Chekhov's home, for outside the double-glazed windows of the first-floor consulting room was a cat, or more precisely, a half-kitten/half-cat, huddled on the window sill, in the rain and sleet, crying bloody murder to be let in. His great-great-grandfather must have carried on the same way when demanding his warm spot next to the hearth.

How alive it all was, but, as I say, it was not where I found the answer.

Not to digress, but because the paths of life are seldom straight, the purpose of my visit to Moscow enters the tale. For a number of years, I had been interested in the development of the new Soviet medical oath. After the October 1917 Revolution, medical oaths were discarded until 1960, when Soviet physicians began again to witness to their medical beliefs. In 1971, the present oath was promulgated and I journeyed to Russia under the aegis of the U.S.-U.S.S.R. Health Exchange program to study the "why" and the "how" of the new oath.

During my stay I talked with many serious scholars who have concerned themselves with the goals and development of the medical profession. The problems of teaching and learning ethics, the conceptualization of the patient-doctor relationship, the complexities of intra-professional relationships were dealt with directly and in depth. Sometimes our sessions ended over caviar and cognac, sometimes over sugar-cake and tea. Always I felt a deep hospitality, a simpatico; that is, on all but one point. Strangely, it was compassion which raised a discordant note.

Compassion, shared suffering, is one of the real human experiences, yet it is most elusive. In medicine compassion may occur unpredictably, but as a physician gains professional strength fully to meet the demands of his patients' serious illnesses he must come to experience it. Compassion is woven so deeply, so intrinsically, into the fibers of medical practice that though it may not be handled, measured, nor prescribed, it is nevertheless indispensable to the nature of any mature physician. Yet when the subject surfaced, invariably my Russian friends winced.

The mere mention of *sostradanya,* literally "co-suffering," set Russian physicians on edge. Their pupils widened, bodies grew tense, and voices sharpened. The most frequent immediate response was to label compassion as a religious idea belonging to a dishonored past. In tones of disdain and repugnance, they explained that there was nothing illicit or illegal about the word, but it was not acceptable, the concept simply had withered. Compassion had been replaced by something better, a national striving for the highest Communist ethic. One man illustrated by describing the terribly hard times for children who had been abandoned or left orphans after the Civil War. Good people, out of the kindness of their hearts, took these waifs into their homes and reared them along with their own children. "Some might call this *sostradanya*, but it really was the emerging higher ideals of the New State." Other physicians quoted Gorky, a great hero of their Revolution, "Suffering is my enemy; I hate suffering and I argue with those who accept suffering." Others pointed out that Lenin hated suffering and shared Gorky's sentiments. Succinctly, I discovered a phenomenon that may not be limited to the Soviet Union, but also appears to be included in the collective plans for a future world: compassion is considered unnecessary.

Compounding my surprise was the final observation with which most if not all these physicians closed our discussions, the recognition that compassion is an essential element of every physician. They did not say empathy, sympathy, or pity. They said *sostradanya*, and as one man put it, "But, of course, without *sostradanya* no man is a doctor. A doctor must give a portion of his heart to each patient."

While this perplexing development had me ruminating, I pursued the shadow of Chekhov. His grave is in the Novodevichy Cemetery, which is in the Arbat, the old city, in the curve of Moscow River, one or two miles south of the Kremlin. On a threatening, gray day after my guide and I searched out a rose, a remarkably rare item in a Moscow winter, we drove through a bleak drizzle to the cemetery. From the north the sanctified grounds are first announced by the tall golden Byzantine spires of the Novodevichy Nunnery, around which cluster the graves of the rich and renowned, a Russian pantheon. The cab left us at a gate in the high brick wall surrounding the cemetery and, shouldering our way through the small doors of battered wood, we were in the village of the dead.

While my guide sought the custodian and directions to Chekhov's grave, I wandered ahead. Intersecting paths marked off the countless small crowded plots which stretched away to the west and the banks of the Moscow River. Fir trees, some standing alone, like white-capped mourners, others in silent, respectful groves, shared with the graves the soft benediction of the misty rain.

Despite the intimations of life, the jackdaws arguing in the trees, the slow pitch of a grave-digger, the clouds of steaming breath from plodding mourners, it was a scene of overwhelming frozen chaos. The damp, deadly cold penetrated bone deep, and unlike other cemeteries I have visited with their clutter of faded flowers, marble crosses, and chipped angels, this was chaos as I had never seen it; eerie, almost pagan. Here, a large, absolutely square block of red marble, six feet by six feet, sitting on four legs like a gigantic butcher's block, there a bust of a movie director, staring imperiously from beneath a wig of wet snow, while behind him a larger-than-life bronze statue of an astronaut framed by a great ring of tarnished metal. One tremendous block of marble memorialized an animal trainer, beloved by children, while on the wall beside me were pictures, presumably of some hardy aeronauts who had flown to the North Pole, for above the pictures set in their neat row of niches sailed an immense metal silhouette of a dirigible. On it went, seemingly endless, with the bust of an automobile manufacturer and a flat slab for a forgotten wife; a maelstrom of stones, inchoate shambles of frustrated immortality.

By now my guide had secured the directions and overtaken me. We sloshed through the mud and snow down a long path and around a dividing wall into yet another area where gravestones stretched in every direction. As we paused, I spied ahead a most arresting marker that seemed to spring from the ground, alive. It was shaped almost like a small house, a troll's house. Its light-brown stone was capped with a metal roof resembling an ancient bronze helmet, with flowing curves, fluted edges, culminating in a trinity of Muscovite spires. Altogether the gravestone had a stunning, mysterious human charm, the incarnation of some forgotten myth. I looked closer. It was Chekhov's grave and set into the stone was an icon of Christ, dead on the cross. (Only later did I put together the date 1904 and the style. The marker is a consummate example of Art Nouveau.)

I paused, thinking, if the man of *sostradanya* was buried here, was the Russian spirit of compassion as well? I hesitated then cast the rose upon the snow-burdened ferns covering his grave. Strangely moved, uncomfortable, yet not knowing why, I waited, then turned and left. Was this all there was to my quest?

A few days later, more of the answer was revealed. I had spent the afternoon with a medical historian and before leaving I broached the subject of *sostradanya*. He responded with the predictable start, yet it was somehow different.

The medical historian occupied the principal's office of an old public school which had been converted into a research institute. The office, which, like most offices, described the man better than a photograph, was an inner sanctum at the end of a long hall, twice barred by swinging doors. His office proper was entered through an anteroom where two smiling assistants benignly guarded my colleague from detail and distraction. Inside, the office was a bit of a squeeze, with chairs, charts, and settee on one side of the desk, while an old, overburdened coat rack, slightly askew, like a superannuated family retainer, guarded the final route round the desk to his chair. The office walls were lined with crowded bookshelves, cupboards, and glass cabinets. Papers, journals, and books clung together precariously in two small hills on his desk while the valley between was filled with ink stand, desk lamp, and the promise of our party, cake, cognac, tea glasses, plates, knives and forks. The early winter evening was fast upon us so that the dark-green shaded desk lamp cast a sharp circle of light on the three of us. "*Sostradanya*," he said with a half whistle, "that is what you are interested in." He pulled back out of the light, swirling his chair, and with his profile silhouetted against the wan winter light of the window he dropped into thought.

After a few minutes, during which he was obviously collecting his thoughts, he spoke, this time to the wall, for he did not return to his former position.

"Humanism is not an abstraction. It is an experience." He paused again, not for a reply but to muster his strength. "You learn this at the Front. I am a man who feels pain when I see a dog struck. In the war I saw great numbers of wounded. We were just a few surgeons and after one battle they brought in wounded, day and night, for three days. You feel sorrow. You see them all as fellow men, as Russians. Then suddenly you see there are Germans too, hundreds of Germans dying before you. You must decide ethically who is to be treated, for they are all human beings. But when you look at the Germans you remember the villages in Byelorussia, ruined villages, burned villages. There was a village where we came upon a well filled with children. I remember one child…" He went on in Russian but the translation ceased. My interpreter, ashen-faced, faltered, murmuring, "It is too terrible."

"Try," was all I could say.

"One child, he was at the bottom of the well, beneath all the rest. We dragged him out feet first. He had been under water for a long time. His body swollen with water. I see his face, upside down, swollen, swollen." He broke off. It was too much, and in that instant I knew I was listening to Chekhov's old man grieving for his son. The room grew silent. He turned to me and said once more, "*Sostradanya* is not an abstraction." We had gone as far as we could go, and with his return to our circle of light the subject changed.

One more experience was necessary for me to understand. Later in the trip, while in Leningrad, I asked to see the memorial for those who had died during the Siege. It was a cold, dark, snowy late afternoon, so dark the street lights were already on, and before entering the grounds we visited the museum which tells the story of the Siege. The great doors of the building did not close tightly on their worn hinges and snow had drifted into the unheated stone room where it lay squeaking underfoot. Here were pictures, statistics, and a dead child's record of approaching death. Each page of her diary had its entry and some were heartrending: "Brother Sergie died today." "Grandma is dead." "Mother died," with the final entry, as death was about to grasp her hand, "and now I am all alone."

We left the building and began walking the quarter of a mile through the blowing snow to the monument. Along the way we passed hundreds of great mounds, each mound containing thousands of bodies, six hundred thousand in all.

As the cruel wind cut across my face, I knew I had heard Chekhov's child answering the old man, with "and now I am all alone." The mystery was falling away. How to be compassionate for one hundred dead? How for a thousand, for a million, for the twenty million sons and daughters of Russia who died violently in the last war? No, it is not indifference nor government policy that makes *sostradanya* difficult and complex for the Russian people. Neither is it the memory of a church which inverted human suffering into a perverted strength, nor is it any man's defiant cry. What draws men back from the full consciousness of his fellow man is not the other man's misery but the intimation of the colossal sea of suffering which surrounds each and every man. To look at that boundless ocean of horror shrinks the soul. To experience it, for surely *sostradanya* is not an abstraction, is to drown.

What I feel for Iona Potava and his child is but the slim sorrow of a distant man. My feeling is to their experience as the least fleck of foam to a bottomless sea. What I have learned, dear Anton, is that the human heart has limits, frightfully real limits, which if exceeded lead to mysticism or madness or, yes, even death. The warmth of every heart must be protected from elemental, cold despair. Love is made to share, but experience teaches each man how much and with whom, until intuitively we all learn our limits, beyond which we dare not venture. Nor can any man judge those boundaries for his brother.

So the rose, symbol of the living spirit, did not rest on Chekhov's grave in vain. I heard the old man talking to me about his dead child. "It was too terrible," that is what I heard, the fear of sharing, the fear of driving me away, yet despite the fear, sharing was ventured. Incomplete, disjointed sharing; beyond my limits, even so the old man reached out, hoping perhaps "that a good doctor should give a part of his heart to his patient."

Endnotes

Reprinted from *Prism* 2 #10(1974): 9-11, with permission. Copyrighted 1974, American Medical Association.

José Rizal

To shoot men is very easy; the difficult thing is not to do it.
—José Rizal (1861-1896)

I have a colleague in the Philippines who thinks me a madman. He is too much a friend to say so directly, but he hints with remarks about head in the clouds when it comes to my search for the idealistic in the practice of medicine. Yet, this friend has directly aggravated my madness, and acutely so, by sending me a biography of José Rizal, the father of the Philippine Republic. If you do not know of Dr. Rizal you should, for then you may better judge a madness I shamelessly would spread to all my colleagues.

On June 19, 1861, José Protasio Rizal Mercado y Alonso Realonda was born in a provincial town of Luzon where his father, a merchant, was an "indo," that is, native Filipino. It was a strict Catholic family in the only Asian country that is Christian. José proved to be a bright boy who swiftly outdistanced his teachers in Calamba, Manila, and went on to study ophthalmology in Madrid, Paris, and Heidelberg. His surgical skill was such that he was considered a miracle worker but he never made much of his practice, seeing it primarily as a way of directly serving his people while he went about the business of creating a nation.

The ultimate genius of the man lies in his understanding of mankind's need for freedom, conversely his grasp of the horror of exploitation in any guise. To comprehend how far he had to come in his thinking, it is necessary, a task perhaps impossible for free men, to appreciate the absolute tyranny within which he was reared.

In 1861 the Philippines had been a colony of Spain for three hundred years, so unimportant that it was administered through Mexico. The entire country was held in thrall by the Spanish friars who controlled government, education, agriculture, and, of course, the church through a tyranny perfected during the Spanish Inquisition of the Middle Ages. The land was owned in vast estates by the Dominican, Augustinian, and Franciscan orders and rented to the natives at usurious rates. Nor was it then possible for anyone to conceive of another way since there were no books or newspapers, no guns or force, no thoughts or words permitted which lacked the friars' express approval. Through the confessional the friars heard all and through the courts they oppressed any who displeased them. Such a state of abject ignorance is difficult to imagine, for the friars kept the Philippines totally sealed from outside influence where today radio, television, fax, and e-mail, with wide-ranging news and ideas, penetrate even the most censored countries.

Rizal had many early encounters with empowered iniquity. When he was a ten-year-old boy, his mother, a devout and obedient Catholic, was arrested and imprisoned without trial for two and a half years on charges which were never made clear. Though conjecture, the most probable cause was that her other son, Paciano, had mentioned to friends, including an informer, that Philippine natives of intelligence and education should be permitted to become friars, heresy to the Spanish friars. That lesson of enforced secrecy was not lost on the family who never spoke of politics except privately to each other nor committed even the least thought of their state of mind to writing.

Despite this intellectual vacuum, Rizal, as a lad, thought out the future political development which would not destroy the oppressors but would bring about peaceful change in a frozen society. He was not a politician but came to politics through necessity, always applying the principles of peaceful change which later his contemporary in India, Mahatma Gandhi, developed as the political science of nonviolence.

Rizal was a scholar and a scientist; there are a number of species of animal life discovered by him in the Philippines and which bear his name. With implacable honesty he applied his scholarship to rousing his people from their stupor. In 1882, permitted to go to Europe to complete his medical training, he blossomed. A polymath, he wrote a grammar for the Tagalog language of the islands, spoke six European languages fluently, discussed anthropology with Rudolph Virchow, became a member of the Berlin Anthropological Society, and turned to literature with the insight of Anton Chekhov and the sharp humor of Rabelais to write two novels, *Noli Me Tangere* and *El Filibusterismo,* which opened the minds of his people to their capacity to become a nation.

Nor was he a recluse, for he held with the Greek belief, *mens sane in corpore sane.* He exercised regularly, at a time when it was considered beneath the dignity of a gentleman; he taught school, practiced outstanding medicine, remained deeply religious, loved women, never faltered in his respect of his family, and fought off despair and cynicism in hopeless circumstances which eventually led to his execution by a Philippine firing squad (the Spaniards had two firing squads, one of Filipinos to kill Rizal and another of Spaniards to kill the Filipino squad if they hesitated to kill their leader), with a generosity and nobility that lives in the Filipino nation to this day. He was a man who sought to be all that he might be.

So now you can see my madness. It is not that I aspire to Dr. Rizal's greatness, I am not that mad, but I search for men like him who are alive and unselfishly struggling with the needs of people all over our world. Though my friend does not say so, many, many do insist that nothing can be done. Nations are too set in their ways, institutions in their mindless momentum crush the future with their dead past. These realists insist on seeing things as they are, sordid, deteriorating, and inhumane, yet madman that I am I stand on the example of Dr. Rizal to look over their heads to what may be, a commonwealth of understanding where power is servant to need while expressed love is the implicit goal of men's and women's behavior, a world in which thought has become understanding and passion become compassion. It is the madness which lies at the soul of medicine.

Endnotes

Reprinted from *Journal of Chronic Disease* 37(1984): 311-312. Original title: "José Rizal (1861-1898)."

Witness to War
A Book Review

Help, me, O God, when Death is near
To mock the haggard face of fear
That when I fall—if fall I must—
My Soul triumph in the dust.

—Anonymous
Found in a slit trench during the
British North African campaign of 1942.

Beware of book reviews written by a friend of the author—and Dr. Charles Clements is a friend—but in this case you can check most if not all of what is reported here against an impeccable source, Dr. Alfred Gellhorn's "Medical Mission Report on El Salvador" in the April 28, 1983, issue of the *New England Journal of Medicine*. In Central America these were parlous times for physicians and their patients, as *Witness to War*[1] makes abundantly clear.

As a family practitioner in a small clinic in Salinas, California, Dr. Clements became disturbed by the strange condition of some of his patients: men who had been deliberately tortured with cigarette burns, women with their breast cut off, many with their minds tormented into numbness. The question rose in Dr. Clements's mind about the effectiveness of what he was doing for these people, refugees from El Salvador. He sought an answer, as a thinking physician must, at the source of his dis-ease, and here hangs a tale which bears a thousand tellings.

The style of his account is balanced, neither romanticizing the plight of the Salvadoran people nor his work with them even though there is enough derring-do to fill a Hemingway novel. The theme, which evolves almost inadvertently, focuses on psychological and spiritual violence, rather than on the all-too-prevalent physical violence, deprivation, and war, and becomes understandable when considered against the doctor's background. Though second in his class at the Air Force Academy, Clements was disillusioned by military flying in Vietnam and left the military. After years of searching as a teacher, sailor, and salvage diver, he entered medical school at the University of Washington hoping to find himself as a family practitioner. However, it was not until he was serving civilians under fire, not as a combat revolutionary but as a Quaker doctor, that he found his calling. Then, despite his internal conflict about taking arms against brutal injustice in El Salvador, he remains true to his larger sense of human tragedy. Sustained by his practiced sense of will, he serves all sufferers as a pacifist doctor, binding wounds, not wounding.

In February 1982, Dr. Clements entered El Salvador by a devious route through Mexico, Nicaragua, and Honduras that eventually brought him twenty-five miles northeast of San Salvador, the capital, in a "controlled area" held by insurgents against an army equipped with the most modern arms and training. For a year he lived with the people, sharing their dread oppression, hunger, and illness. At times he was his own best patient with dengue fever, malaria, malnutrition, intestinal parasites, and the thousand fears and fatigues that a one-man practice for ten thousand people in the jungle is open to.

With an experienced feel for people, he catches the spirit of the campesinos, the guerrillas, as well as the farmers and their families who first brand him a "bleeding heart" gringo but finally accept him as a respected doctor with whom they share more than just a dollop of their life-sustaining honey. But the real honey is the spirit of survival within the people, survival of family values, free of revenge despite the atrocities perpetrated on one and all. They band together to save both the lives of their loved ones and their values as human beings. This, despite every kind of assault ranging from betrayal from within to a napalm-armed A-37 jet diving down from above. They display the strength of spirit that withstands the assault of discovering a slaughtered young woman in the brush being devoured by vultures. Overcoming the desire to run and hide, they drive the creatures off and bury the faceless body. Such spirit rises above pain, suffering and, most unusual in our secular world, politics.

Medical history has its revolutionary heroes, but Dr. Charles Clements is a step beyond. Though medical thinking breeds conservative men who generally prefer their patients survive rather than their political theories triumph, there is a bedrock cadre of radical physicians who have taken to arms in the name of revolution. Benjamin Rush in the American Revolution and Thomas Sydenham in England's Civil War stand with such other notables as J.P. Marat, D.J. Larrey, Norman Bethune, and Frantz Fanon.[2] However, Charles Clements is for a new revolution, or perhaps a very old one, which forswears violence in any form or for any cause. Unlike Thomas Sydenham who used a broadsword to deadly advantage, he refused to carry arms. Dr. Clements was no crusader, for in his bones he understood the disease of politics, and he used the balm supreme in treating those obsessed with power—acceptance and tolerance.

Dr. Clements is repeatedly tested by those who first consider him a coward and only slowly come to accept him on his own terms. Service by healing not harming, his belief is tested repeatedly but is also respected by those who know better than he the violence that can be done to the spirit. Gabriel, a field worker, asked him why the North Americans are so concerned about physical violence. He then described how he felt working on a hacienda where his job was caring for the landowner's prized dogs who ate better than he. Gabriel saw his children die of untreated illness aggravated by malnutrition while the boss's sick or injured dogs were driven in a car to the veterinarian in San Salvador. It is a modern form of "Let them eat cake" and it does not take a highly trained mind to appreciate the corrosion of this violence of the human spirit.

Read *Witness to War* and feel in your bones how all physicians must choose between healing and violence. For what Dr. Clements has done with his personal example of sustained courage—refraining from striking back in the face of unbelievable provocation—is to strip each of us of our comfortable rationalization that as long as we are on the side of the good we need not choose but simply remain in step with the "good crowd." Read *Witness to War* to reaffirm the unhappy but human truth that a physician must choose every day to be for or against healing. There is no temporizing. There is no creed, party, or government that can make it otherwise. And if the physician is for healing, then he must stand strong for healing all the sick, not just some, as there is no middle ground to human suffering. Here in the spirit of shared suffering, as Dr. Clements shows us, physicians find their deepest purpose.

Endnotes

1. C. Clements, *Witness to War* (New York: Bantam Books, 1984).
2. R. Crawshaw, "Célébration des Médecins en Révolte," *Medecine et Hygiene*, no. 1203 (July 1976): 1125.

Obituary:
Carroll Dean Henry Behrhorst, M.D.

A doctor, in the truest sense of the word, is to be not only a wise man but, above all, a good man.
—Felix Martin-Ibanez (1911-1972)
To Be a Doctor

Carroll Dean Henry Behrhorst, M.D., founder of the Behrhorst Clinic, Chimaltenango, Guatemala, died on May 7, 1990, in Chimaltenango. He was sixty-seven years old. To make rounds with "Doc" Behrhorst was to learn from a complete physician. Intelligent, courageous, compassionate, he entered the world of the sick and powerless as only a deeply caring physician can.

Carroll Behrhorst was a native of rural Kansas. After graduating from Washington University School of Medicine, St. Louis, Missouri, in 1947, he continued his training in family medicine at the University of Cincinnati Hospitals, St. Louis City Hospital, and St. Joseph's Hospital in Alton, Illinois. He served in the U.S. Navy as a medical officer with the marines. He returned to Kansas to establish a family medicine practice in Winfield.

With a perspective that went beyond the borders of his state and nation, Dr. Behrhorst made a number of trips to Guatemala in the 1950s, originally under the auspices of a religious organization but later independently. By 1962 he was so moved by the miserable health care of the native Guatemalans that he closed his Kansas practice to move, with his family, to the Guatemalan highlands. They settled in a town of twenty thousand, Chimaltenango, which lacked any health care facilities.

Dr. Behrhorst was confronted with medical needs that could overwhelm any but the strongest of physicians. With his philosophy of care, "Help those who need help to help themselves," he practiced what he preached for twenty-eight years. One of his favorite maxims was, "The man who does not plan ways of doing himself out of a job is not doing his job." Early on he set about doing himself out of his job by focusing on the larger health care needs of the people—needs associated with malnutrition, dehydration, violence, respiratory infections, parasitic diseases, and contaminated water supply. He was determined to help them by teaching them to manage their problems within their resources.

His small clinic in Chimaltenango has remained small—two physicians and a dozen nurses—yet it flourishes as a teaching establishment developing a whole new breed of indigenous health workers, the health promoters. These Guatemalans are selected by their village to receive rudimentary medical education at the clinic and then work directly in their villages. Dr. Behrhorst staunchly resisted the temptation to appeal to outside help in the form of advanced Western medicine, choosing instead to develop techniques that would allow the emerging indigenous health provision system to grow on its own.

A hospital developed with his clinic, also with the goal of raising health standards. The families of the sick were brought directly to the small hospital of seventy beds to help with the care of their sick relatives. The staff used this "opportunity" to teach the people elemental health practices, such as using contraceptives, dressing wounds, digging latrines, boiling drinking water, growing nutritious vegetables, and washing their hands before eating. This work won recognition from the World Health Organization, which established a worldwide program replicating Dr. Behrhorst's model.

In 1980, the Behrhorst Clinic evolved into the Behrhorst Development Foundation. The foundation continues the work of Dr. Behrhorst, seeking ways to break the age-old cycle of disease and poverty. Water projects and land ownership through small repayable loans enable increasing numbers of Guatemalan Indians to reclaim their health and dignity.

Dr. Behrhorst maintained his contact with the whole world of medical science. He was an active faculty member of the University of San Carlos in Guatemala City. Starting in 1982, he spent a number of months each year at Tulane University School of Public Health and Tropical Medicine in New Orleans, Louisiana, inspiring medical students to the rewards of service in less-developed countries.

The great plague of the twentieth century, violence, proved to be one of Dr. Behrhorst's most daunting problems. Guatemala was, and is, a benighted land of violent political turmoil. For years, government troops and armed guerrillas have struggled for control of the countryside. In the oldest tradition of the medical profession, Dr. Behrhorst remained strictly neutral in the political struggles. The political beliefs of the wounded went unnoticed while casualties from both sides were treated in the hospital.

Neutrality, however, never exempted Dr. Behrhorst or his staff from the threat of death. In 1983, an unidentified combatant gunned down one of the hospital physicians. In the same year, only eighteen of forty-five trained health promoters were alive and accounted for. Although all the international agencies recalled their medical teams from Guatemala, Dr. Behrhorst carried on. Each evening, unarmed, he calmly walked the entire length of the town to let everyone know that the clinic staff was not intimidated and would carry on despite the dangers.

Dr. Behrhorst's compassion was never better shown than through his positive effect on frightened, isolated people. In 1985, during a temporary pause in the "troubles," he journeyed into the back country to visit some of his surviving health promoters. After stepping down from his jeep to signal to a distant figure that he was unarmed, there was a pause. Within moments, he was greeted by a joyous, tearful, and breathless man running to his side to embrace him. Dr. Behrhorst was a sentinel of hope to the oppressed. They responded with the passion of the saved. He was led to a humble home, where his arrival was celebrated by a feast of corn cakes and coffee prepared by the family. While acclaimed in their praise, he was consulted in their need.

Endnotes

Reprinted from the *Journal of the American Medical Association* 264(1990): 2132, with permission. Copyrighted 1990, American Medical Association.

Undrained Brains

The separation from wife and children, the breaking up of a settled establishment, and the going from the certain to the uncertain—all this was for the moment painful, but I had inured myself to an uncertain life.
—Mohandas Gandhi (1869-1948)
Gandhi, An Autobiography

Most physicians are aware of the "brain drain," which siphons off trained physicians from developing countries into the manpower pool of developed countries, but unfortunately, few physicians appreciate the role of undrained brains—the bright, dedicated, highly trained physicians of the Third World who have chosen to remain and practice scientific medicine under the often daunting conditions of their native land. Unwittingly, physicians of the prosperous countries may even mistake undrained brains for fools or failures, confusing their high professional dedication with parochial ignorance. In any case, physicians in developed countries can properly recognize the contributions of their undrained colleagues through a proposed program.

A project of the Club of Kos, a nongovernmental agency for international health policy, led me through eight developing countries (Sri Lanka, India, Greece, Egypt, Thailand, Pakistan, the Philippines, and Fiji) to evaluate health services from the patient-doctor perspective. This journey provided considerable contact with undrained brains: men and women of superior medical training, often including years of study abroad, motivated by a deep concern for health care in their native land that has made them central figures in the events of their local and national communities. They are bright enough, socially as well as intellectually, to have had an opportunity to emigrate, but instead they chose to remain to serve the sick and needy of their own land. Of course, not all the physicians in developing countries qualify as undrained brains; some lack the intelligence or drive to find opportunities abroad. They never face the critical choice.

In judging the dedication of undrained brains, a clear distinction should be made between them and medical missionaries or secular medical heroes, such as Dr. Tom Dooley or Dr. Norman Bethune. Although all confront similar problems of incredible medical needs, undrained brains are never foreign to the destitution in which they live. They have neither the memory of better times with its promise of eventual return to an easier life nor the vital support systems from "the people back home" that sustain so many secular and religious medical missionaries. Because of birth and rearing, undrained brains are one with their cultural background. Virtue is their only reward, and they are seldom recognized for their essential contribution to world health.

Many of the professional problems faced by undrained brains are common to the practices of all physicians striving for high-quality care. Economic constraints, technologic obsolescence, ethical dilemmas, political uncertainties, and social disfavor are ever present, but the magnitude of the problems is so different from that in the developed world that they appear to be created in a separate hell.

Economic strictures, for example, are immediately apparent to a visitor met at the airport by a native colleague, who quickly explains that the car is borrowed, generally from the ministry of health, since no doctor in the country can ever expect to earn enough money to own an automobile. More serious is how fluctuations in foreign exchange have increased the cost of some drugs which, consequently, are no longer affordable by most patients. Luckily, the cost of a year's treatment of leprosy with sulfones remains in the range of $0.50, but even this cost proves prohibitive for many patients. In such countries full-time professors of psychiatry earn the equivalent of $120 a month, while the chancellor of a medical science center with a four thousand-bed hospital is paid the equivalent of $4.00 an hour ($840 a month). There are no discretionary funds in the life of an undrained brain.

Medical teamwork becomes difficult in this setting, since team members must have a second job to survive, and once the team member is well trained, he or she is apt to be recruited elsewhere. Trained nurses in India know they can make ten times as much for shorter hours and easier work in a Middle Eastern hospital. The surgeon in charge of a ward must be prepared at a moment's notice to carry out every procedure personally, but also to carry the only set of keys for access to drugs and valuable equipment, such as paper for an electroencephalography machine; any transportable object of value may be traded for food.

Probably the most corrosive economic deprivation is the lack of foreign exchange. All currency except the national one is forbidden to the undrained brain, who must depend on friends in other countries to forward old medical journals to which he cannot subscribe. These foreign friends cannot send audio or video cassettes; the import duty on anything remotely electronic in countries attempting to protect their embryonic industries may be five times the original cost in a developed country. The undrained brain can never look forward to attending a medical convention or receiving refresher training abroad. The cost of personal travel is prohibitive. Once he has completed his training in a developed country, often at his government's expense, he must remain in his native country unless someone abroad will pay for his travel, an unlikely occurrence. For the undrained brain, staying alive professionally is a grim and continuous struggle.

The political uncertainties of practice in a developing country are astonishing. "Show" hospitals are maintained by political leaders for national prestige, just as impractical and expensive international airlines may be maintained to fly the flag. Show hospitals often serve to conceal pressing immediate problems. Close examination reveals much of the equipment in show hospitals to be second-hand foreign discards, incompatible with irregular local electrical voltages, bereft of replacement parts, and lacking technicians from the other side of the world for proper calibration. Although such instruments may prove unworkable, it is not unusual for 85 percent of a national health budget to go for such "advanced" efforts. Particularly aggravating conditions ensue if a political leader or a member of his family contracts a particular disease; in one country an entire cardiovascular wing was added to the central hospital in response to just such a political "necessity." More immediate problems arise in maintaining a sterile operating room, when an imperious politician wishes to be photographed "serving the people" or when his minions wish to inspect anything and everything, including the contents of an autoclave. A confrontation over such issues calling for immense tact and incorruptible morals is not always successful.

Perhaps the gravest political problem is the lack of a free press to report the health problems of the community. If the political leader proclaims that leprosy will be eliminated in ten years and the doctor sees five thousand new patients with leprosy each year, there is political danger for the doctor who speaks out. Some undrained brains go to jail for attempting to carry out a scientific medical practice that is relevant to the needs of their community. In one case, an arrested physician was released without reason after the people of his community in mute protest marched around the jail for ten days.

Undrained brains accept with pride successful emigrant colleagues as people who march to a different drummer. These classmates become irksome, however, when they return to visit and boast of lucrative medical practices that produce fine homes, superior education for their children, and improved personal health—all in an atmosphere of political freedom. They become unbearable when they extol the unlimited educational opportunities available to them and their children. Perhaps unwittingly, the successful emigré reminds the undrained brain of the many sacrifices his family must make as a consequence of his choice to remain on the firing line.

Why do undrained brains do it? A professor of medicine in a developing country replied, "That is a good question. Why should a physician climb five flights in a Bombay slum for 15 rupees he will probably never collect?" Pausing, the professor answered his own question, "Well, first, we are scientists. We want to know….But then did not Alexander Pope put it best with 'No finer aim can man attain than to alleviate another's pain'?" A different answer came from a high official in another country: "How many people in this world share in the possibility of nation building?" They do it because they are dedicated, and though they may suffer from disappointment, discouragement, and even despair, they do not suffer from a lack of constructive action.

Fortunately, one can do more than simply sing the praises of these distant heroes. Physicians in prosperous countries can act to reinforce the contributions of undrained brains by contributing on their own. I recommend that every medical-specialty society in every developed nation add to its members' yearly billing a chance to check off a contribution equivalent to one dollar, to be used by the society to finance the attendance of an undrained brain of their specialty at their annual meeting. Such travel fellowships could be of great value to the receiver and also to the donor.

The American Society of Internal Medicine, the Société Française de Pediatrie, the Norsk Kirurgisk Forening, the Canadian Public Health Association, and the Deutsche Gesellschaft für Neurochirurgie, for example, could reach out directly to like-minded undrained brains, men and women of unquestioned good will, who carry a disproportionate share of mankind's medical burden. This reaching out, which for a family practitioner in the United States would represent less than 1/100,000 of his annual income, would be direct, personal, immensely productive, and free of governmental interference, remaining within the functional organization of a medical society. Each year such donations could bring a small but important number of undrained brains into the forefront of their scientific specialty for a pause that would do more than refresh.

To coordinate this effort, the World Medical Association should tactfully but forcefully inform every medical-specialty society in the developed world of the possibility, while offering channels for selecting candidates and practical advice to the specialty society on administering the funds.

Such travel fellowships should not be considered simply a reward or an honorarium to be granted to undrained brains in appreciation of their unselfish devotion to duty. Rather, the award should be seen as equally rewarding to the donors, who would be revitalized by the inspiration and determination of their guests. The quid pro quo for physicians in developed countries would be the reinforcement of their personal commitment to service, as they directly experience the humanitarian imperative in the life of the visiting undrained brain.

Endnotes

Reprinted from the *New England Journal of Medicine* 306(1982): 99-101, with permission. Copyright ©1982 Massachusetts Medical Society. All rights reserved. Original title: "Undrained Brains—a modest proposal to recognize some contemporary medical heroes."

Dr. Karl's Finest Colloquium

A physician must be a Philosopher; that is to say, he must dare to use his own reason and not cling to antiquated opinions and book-authorities. He must above all be in possession of that faculty which is called Intuition, and which cannot be acquired by blindly following the footsteps of another. He must be able to see his own way.
—Paracelsus (1493-1541)
Medicine

The unique *joie de vivre* of the Menninger School of Psychiatry in Topeka, Kansas, during the immediate post-war years, is best reflected for me in Dr. Karl's colloquium. He intoxicated us with the discovery of possible and elemental change in ourselves, in our world, in the soul of our culture. As he led the way, we felt the earth shift beneath us. We were young, serious men and women, imbued with the bedrock belief that we were about to make a significant contribution to mankind's health. Day and night we ate, slept, and sweated psychiatry. These times may be recollected, but it remains difficult for many to believe that one man could inspire so many students to reach for the highest ideals of service to the suffering. We rallied to Dr. Karl's leadership each Saturday morning in Hawley Hall.

What I have to say is qualified for two reasons. First, all I have are memories without a shred of written record. Second, my limited role in these events was simply as a student among students. I was not analyzed nor supervised by Dr. Karl, never a member of the inner circle working with Dr. Karl on papers, books, educational programs, or research. What follows are one student's reflections garnered from his lectures, learning from his response to others' lectures, consulting with him over personal professional concerns (his and mine), and later serving as his sometimes host in Portland, Oregon.

For me, Dr. Karl's finest colloquium came in 1981. It reinforced the vivid memory of my first colloquium, July 10, 1948, thirty-six years before. This was before there was an adequate lecture hall. We met in a classroom in Winter Veterans Administration Hospital, a dark, hot closet, with a six-foot, floor-to-ceiling air conditioner that roared, blew, yet hardly cooled. Back then effective air conditioning was a sign of administrative rank, limited to the office of Dr. J. Frank Casey, Winter Hospital manager.

Dr. Robert Knight had just left the Foundation to establish a new clinic at Stockbridge, Massachusetts. Dr. David Rapaport was leaving and said goodbye at that colloquium by way of outlining the dawning future of advanced psychological research. His ideas were too complex to remain in my memory. In contrast Dr. Karl's remarks live in my mind. He focused on the dangers of nonprofessional counseling and therapy, recounting his concerns about Carl Rogers's nondirective therapy. My imagination was fired by Dr. Karl's connection between nondirective therapy and the plague of rabbits in Australia, a subject then on his mind. The link, as I recall it, was our need, the residents' need, to carefully consider what it means to do good, indiscriminate "good," such as introducing new species into environments unprepared to accept them. His vision of a plague of "do-good" therapies with "done-bad" outcomes unfortunately proved correct.

An accurate account of the subjects of Dr. Karl's colloquia, including what I believe his finest, is the task of a learned historian. Should it be undertaken, the account should never omit the essential ingredient, Dr. Karl's unique style.

For me, his style is interwoven in memory with the principal scene of action, Hawley Hall, a converted army barrack furnished with rows of government-issue wooden chairs, twelve to a row, with an aisle down the middle. The space between the first row and the stage, the pit in a conventional auditorium, was occupied by a worn, varnished table, two straight-back chairs and an unstable, portable blackboard. We entered through a recalcitrant screen door at the rear which announced each arrival with a loud slam.

Suddenly yet on time, Dr. Karl would appear swathed in a fresh white coat. He would march down the aisle leading a parade of guests, staff members, and just plain folks. Arriving at the front table he would deposit an ungainly armful of papers, reprints, magazines, journals, and books—material he might and might not refer to later. Then, with a stern frown of suspended judgment, he would turn to consider the audience. None could doubt that Zeus had assumed his throne.

The frown never lasted long, for as he recognized someone in the first few rows his face would break into a smile as he asked, not very privately, if they had read somebody's book on the plight of New Mexico's Native Americans or another on the threat to New Zealand's hummingbirds. The inevitable "No" would disappoint him but only momentarily. Though his initial question was startling, in retrospect I see it not as cavalier, but his way of establishing a link between his mind-set and the audience. He assumed all minds worked with the breadth, speed, and incisiveness of his own. "No" simply came as another challenge to raise us to his caliber of thinking.

As a hush fell over the eager audience, we were treated to his use of the pause. He would stand before us with a quizzical smile. What is he about to say? It must be important for him to wait so long, for him to turn and gaze out the window. Only after we experienced a twinge of anxiety that we had been lost to him in his meditation would he begin—always with something unexpected, such as "I see no one has brought paper and pen to take notes." Then there would be an audible rustle of notebooks opening, for we knew we were at the one place on earth where students of the human condition had such a rich diet, such an open forum, such sophisticated stimulation, such reinforcement of purpose, such hope that we could actually believe the mentally ill were treatable, even curable. With his intellectual vigor, unfailing honesty, his ranging curiosity, Dr. Karl never disappointed us.

What a distinguished assembly of guests he introduced to us, and always as accepted members of our family, fellow students of the human condition. What a list, the best and brightest in psychiatry, Paul Federen, Anna Freud, luminaries from all parts of the world, including Eleanor Roosevelt, Margaret Mead, Aldous Huxley, Norbert Wiener. The variety of subjects was limitless, with Dr. Karl's delight knowing no bounds at the demonstration of a research servo mechanism scooting about Hawley Hall like a mouse attempting to escape a cat. For us, it was a miraculous experience to watch Helen Keller palpate Dr. Karl's head from chin to crown and then turn to the assembled residents and through her interlocutor, Polly, proclaim, "A lofty brow." We cheered!

His style, to use a word he coined, was transcillient, amazingly blended to the immediate yet immiscible with the common. If the guest speaker, and I remember this more at symposiums and seminars, lost him or worse, bored him, his body seethed with restlessness. Seated on the Hawley Hall stage, which was used for presentations by distinguished guests but not for colloquia, he would first fidget, then pass messages, verbal and written, to people in the audience. If that did not stir the speaker to get on with the point, he would rise and adjust the microphone, though it needed precious little adjustment. In the extreme, he would simply start the question period right then and there, with little regard to where the speaker's address might have wandered.

His style colored consultations. Visiting him in his office to discuss the diagnosis of a movie-star patient might find a quarter of an hour devoted to his problem in securing proper funding from the Veterans Administration for the resident training program. There was no predicting what might occur, for in the middle of a presentation he might interrupt to offer the speaker a sweet from a box of chocolates stored in his desk's top drawer or, as reported to me by my analyst, exasperate the members of the Psychoanalytic Institute by arriving at a meeting with two quarts of strawberry ice cream and dishing it out during an intense discussion of the place of the id in the process of identification.

Again, there was nothing supercilious in his failure to "stick to business." At times it was poignant. I remember in 1953 consulting him in a Washington, D.C., hotel room. It was late at night after he had experienced a trying day of work at a professional meeting. I sought his help for a personal problem. My life was in disarray from psychological wounds experienced in the Korean War. I wished his wisdom in searching for a way to resume my interrupted career. He listened intently and then, with much feeling, began recounting his here-and-now trials and suffering with his father's, C.F. Menninger's, terminal illness. He asked us both the searching question, "What does it mean to be a good son?" Looking back I now see how my tale had touched a deep chord in his being, leaving him resonating openly and directly, his pain in concert with mine. Though not elaborate, his heartfelt advice proved all the difference for me. Dr. Karl's style was completely the man.

But I promised to tell you what I believe to be his greatest colloquium. It took place on January 15, 1981. By then I was established in Portland and though distant we maintained correspondence and visits back and forth. In 1980, our local psychiatric hospital embarked on an expansion of beds and I invited Dr. Karl to dedicate the new wing. He accepted a year in advance. He said he would and as it turned out his word was his bond.

Earlier in the morning of the 15th, he had consulted with Portland's city fathers about a new jail they were planning to erect. He arrived at the hospital somber, sore pressed by what he had heard. Once he was settled before the audience of several hundred concerned citizens he turned us into students of the human condition as he passionately addressed Portland's example of man's inhumanity to man.

Age had taken its toll on his body but not his verve. It never touched the sparkle in his eyes. He paused, as ever, and then surprised the audience with, "What kind of prison do you wish for your city?" He was unhappy with what he had heard and charged us with our part in man's inhumanity to man, with the fearful responsibility to do more than good—to be thoughtful, deep, and ceaseless in searching for meaning in the suffering of others. He led us to consider the place of forgiveness, the need for hope, compassion for the less fortunate. He dedicated us as much as the new psychiatric wing of Holladay Park Hospital.

You ask how this was Dr. Karl's finest colloquium, so far from Topeka? The fineness lies more in the circumstance than in the content.

Unbeknownst to us the President of the United States, President Jimmy Carter, had summoned Dr. Karl to be at the White House on that selfsame day. But the President's summons arrived too late. Dr. Karl had committed himself to us and our concern for the mentally ill. He would not be diverted from his commitment. He chose to speak to us rather than receive the highest civilian award of the nation, the Freedom Medal, personally, from the President of the United States.

Can any doubt this was his finest colloquium? Could there be a clearer way of establishing his soul-deep belief that the proper place for a physician is serving the sick? Could there be a better way to inform our frontline work with meaning? Could there be a more powerful example that, despite any lure of fame and fortune, our goal should be offering meaning to human suffering through scientific understanding and shared recognition?

Once again, Dr. Karl had woven seemingly disparate themes into a coherent, inspiring event. He lived his conviction that he had meaning and that each of us has a significance that we can appreciate only as we grow in mind and spirit.

The lesson of Dr. Karl's colloquia, at least for me, has been to seek meaning in the suffering that inevitably accompanies life, to seek it in my life and the lives of others. Seek meaning steadfastly, relentlessly, and always with hope.

A Psychiatrist for a Troubled World
A Book Review

For the subject of inquiry and discussion is simply and solely the sufferings of these same ordinary folks when they are sick and in pain. Now to learn by themselves how their own sufferings come about and cease, and the reasons why they get worse and better, is not an easy task for ordinary folk; but when these things have been discovered and set forth by another, it is simple.
—Hippocrates (ca 460 B.C. - ca 377 B.C.)
Ancient Medicine II

William Menninger was my teacher, my mentor. He was a man who burst into smile when we met and would throw his arms about my shoulders to give me a hug. For me, years later, his death is but yesterday. I mourn his passing. Do not expect an objective view from me.

It is a responsibility of every reviewer to either recommend or reject the book examined, and to do so on the basis of content and intent. I recommend *A Psychiatrist for a Troubled World* [1] on both counts.

The content is fine, for here is first of all a working textbook of modern psychiatry. By collecting Dr. Will's papers, the editors assembled ideas that are contemporary, pertinent, and understandable—points of reference in the day-to-day practice of the general practitioner and of the psychiatrist. No wordy flights of theory, rather practical accounts of his thoughts drawn from his broad experience. As a consultant with welfare workers, juvenile court workers, public health nurses, and colleagues, I have used for clinical teaching the series of lectures given by Dr. Will and carried in this volume as "Teaching Outlines of Psychiatry for Nurses and Attendants."

Not only is there much to be learned directly from the content, but indirectly much to be gleaned from Dr. Will's style of writing. His words flow smoothly, with the essentials every physician should master—clarity, precision, development, coherence, and the rare elixir of tempered feeling. He wrote as though it were easy, and perhaps it was, but I suspect that considered thinking and careful editing contributed to his style. Certainly his manner of presentation would enhance understanding of clinical history.

What of the intent of the editors and the author? The editors worked to honor the man and did so better than they know. Though I do not speak for myself, I know that silent tears have been shed by some, reading back through the pages to times bygone. Remembering William Menninger, through his own words, summons nobility in all of us. He was the complete physician. He knew his field; he knew his patients; he knew his community.

He became the complete physician by starting at the beginning, with details, with the microscope, with leukocytes in the spinal fluid (1923), and through the course of his life, as measured in the chronology of this book, he grew, moving always to broader views, increased responsibility, and deeper insights. The path is marked out in the table of contents: neurology in the 1920s, psychiatry in the 1930s, psychoanalysis after psychiatry, community psychiatry in the best sense of the words—first with military psychiatry in the 1940s, then moving to industrial psychiatry in the 1950s, and finally to medical statesmanship—a national voice speaking out for the mentally ill as he addressed twenty-two different state legislatures.

The course of the man toward progressively more public service contradicts the presently fashionable opinion that locates the psychiatrist socially isolated behind a couch. Dr. Will's work reveals the emptiness of the "modern discovery" that every psychiatrist must relate to his community. His career shows that for decades psychiatrists have been in the community. I know, for in 1949 I attended his seminars on social psychiatry.

The editors do more than honor Dr. Will. They contribute to his myth. Do not shrink from the idea, for nothing demeaning is intended. Rather, what is meant is myth as a great social vehicle for conveying attitudes, beliefs, and values from age to age, keeping alive the best in man. And the saga of our times is as great as the sagas of times past. Recognized or not, we are all struggling at Thermopylae and each of us has value, but our heroes are inestimable, a standard to be kept before us. As myth develops, it follows a repetitive course—first act, then anecdote, legend, and finally myth. If it is nurtured by the usage of years it becomes a saga. With the ultimate touch of genius from the poet, it becomes an epic.

The book will have contributed mightily to the early form of myth by crystallizing oral and written records into lasting form. I look to the next step—a definitive biography—largely because the editors will then have greater literary license to allow even more of the light of the man to show through.

Additional insight into his strength is gained by reading his letters. He wrote in a personal manner that carried impact. To receive a letter from him meant you had been thought about. He wrote to a defined person, you, and you knew it. The flow of these letters was phenomenal. It was not unusual, his secretary reported, for him to dictate one hundred personal letters a day. Perhaps it was outside the scope of this volume to include letters, along with a sample of the unique yearly Christmas card, but they are of value and should not be passed over in a future work. Such a biography could probably outreach *Doctors Mayo* and should match Cushing's *Life of Sir William Osler* or Jones's *Life and Work of Sigmund Freud*. Everything is here for a masterpiece of humanness, perhaps even an epic.

Truthful Tale

What of the author's intent? I can best approach that question with an anecdote, which, although possibly apocryphal, says so much about

Dr. Will that it would be true even if it never happened. The tale was related to me during my residency at the Menninger Foundation, on one of those occasions that are familiar to all physicians. Late one night there had been an emergency at the hospital, and after caring for the patient I retreated to the ward kitchen with those on night duty who could get away. Coffee and camaraderie were in order. As those late-at-night conversations often do, the talk turned to "those good old days when times were really rough," and a veteran aide spun out the following:

Back in the thirties there was a paretic patient who had a particularly well-developed hate for his doctor, a resident. The patient was six foot three and two hundred and thirty pounds of muscle, while the resident was just a little over five feet—and that a slight five feet. The patient's hate was matched by the resident's fear. The resident became so intimidated that he would only visit the patient while the patient was shrouded in his daily sedative wet-sheet pack. It became a quiet joke among the ward staff that the pack did as much for the resident as it did for the restrained patient.

One day during a bedside visit, the patient, in a frenzy of rage, burst from his restraint. The resident bolted from the room, fled across the hall, and hopped into a janitor's closet. There was barely enough space for him to crouch in the sink as he pulled the door closed behind him. The patient, in hot pursuit, picked up a chair and began breaking down the door. He had smashed the door panels apart by the time a covey of aides caught up with him.

Despite the struggle, the resident hopped out of the sink, through the broken door, scooted between the patient's legs, down the hall, out the front door, and across the lawn to the clinic office building, where he burst into Dr. Will's office crying the horrible news that Mr. X was loose and destroying the hospital. Dr. Will looked up from his desk and, after an instant's pause, commented: "Well, what are you doing here? Go take care of your patient."

Menninger's intent, in all that I have read and known of him, is to ask us, "What are we doing here?" In the warmest, friendliest, firmest manner he has asked, by his thought, by his writing, and by his actions, "What are you doing here?"

Perhaps one more anecdote can illuminate how real was his question. In the late spring of 1952, I was a Navy psychiatrist stationed with the Marine Corps at Parris Island. Late spring in that part of South Carolina is remarkably like humid midsummer in almost any other place in this country, and when word filtered down that a Presidential Fact Finding Committee on Military Manpower was shortly to arrive on the base I could not have cared less. That is, until I learned that the chairman was Dr. Will.

Again the Question

A week later, at dawn, the committee descended in their own plane, like gods in an ancient Greek drama. They were quickly surrounded by all the local brass and squired from point to point to observe the problems of inept trainees. The men in question were of low IQ, with little education, unable to speak English, socially deprived, and emotionally impaired. (One platoon had been so inept that while firing at targets on the rifle range they had shot away all the benches and drinking fountains for one hundred yards around.) Dr. Will talked with the men and their leaders and considered the problem.

Late that afternoon, he attended a reception given by the commanding general. He had heard I was on the base and asked that I be invited. The air-conditioned atmosphere was one of mutual goodwill. Bending elbows with the brass can be exhilarating. Dr. Will said a few words laudatory of the war effort and the hopes of the committee. Then he bade us goodbye, and as he left for his plane he drew me aside and asked, "What are we going to do about all these men? How are we going to make them useful?" I was dumbfounded, for he had questioned me directly. It was a while before the words sank home, "Well, what are you doing here?"

If you wish to know the honor of this man, seek out and read *A Psychiatrist for a Troubled World*. If you wish to share the honor he gave to his profession, take his work to heart and answer with your own effort his question, "What are you doing here?"

Endnotes

1. W.C. Menninger, *A Psychiatrist for a Troubled World: Selected Papers of William C. Menninger, M.D.*, ed. B.H. Hull (New York: Viking Press, 1967).

Part 7

Compassion in Shadow

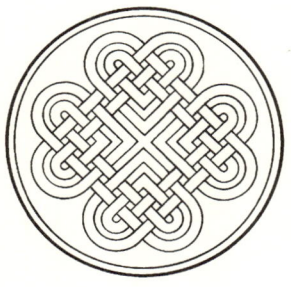

Now I find hidden somewhere in my nature something that tells me that nothing in the whole world is meaningless, and suffering least of all.
                    Oscar Wilde (1854-1900)
                        De Profundis

Overview to Part 7

In a thirst for compassion, let us make certain to taste the full glass including the dregs, residue of man's inhumanity to man. Try but a sip of the potion of compassion denied, if only to test the possibility that I may be denying your feelings.

Your personal suffering, acknowledged or unrecognized, is the precious stock that reflection ferments into soul nourishment. As passive reader, confused patient, preoccupied doctor, harassed citizen, or simply compliant human being, have you been slighted, demeaned, or hurt by this book? Has your compassion been denied? Have I, tangentially, imposed my experience and interpretation of life on you; in some way lessened your consideration of human suffering as a shared sacrament?

To understand how judgmental we can and should be in matters of personal being, let us hold a magnifying glass on how you and I relate, the better to understand the part compassion may play or fail to play in ventured humanness. Ostensibly, *Compassion's Way* reflects my unflagging respect for your sense of discovery, a premise easy to assume, difficult to judge. But then in another chamber of my heart, I may conceal personal motives closer to my bank account than your concerns. Judge my profession of shared compassion with the intuitive suspicion proffered intimacy invariably invites. Certainly, beware of tidings of unsolicited empathy announced prior to an encounter. Wisely withhold belief until experience validates your trust.

Trumpeting specious concern, Wiseman's film **Welfare** unintentionally strikes at the heart of the wisdom-in-compassion issue. With heedless insistence, a bullying know-it-all, the film floods the viewer's judgment of the nature and degree of suffering borne by the poor. Overwhelmed by a litany of social wrongs, the audience's capacity for experienced compassion is degraded into a mishmash of perverse sentimentality, "entertainment."

Reader, be suspicious should this book become an entertaining read. Any tickle of vicarious pleasure in considering the suffering of a fellow human being can be evidence of counterfeit concern. Beware of any literary form of the Genovese phenomenon, the condoning bystander.

Ms. Kitty Genovese was a young, New York woman who was attacked in front of her apartment house by a lurking, rejected lover. When she cried out for help to at least twenty neighbors, onlookers from the safety of their apartment windows, not one called the police as she was methodically beaten to death. Later, when asked why they did nothing, most explained they did not wish to be involved. Spectators in the "balcony" were so thoroughly entertained by the unfolding horror of a young woman's murder they did nothing to interrupt "the show."

We, you and I, should remain acutely aware of how I might, despite remonstrations to the contrary, mislead you into becoming a passive onlooker, a bystander beguiled by the destruction of dignity if not the person of another. As windows on our world, books as much as television and movies can insidiously fashion us into an audience entertained by trivialized human suffering. We risk our souls as a people, much as spectators of a Roman circus did, by remaking the suffering of another into vicarious entertainment: "virtual" pity.

"Entertainment" is a loaded word, derived from the French, meaning to stand between, to be uninvolved, a position that can place the viewer's moral agency at risk. The suffering of another becomes pornography when used as ersatz catharsis, a cheap response devoid of emotional commitment. If by even a glimpse of another's horror I offer you a "good" read by enabling you to distance yourself from reflecting on how that misery may resonate with your personal moral destiny, perforce I become your subtle enemy rather than trusted companion.

Since childhood is so likely to inform adulthood, consider again the little girl shoved to the end of the line, the boy with a lisp being mocked for sounding different, the bright scholar—an adolescent lass—ostracized by a covey of gossiping girls for achieving where others fail, the "dumb" kid set up as scapegoat for a teacher's unjust reprimand by a chorus of "Johnny did it!" Remember, if you will, your bystander's reaction of not wishing to be involved.

I share and respect your recollection, acknowledging how I too tolerate evil, yes, as an adult as well. How, too often, I pass by, leaving small evils unremarked, dismissed without reaction, or worse, with the vicarious satisfaction that some passing injustice is not my lot. Let us frankly share our moral vulnerabilities, mine and yours, the better to trust each other.

The memory of evil unrequited, harsh as it may be, heals as it reveals the beam in our eye. History proves a balm for those who recognize it as a window on the present.

The Tattletape Tale recounts how doctors perniciously ladle out doses of scorn from "black bottles" of indignity. I acknowledge that these "black bottles" of social poison flourish with my passive tolerance, tacit approval, in a social atmosphere sodden by a very fine drizzle of sleaze.

Marketplace of Pain and Suffering attempts to explicate the grip of economic forces on medical care, underlining the implacable power that organizations demand of physicians, even preempting professional goals.

Hold close your school yard recollections as a talisman of mercy recognized while examining the medical profession for shards of unacknowledged suffering. **Computerized Medicine** is neither a scandalous report nor banal entertainment but reinforcement in valuing patients' suffering. **Who Is Calling the Shots?** exposes a significant beam in my eye, while **Community Mental Health and Psychological Pollution** asks physicians to pause long enough to examine how their scientific facts, if not their behaviors, may implicitly displace compassionate relationships with patients.

A darker side to medical curiosity appears when good intentions are publicly construed as self-serving. Destruction of a sense of caring is laid out in **Reflections of a Director on Resigning from a Mental Health Clinic**. Here the shards of a morning dream, a fancy of my medical imagination, are examined in the stark daylight of a ruthless political world, ignorant, if not uncaring, for another's suffering.

Positioned as the medical profession is on the edge of unseemly wealth, a physician's recognition of possible self-interest is seen as politically incorrect and treated as ludicrous in **They All Laughed When I Spoke of Greedy Doctors**.

For a different view of reimbursement for medical treatment, one that deals directly with the possibility of selfish gain, **Fee for Service from the Poor** offers a touch of insight to that difficult facet of the patient-doctor relationship.

The distance of a foreign country, with the remove of an alien culture, not only permits candor about hometown practices but facilitates swallowing down the thick, sometimes unpalatable, elixir of wisdom. **The Cost of Caring** takes us to England, to the side of British nurses, doctors, administrators, dentists—well-meaning, caring people—caught in a confounding professional impasse between patients' needs and collective denial of those needs. They speak to how prolonged, unrequited exposure to aggravated human suffering against limited resources eventually exhausts their vocation to compassion. Their loss of hope in ever achieving their chosen role of personal service, their experienced despair, reminds us how caring has both personal and civic limits.

At this point, you may better understand my concern that you might see Wiseman's *Welfare* as an account of man's inhumanity rather than what it is, macabre entertainment, promiscuously scattering the viewer's attention in every direction but inward. Sorting out a significant message from its confusion of startling images calls for, among other things, precise acuity of personal values, differentiating human spirit from cultural gossip.

These shared accounts of compassion denied are intended to activate awareness of possible dereliction of personal honor, the better to recognize omissions of moral courage in your encounters with the world. Experience suggests that when drinking from the cup of wisdom, sip slowly until you have a taste for pungent reality seasoned with the spice of moral will.

Welfare
A Film Review

The end of the human race will be that it will eventually die of civilization.
                              —Ralph Waldo Emerson (1803-1882)

In the heat of battle between a welfare recipient and a caseworker, the recipient turns to her friend for reinforcement and is told, "Two plus two ain't twenty-two." I wish that Mr. Wiseman, who filmed this documentary, had a friend who had whispered into his ear, "Camera plus *verité* ain't a true picture." But then perhaps Mr. Wiseman is not interested in a true picture.

In reviewing this film I had three options: to review the content, to review what the content was not, or to review Mr. Wiseman. In any case, my advice is to avoid seeing the film. Since Zipporah Films, which produces Mr. Wiseman's films, has liked some of my remarks about some of Mr. Wiseman's fine and not-so-fine previous films, they graciously sent along a print of his latest documentary for local showing. We presented it at our neighborhood hospital after a good dose of publicity, to insure a receptive audience. About two hundred people attended, and we set to with a will. Nonetheless, at the end of reel two—we only had one projector going that evening—I stood up and announced that we were two down and three reels to go (one and a half hours more), and I wondered what the sentiment of the group might be. The vote was approximately 10 to 1 to skip reels three and four and go directly to the closing reel, number five. Admitting this hiatus, what follows is a three-fifths review.

First, why was the audience willing to forego two of the five reels? Were the viewing circumstances poor? No, admittedly there was no popcorn, but the hospital auditorium is a modern, air-conditioned building, with all the amenities for good viewing and no squalling babies. Was it because the audience was made up of a bunch of nincompoops, anxious for the good guys to get on with wiping out the bad guys? Hardly; the group was a cross section of well-motivated professionals (including caseworkers) and involved citizens, some on welfare. It was the film that turned the audience off. Why?

One reason was its horror. There was more hysterical tittering through the showing than I have heard since Olivia de Havilland writhed through *The Snake Pit*. For those who never saw that film—it was a 1948 exposé of the state hospital system, a madness of abuse and neglect. The laughter at Wiseman's documentary came in connection with the inept and helpless struggles of the welfare recipients. During the discussion that followed the film, some of the caseworkers acknowledged themselves as "laughers," accounting for their reaction as overidentification with the subjects of the film.

If overidentification is the cause for being turned off then the audience did fail the film, but I had another reaction, which was not overidentification, though I did identify with a portion of the overdramatized struggle. For my induction into the Army as a private in 1941, I had been sent to an address at 39 Broadway, in New York City, the very same place to which the hapless recipients in this film are sent; presumably the building is no longer an Army processing center but has evolved as a welfare processing center.

But let me briefly outline what *Welfare* is all about. Mr. Wiseman took his crew and cameras into a New York City welfare office and ran off a couple of miles of film in the faces and over the shoulders of the workers and recipients. The result is a tediously long record of a day in the existence of souls ground at the interface between the haves and have-nots. *Welfare* begins with long shots of dirty, cold, city streets and huddled lines of shivering people waiting outside a large building. Then follows close shots of people—black, white, yellow, and red, large and small, fat and thin—with the blank drab expression that comes with chronic waiting, having their Polaroid pictures taken for identification purposes, the "packaging" machinery for fitting humans into an inhuman system. Next are "emergency" interviews: people who lost their food stamps, or lack housing. Some look alert and some look drugged (here there was much tittering). The communication system between humans is primitive. Questions are repeated many times, and answers are given just about as frequently.

"You lost your food stamps?"
"Yes, I lost my food stamps."
"They are lost?"
"They are lost."
"Have you checked your mail box?"
"I checked the mail box and with the 'super.'"

So it goes. Some get help and some do not. Most get a runaround that anyone who has been in the military will immediately recognize as "the system."

The camera moves upstairs to the housing section on the fourth floor. It is much the same.

"Have you a certified and notarized copy of the doctor's request that you be moved to a place where your child will not be bitten by rats?"

"Ya. I have…. [etc.]"

"Well, it won't work the way it is set up. Despite what legal aid [or some other agency] says, it takes one and a half years for the building inspector to make a visit, so I will give you a note to the Social Security [or some other agency] to get you out of the place."

"Thank you, but I have been to the Social Security [or other place], and they sent me here."

Then the disclaimer that the agency is as helpless as the welfare recipient.

Some of the workers are polite, some are rude, just as some recipients are polite and some rude. Wiseman likes the combination of a hostile worker (innately mean or in a frenzy of exhaustion) and the hostile recipient (innately hostile or exasperated beyond endurance). When the camera has located this combination it goes on and on, uninterrupted by intervening supervisors, police, or lack of sufficient film in the camera magazine.

Inadvertently, the solution to these confrontations is revealed. It is the only valid solution possible when one person (a sadist) is using the system to vent his anger on another, or one person is using the system to have his self-esteem crushed (a masochist). A third person appears and offers to lift the pummeled one out of the system's routine to get resolution. In this case, a bystander recipient says, "Come on, I'll take you downstairs to see Miss Perry. She will work it out." How many times in the Army is it a sergeant in the back office of the supply room who gets the guns out to the fighting men in spite of the paperwork? In fact, General George Patton used his own money to buy parts for his tanks from Sears Roebuck to keep his outfit moving on maneuvers in the United States. But Wiseman's camera just shifts to another hostile encounter.

Please do not hear this as an apology for our present welfare system; it is not. The point here is that if you wish you can take a camera anyplace and make it look like hell. A movie tour of Europe can, at the discretion of the director, focus on the auto wrecking yards in twelve different countries, and that is what the film will say.

I voted against the two omitted reels because Wiseman was reporting trivia. It is a strange paradox when I must call the following trivia:

"My mother won't help. She told me to go hang myself."

"Who says you're pregnant? You need a doctor's certificate."

"I'm being rejected again."

"How can you save something on eleven cents?"

"You need a letter from your shrink to say you ain't crazy."

"Everybody is your boss when you are destitute."

"Bullshit, you cannot have an apartment if you are under twenty-one."

"You must sign your house over to Welfare."

"I'm not yelling, and there is no reason for you to continue to yell."

"I do not have the money to buy what I need to steal."

It can go on and on, and the film does. If I call it trivia I am in danger of indicting myself as an "inhuman, callous, rich doctor" who does not give a damn about the suffering of others. I suspect that is how Wiseman gets the critic, or at least how he might get some critics, to sit through the five reels. I am not any more inhuman for not watching this suffering than I am for not choosing to watch napalmed children on television. Man's inhumanity to man is hardly news and certainly not entertainment. But the modern media, armed with their technology, can turn any amount of suffering into trivia, as Wiseman has. He simply does not picture the real horror in the life of a welfare recipient, a particular man, a particular woman.

Merely showing battle casualty after battle casualty does little else but fill the viewer with a revulsion against war. It does nothing to help the viewer understand causes of the horror. It is not artillery brigades that cause war any more than missent Social Security checks cause destitution.

The result of the viewing, as brought out by some in the discussion after the film, was revulsion and the simplistic conclusion that "the system has got to change." If someone had entered the auditorium with a Molotov cocktail to hurl against the local welfare building, or a letter bomb to send off to the national Social Security computer, I am afraid some of the audience would have volunteered for the job. It was ancient cliché in spades: since this system won't work, "back to the drafting boards"—as if systems can ever be made human.

The horror of welfare, which cries out to be made explicit, is the belief of so many that systems care for our less-than-able siblings. Not that there should be any call for a return to the "good old days," but our welfare system was developed as an expedient of government and has remained so ever since.

Our welfare system stems from the English Poor Laws, which Parliament pushed through in the 1500s at the behest of Queen Elizabeth. She was revulsed by the sight of paupers and the reek of the dying when she rode through her realm. Contemporary lawmakers put the need for Poor Laws down to the immigration of Flemish wool workers (Vietnamese refugees will take jobs away from our people), but the grim fact was that Elizabeth's father, Henry, was at fault. He had a few political problems with another system and with a heavy hand eliminated the Catholic Church, and, with it, most of the existing eleemosynary institutions. He left the poor and sick to care for themselves, and, predictably, they did a miserable job of it, so miserable that the state was forced to pick up the bill or face a revolution.

With Poor Laws, welfare replaced charity. In the process and ever since, the giving agent has been the unfeeling, reluctant state, intent upon making people feel well (welfare), no longer a church or religious order, with the hope of engendering love (charity). The absence of the intent to love makes for the horror of welfare.

Feeling the sense of lovelessness in the film, I brought it up for discussion afterwards by remarking that we might well be looking at the future of medicine. With a state intent upon getting and keeping people well, the love implicit in the patient-doctor relationship was almost certain to be squeezed out. If I had brought up Henry VIII's destruction of the Church to protesting sixteenth-century Englishmen, I could not have been less successful. I am sure there would have been some stalwart yeomen who would have stood up and pointed out that the Church was riddled with rip-off friars and fat abbots who could not tell an act of love from a pitcher of ale. One earnest young man from this audience who identified himself as working on Walter Reuther's Committee of 100, an outfit intent upon doing over our health delivery system, cornered me after the others had left. There was no appeasing his god of systems. He could only see that a "more equal access to the health delivery system" was imperative. Was I really still thinking that the American nonsystem of health care had a future? There was no altering this "true believer's" conviction, so I quickly gave up. Men are intoxicated with systems. As Thoreau put it, "Men do not live by bread—they live by words."

Walking home I could not help thinking that a future Big Brother would be hiring, at a handsome salary, some future Wiseman to film the horrors of Big Brother's inhuman system to be shown at psychologically determined times and durations (perhaps fifteen minutes a week) so that people of a future Orwellian world might become properly aroused and then, after full and proper discharge of their packaged indignation, subside, one and all, back into the great social slough of a technological future. It was difficult for me to sleep that night not because of my thoughts about *Welfare*, but because my mind fixed on the hypocrisy implicit in a system of filming that brutalizes the audience in the name of truth.

Endnotes

Reprinted from *The Pharos* 39(Spring 1976): 74-96, with permission.

The Tattletape Tale

The younger generation is only worth as much as the goal set before it: that was Napoleon's secret of the marshal's baton in every soldier's knapsack.
—Oswald Spengler (1880-1936)
Neubau des Deutschen Reiches

Physicians treat cynicism in medicine much as they do the weather, with much talk and little action. Yet, unlike the weather, cynicism can be a predictable, constructive force, especially when used to focus moral light on an existing evil. In fact, physicians could go so far as to teach medical students positive cynicism, the examination of human values, the sharing of the self-evident truth that no thinking physician successfully completes his daily rounds without some touch of that special cast of mind, and the sharp vision of things as they are, which a proper cynic uses to clarify social values.

A Shrine to Disbelief

An example of constructive cynicism in the service of higher professional standards occurred when a shrine of disbelief in positive human values was erected on our local health science campus. It is an archway under which all students and faculty must pass, genuflecting in token of real or fancied dishonesty. Moreover, each and every one bends the knee without objection, all in thoughtless obeisance. This ritual of our conventional culture, the modern world of electronic ignorance, is so thoroughly ingrained that, as yet, none suspect, let alone protest that they are judged guilty until proven innocent.

Our shrine of guilt stands inside the door of the medical school library. It was erected when the library staff ascertained that seventeen percent of the library's books had disappeared over the previous three years. As the shrine stands, students and faculty pass beneath this steel and plastic arch bending their knees to release the polished stainless steel gate. The shrine demands acknowledgment twice, once when entering the sanctum of the library and again when leaving. Unless the shrine's requirements are fulfilled, there is a quick and certain value judgment when an alarm buzzer loudly proclaims sin to the entire library. No saints at this shrine, only sinners, for, as the name implies, the Tattletape System focuses on offenders. It has been searching every patron since the loss of six thousand volumes on the assumption that all are guilty thieves unless proven otherwise. As far as I can ascertain, aside from myself, not a soul has objected to its insinuation of dishonesty. By complete tacit approval of personal electronic surveillance, all agree, individually and collectively, that we are dishonest men and women.

The point is not that books are stolen from the library, but that students and faculty are dishonored and no one protests. A potential for thievery exists in all men, but much more potent and much more prevalent is mankind's potential for bondage, particularly for contemporary electronic bondage. No, the horrendous point is that being an honorable man or woman apparently has become secondary to being a physician. Developing and maintaining a personal ethic seems incidental to accumulating books and book learning. At best, personal moral excellence appears as a metaphysical abstraction without visible relationship to collegiate lives, certainly as exemplified by the failure of faculty and student body to react to the Tattletape System.

Whatever Happened to the Honor System?

Self-deception about moral issues seems almost expected, for when I shared my disgust at kowtowing to the Tattletape System's shrine with the library staff, I was asked, "But, what can we do? The only alternative is personal search." I grunted while the rejoinder continued: "To post somebody at the door to check every person as they leave is demeaning. It would be personally degrading to them." I grunted again, no recognition of electronic degradation here nor of any alternative leading to an elevating experience. Inherently, I am suspicious and diffident about all systems; yet, there was a time when an honor system was at least debatable. Who now is interested enough in honor to discuss it? It is lock-step conformity with technology.

Though failing to establish a dialogue concerning honor may tempt the instructor of medical morals to leave his passive listeners with the consolation of philosophy, a prod or two from cynicism's gifted younger brother, stoicism, may stir the students if not the faculty. Students, in your health and vigor, are passing grades your only goal? Have you abandoned thoughts of freedom? Books were chained to the walls in the repressive scholastic world of the Middle Ages. Do I hear someone murmur, "Well, at least that was better than the Nazis who burned books"? Ugh, where are the scholar's moral and political ideals? Are ideals no more than a bookworm's dream feasting on the guts of knowledge and adding nothing to the dignity of man? Is liberty too expensive, and like the books, do students feel safest when linked in conforming electronic modules, when channeled to some distant moralizing computer, when playing children's games in a world without moral maturity?

Yes, you moral sluggards, you have nothing to lose but your apathy! Your failure to confront the Tattletape System means the malignant possibility that future patients will be treated as real or potential deviates from some crazy, depersonalized system of health. Future patients will be regulated and checked, not for stealing, but for physiological or psychological noncompliance. Then it will not be the librarians who are the guardians of the gates, but today's students, tomorrow's practitioners of some Tattlesick System. Are medical students learning to become healers or unthinking agents of compliance and prescribed pleasure—the custodians of some future Tattletale Drug System?

Life With Dignity

It is not just cynicism that I suggest students consider, but the result of constructive thought through cynicism. Then, as the student becomes a practicing physician, this penetrating appurtenance of the philosophy of medicine will also be part of a philosophy of life. So much talk of death with dignity. Does the patient have to be at death's door for the subject to be broached? How often do the faculty and students consider life with dignity? I mean aloud, direct consideration, a dialogue between student and patient about dignity and grace based on a lived philosophy. Is the student taught to treat his patient by relying on his own judgment or depending on the rules of the system? And if he relies on his own judgment, will the patient have a physician who knows the value of freedom? Only as the student evolves a personal philosophy of medicine can human values prevail. Diogenes searched the streets of Athens for an honest man. Patients search our wards and clinics for a fully valued physician. Students, listen carefully to constructive cynicism's admonition that comes with experienced intelligence, "Physician, examine your values well."

Endnotes

Reprinted from the *Journal of the American Medical Association* 239(1978): 621-622, with permission. Copyrighted 1978, American Medical Association.

Marketplace of Pain and Suffering

> *My God, ny God, look upon me; why hast thou forsaken me: and art so far from my health, and from the voice of my complaint?*
>
> —Psalms 22:1

As I was returning from a visit with a friend convalescing at home, his continuing complaint set in motion a cascade of reflections about the present state of health care delivery.

My friend, a seventy-eight-year-old retired attorney, had spent a week in a local medical center undergoing diagnostic evaluation of persistent weakness which turned out to have its source in an intestinal malignancy. He recounted how he had but one inadequate bowel movement during the hospitalization, yet despite reporting his condition, was discharged with the advice that his bowels would empty once he was home. At home his discomfort grew with the passage of little but time. On the second day home his distress necessitated calling in a visiting nurse who to the patient's gratitude and satisfaction physically removed a fecal impaction. At home his complaint was no longer considered irrelevant or insignificant, but responded to as pertinent and important.

While listening to him, in my mind's eye I paged through his hospital chart which in all probability recorded everything that medical science had done, everything except allay the patient's real and immediate suffering. Subsequently, my thinking made an odd association between his condition and that of the nation's ongoing yet unsuccessful national health care debate, painful obstruction of a natural process to the point of impaction.

Like the hospital, the nation's leaders in politics, economics, and health professions fail to pay heed to the public's pain as they busily concentrate on the nation's malignant health care cost crisis. The parallels open a possible perspective on both my friend's and the nation's problem, the replacement of the marketplace of pain and suffering by a commodities market in health care. Focusing on the marketplace of pain and suffering clarifies and perhaps offers a path to conciliation among contesting parties in a renewed and possibly successful health care debate.

It took some time to assemble my thoughts into passable logic that starts with how experts account for the diminishment of the national health care debate of 1994. Each of the experts' points—unfettered choice, promoting health maintenance organizations (HMOs), collective versus individual rights, research and education, and intergovernmental relationships—is important, yet the list omits a fundamental problem the public seeks to debate, the place of bodily pain and personal suffering in health care.

The marketplace of pain and suffering has operated since ancient cultures first proposed propitiating their gods through sacrifice of a valuable object or person. Abraham's willingness to sacrifice Jacob to Jehovah serves as a surpassing example of the high price placed on such transactions. In the exchange, the degree of expected reward of relief from pain and suffering is proportional to the value of the gift. During the Middle Ages an active, open market in solacing pain and suffering, including published price lists, developed when the Church commercialized the granting of indulgences.

There is little new about the marketplace of pain and suffering as it embraces health care with the patient's demand for solace and support from medical science. In return the patient offers to pay for the health care commodity, the skill and experience supplied by the doctor, nurse, and/or technician. Until recently, the marketplace was governed by a tacitly established rate of exchange, "usual and customary," an amount intended to afford providers with a comfortable, though not extravagant, lifestyle.

Fifty years ago, medical education made little direct reference to the marketplace of pain and suffering and none to the commercial health care market. It was a time when medical advertising was illegal and my training tacitly directed me towards the marketplace of pain and suffering with the implicit admonition to do well by doing good.

I was taught there were two components to quality service, the science and art of medicine. Science addressed patients' pain while the art of medicine addressed their suffering. By offering the patient an immediately accountable and understandable commodity, health care services, the competent physician proved proficient in both science and art.

In the last fifteen years, the concept of a marketplace for pain and suffering has faded from the minds of most participants to be replaced by a preoccupation with cost of care. The ensuing uproar, sometimes reaching hysterical proportions, has insurance companies spending vast sums advertising the advantages of the evolving system of cost effectiveness while large industrial corporations cry havoc over a professed inability to survive because of excessive health care costs, and together they tout the need for a commercial marketplace for health care. Consequently, the marketplace of pain and suffering is being recast, if not replaced, by a new concept of exchange between patient and healer.

While focusing on the patient's bodily pain and psychic suffering, the marketplace of pain and suffering recognizes the realities of economic and political forces but holds them secondary to the process of healing. The present stewards of health care no longer are healers but employees of organizations whose mission is economic return and political viability. Their mission statements do not deny the existence of patients' pain and suffering but hold them secondary to the pursuit of their organizations' primary goal, profit.

While self-interest of some of the former stewards of health care set them to exploiting their economic advantage, the majority of physicians entered the marketplace of pain and suffering professing to offer yet another element, their vocation, the need to be needed through service to others.

In the past the complete physician was expected to use vocation prudently to balance elements of economics, politics, culture, and technical skills when addressing the patient's pain and suffering together with the community's concern for health. Vocation no longer is audible in the health care debate, now a faint murmur in the hubbub over the cost of care.

Predictably, the marketplace of pain and suffering places relatively high value on vocation, as displayed in the healer's proficiency of professional skills and ability to relate to a unique and understandable human being, the patient. The latter point matches consumers' implicit and high demand for recognized dignity when entering the marketplace as a vulnerable patient. This agreed upon marketplace commodity, the patient-doctor and/or the nurse-patient relationship, is presently being "downsized," though not excluded, by health industry organizations operating in the health care marketplace.

A few simple examples of how the present commercial health care marketplace devalues and constricts, if not obstructs, vocation-directed behavior of doctors and nurses lends understanding to the pervasive effect of marketplace motives on patients. Nurses, never noted for overpayment, now face the prospect of decreased pay coupled with a loss of vocation. The change goes by such names as "reskilling" or "reengineering" and results from efficiency studies of hospital nurses making rounds. Their professional activities have been broken down into a set of tasks, each task demanding its distinct level of training, skill, and judgment. The registered nurse (RN) is expected to be proficient in the full armamentarium of high professional skills—detecting a failing heart by subtle signs of cardiac decompensation; moderate level skills such as administering medications in a timely and appropriate fashion; low level skills such as knowing how to make a patient comfortable in a hospital bed.

Administrators see economy in reducing the number of fully trained nurses by delegating lesser skills to lesser paid employees, the licensed practical nurse (LPN) and the certified nursing assistant (CNA). Understandably, no organization wishes to pay nursing salaries for housekeeping duties, but as the nurse is gradually removed, distanced from the patient to become a personnel officer, overseeing a work gang, nurses' sense of vocation perceptibly diminishes. Then the nurse is restricted to the most critically ill patients with time for others only as administrative duties permit. Consequently, the patient, as my friend can attest, no longer has a healing nurse to communicate his pain to, only a surrogate who will "pass the word along."

Similar distortions of vocation target the physician. One example suffices: the requirement for the practitioner to limit examination time with outpatients to a standardized norm. This stricture forces doctors, despite any unique needs of the patient, to limit the patient-doctor contact during medical encounters. In some cases the allocated time is eight minutes, in others perhaps twenty. During that period of time the doctor reviews the patient's record, listens to the patient's account, assesses the need with a focused physical examination, prescribes a course of action, and responds to the patient's questions. Meanwhile, the office nurse has been instructed by the administrator to knock on the door once the "normal" time limit has elapsed. Doctor reskilling is similar to nurse reskilling: profits up, vocational esteem down.

These recent marketplace changes frequently confound patients. They find upon entering the new marketplace that the initial question is not about their medical complaint, but about their economic status of eligibility. The next discordance arises upon discovering the number of ancillary people, nurses, and business personnel employed to limit access to the doctor. The change that provokes patients most is limited time with the doctor, often seen as inadequate to discuss their plight. For the patient, fears of pain and suffering are converted by the new marketplace into fear of the health delivery system itself.

The consequent level of confidence the public holds for the medical profession may be measured indirectly by the increasing incidence of malpractice suits and directly by opinion polls. Perhaps coincidental, but certainly parallel with the development of the commodities health care marketplace, public confidence slipped from 73 percent in the 1960s to 22 percent in 1993. Yet another measure of public dismay with medical care can be measured by the 10.3 billion dollars spent out of pocket by patients for alternative therapies that minister to their pain and suffering, compared with 23.5 billion spent out of pocket on conventional medical care.[1] Here is a clear case of patients voting with their feet. Taken together, patient, nurse, and doctor experience a profound loss of shared trust.

Nor do the reasons for the diminished trust lie with a shift in personnel, medical philosophy, or unreasonable patient demands but with the elimination of vocation-directed service within the present marketplace. Restructuring, explained by proponents of the commercial health care marketplace as an economy of expanding scale and necessary efficiency, is actually an implacable process of subordinating human values to system demands.

It is too easy and wrong to cast the present stewards of the health care marketplace as unfeeling mercenaries. In fact, they are fellow human beings who bleed when cut, sorrow at loss. In the main they are individuals who wish to feel they contribute something good to the world. Nor are they opponents or villains but individuals carrying out the mission of their organization, much as dedicated members of clinics, churches, and schools carry out their organizations' missions.

However, as noted, the present purveyors of health care have a significantly different mission from that of the former stewards. Theirs is primarily economic profit in the process of curing patients. Their idea of doing well is driving out inefficient competitors by efficient methods that assure sustained profits for their stockholders. Nor is there anything remarkable in the commonplace pursuit of profit except as it refashions the marketplace of pain and suffering of human beings into a commercial marketplace, similar to that for shoes or automobiles, a marketplace which ignores overarching needs of customers.

The reason for the failure lies in an elemental contradiction between the two marketplaces. The present one deals in "hard," hands-on products, which can be measured and controlled. Though the former marketplace also deals in "hard" products, it has a place for "soft" ones, pain and suffering, as well. However, the production of "soft" products frustrates the new stewards, for "soft" commodities prove too variable and individual to standardize or quantify for "bottom line" evaluation.

An example of the present marketplace omission of a "soft" product is found in the commercial vendors' response to the frequent health care market demand for relief of anxiety. The anxious patient suffers from a condition that defies easy quantification. Unlike appendicitis, the diagnosis and treatment of anxiety reactions do not fit the economic discipline of efficient organizations, first numbers, then accounting, followed by control. Unlike an appendectomy, a "hard" product where an offending organ is surgically removed from a passive patient, treatment for anxiety reactions involves *patients* in altering their lifestyle, sometimes in a profound way. However, treatment for anxiety reactions, as innumerable psychiatrists will attest, is turned into a "hard" product by management fiat to efficiently remove the symptom through pharmacological means rather than treat the cause through difficult-to-account-for investigative counseling leading to insight. Too often, anxious patients are given a prescription for an antianxiety drug and sent on their way, for though mental health services are available in the contract, healing is not.

A subtle process of altering accepted language accompanies market restructuring. "Health care" becomes a noun designating a commodity, no longer a verb for compassionate care. The same implacable commercial jargon relentlessly translates "doctor" into "provider" and "patient" into "consumer." Nor is the change limited to language, for concepts and behaviors are also refashioned by Procrustean commercial standards.

The primary strategy of restructuring uses vast capital reserves of giant corporations to drive small retailers of health care from the marketplace. Some health care corporations go so far to control the marketplace by purchasing schools of nursing and medicine. The shrinking space left in the marketplace for cottage industry providers, fee-for-service doctors, is on the periphery, that is, rural and "boutique" practices. The restructured marketplace increasingly offers mass products for mass buying, HMOs marketing to large employers at reduced prices. The wholesale buyer is promised reduced prices, resulting in downsizing for health care workers with the elimination of many vocation-oriented services, including eliminating hospital chaplains and social workers.

The customer, the potential patient, is as well refashioned for better control through product advertising, billboards proclaiming how "We Really Care" at a local HMO, and television spots inviting pregnant women to inspect the new, redecorated obstetrical suites, complete with Jacuzzis.

Powerful refashioning appears in contractual agreements. Insensibly, the marketplace of pain and suffering recedes from public consciousness as the future care of patients is determined by marketplace "decision makers." These are the agents of employers, often benefits officers, who bargain for their employees' health plan. By displacing the patient as buyer and doctor as seller, the industry agent bargains for the most prudent, if not cheapest, insurance package from the seller, a health insurance organization sales staff. As bystanders, the patient, nurse, and doctor continue to confront pain and suffering as they have in the past, but their concerns have less and less influence on the quality of care they pursue. Authentic patient choice has been eliminated.

The Overall View

When the 103rd Congress ground down to gridlock on health care reform, the health care industry set out to establish the present "competitive" health care marketplace. At that point the government's role in health reform became peripheral to profit forces in a trillion dollar industry. "Downsized" government is now but one among many purchasers, largely for the poor and the elderly.

Despite profound changes, the marketplace of pain and suffering will never disappear. Even in the dark years of Soviet domination I discovered an active marketplace for pain and suffering operating *underground* in Russia. This will not occur here, for like the sick in the People's Republic of China, our pained and poor patients are likely to increasingly resort to nonscientific, alternative care with its ability to respond to their basic demand.

The profession's task is to articulate the marketplace's responsibility to meet fully patients' needs with a beyond-profit, moral understanding of scientific, humane health care. We need to explore a program of "Prudent Consumer Meets Prudent Provider" that leads to trust through consensus of values. The issue of quality of care is to be reframed as an issue of quality of life not of contract.

Real and present dangers exist if policies encourage ruthless competition, short-term profits rule, and unaccountable wealth accumulates through new technologies independent of their place in the social and health scheme of society. Civic, industrial, and professional leaders need broad support in recognizing that the highest rewards are long-term, achievable to the degree all parties trust each other.

It is essential for participants in the delivery of health care to understand and articulate that the dynamic of profit exists within a larger context, defined by the public's values. To make the point, physicians must reach the public in an organized manner, clarifying through public discussion the unrecognized demand for humane care. Then, in a spirit of collaboration rather than confrontation, these findings become values understandable and, most important, considered carefully by all concerned.

Short of religion, the ultimate reality for human beings is death, a feared destination many approach along a thorny path of pain and suffering.

Against the present delivery of health care this truth demands a new strategy for identifying public values in the delivery of health care. In turn, the findings will undergird a functional marketplace of pain and suffering for healing as well as curing patients, their "voice of complaint" heard and responded to.

Endnotes

1. D. Eisenberg, R. Kessler, C. Foster, F. Norlock, D. Calkins, and T. Delbanco, "Unconventional Medicine in the United States," *New England Journal of Medicine* 328(4): 250.

Computerized Medicine

Expedit esse deos, et, ut expedit, esse putemus.
—Ovid (43 B.C. - ? A.D.)
Ars amatoria
(It is convenient that there should be gods, and that we should think they exist.)

Graciousness, rather than insight, characterized an invitation from Dr. Stephen Yarnall to attend the Washington/Alaska Regional Medical Plan's Conference on Medical Communications. Dr. Yarnall, professor of medicine at the University of Washington, put together a smack-dab, up-to-date to-do on satellite communications, remote health care for manned spacecraft, emergency communications, health data storage, two-way television communication, and remote electrocardiograph (ECG) monitoring networks. Unfortunately, all I had to contribute was the angst of a solo practitioner, a voice crying in the electronic wilderness.

But, then, the setting was superb—the Seattle Science Center, that startling window on the future. The site of the Seattle World's Fair appeals to me, for it was there in 1962 that I discovered *the* religion of the twentieth century. The insight seemed to burst from the blue but, as most insights, was simply a case of stumbling upon the obvious.

While strolling along the serene, cloistered walks about the fountained court and through the towering, white arches of the Science Center, a religious feeling gradually replaced the excitement of the moment. As

I wandered past altar after altar, each shining computer—with flashing, electric, votive lights, spinning prayer wheels of memory drums, and triptych of hardware—reinforced the sense of church. Suddenly, it dawned on me that the new idols were being worshipped as the old. For an awful moment, I was tempted to call down a latter-day Moses from the slopes of Mount Rainier to smash these chrome and plastic idols, these baals that measure the price of everything yet know the value of nothing. No question, the helix threatens to replace the cross.

Fold, Spindle, or Mutilate

However, I immediately squashed the idea. My place is not in the holy flames of a modern heretic's bonfire. Hallelujah, brother! Let the record show that I neither fold, spindle, nor hack but join in the sacred chant, "Hail to IBM, Microsoft, and DNA—godfathers to us all." Clearly, my return to the Science Center was a nostalgic retreat to wrestle with the devil of ignorance.

Dr. Yarnall, who moderated the conference, has a fine, direct manner, and his open smile is only faintly shaded by the lined tracery which comes in a man's career when he realizes it is not the world he has by the tail but a tiger. Dr. Yarnall's tiger is a royal Bengal beauty answering to the name of "Computerized Medicine"—the kind of beast which may well take a lifetime to tame.

The papers followed swiftly, one upon the other, with the same invariable preamble to each and every one: "This advance in technology is intended to assist the doctor in his work and in no way to interfere with the patient-doctor relationship." Why the repeated protestation? Like Gertrude, once Queen of Denmark, methought they didst protest too much.

"Confidential" Reply

My suspicions were heightened, with a whiff of something rotten in the state of Washington, by a "humorous" remark from an anonymous avant-garde spokesman of information control who interrupted Dr. Edward Rosenow, executive vice president of the American College of Physicians. Dr. Rosenow was illustrating the physician's increasing drive toward self-improvement by citing the college's experience with self-assessment tests. When the college expected two thousand physicians to take the tests, twelve thousand responded. At this point, the man of the future "humorously" interjected from the floor that these tests were extremely useful if corrected by a computer. The computer could not only send the doctor a "confidential" reply but simultaneously supply the college with a breakdown on his performance. No laughter from me on that, simply a mental note to do my own correcting on any future self-assessment tests.

The clincher for my suspicions came with a slide used to illustrate the last paper of the day. The slide was a cartoon, in remarkably bad taste, of naked patients strung upon a conveyor belt carrying them to an automated hand that was prearranged to dip into K-Y jelly and perform a rectal examination, with a readout from an elaborate machine. At that point, doubt left my mind about who was getting what with the electronic wave of the future.

Lest it seem ill winds blew from but one quarter, the tale of a biophysicist bears repeating. During the preprandial cocktail party, a biophysicist elaborated on his difficulty in appreciating the sacredness of the patient-doctor relationship. A friend of his, a service engineer with a medical technology company, had installed an elaborate ECG machine for a local cardiologist. A day or two later, the technician received an irate phone call from the physician, who berated him because the "lousy" machine could do no more than draw a straight line. The cardiologist fumed and demanded instant action, since he was in the middle of an important examination.

The technician immediately rushed to the doctor's office only to discover that the machine was indeed straightlining. Starting with the stylus, the technician began working his way back through the system searching for the trouble. Each component checked out perfectly; so he followed the lead wire off the machine through the wall to the patient's examining room. When checked, the lead contacts with the patient were OK, but the patient turned out to be remarkably cold, an input problem, since the patient was dead. Here was no heartwarming tale of the patient-doctor relationship; rather, it was a chilling case of the doctor-organ relationship, with the patient lost as a person. Luckily, dinner was served before I could reluctantly and honestly voice my despair for a physician turned zealot.

The theological theme of the meeting surfaced again at the delicious dinner when Mr. William Holm, curator of Northwest Coast Indian Art at the University of Washington, gave a slide presentation on communication through Indian art. Following his educated eyes into a profound world of medical lore was particularly revealing. The shaman's green bug rattles for communication, his carved, black boxes for the storage of secret knowledge, his antennae-like, grizzly clawed headdress for contact with the spirit world were all together a harmonious counterpoint to the melody of the conference. There is simply nothing like the patient-doctor relationship to bring out the magic in man. For a few minutes, the persuasive spirit of this lost culture had me considering the purchase of an elk-hide apron, fringed with puffin-bill rattles, rather than buying a more improved computer for the office.

A panel discussion the next day attempted to summarize the proceedings, but, in my opinion, the task was too great. Though unannounced, two agenda competed for attention throughout the conference: one, communication of medical data; the other, storage of medical data. The topics proved so disparate in content and direction that a full morning's work by even the most acutely perceptive experts in the world could not have synthesized them.

However, the panel did a fine job with the communication of data by pointing out how physicians have resisted any change in style since time immemorial. The present resistance to new techniques in communicating data parallels in nature, if not in time, the introduction of earlier instruments of medical communication.

The stethoscope is as good an example as a remote ECG monitoring network for the resistance and confusion stirred up by a new data collection device. The thoroughly modern physician of 1820 was swift to add Laennec's wooden tube to his armamentarium, while his conservative colleague never allowed this "work of the devil" to come between him and his patient. Even into the twentieth century, some diagnosticians disdained mechanical devices for auscultation insisting that the silk handkerchief was the only proper "instrument" to place upon the patient's chest before directly applying the doctor's ear. Techniques of data communication still, and probably always will, have to contend with the physician's classic resistance to change.

However, the storage of data appears to be a very different matter. Unlike communication, where the autonomy of the medical ethic is unquestioned, the new medical data banks have an ethic which is unlike any previous medical innovation. They stand outside the medical ethic.

Code of Values

Dr. E.R. Gabrieli, an expert on medical records from Buffalo, New York, made this point, but the audience failed to respond. He described his role in developing a code of values for the emerging profession of computer technicians. The code is forming with little help from the medical profession. His attempts to enlist the aid of the American Medical Association have come to naught, though sources there tell me that they, too, are wrestling with this ever so important and complex problem. Whatever the reason, the serious problem of extending the medical ethic over data storage banks goes unresolved.

The immense computers of the Department of Health, Education, and Welfare are under the government's ethic (that is, the party in office), while the vast, central insurance company computer, which can, without your knowledge, strike you off as a double risk for simply failing to follow through on an insurance application, has its ethic firmly entrenched in *caveat emptor* ("let the buyer beware").

I am grateful to the Seattle conference for making clear to me, if not to others, the horrendous problem of medical data storage. It is vastly different from the jurisdictional and territorial battles precipitated by new techniques of medical data communication. Medical data storage problems are a magnitude greater and are not to be solved by political manipulation. Our fundamental philosophy of individual medical care is on the line with this problem. Knowledge is power, and hard knowledge about specific people is power over those people despite a thousand disclaimers.

He who controls the medical data storage banks will control the health care processes, for he who controls what information enters into a decision controls the decision. At the Seattle conference, it suddenly became clear that a new philosophy of human interrelatedness in health care was being considered by the introduction of new agents into the *decision*-making process.

When it comes to the control of medical data, this is not an extension of the stethoscope. It is an extension of the medical records library and can come to turning over the medical records of all the physicians' offices and the hospitals throughout the country to industry and government. With the present trend in computer programming, the physician of the future may have as much chance of getting and keeping the records of a patient as a British general practitioner now has of following his patient's condition once hospitalized.

Medical Data Storage Banks

Again, the illustration may sound jurisdictional, but it is ethical. Unlike the British National Health Service hospital, which is run by specialist physicians, the medical data storage banks will be run by computer technicians, good people, perhaps, but versed in controlling flow through a system, not in the art of helping individuals into, through, and out of this world.

The computer technician has wrapped himself in the ultimate scientific illusion, verging on an article of faith, if he believes that he can treat the *content* of his medical storage system as a simple scientific object, much as a bacteriologist treats a tuberculosis bacillus in a test tube. Content is not just a byte (electronic lingo for that part of a message packet which contains eight binary bits and is processed by the computer as a unit) that the technician has in his storage system. No, what he has in there is human nature; the most contrary, logic-defying, exasperating, and indispensable part of keeping us all human, and, hopefully, humane.

Apparently, the technician and the doctor-technician do not want to know, feel, or believe they have encapsulated a direct extension of a human being. In contrast to believing, they wish to have their belief affirmed, for then they can play out a power game with those who believe the medical record is an extension of the individual. The technician's response is predictable, "Well, Doctor, you are right, of course, but in time we will quantify your 'handholding' information as well," but all the time he is thinking or has literally been saying to me in Portland, "After we outlive the present generation of doctors, we will train the new ones to fit our computer logic."

Clearly, the time is close at hand when the physician must relate primarily to the computer and only secondarily to the individual patient. Little adjustment appears necessary, since the patient and the computer are becoming synonymous. The control of the computer is in the hands of the technician who does not want to know, feel, or believe that he has power and consequent responsibility. How could he sleep nights if he knew he had spun out a system that ensnares us all?

Perhaps it was asking too much of any single conference to wrestle with the enormous problem of the ethics of medical data storage. However, it is not a new subject, for the British, with their elegant sensitivity to individual rights, have already proposed that personal information become legal property and receive the full protection of the law. They are also asking that medical data banks be licensed and have integrity officers, much as mines have safety officers. No doubt about it, the subject needs a thorough airing.

These thoughts were much on my mind as I drove home from the conference, and as I crossed over the mighty Columbia River from Washington into Oregon, they began to fall into commonsensical order. Reaching secure ground, I again knew that no matter how efficient the great new sacred Interstellar-National-Computerized-Therapeutic-United States of American-Community-Health-Delivery-System might become, there just is never *ever* going to be a substitute for the simple satisfaction, yes, joy, of patient and physician talking together.

Endnotes

Reprinted from *Prism* 1 #6(1973): 9-11, 48-49, with permission. Copyrighted 1973, American Medical Association.

Who Is Calling the Shots?

Give me librium or give me meth
—Graffiti scrawled on a Greenwich Village wall

There is no sense dissembling or fancying it up, I have some harsh things to say about the doctor-drug firm relationship. Relating to drug firms has been a longtime problem for me and I gather for some others in the medical profession as well. Looking back over the years, I can remember experiences with drug houses which sent my blood pressure high enough to merit a dose of intravenous Valium. I am not talking of the simple inanity of finding a tin oil can in the morning mail containing some medication intended, as the brochure announced, "to oil up the joints" of my arthritis patients. The long-departed Senator Kefauver set the style for media-highlighted congressional investigations which document such minor shenanigans. What catches in my craw are the major encroachments on my ethical relationship with my patients.

One flare-up should serve as an example. Since I am afflicted with strong judgments, prone to somatic expression, and am often at a loss for that dispassionate calm of the confirmed bystander, when I received a set of recordings of classical music from Pfizer Laboratories with some propaganda about "tranquil" Sinequan, I froze, heart, soul, and body. The timing did it, for the recordings arrived precisely as I ushered a deserving woman from my office for whom I had just written a prescription for Sinequan. It was what she needed, a sedative antidepressant effect which might take enough of the sting out of her nerves to allow her to think yet not befuddle her. The prescription was a little hard on her purse. Not impossibly hard, but expensive enough for the two of us to recognize that she would check the cost against her budget. The synchronization of the prescription and the unsolicited gift made a "cause and effect" conclusion inevitable. My patient was buying me pleasure along with her medication. As soon as I had the opportunity, I called the detail man and asked him to drop me from his firm's mailing list. He assured me it would be done.

As happens, it was not done and when I received yet another recording in the series I put a call in for the president of Pfizer and had a brief and pointed discussion with his executive assistant. A week later a polite and forthright letter showed up from the president thanking me for the call and stating that he had immediately directed his assistant, the man I had spoken with, to visit the corporation owning the computer which controlled deliveries and have my name removed from its innards the same day. The action pleased and surprised me, for on being expunged from that electronic genie I subsequently ceased to receive about a pound of unnecessary mail a day. Evidently the computer controlled more than one account and out of spite or idiocy, severed me from all the pharmaceutical corporations in the country.

This example is not one of the harsh things I have to say about the doctor-drug firm relationship. It is simply to illustrate my sometimes feelings. Not all my feelings toward drug firms are negative. Some gifts which have come my way, Frank Netter's anatomical drawings, for instance, which the Ciba Corporation sent me when I was a student, helped me as no other illustrations could to visualize the universe that is the human body.

It comes to mind too that yet another gift from a drug firm helped and in a most unpredictable way. When I graduated from medical school, too long ago, Mr. Eli Lilly sent a copy of Sir William Osler's *Aequanimitas* to me and each of my classmates. Mr. Lilly's faded letter of congratulations is still folded into the first page of this book that has seen some strange voyages. Perhaps the strangest began late one night when, as the resident with the duty, I was called to help a panic-stricken patient. She was a young nurse, a patient on a closed psychiatric ward, with whom I was unacquainted. She was terrified, believing that she was about to die. Earlier in the evening she had been given a sedative, which had not acted, at least not as planned, for it increased her restlessness. Following standing orders, the medication was repeated and the effect, an idiosyncratic reaction which happens to a significant number of patients, excited her even more. When I arrived she was sitting bolt upright looking as if she expected a bomb to go off under her bed. I cleared the room of attendants, turned off the overhead lights, and in the subdued glow of the bedside lamp sat down to find out who she was and what she expected from life. Gradually as we talked, and how it came about I do not know; vaguely I remember she recounted that she came from Canada, from near the birthplace of Sir William Osler. I shared my fondness of *Aequanimitas* and, as she had not read it, I spun out why, as much as I could easily recollect. Later, I realized, I must have been repeating what some parent had once done for her years before, only then with a fairy tale. She went to sleep and the next morning she was still sleeping when I made rounds, so rather than disturb her, I left my copy of *Aequanimitas*, which I had brought along, on her bedside table.

I never saw her again and probably would have forgotten the incident, since I had replaced that copy of Sir William's classic with another, if a package had not arrived in the mail years later. It contained the book, only how it had changed. She had carefully rebound it by hand, tooling a beautiful design with my initials across a soft morocco cover. Inside was a brief note of thanks tucked alongside Mr. Lilly's letter. Ah, what wonderful medicine he had given me to prescribe. How could I be anything but grateful to both such generous benefactors.

But I digress, for I wish to say some harsh things about the doctor-drug firm relationship. An encounter with Geigy Pharmaceuticals threw it all into perspective. Mr. Robert Elsner, the enterprising executive director of our county medical society, mentioned that Mr. Gerald McCutcheon of the Geigy concern had suggested that we participate in a symposium for the local doctors. My natural suspicions immediately surfaced, but then if it would help patients I was for it. Over a period of months a correspondence developed in which Mr. McCutcheon offered more and more, carrying the plans for the symposium along. He suggested many topics but left the determination to me, Depression Accompanying Family Crises. He suggested speakers yet left the selection to me. He arranged for the hall, for the reception, for the transportation, and honorariums of the faculty, for the announcements, for the tickets, for every detail. My suspicions were acute yet controlled.

When he flew into town before the symposium this pleasant man was concerned about the complex coordination of the slides, speakers, recordings, every detail of the mechanics of the occasion, down to the proper temperature for the meeting hall. My suspicions remained, though muted by the natural anxiety generated by my role as symposium moderator. The symposium came and went. By many accounts it was a success, yet my suspicions remained unresolved: What is in it for Geigy?

There were no detail men hawking Tofranil in the halls, no profusion of colorfully lettered ballpoint pens, no Geigy balloons for the kiddies, no well-placed cards in the program suggesting that Geigy had the answer to depression and would be ready to call at the "doctor's convenience" to explain the value of their miracle drug. In fact, the only evidence of Geigy's role in the whole affair was a brief statement at the bottom of the program, acknowledging their sponsorship, and their expressed thanks to me and other speakers for sharing our thoughts with so large and thoughtful a group of people concerned with the care of patients.

Geigy's representatives never did say what was in it for them, they were too busy making sure we could say what we wished and the audience could hear what they wanted to. In fact, when it was all over and Mr. McCutcheon had returned across the country to Ardsley, New York, the only thing left to be cleaned up was a mass of dirty, misplaced suspicions in my mind.

Once again I had the dreary job of figuring out what had gone wrong with my thinking, so a few days later I asked Mr. Elsner, the spark that started the productive fire, what want wrong. For a few minutes he did not understand my question.

"Why, they are gentlemen. Perhaps you could call it goodwill. I can not say for them but as I see it they are genuinely interested in helping doctors get on with their work."

He realized I was still bemused, "Oh, I see what you are thinking of, the color TV sets that doctors get. Swilling down the free booze on hospitality trips to get the doctors to prescribe their brand of drug. Reputable drug firms are not interested in that."

And now I began to see the harsh side of the doctor-drug firm relationship. If the drug firms are not interested in ladling out free booze how come it gets ladled out? The answer is atrocious. No one had to spell it out. I figured it out for myself. The free goodies (or in some cases, baddies) which have nothing to do with patient care, are given because they are expected, expected by doctors. It is the doctor who literally carries a shopping bag through the convention exhibits to fill his wants, not the patients' needs. Are the drug firms to say "No" to doctors' expectations? If the doctor sends one hundred carbons of filled prescriptions of a drug to the firm that manufactures it and says he expects a color television set to keep up his work, should the drug firm question his treatment?

The ugly analogy finally became clear to me when I reflected on Oregon's law that makes both parties liable in an act of prostitution. Unfortunately, for too long I have been thinking that the proper treatment for the social problem was to get the apparent problem off the streets. The fact of the matter is, if there is a law against tangoing, and it takes two to tango, we better not restrict ourselves to berating the dancer who is following the lead while ignoring the one who sets the tempo.

Now do not for a minute hear me going on the stump to outlaw the tango, ladies and gentlemen of the night, drug firms, or doctors. The only law I am genuinely interested in seeing passed is a law against the passage of so many persnickety, inconsequential laws. What I am for is a little more order and logic in the strong judgments I am afflicted with. So the next time I am overcome with the urge to get the president of some drug firm on the horn to complain of the outrageous seduction he is perpetrating on me I think I better phone around to a few of my colleagues and find out how they are responding to the seduction. Specifically, to ask my friends how they savor the liquor of the hospitality room when they know, as they might, and certainly will if I have my way, that the bill is coming out of a sick man's pocket.

Perhaps there is a possibility of a dialogue among physicians as to what is the proper gift for them, in their position as a healer of the sick, to accept from a drug firm, or for that matter, any firm. My premise in initiating the dialogue would be, any gift which directly and appreciably enhances my ability to serve patients is acceptable, all others make a prostitute of me.

When I tried this idea out on a detail man of my acquaintance, he looked quizzical, paused, and dryly commented, "You are about to become remarkably unpopular with your colleagues." There is just no two ways about it, life just goes on getting difficulter, and difficulter.

Endnotes

Reprinted from *Portland Physician* 32(1975): 18-19, with permission.

Community Mental Health and Psychological Pollution

No hand be laid upon the works of the commune without the intention of making them correspond to the noble soul which is composed of all the souls of all its citizens united in one will.
—The commission to build the Duomo, great cathedral of Florence, 1294

Instant crusades are fashionable, and the simplicity of their origin, a cause and a cry, doubtless explains their popularity. My intention is not to be fashionable but to use a contemporary word, "pollution," to lance the modern form of an ancient evil, iatrogenic illness: air pollution, noise pollution and, now, psychological pollution, the foul and fouling emissions of the mental health technocracy. Nor is it my purpose to condemn the elaborate system of psychosocial treatment that is evolving in our nation. Rather I wish to look, with you, at some of the unexamined side effects of community mental health programs.

By my definition, community mental health is a doctrine of belief, an assertion that the administrative organization delivering medical services to the potentially and actually mentally ill, deviant, or deficient should parallel the political organization of the patient in order to engage and maximize social, economic, and political resources. This movement has a potential for unprecedented social and political power. It is not my purpose to oppose or condemn the concept of community mental health but to examine it openly.

Mental health movements are not a new phenomenon; they have happened before, but without the present punch. One hundred years ago Dorothea Dix engaged in a crusade whose battle cries echo today. I do not wish to detract one iota from the luminosity of her renown, but I wonder whether during her most urgent advocacy of state asylums she ever considered their potential for becoming "snake pits." Certainly she knew that she was convincing legislatures, not of her espoused humanitarian principles, but of the reduced costs that would ensue with centralizing the states' "problem." She was probably aware that under the asylum system physicians might become absorbed in administration and forget to be practitioners of medicine. I am tempted to believe that she knew this only too well yet believed the urgent need for reform warranted the risk. Armed with one hundred years of such hindsight, does present-day psychiatry also wish to assume the risk of planning and manning the snake pits of tomorrow?

Fortunately, state hospital snake pits as a palpable form of psychological pollution are fast becoming a thing of the past. But it should give us pause to reflect that the medical profession was not in the forefront of reforming the snake pits. Rather, in many ways the physicians of the 1920s, 1930s, and 1940s contributed to the pollution. By tacit approval, informed neglect, narrow-minded zeal, and bureaucratic servility, they failed to offer an adequate account of patients' treatment. But we should not single out the state hospital physicians as villains; for in snake pit after snake pit, and in state after state, always it was the state medical society that condoned and approved. No physician should ever forget that the Nazi system of human experimentation was carried out with the approval of the national medical societies of Germany who used as justification U.S. medicine's research, devoid as it was of informed consent.

I reiterate: This is not a scientific paper, wielding finely honed logic to prove a point. It is rather an attempt to reverse the glass, to see ourselves as psychiatrists in a world of increasing psychological pollution. To that end, permit me to cite a few experiences designed to highlight three major forms of psychological pollution: the attack on and abuse of privacy, identity, and innovation. Then let us explore with imagination what we can do to stem and eventually clean up the pollution.

My state established a central computer to encode information on all patients in every state-supported mental health service including twenty-six local clinics. The only delineation of responsibility for confidentiality was a verbal assurance, "It won't fall into the wrong hands." These data have been computerized without the permission or even knowledge of the patients and, except for two dissenting votes, with the unanimous approval of the district branch of the American Psychiatric Association. Within a few years, intimate data on 10 percent of the state's families will be on file within the state political system. *Leakage of confidentiality; psychological pollution.*

A governor's task force for increased government efficiency has advocated the use of a universal chart—a common hospital-clinic chart—in conjunction with court records. The task force pointed to duplication of information and paperwork on people in trouble within the state and local governments and stressed the economy of time and effort that would accrue if health charts became part of the court record (without the patient's consent). *Damage to identity; psychological pollution.*

My seventeen-year-old daughter, who volunteers to help elementary students with their arithmetic, was told by her supervisor to read "Jimmy's chart." She said she did not want to become involved in Jimmy's background. The supervisor insisted, saying it would do her good, so she sat down with the chart of the medical school's workup of Jimmy and his family, complete even to the transcription of the psychiatrist's interviews with the parents. *Destruction of privacy; psychological pollution.*

The point in these three examples is that since they happened and are happening we who should be interested in protecting the patient seem by our acquiescence or apathy or both to be abetting those who, no matter how unwittingly, subvert the patient's integrity.

Then there is the subtle pollution that destroys or distorts the physician's identity as well as that of others who are on the mental health firing line. A curious form of quietism, a kind of self-immolation appears to be developing within the profession.

In Oregon, we conducted a careful study of an epidemic of resignations among professional mental health leaders. Though it is statistically difficult to establish a base rate of resignations, the study revealed a consistent breakdown within the professional in his attempt to reconcile his view of himself with the demands of the community.

Before we write this point off simply as poor education or the lack of political or sociological "know-how," let me quote briefly from the *Handbook of Community Psychiatry*.[1] "By letting himself [the community psychiatrist] be manipulated, and at the same time by slightly altering or adding to the assignment, he is often able to turn the situation to his own advantage in a way that lands him a jump ahead of his would-be manipulators." Try that for a few years with city hall.

Or again: "...it is good strategy for a psychiatrist or other mental health worker to accede with good grace to requests that are made of him by accredited representatives of the community, even when the undertaking seems rather useless....those making the request are also placed under some obligation to him, which they may later wish to repay." Surely this is a direct suggestion to prostitute the profession into the use of guilt and guile. *Psychological pollution.*

Along with the professionals, the identities of the other echelons of psychological service are often distorted and destroyed. I was a consultant to the social service department of an agency sponsored by the Office of Economic Opportunity. Consulting with and trying to encourage these workers is a chronic first-aid assignment. After eighteen months of training and supervising "indigent nonprofessionals," not a single worker of the initial staff of eighteen remains.

Under the guise of humanity, the requirements are inhuman in the extreme. "Here is your title as an indigent nonprofessional; now get in there and help your fellow man." Help them, but without the education, stability, finances, and status that the professionals have at their disposal. The task is doomed from the start: No one can help them hold together their shreds of identity when they are thrown into the ghetto to do what cannot be done. *Psychological pollution.*

Then there is the grim reality of the suicide rate among psychiatrists. What steps are being taken and who is trying to disabuse the psychiatric resident of the awful illusion of omniscience in community mental health? Is he trained to say and will he say "Impossible!" when the community demands an easy solution to violence, drugs, or delinquency? Is he ever counseled about the limits of one man's ability to help in the social-psychological problems of his fellow man, or is he given a sword and directed into futile battles with the windmills of our growing anger until, goaded beyond his endurance, he resorts to the vilest of pollution? Suicide is the most malignant form of psychological pollution within the profession.

A third form of psychological pollution is the torrent of innovative, unexamined anodynes that flood the scene. Armed with the doubtful philosophy that new is good and old is bad, physicians and their mental health colleagues sometimes act like soap salesmen, doling out new drugs for old complaints. The "wiggling" child is one miserable human example of what happens when an old problem is "licked" with a new solution. The fidgety child who is unlucky enough to be in a class taught by a teacher burdened beyond reason by the impossible assignment to care for the "whole child" oftentimes finds himself referred for drug therapy. According to one author, "In some of these cases, the parents perceive the child as having deteriorated, even though the testimony of objective observers, such as therapists or teachers, indicates improvement...."[2] The author calls for active intervention to prevent continuation of drugs. Since when has restlessness become a treatable disease? The zealot who treats without knowing is a purveyor of psychological pollution.

The plethora of innovative psychological games, techniques, and therapies espoused by some modern community clinics warrants that something be said about their unsavory side. The divorces, deaths, and psychoses associated with so-called sensitivity training and its ilk contaminate our population and are close kin to the phenomenon of "destructive obedience," the training of people to do evil. Milgram[3] has forthrightly shown how forcefully the act of psychological pollution can be implemented in the name of science. He and his co-workers were shocked at the ease with which college students could be seduced into torturing their fellow students. All that was needed was a white coat, an authoritative air, a scientific "spiel," and impressive equipment. Is there a better name for this black science than psychological pollution?

These are contemporary examples, mind you, not data dredged from some distant dark age. This is not to say that the present community mental health program is necessarily evil but to indicate a powerful social force that should be approached with consummate respect to be controlled with intelligence, not with naive tinkering.

Mental health workers, psychologists, psychoanalysts, social workers, social psychologists, psychiatric nurses, aides, psychiatrists, indigent nonprofessionals, all have an omnipresent and grave responsibility to search for public answers to private problems. We can, and must, do many things now about psychological pollution. The theoreticians have the pressing task of developing a philosophical, metapsychological foundation for community mental health. The psychoanalyst needs to consider psychoanalytic theory within the context of treatment.

One possibility for the theoretician to explore, as some mathematicians are, is proving that some problems are insoluble. Despite appearance to the contrary, this would promote optimism rather than pessimism since it would free workers from trying to solve what is at the moment, at least, insoluble and turn attention to problems which have a solution. Without a thought-through theory to guide us we are blind, stumbling through a dark land.

The insights of the psychologist are needed to understand psychological pollution. We are in the vortex of a vast social turmoil reflecting a subconscious revolt against a pernicious bureaucratization. Ellul[4, 5] has shown government bureaucracy to be an implacable force, "the rule of nobody." Who of us has not seen humaneness gradually squeezed from mental health programs as they develop from research projects to pilot programs, to large service programs, and finally to megaprograms? In a recent article, Dole[6] literally pleads for help against the political pressure that would force him to increase his methadone maintenance program to include twenty-five thousand heroin addicts. He tells of the perils of success in community mental health: "There is however a serious danger that treatment programs will become subordinated to power struggles. So far the programs have been effective because their direction has been medical. The procedure has been developed by physicians with personal experience in treatment of addicts, not by governmental agencies or the medical administrators chosen by them. The success of this treatment in rehabilitation of addicts will decline significantly if methadone programs cease to be medical institutions, and instead become instruments of another bureaucracy." Here is but one example of a current need to direct medical-social processes with psychological insights and knowledge not yet available. The social psychologist can help us to understand our perhaps innocent participation in the destruction of the patients' psychological health. If there be any hardy souls who contemplate themselves managing the treatment of twenty-five thousand heroin addicts, I certainly encourage them to ally themselves immediately with at least one thoughtful social psychologist.

In this context, it is of tremendous theoretical and practical importance that the role of politics be clearly understood and taught. The politics of staff, agency, community, and nation, complete with their interrelatedness to mental health and illness, should be worked through at a theoretical level before the Dr. Jekylls of this generation are engulfed by the Hyde-like evil of bureaucracy. Professionals have an absolute obligation to be scientific, not political. In all the intrigue of coveting staff, nabbing grants, negotiating contracts, wheedling budgets, and placating the public, the ultimate *raison d'etre* should not be forgotten: What is happening to the patient?

So much for theory; for the clinician, psychological pollution abounds. One flagrant form is the "New Custodian," the technician acting as clinician. He is an ensconced dehumanizer, the organization man, the manager, prepared to cross every "t" and dot every "i" no matter at what cost to human emotion or life. He is easily spotted, particularly as programs become counterproductive. Competent clinicians can see beyond the New Custodians' programmed bottom lines to the sometimes crushing reality that though the therapy was efficient the patient committed suicide.

Every psychiatrist and fellow frontline workers must see psychological pollution for what it is. No professional can afford to limit his examination to a narrow personal responsibility. It is not enough to check whether one's own pant cuffs are clean; they probably are. The surrounding conditions may not be; only trained vision can see the contamination for what it is. Vision carries with it a larger responsibility of describing what is seen to those who can hear; a responsibility that consistently avoids condoning acts that pollute the minds of others.

This advice is ancient yet is especially pertinent today, for the forces of pollution are beyond the vision of most and easily denied by all. Certainly the most commonly invoked rationale for participating with institutions on an inexorable destructive course is, "But I have a spouse and two children to think about." However, life is not made up of a series of climactic moments of truth, but of a continuous struggle to choose among innumerable, disconnected petty details which are, nevertheless, subtly demanding an answer: to be or not to be, to think or not to think, to feel or to sink into apathy.

Too often professionals are lost to the moment of truth long before it occurs. Insignificant compromises, ideas half thought through, and abortive convictions pollute standards and ideals. The outcome of psychological pollution is psychological death.

Nor is a list of pollutions in community mental health enough. A plan of positive action and personal imagination is essential. Although almost as many models for community mental health have been suggested as there are communities, one more is offered of the mental health worker seeing him/herself as an individual deeply engaged in a demanding human endeavor. The archetype of community mental health is the cathedral, the sculptured symphony of balanced stress and strain. Those vast social edifices were built with incalculable dimensions of time, effort, money, and thought. The endeavor was for the spirit of man, not material life.

Like the people of the twelfth century, we have embarked on a tremendous community venture that none of us will live to see completed. No one man can conceive either the ancient or modern cathedral's ultimate goal. Neither medieval nor modern man is inspired by a static master plan but builds on a foundation of hope. The analogies are many: both demand the builder live in and grow with his work, both call upon citizens of all classes to volunteer, both seem superhuman in scale yet both are human in detail, even to the mortal expression of the ancient gargoyle and modern gargoylism.

Cathedral building is a worthy model for our times. Chalk and pencil mark too broad a line. Each tiny error, introduced by blurred chalk and pencil lines, would be carried over in the work to multiply as the cathedral grows to final completion. Each mortised joint must be precise, each line of masonry must be absolute, each pillar must bear its load squarely, so ancient craftsmen carried a small knife to mark a precise line with its thin, sharp blade. In building our present-day cathedrals, each mental health worker has just such a fine, sharp instrument—the disciplined mind, with its critical sense open and sharp. All that needs be done is use the instrument.

Finally, the examples of psychological pollution in my own state are cited not because I cherish it less or another more, but because the responsibility of the physician is to experience his immediate world as it is. In Oregon, the clinicians, the legislators, and the administrators have eliminated the universal chart, patients are now informed of the state's computer, steps have been taken to protect the patient's privacy. We wish to build our cathedral precisely, a monument to shared human values. Others help by listening to their children thoughtfully, reading the newspaper intelligently, visiting local agencies regularly, and most of all by honing the mind to latent problems. The physician, like a modern Cato, is responsible for reminding all citizens, all governments, all professions, that not cost, not status, not implementation, not science, but the care of the patient comes first.

Endnotes

Reprinted from Bulletin of the Menninger Clinic 35(1971): 407-415, with permission.
1. L. Bellak, ed., *Handbook of Community Psychiatry and Community Mental Health* (New York: Grune & Stratton, 1964).
2. A. Barcai, "The Emergence of Neurotic Conflict in Some Children after the Successful Administration of Dextroamphetamine," *Journal of Child Psychology and Psychiatry* 10(1969): 269-276.
3. S. Milgram, "Behavioral Study of Obedience," *Journal of Abnormal and Social Psychology* 67(1963): 371-378.
4. J. Ellul, *The Political Illusion* (New York: Knopf, l967).
5. ———, *The Technological Society* (New York: Knopf, 1964).
6. V.P. Dole, "Methadone Maintenance Treatment for 25,000 Heroin Addicts," *Journal of the American Medical Association* 215(1971): 1131-1134.

Reflections of a Director on Resigning from a Mental Health Clinic

Rather than be less,
Car'd not to be at all.
    —John Milton (1608-1674)
    Paradise Lost, Book II, line 47

The one immutable law of life is change, so to every position of responsibility the time comes to step aside and allow someone else to carry on, even as a director of a small community mental health clinic. It is not often that the change is freely made. Too often it is forced by health, by growth, or by the wishes of others. However, in the one particular case as the director of the clinic, I made the choice. I resigned.

This fact in itself merits little attention but the implications for others, particularly for patients in mental health clinics, are important and merit reflection. To know some of the pressures on the clinic staff, the board of directors, and on the director is to know some of the pressures on patients, for if in zeal for community mental health the citizens ignore the selection, care, and development of their instrument (the mental health professional) the nationwide community health program can be at best mediocre.

Briefly, here is a review of the circumstances of the resignation. My contact with the clinic began in 1961 when I was asked to become part-time clinical director. The clinic had just been organized and was intended to serve the county of one hundred thousand inhabitants on the periphery of a modern large city. For five years I worked one and a half days a week as the director of the clinic, which gradually developed into a viable professional entity. Community acceptance was present, but underlying sociological problems, complicated by political ones, gradually narrowed the life of the clinic to a hand-to-mouth existence.

It had always been part of my plan to resign if only to make way for younger and abler minds. However, now it was different. Much as I resisted, I had passed judgment on the failure of my fellow citizens, and voiced my protest in the most potent way I knew, by resigning. My resignation did not in any sense follow the natural growth of the institution, but rather, my judgment of failure in both the institution and myself.

To study the effects of resignation upon the patients and staff of an institution is an extremely complex task. To do so properly would require the services of a historian, anthropologist, social-psychologist, sociologist, and psychoanalyst. What is offered here are largely subjective judgments, yet they may have value in the development of evaluation of mental health programs.

To begin with the effect on patients: This is "old hat" for most psychiatrists who have experienced the effects of telling their patients they are leaving. Regularly, while in training, there are times when psychiatrists must move on from a service, a hospital, or a training program and in the process work through with patients the basic human anxiety stimulated by separation. For my clinic patients there was no difference, as far as I could see, from other situations when I had been forced to terminate treatment. The circumstances were touched on: "I will be leaving the clinic in the near future and a new director will be found who will be your therapist." The transference was, as always, directed to the institution until another therapist could resume the psychotherapy. Meanwhile, the personal implications of separation for each patient were worked through in terms of the patient's particular personality dynamics.

There was, however, a difference for other patients of other therapists in the clinic. News of my resignation found its way into the local newspaper as a brief note on a back page. The information also passed by word of mouth through the community, stimulating concern in patients of other staff members. Frequently, staff members were called upon to clarify that though the director was leaving their patients' therapy was not in jeopardy. Each staff member remained alert to the implications. Was the patient's remark a plea for help? Was it a manifestation of resistance? Was it an opportunity for the therapist to displace personal feelings onto the patient? All of these possibilities were of immediate moment, reverberating in the therapy of most clinic patients.

One gross, statistical measure of the effect of the resignation on patients emerged by comparing the number of cancelled appointment hours per month at the clinic. The gross level of attendance of patients at our clinic had remained at 92 percent month in and month out over the years. However, in the month that followed the announcement of the resignation, there was a drop to 86 percent. When this figure is examined as a 100 percent increase in the rate of cancellation, its significance can be appreciated. In a sales program, a business manager would be appalled at a 50 percent decrease in orders. We were not appalled, largely, I think, because of our failure at measuring our effectiveness. When the director resigns, patients' identification with the institution diminishes.

The staff since its beginnings had a spirit of camaraderie built upon open, accepted dissension. The resignation had its effect on staff morale. Before dealing with patients, each staff member was given opportunity to carefully work through feelings of separation and anger to avoid displacing these complicating facts of staff life onto the patients. The working-through process was done through formal groups (such as staff conferences), through supervisor-supervisee conferences, and through informal after-hours contacts and schedule breaks.

Each supervisor was called into the director's office and told firsthand of the resignation. The information was from the director himself and emotions stirred were real. Surprise–denial–anger and beginning acceptance developed, after the flurry of resentment such as, "Oh, you M.D.s are all alike. You have your private practice to retreat to." Then each supervisor in turn directly told each of his staff members. There were no "leaks" and everyone learned of the fact in a place and time to work on it. Finally, the whole staff was told that it was expected that time would be necessary to work through the reactions of the change.

As matters developed, each staff member had to answer the questions, "What does this mean to me?" and "If the director does not stay with the institution, should I?" Questions of loyalty, finance, and career surfaced precipitously; first, as a hurt or anger, gradually in a realistic appraisal of the situation at hand. It appeared that the staff decided to "wait and see." Panic and confusion, the "mass resignation" reaction, were replaced by consideration and patience. One staff member wrote a telling paper on the psychological process of choice. Another addressed a long-delayed writing project, and a third undertook a research project on an "epidemic" of resignations of directors occurring throughout the state mental health system.[1] Without exception, they remained at their post, continuing their work.

One staff member, a psychologist, put it: "My most important reflections to date have led me to conclude that there are two different kinds of reactions or consequences to such a resignation. One is the ritualistic or stereotyped gestures that are made when anyone who has been around passes from the scene. I don't think these gestures penetrate too deeply into the people involved, but they are certainly necessary, and are like the shocked sobbing of the traumatically bereaved, or the ceremony in which a watch is given to an old employee.

"The other set of reactions is individualized, though probably predictable along some type of tangible gradient. It seems to depend upon how much the leader was really 'with' the organization and the people in it. 'With' is in the existential sense, meaning did the leader come across to the people as a person, and also, how much the other people involved in the organization were 'with' the organization or 'with' the leader in a most personal sense.

"These individualized reactions need time to unfold. The working through is not stereotyped. It seems to me that those left behind find themselves having to withdraw somewhat from the institution as they measure in some way the extent to which the institution contains manifestations of the resignee. The remainees must realize that they are going to have to separate from the residue of the person who resigned before they can invest something of themselves in a newly constituted institution."

The most important effect was the integration of the staff in considering the resignation. Rather than centering on feelings of anger and abandonment, they addressed themselves to "what should be done," and out of the staff considerations (not the director's) came a plan for better clinic organization, avoiding the past dilemmas. The impossibility of continuing the director's position in its existing part-time form was recognized, and the staff proposed that rather than accept the resignation as a defeat, to learn by the experience and reorganize in such a fashion that funds could be available for a full-time, rather than a part-time, director. It was also recognized that the services of a business administrator were needed for administrative structure, a concerted public relations program, and a sustained board action. In the weeks following the resignation the plan was honed and eventually placed before the board.

In considering the resignation with the board of directors, the effect was unpleasant. The president of the board withheld the knowledge of the resignation from fellow board members in the hopes that it would be reconsidered. The board president's delay made for intense unhappiness among the members. Some of the board members learned secondhand, either from neighbors or employees, with their surprise compounded by a sharp hurt of being considered secondary, incidental to what was occurring. Not until the reasons for the delayed communication surfaced at a stormy board session was there a reduction in immediate anger.

Gradually, the board worked through their surprise and began addressing the problem of the replacement. One board member, without authorization of the board, went to local county government with an offer to relinquish the clinic. This act of the board member echoes a mass resignation phenomenon. The act was looked on askance by other board members but the significance was never considered by them as a body. Eventually, the board approved the staff's plan to increase functional time for a director together with a business manager.

Board members appeared to lack understanding of the emotional impact the changes had on patients. Attempts were made to focus board members on consideration of similar situations in the medical literature. Repeatedly, board members were encouraged to read *The Life and Death of a Mental Hospital*[2] for a clear account of the effects of board action on mental health patients, to no effect.

The impact on the community was difficult to judge. Many members of the community remarked to me on the resignation, some with embarrassment. Few asked why. Not that I was reticent in giving reasons, but there seemed to be an uncomfortable air about the subject, the aroma of "let sleeping dogs lie." However, former patients in the community addressed the problem differently. Whether I happened to encounter them in a gas station or on a ski slope, they asked directly if I was leaving the community. When I told them that I was not but was simply leaving the position, they seemed satisfied.

One local agency director (who was not a social worker) sighed in relief to a clinic staff member, "Now that he is out, why don't you take over and we will have a social worker running the clinic." The implication was that social workers cause less trouble in the community than physicians. The local health department made no direct attempt to evaluate the situation, though the clinic is the only public mental health facility in the community. The people in local government who responded with concern were the "little" ones who had worked with the clinic staff on patient problems, who had come to staff meetings, who had directly experienced the clinic as a help in their work. Court workers, public health nurses, and welfare workers (those on the front lines) uniformly expressed different degrees of regret at the impending change.

The professional community by and large took immediate interest in the resignation, wondering if I would have time to accept more referrals of private patients. The state mental health division was surprised by the resignation and informally remarked, "We thought we had you *hooked* and that all the talk about difficulties would never bring you to resign."

Some of the professionals adopted a "Now that you are no longer working there, you can let me in on what has been *really* going on" approach. It was pointed out to them that the situation at the clinic had been fairly well documented in fifteen papers published by the staff but that if they had any questions after they had studied the material, someone would be glad to go over the questions with them. With this they usually withdrew, remarking on professionals' cynicism. Feelers came to staff members about other jobs: "I heard of the resignation and since you will be looking around, I thought—." It had a tinge of the macabre, like those postcards that come after a death in the family offering to buy the "dear one's" clothes. The only individual who knowingly asked "why" about the resignation was the clinic's director of research. He addressed himself to this question with all of his scientific curiosity and know-how.[1]

Lastly comes the question of the effect of the resignation on myself. Though the act was not a surprise, not an impulsive act, personal emotions generated were no different than for others who cared about the resignation: hurt, anger, and gradually a realistic appraisal. I, too, had to answer: "What does this mean to me?" My first response was to cheerfully deny my feelings with the inane requiem, "You cannot win them all." My next temptation was to indulge in self-pity and recrimination. The desire was strong to document my growing suspicion that my abiding sin of "talking down" to some people in the community came from their not being on the level with me. What that would come to would be simply another scabrous letter in the newspaper—a too-common spectacle.

Another temptation was to fly to compulsive intellectualization with a series of papers on: (1) Semantic Blocks Between the Layman and the Professional in Mental Health Programs, (2) Transference and Countertransference in Community Psychiatry, (3) Human Values and Their Application in a Small Mental Health Clinic, (4) The Cyclic Nature of Public Response to the Mental Health Movement, (5) Systems Theory and Sibling Rivalry Among Board, Staff, and Patients.

None of this could do—rationalization, projection, intellectualization —all thin gruel for a full understanding, and yet to be objective is not enough. As my thoughts no longer withdrew from but adjusted to the idea of resigning, a broad personal view of the change opened. The working through began to fix with lifelong memories the quicksilver of experience. The last great defense against change is memory.

To know the meaning of the resignation to the director is to know something of his working through the problem. Though it may be difficult to believe, such information might have scientific value. Perhaps it does, for how more profoundly can the character of the mental health establishment be judged than in the thoughts of its members? With this in mind I quote some notes made after the resignation.

"The image of Arrowsmith swirls back, the adolescent dream of a physician. But yet a finer net seines up the form of Don Quixote. It is as though all that happened was a flight of fancy, a thought of Cervantes, and I, a sort of Don Quixote and Sancho Panza combined. For did I not rule an island such as Sancho Panza with as little training and less wit? Those sometimes bumptious staff meetings when we laughed until the tears came—oh, shades of Sancho! Did I not tilt with windmills of a county government? And, oh, the quixotic castles I built!"

"I remember so well a rainy morning during coffee break, over a steaming cup, squiring a fellow-worker through the fantasy halls of what a new clinic building might be. The quiet, carpeted halls led past bright playrooms for children, around a cloistered garden where reflection and meditation sprang from the very atmosphere, where serenity and veneration flourished. And over the doorway of that cloudland clinic I even inscribed a motto: 'Regain your hope.' Ah, what madness (and madness it has been called by my kind friends who gently counseled me against seeing the work for more than it was)."

"Only now I see. The madness falls away and in the light of saying 'goodbye' things appear as they are. All I can say are the words of that gentleman from La Mancha when at last his sanity returned: 'Forgive me, my friends, for having caused you to appear as mad as I by leading you to fall into the same error, that of believing that there are still knights-errant in the world.'"

The resignation of the director had an effect on all members of the institution: board, staff, and patients. For some it was superficial, for some profound. The effect was statistically evidenced in the patient attendance rate. For those, from patient to chairman of the board, who saw it as a real event in their relationship to the institution and worked through consequent emotions, growth was discernible. For those who held the event and consequent emotions beyond the circle of their lives, who did not work it through for what it meant to them, it was a defeat; at best a loss, dealt with by a proportionate denial of their involvement in the institution. An institution, such as a small mental health clinic, survives as its members are prepared to give to it. An institution lives as its members are prepared to breathe life into it by incorporating it into their lives.

Endnotes

Reprinted from *The General Practice of Community Psychiatry*, Beaverton, Oregon, Benjamin Rush Foundation, 1969, 239-248, with permission.

1. M. Greenbaum, "A Study of a Mild Epidemic of Resignations among Professional Mental Health Leaders," *Archives of General Psychiatry* 19(1968): 266-280.
2. E. Stotland and A. Kobler, *The Life and Death of a Mental Hospital* (Seattle: University of Washington, 1965).

They All Laughed When I Spoke of Greedy Doctors

Now they were come upon the hill Lucre, where the silver mine was which took Demas off from his pilgrimage, and into which, as some think, By-ends fell and perished....they marvelled...that men of such knowledge and ripeness of wit...should be so blinded to turn aside here.
—John Bunyan (1628-1688)
The Pilgrim's Progress

At an annual meeting of the Oregon Medical Association, a respected colleague proposed that the state medical association join him in deploring the unreasonably high fees of some physicians. It seemed like an appropriate idea to me and I made a point to be present at the reference committee meeting to take part in the general testimony.

Consideration of the resolution followed a heated debate on cognitive versus procedural reimbursement. This involuntarily gave a slant to the discussion concerning reasonable fees, for when introducing his resolution my colleague contrasted the reimbursement of a pediatrician working up a child for an appendectomy with that of the surgeon who removed the offending organ. Any merit I had given his resolution began evaporating as the debate focused on who was to get the most, the pediatrician or the surgeon. What had brought me to the hearing was the problem of greed within the profession, independent of specialty, in which a small proportion of the practitioners lack moral compunction about charging all that the traffic can bear. As one physician put it, perhaps as a slip of the tongue, "They practice money and make medicine."

The words about relative reimbursement began sounding like growling dogs over a bone, devoid of concern for the carcass the bone came from. Hoping to focus the problem on causes deeper than relative reimbursement, I took my place in the line at the microphone and when my turn came declared, "I speak in favor of the resolution since it addresses one of the critical problems of the medical profession, physician greed. I suggest the reference committee refer this problem to the Impaired Physicians Committee for study and action."

The room broke into laughter, and when the hooting and hollering subsided I went on, "Look, today the central clinical problem we physicians face in practice is appetite control. Patients seem insatiably hungry for cigarettes, food, sex, money, work, love, and pills. Are we so different from our patients? Consider what we have been able to do through the Impaired Physicians Committee for doctors with a malignant appetite for alcohol and other mind-altering drugs. We have an incidence of drug addiction that runs one hundred times higher than that for a comparable lay population. This is because we work hard and have practically unlimited access to mind-altering drugs. Does the same not apply to money? With hard work and inflation we are exposed to the danger of greed as never before. I think the Impaired Physicians Committee should take a look at what is going on with these skyhigh-fee practitioners."

Well, the chuckles continued as I sat down and I well know what it is to be "the laughingstock of your peers," but if anyone took a close look at a money-impaired physician, I doubt that the smiles would last. There he is, never seeing patients, only customers. No free care given by him. The poor receive a no-nonsense command to go elsewhere. With his lust for a buck, the money-impaired doctor is a menace to the profession.

However, the subject proved moot and unactionable since the Association's attorney took the floor as a point of order and informed us we were acting illegally according to Federal Trade Commission regulations in raising the subject of particular fees in an organized professional meeting. The subject was immediately dropped but left me thinking that someplace in Washington, D.C., there must be a mighty powerful rich man's lobby at work, since now it is against the law to talk about pirates.

Endnotes

Reprinted from *Western Journal of Medicine* 142(1985): 267, with permission.

Fee for Service from the Poor

Hell hath no fury like a spurned philanthropist and yet I do not know which is the more regrettable—a donor who is ignored or a recipient who takes a grant for granted....

—Alan Gregg
in P. Wilder, *The Difficult Art of Giving: The Epic of Alan Gregg*

A dilemma arising in any charitable enterprise is the recipient's potential loss of self-esteem in the give-and-take transaction. Frequently, institutions becloud rather than clarify the problem of human feelings, and only by direct personal confrontation can a charitable enterprise be explicitly worked through as a mutual give-and-take process.[1-3] By asking the poor to pay a fee for service, one may enhance their knowledge and participation in a human exchange.

Such a confrontation occurred between a psychiatrist and the social service staff of a Head Start child care center. With mixed motives of civic-mindedness and personal gain, the psychiatrist volunteered to assist the staff of a child care center in a depressed area; the center was funded inadequately by the federal government. The agency director assigned him to the social work department, which was staffed by one graduate social worker, approximately four paid staff workers, and ten trainees, some from a twelve-week poverty program. The word "approximately" refers to the flux and instability in staffing this agency, a situation shared by most first-line agencies in depressed communities.

The Staff versus the Consultant

The first step toward achieving a working relationship with the staff members was determining their needs. Group techniques quickly established their wish to know "if any of these people (clients) are crazy" (clinical appraisal); "What are we supposed to say if someone calls up and says that he is going to shoot himself?" (interviewing techniques), and "How am I supposed to get along with some fussy people around here?" (staff interaction). The psychiatrist acknowledged he might help with these problems, offered to consult with the staff members half a day every two weeks, and then wondered what he could expect in return.

The response was immediate and loud. At first, his question was treated as a joke: "Come on, you're rich and we're poor." The consultant acknowledged that he was well off by most standards but that he looked for rewards as others did, emphasizing that he would be less than honest if he claimed he did not.

Another worker said: "It's a privilege to work with us; we are poor. In fact, we have degrees in being poor."

"Yes," the psychiatrist replied, "but why shouldn't I work with another group down the block? What is in it for me here?"

"Money?" asked a worker. "We don't have none, see the boss."

"No, if I wanted money I would go to paid agency work, where I would expect the going rate for psychiatrists' time," was the consultant's reply, and minds began calculating a potential income. The consultant continued, "No, my rewards are two: the pleasure of working with concerned people and the assurance that I am doing a constructive job. In private practice, the patient's payment of a fee represents his belief that I am doing the right kind of job for him. Here I propose you reassure me that I am doing a constructive job by paying me at the end of the year with the documented proof that I have helped ten children, one a month."

"Get off it, you aren't serious," exclaimed another worker.

"Yes, I am! You look like nice people but I am not here to socialize. I want my time, eight hours a month, to pay off for me—and the payoff I want is to know that ten children have had a better break, no matter how small it might be."

Another, more sophisticated member said with evident disgust, "Why, you're just trading with people." Acknowledging this truth, the consultant went on to point out that "the name of the game," whether social rehabilitation, psychiatric treatment, or economic opportunity, was dealing with people. What mattered was the motive: "Predominantly, my motive is to help others, but it is lying not to say I want something for myself." Reluctantly, the group agreed to a contract.

Achieving a Modus Operandi

Once established, this open, mutually confident exchange continued between the staff members and the consultant. They were free to ask questions and to expose feelings that they might hide from the "visiting dignitary" but that were open to their employee. During the year, many subjects were covered. The question "What are we here to do?" resulted in hammering out the first operational job description they had ever had. "How much can one really help?" offered realistic limits to the overextended, uninitiated worker. "How does race affect work?" brought the group to the realistic conclusion that saying that they were all brothers and sisters did not make it that way. Interpersonal staff problems were constructively considered in open meetings.

At the end of the year, one session was devoted to the payoff. In response to the consultant's request for ten cases, generalities were used, "Sure, sure, you were a big help," but generalities were not accepted. The consultant held the group to specifics. Over the course of the morning, the group, with alternate groans and shouts of glee, paid off; they named ten children and the time, place, and manner of help—a worker who learned how not to make matters worse for a battered child; a worker who was free to hold a child when immediate limits were needed. It was the staff's reward and their payoff as well, and with joy the session closed on, "Oh, wait 'til we get you on the next contract."

Evaluating the self-esteem of the recipient in a charitable encounter is difficult, and attributing influence to a specific act, such as personal candor, is next to impossible. However, with this experience, hunch became opinion that, for people who are leery of promises or suspicious of programs, frankness is vital. Opinion became conviction; this was seen in the high attendance and animated involvement at all of the meetings, in the workers' private requests for help for themselves and their children, in a request to contribute to another community project (a clinic established by a radical political minority), and in personal thanks. The personal thanks ranged from letters to direct affirmations of the value received, to a most tender encounter with an older worker, who, on her last day on the job, caught the consultant at the door as he was leaving. She spoke of her conflict in leaving, her fears of what was ahead, and her thanks for what had happened in the group. Then, with a big hug and a kiss she murmured, "Bless you, child, bless you." It is not often that a psychiatrist finds such rich secondary rewards. The primary reward remains the solid knowledge that ten children were helped.

Endnotes

Reprinted from *American Journal of Psychiatry* 128(1971): 230-232.
1. R. Crawshaw, "The Experience of Giving," *Medical Opinion and Review* 2(1966): 16-23.
2. R. Crawshaw, "The New Custodians," *Medical Opinion and Review*

4(1968): 63-67. This essay can be found in part 8 of *Compassion's Way*.
3. R. Crawshaw, "The Other Side of Charity," *The Pharos* 34(1971): 75-78. This essay appears in part 1 of *Compassion's Way*.

The Cost of Caring: A View of Britain's Delivery of Health Care

Any social hope that is going to be any use against the darkness ahead will have to be based upon a knowledge of the worst: the worst of practical facts, the worst in ourselves.
—C.P. Snow (1905-1980)
The State of Siege

That everyone cannot have everything is a commonplace of our world, yet, as any government leader knows, this reality turns to political poison when applied to the delivery of health care. Curious to learn how British political and medical leaders do or do not deal with this social toxin, I embarked on a week of talk, observation, and reflection with them, the better to understand how Oregonians might face the "everybody/everything" issue.

The Oregon Health Plan is a civic consensus on the makeup of a prudent though somewhat limited package of health care services developed by combining citizens' health values, generated through statewide community discussion, with the best available health care facts medical experts could offer. The resulting basic health care package eliminates unnecessary, futile, and unproved procedures while offering access to care for an additional 140,000 Oregonians.

In 1994, three separate delegations of the British Parliament visited my state of Oregon to observe how we ration health care. On leaving, they proffered a continuing dialogue together with a firsthand look at the United Kingdom health delivery system. As a founder of Oregon Health Decisions, a civic organization that helped frame our health plan by securing citizens' grass roots health values, I grasped the opportunity to compare our experience with that of the British.

More than the Foreign Office's generous invitation hastened me from Heathrow Airport through the November rain squalls to St. John's and St. Elizabeth's Hospice in North London, to the bedside of a dying friend. Later that sad day, another personal need again brought me under the aegis of the National Health Service (NHS). In transit from the States, damage was sustained by my C-PAP machine, an electronic device for delivering pressured air to my lungs at night, to relieve a chronic obstructive sleep apnea.

After an unsatisfactory attempt to reach the C-PAP manufacturer in Kansas, I resorted, wisely as it turns out, to the Casualty Ward of the Royal Free Hospital. After a reasonable wait the busy triage nurse heard my complaint. She paused long enough to compliment me on the weave of my jacket and then summoned the hospital's standby electronic engineer. This self-effacing man made off with my sick machine, disappearing into the bowels of the hospital, only to return in a half hour with it fully functioning. The staff and clinic clerk refused any offer of payment. In both encounters the NHS worked, in my judgment, as well as or better than U.S. standards of care.

Yet I did not leave the Royal Free without a subtle reminder that the attentive nurse was far from carefree. Over her shoulder, taped to the wall of the nurses' "break room," could be glimpsed a tattered headline, "More Managers, No Nurses." It was the first of my "snapshots" of the United Kingdom's health delivery system.

The Rt. Hon. Mrs. Marion Roe, Member of Parliament (MP), the chair of Parliament's Select Committee on Health, was kind enough to see me early Monday morning. Outlining the government's path to health care reform, she graciously explained how in health reform the British people are not directly confounded, as U.S. citizens are, with political gridlock. The flow of legislative initiatives for reform begins with trial balloons, wishes tied to practicality by way of Green Papers. These announce what the ruling party would like to accomplish. After public hearings and responses from party members, experts, and "ordinary people" (in U.S. parlance, "citizens"), the Green Paper is superseded by a White Paper pinpointing what the government intends to do.

In response to my question of possible legislative distortion through pressure from special interest groups, the bane of U.S. health reform,

Mrs. Roe elaborated on Parliament's insulation from lobbying pressure by short election campaigns with small budgets limiting political advertising. Later, from another source, I learned how British tobacco interests attempt to sway elections by relinquishing their numerous billboards to Conservative Party members during the six-week campaign. Another source detailed the workings of the private corporation that answers only to Mr. John Major, the prime minister, as it collects and distributes political contributions. Given a few such discrepancies, the description of the British legislative approach to health reform sounded more reasonable than the ineffectual scramble of the U.S. Congress.

The next day, Labor's shadow minister for health, The Rt. Hon. Mrs. Margaret Beckett, MP, shared her commitment to the Labor Party's health care reform program to follow their expected victory in the next general election. Put simply, the Labor Party stands solid for the present one-tiered health care system as the most essential protection of the health of the underclass. It is completely against the present trend toward a two-tiered marketplace system with privatized health care through fund holding.

Mrs. Beckett, a psychologist by profession, expressed dismay at the failure of some doctors to appreciate the significance of social sources of illness. During a national meeting on homelessness, doctors walked out on her presentation when she pointed to the need for jobs, shelter, and nutrition in dealing with hypothermia. Subsequently, these doctors went out of their way to hector her for "bringing politics into medicine."

A leisurely breakfast with Mr. Hugh Bayley, MP, back-bencher for Labor, was a delight of informal candor. He openly shared his sense of concern at what the future holds as his nation confronts the central dilemma of health care, the "everybody/everything" problem. He said he sees the problem becoming a local one of painful concessions. The inevitable trade-offs will be worked out as votes about the health care system and how accountable it is for its mission statement. The votes may be expected to revolve about medical outcome measures and the undeniable role of social determinants in health. Like the other legislators, however, he offered no suggestions on how these inevitable trade-offs might be articulated by political leaders or how the British people will react to them.

The British press offers a perhaps distorted, certainly hysterical counterpoint to the sane talk of the Members of Parliament. As in newspapers around the world, London's headlines trumpet failure and corruption, there referred to as "sleaze." Examples during the course of a week's visit were: "Top Hospital in Hoax Row" (*Evening Standard*);[1] "Put Patients Last, NHS Manager Tells Doctors" (*Sunday Telegraph*);[2] "Doctors Accuse Trust Chief" (*Times*);[3] "Uproar over TV Scare on Baby Deaths—50,000...Call Helpline" (*Daily Telegraph*);[4] "Hippocratic Trusts: The BMA Spits Out Its Managers' Medicine" (*Times*);[5] "Ministers Reject Pay Raise for Health Workers" (*Times*).[6] In addition, letters to the editor and articles rang with unrequited angst: "Doctors Forced into Rationing Care" (*Observer*);[7] "Who Do They Think They Are?" with a bold-print lead-in: "You want a career in medicine? Forget medical school—become a manager. Five years ago the London areas NHS had 1,180 managers. By last year there were nearly 5,000" (*Evening Standard*).[8]

Sleaze is keenly appreciated by the British Medical Association (BMA). An encounter with the editor of the *British Medical Journal* began with him asking me what I was up to in England. My blurted reply, "Seeking the truth," immediately prompted his question about the truth of alleged scientific misrepresentations by Dr. John Malcolm Pearce, consultant obstetrician and gynecologist at St. George's Hospital. That doctor had been charged with publishing two case reports in the *British Journal of Obstetrics and Gynecology* of procedures that never took place, a possible case of scientific sleaze, if not outright medical malpractice. Our luncheon conversation revolved closely around this case and the profession's task in determining, explicating, and pursuing sustaining core values.

Conversation with the chairman of the British Medical Service Council and its secretary flowed in the same direction, with a forceful account of a recent BMA summit meeting. For the first time in thirty years, leaders of British medicine had assembled to establish their nonnegotiable standards for future patient-doctor relationships. The BMA was responding to the counterproductive elements of health reform by moving to first principles, empowering the medical profession in a direct, proactive alliance with patients. Thus, doctors hoped to counter the threat of health industry commercialism, fund holding, the British counterpart to U.S. managed care. The question is, will general practitioners, some of whom are miserably disheartened, buy into the core values?[9]

Moving to the front lines of health care delivery took me to Colchester and into a familiar collegiality with hands-on clinicians. In their preoccupation with a world of diminishing resources, quantitative considerations of economy inadvertently outweigh qualitative issues of caring.

On the front lines the tyranny of new medical technologies is blatant. British doctors face relentless political demands to offer the best, demands underlined by a recent "medical scandal" in which British children suffering from brain tumors were flown to the United States for surgery. British pediatric neurosurgeons countered "the very good publicity machine at the New York medical center" (*Sunday Telegraph*)[10] with news releases proclaiming their high skills and world-class equipment.

Shifts of resources intended to keep up with the medical technology "arms race" play out as severe attrition for other services, particularly chronic care. The loss to chronic care is more than building new efficient hospitals for acute care while leaving old dilapidated hospitals for chronic care. There is a palpable loss of quality in the direct care of many chronically ill patients. In a *Sunday Telegraph* article, "Long on Age, Short on Care," William Lang, a health economist, predicted, "Ultimately, in such a 'doomsday' scenario [unlimited high medical technology], the resulting burden of care might be contained only by withdrawing from old people the right to medical treatment." As frontline workers struggle with diminished resources, Mr. Lang's prediction becomes but a daily reality.

Dr. Geoffrey Carroll, Director of Public Health, North Essex Health Authority, forthrightly faced the "everybody/everything" problem by taking it to local ordinary people. Starting public discussion with questions such as, "Where do sex change operations costing between £5,000 ($8,000) and £10,000 ($16,000) fit into a tight community budget?" he has secured a preliminary public priority ranking for mid-Essex health expenditures. Not surprisingly, his development of grass roots health values ranks prevention first and in vitro fertilization last.[11]

On the front lines of Britain's present delivery system there is no mistaking who, aside from patients, suffer most. It is the nurses. Whether in a rural psychiatric facility or a community hospital, nurses are daily confronted with the tragic task of denying full care to patients. As one suburban nurse explained, "As head nurse I have made my ward an island unto itself. We do the best we can, knowing we can never care as we were trained to care." An urban nurse was more direct: "If a consultant refers a patient in renal failure to my dialysis service when it is full, I simply say, 'Do not bother—we cannot take another patient.' I will not sacrifice quality for quantity."

Ms. Liz Winder, director of nursing policy and practice for the Royal College of Nursing (RCN), is a candid, thoughtful woman who conveys a sense of active caring. She visibly paused as I recounted hearing offhand remarks of nurses described as "whinges" (whines). "Yes, I know. Those same people cry 'nurseynursey' when we speak up at hospital administration meetings." Then she thoughtfully explored how this biased view of nurses grows with "reskilling," the searing transition her profession is presently immersed in, leaving others to judge that the nurses suffer from a case of the victim being held responsible for her victimization.

Increasingly, nurses find themselves shifted, under guise of a more efficient nursing profession, from patient care to management positions. In effect, their nursing skills are being delegated to low-paid staff who regularly function without training or supervision. Management responsibilities for nurses now center on administration budgets and personnel assignments, which call for skills vastly different from the bedside patient care that attracted most nurses to their vocation. Consequently, caring skills atrophy while the rewards of the nurse-patient relationship no longer sustain and reward the nurse.

"Reskilling" echoes to a similar process in the United States, which goes without a generic name. Characteristically, when a U.S. health industry corporation takes over a nonprofit hospital, "unnecessary" staff are declared redundant, too expensive to be retained. Chaplains are fired, social work staff decimated, and nurses converted to piece workers deprived of professional status and job security. As with U.K. nurses, their patient care responsibilities are reassigned to untrained workers, including housekeeping staff. Resulting redirection of professional staff members from their clinical mission with patients appears in institutional reports as "bottom-line" profit, without mention of the consequent loss to patients.

Limited contracts with a few NHS managers affords but a narrow, circumspect view of their situation. Those with whom I talked hammered out a single-minded complaint, their sense of being despised by the general public. A plausible explanation of the managers' plight was offered by a concerned lay person. "It is not so much the sleaze factor, the discovery of corruption in dishonest public health officials, as it is the general recognition that the system has so many political traps and institutional barriers that it is close to inconceivable that a person of integrity might serve in a principled way."

Though managers, like others, warned, "Don't believe the statistics," a faint unpleasant whiff, not of disinformation but misinformation, hung in the air. The low-level grumble that the government is willfully avoiding a debate on health care reform adds to a fetid suspicion that the government is less than candid in reporting its performance, relying on delay and information murkiness to cover painful gaps in service and policy.

"Friction" in the transfer of official information surfaces with a close reading of the covers of Parliamentary documents. These paperbacks carry unusual price tags, £36 (U.S. $60), while photocopies of government documents are available at a charge of £80 (U.S. $130) a page. Freedom of information in Britain proves prohibitively expensive. On one occasion, frank opacity of information clouded a discussion when my informant, to confirm his testimony before a Parliamentary committee, paged through a copy of the record only to discover his testimony omitted.

Concern over information opacity surfaces in British science journals.[12] *New Scientist* carried outright charges that secrecy in the British medicine's control system inhibits the care of ordinary people. In answer, Minister of Health Tom Sackville stated that it [the secrecy clause of Section 118 of the 1968 Medicines Act] "by no means excludes proper implementation of the general duty to safeguard the public health."[13]

A subtler if not insidious barrier to the free flow of medical information explains the dearth of medical malpractice suits in the United Kingdom. British doctors often countersue patients for libel in the event of a malpractice complaint. Under common law, libel charges immediately seal pertinent medical records from public disclosure while eliminating confidentiality for complainants, as libel lawyers enjoy full discovery. Consequently, anyone considering blowing a whistle on a sleazy medical activity is intimidated by the cost of legal fees. According to some informants, silence prevails where complaints should be voiced about unprofessional behavior. Clearly, the resolve of patients suffering offense or injury at the hands of blameworthy staff is neither high nor reinforced.

Taken with the "warning on the label," the present position of the patient in the NHS might be left at the level of government surveys showing a high level of satisfaction.[14] Undeniable validation of patient satisfaction, however, is heard in personal accounts, one in particular from a civil servant, a former U.S. citizen, who, with bright-eyed gratitude, recounted his lifesaving, career-restoring, NHS, successful kidney transplant for chronic renal failure.

In the United States, the "noncompliant" patient, often a neurotic individual with physical complaints needing psychiatric attention, who persistently asks questions, reluctantly follows medical instructions, seeks second opinions, and declines the passive role in his or her health care, is relegated to a rough road on the periphery of the health care system. In the United Kingdom, where an estimated thirty thousand patients are being removed from doctors' lists every year, the "stroppy" (obstreperous) patient plods a parallel path.[15] Some suggest the number of "delisted" patients more likely reflects the cost of their caring rather than difficulty in relating to doctors, since fund-holding doctors have an implicit financial incentive for delisting and shifting costly patients to the NHS, inasmuch as they have a direct interest in saving the funds allotted to them. A somewhat similar phenomenon has appeared in the United States with health maintenance organizations and insurance plans "cherry picking" a young, healthy clientele.

As the presence of professional nursing at the bedside diminishes, a most serious plight befalls the incapacitated elderly. Attentive relatives are frequently dissatisfied with the quality of care the elderly receive in chronic care facilities. Making common cause of their concerns, relatives sometimes band together under the aegis of a local Community Health Council (CHC), which is intended to represent ordinary people's health care interests. Their activity was categorized by one CHC staff member as guerrilla activity in the warfare between the doctors and the managers. In effect, the CHC reports on the considerable gap between health services and social services. Though CHCs have limited position and less power, they hear a host of complaints and suggestions.

CHCs deal directly with the immediate trade-offs in care, for example, the bureaucratically mandated centralization of three small community hospitals into one large facility. They maintain the "casualty counts" in the internecine health establishment warfare by responding to public questions about rising numbers of unexplained deaths among geriatric patients. The latter issue carries with it considerable information opacity, as investigation of unusual deaths often leads to a muddle of lost institution records, indecipherable medical reports, and overworked registrars demanding to know how anyone might reasonably expect accurate records in the face of their intolerably heavy caseloads.

My week concluded with dinner at London's Printer's Pot with Mr. Alan Crystall, a Liberal Party East London borough councilman. He offered a startlingly new perspective on the "everybody/everything" problem. Commencing with a common tale of professional disillusionment ("The brightest day in my life dawned the day I retired from dental practice in NHS"), he recounted how over the years his commitment has waned as he has watched colleagues forsake quality dental care in order to convert their practices into high-turnover money machines.

Nor was my dinner companion sanguine about the future of health care, for he concluded with a question that would cause a wise owl to blink, "Do you think we can afford civilization any longer?" He suggested an alternative to the difficult "everybody/everything" problem I had never considered: abandon pursuit of community. A workable commonality is just too expensive!

So many men and women of goodwill were speaking with such trusting candor. In matching candor, I acknowledge encountering not a single villain, not even a cynic, none who did not wish to care. Yet there was such a pervasive sense of loss of direction. Like a ship with a defective compass, the British health care delivery establishment sets a course for a port the crew despairs of reaching.

Such trust in me, a transient passerby, can only be a measure of their palpable suffering, individual and collective, personal and institutional. They spoke as they did, trusting I would understand. Two facts came through clearly. To the degree that I understand, I hesitate to offer any advice about the British way to health care; rather, I am moved to reflect on the profound confusion we share. A multitude of well-meaning people on both sides of the Atlantic are infected with an insidious apprehension, born of unexamined fear, that they may be unable to serve the sick and yet remain caring human beings.

At heart lies our unspoken fear of the sick person, fearful not of his or her illness but fearful of what the sick person has come to mean, a dehumanized unit of work. Unwittingly, the sick person in our advanced health care system has evolved into a highly infectious carrier of soul sickness, the frightful, spirit-draining ennui of bureaucracy. We find ourselves in a dilemma. By attempting to care, do we empower the contagious soul sickness of complex social, intellectual, civic, and economic perplexities? Should health professionals, like anchorites of old, abandon this world of care and retreat to a modern monastery, a research center? Should we abandon the bedside to chance and the devil who lives nearby the "bottom line"? Or should we respond to the challenge of the sick and disabled who in their suffering ask us if we are civilized?

Asking what to do returns to how the "everybody/everything" issue impacts my state of Oregon. I returned with two powerful observations:

1. Britain has a health delivery system that, though stumbling in its search, professes to be for everyone. Until Oregonians profess the same, we are blatantly uncivilized, willfully ignoring the 120,000 Oregon children who presently lack access to health care. What we profess is an immoral system that exploits the working poor.
2. The cost of caring, much as the cost of medical supplies, must become a commonplace consideration in the planning and maintenance of Oregon's health services.

Unwittingly, a weary British nurse said it for all of us. "When the day is done I look around the ward and think, no one has died, the ward is pretty much together, but, oh, there has been no time for caring." Her tacit question, mine, and, I hope, that of all health professionals, is, When do we face the cost of caring?

Endnotes

Reprinted from The Pharos 59(Winter 1996): 11-15, with permission.
1. G. Smith, "Top Hospital in Hoax Row," *Evening Standard,* 17 Nov. 1994, 1, 2.
2. V. Macdonald, "Put Patients Last, NHS Manager Tells Doctors," *Sunday Telegraph,* 13 Nov. 1994, 1.
3. J. Laurance, "Doctors Accuse Trust Chief Who Told Them to Put Patients Last," *Times,* 14 Nov. 1994, 6, 19.
4. R. Highfield, T. Harnden, and R. Spencer, "Uproar over TV Scare on Baby Deaths," *Daily Telegraph,* 19 Nov. 1994, 1, 2.
5. "Hippocratic Trusts: The B[ritish]M[edical]A[ssociation] Spits Out Its Managers' Medicine, editorial, *Times,* 14 Nov. 1994, 19.
6. A. Leathley and J. Laurance, "Ministers Reject Pay Rise for Health Workers," *Times,* 14 Nov. 1994, 1.
7. M. Benson, "Doctors Forced into Rationing Care," Letter to the Editor, *Observer,* 13 Nov. 1994, 24.
8. J. Revill and F. Lynch, "Who Do They Think They Are?" *Evening Standard,* 9 Nov. 1994, 12.
9. L. Dillner, "Doctors are More Miserable than Ever, Says Report," *British Medical Journal* 309(1994): 1529.
10. V. Macdonald, "Surgeons Challenge Lure of U.S.," *Sunday Telegraph,* 13 Nov. 1994, 14.
11. *Rationing in Action.* (London, BMJ Publishing Group, 1993).
12. A. Tonks, "Stop Drug Secrecy, Says Government Watchdog," *British Medical Journal* 309(1994): 831.
13. M. Frankel, "Medicinal Secrets," Letter to the Editor, *New Scientist,* 3 Dec. 1994, 51.
14. S. Bruster, B. Jarman, N. Bosanquet, "National Survey of Hospital Patients," *British Medical Journal* 309(1994): 1542-1546.
15. "BMA issues guidance on removing patients from lists," *British Medical Journal* 309 (1994): 1111-1116.

Part 8

Compassion's Cruel Companions

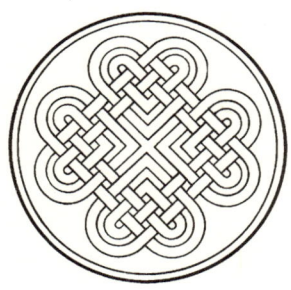

I think it was a great medieval philosopher who said that all evil comes from enjoying what we ought to be using and using what we ought to enjoy. Progress and efficiency by their very titles are only tools. Goodness and happiness by their very titles are a fruition; the fruits that are to be produced by the tools. Yet how often the fruits are treated as fancies of sentimentalism and only the tools are facts of sense. It is as if a starving man were to give away the turnip in order to eat the spade; or as if men said there need not be any fish, so long as there are plenty of fishing rods.

G.K. Chesterton (1874-1936)
in Marcus G. Singer, *Morals and Values*

Overview to Part 8

The residue of man's inhumanity to man contains not only compassion denied but compassion ignored. To understand the full measure of compassion, other human beings must be accepted as we accept ourselves, ignorant of our full nature, ignorant of our inherent barbarism, sometimes concealed, sometimes blatant.

We are all ignorant, to different degrees and in various ways, so the fact of ignorance does not account for a lack of compassion. Low IQ may limit scope of reason but carries with it no expectation of lessened humanity. But how different is the manner of ignorance from the fact in circumscribing compassion?

Ignorance is the seed of compassion when occasion for curiosity, cause for investigating an unknown other. However, when ignorance is joined with the use of power to control an "unknown" other, cruelty flourishes, albeit often disguised as "only trying to get the job done."

An example of cruelty when curiosity is extinguished by unfeeling power surfaced in the anguish of a grieving mother recounting how her twenty-five-year-old son was diagnosed with terminal leukemia and when he asked his oncologist how long he had to live, the oncologist snapped back, "Not long enough for us to get on a first name basis." The patient's curiosity was cruelly cut dead when it failed to serve power needs, presumably the treatment regime established by an emotionally ignorant physician. White-coated in our starched garb of righteous cleanliness, physicians, sometimes inadvertently, sometimes willfully, mark the sufferer as one apart, subject of their power.

The review *Shoah* examines this phenomenon at higher magnification. But first reflect on the wide-angle dimensions of human ignominy revealed in the essay **African Slavery and Western Medicine**. Consider, if you will, the number of physicians who, for four hundred years, "treated" slaves at collection points in Africa, there to certify the worth of human beings as healthy commodities, then as slave-ship doctors to ensure the cargo arrived in salable condition, and those doctors who on the plantations of the New World, including the United States, enabled the proprietor to maximize his return on investment. How was it possible that for four hundred years the organized medical profession participated in a holocaust that stole fifteen million Africans from their homes, killing two million in transit to slavery, without raising a whisper of concern for this monstrosity of inhumanity? Consider the dimensions of this ignorance and how it played out again in Nazi medicine during the worst of the twentieth century's holocausts, then wonder with me, how well informed we are today with our knowledge of the "other"?

Nor are the dynamics of slave doctors' ignominy any different from that of the oncologist's with his vicious rejoinder to his patient. The slave doctor did not think of slaves as "other." Slaves were willfully denied identity. The slave doctor, concentration camp doctor, and the ignorant oncologist share a sustained state of mind which devalues not only the humanity of others but theirs as well.

The idea of medical cruelty is counterintuitive, often considered a bygone phenomenon, like prescribed blood letting, venipuncture, that finished off President George Washington or the medical abuse Sigmund Freud experienced as treatment for his oral cancer. Medical cruelty is dismissed as medical history of former times and foreign cultures. For example, what could be more foreign than the German medical profession's participation in the Nazi program of racial purification? The review of the film ***Shoah*** attempts to develop perspective on the ghastly holocaust the better to determine compassion stillborn, how we may ignore compassion today.

How physicians have avoided, if not ignored, compassion for colleagues is documented in **An Epidemic of Suicide among Physicians on Probation**. Only with unceasing moral inquiry, self-examination by the doctor, by our medical organizations, by our profession, do physicians merit recognition as healers.

Are mind-bound bureaucrats progressively leading physicians to heartless compliance with amoral organizations? The op-ed **Stalinization of Health Care** poses a seldom-asked question, Is the medical profession safe from incremental accommodation to moral subordination?

Academic Sanction approaches medical ignorance from an international perspective, recounting the desperate straits of good physicians unjustly held accountable for evil circumstances. It is well to judge this account, albeit on a global scale, against your personal experience. What was your position on withholding economic and cultural support from South Africa because of apartheid? Was your reaction similar to the school room Johnny-did-it phenomenon? Did you count the cost of banishing to intellectual purgatory *all* the inhabitants of a foreign nation, including those struggling against an abomination loose in their land?

For many years, preemptive technology has been at work inadvertently dehumanizing our way of life through tacit moral accommodations. Set in the 1960s, prior to the advent of "virtual" human interaction through answering machines, "automated" bank tellers, and programmed shopping mall clerks, **The New Custodians** identifies a common nidus of "inconsequential," bureaucratic brutality, "Sorry, but this is not our policy." Here is license for personal irresponsibility, which implicitly encourages others to join in mindless evil. Semblance of personal moral identity evaporates with the classical denial of personal involvement, "The boss [the Camp Commandant] told me to…."

Sometimes fellow feeling is ignored by leaders of a tribe, even as elite a clan as the national leaders of American medicine. Here, distance offers the curious phenomenon of acting as a sounding board by amplifying the hypocrisy among unguarded leaders declaiming far from native ears. Listen for any fellow feeling among the 1971 leaders of American medicine as they hold forth before a London audience in **Is There a Doctor in the Nation?** How dedicated to the commonweal do they sound as they play "hard ball" for personal recognition on a "neutral" court?

The demand for profit in delivering health care, often ill-disguised as efficiency, willfully confuses corporate policy as moral agency. **A Modest Policy Proposal: The National Health Selective Disservice** aims at comic relief, yet over a decade later its satire seems too close to the bone when respected economists propose social policy to contain, if not eliminate, hundreds of millions of "superfluous people" on earth, those who can not afford to actively participate in the world economy. Our ability to mass produce black bottles of poisonous conformity exceeds imagination.

Compassion is not particular, reverberating as it does through the full spectrum of human passion, even resonating to the hate that is an inseparable part of suffering. An unexpected conclusion follows that to know compassion one must know hate. If this observation fails to find an intuitive niche, consider the quality of compassion to be expected from a dispassionate someone who has never loved, who has never felt the urge to strike out in anger. Passion is not learned as a discipline. Passion spontaneously forms from personal experience to appear unconditionally and whole.

Expression of lesser feelings carries with it ambiguous possibility of conditional love and/or disguised hate. To filter out resonating hatred from an awareness of another's turmoil fatally compromises the compassionate encounter while invariably diminishing sense of sharing. We should never remain ignorant of our hate, remembering how rage, hate's older brother, can speak for virtue. Accepting the reality of hate, even inchoate hate, is the burden of **Nurturing Hate in Psychotherapy.**

Though we may wish comfort in believing man's inhumanity to man is distant in time and place, taken together these essays recognize cruelty's everyday roots in the nature of man. Consequently, we have a Sisyphean task of controlling in ourselves, in our relationships with loved ones, cruelty's twin brother, hate. Then, as it is possible, we understand hate's origin, message, and effect on those who struggle against its evil purpose, enforced impotency of another. Anything less than full recognition of our personal capacity to hate diminishes our value as an individual, patient and physician. Though ignored, compassion need never be forgotten, if only remembered as counterpart to hate.

African Slavery and Western Medicine

> *Don't be no rougher on him than you're obleeged to, because he ain't a bad nigger.*
> —The old doctor
> in Mark Twain, *The Adventures of Huckleberry Finn*

Strange how seldom we find in life what we seek, yet stranger still how often our discoveries surpass imagination. My wife and I fell into just such a paradox on a voyage across the South Atlantic. We set out to view Halley's comet at its brightest from the Southern Hemisphere, only for me to inadvertently discover a dark side of medical history: the medical profession's role in that movable holocaust, the African slave trade.

Our five-thousand-ton, sleek, white cruise ship embarked from the West Indian island of Barbados. The complement of 185 passengers included an eminent astronomer to point out Halley's comet, which incidentally proved to be a disappointing smudge in the night sky. An oceanographer was also aboard for us to understand better the seas we crossed. Our first port of call was Devil's Island—nefarious, hot, and isolated.

Devil's Island is actually one of three islands, the Îles du Salut, six miles off the coast of French Guiana. The main isle is disfigured with jungle-covered, crumbling remains of the abandoned penal colony. The oppressive heat made climbing the steep road from the landing a sweaty job; haunted too, much as visiting a long-deserted graveyard, with uprooted stones, unhinged gates, scattered shards of broken glass, strange whirring insects, twitching lizards, feral pigs, and unseen things scurrying about in the thick overgrowth, emanating an eerie sense of pervasive malevolence. On the island's plateau, skeletons of cell blocks stretched, row on row, engulfed by twisting vines and immense tropical trees. Two corroded iron rails ran down the sides of each ruined cell block, marking what remains of the bed rails to which prisoners' ankles were fettered each nightly lockup. When I stretched out on the remains of one rusty bed my ankles fit the rail stocks snugly. Certainly, hell provides room enough for all of us.

On the island's highest bluff, positioned to catch any suggestion of a breeze, stands the ruin of the prison hospital; a decaying, two-story shell with an unnecessary sign, echoing Dante's admonition in three languages,

"Extreme Danger — Do Not Enter." This first island tour proved disheartening.

Back aboard, after a welcome shower I made for the ship's air-conditioned saloon and the solace of a tall gin and tonic. Yet the experience was not easily put out of mind, for I found myself wondering what tales the long-gone prison doctors of Devil's Island might have spun. What had they seen, heard, and thought of duty in this overheated purgatory? What had they made of treating condemned bodies and shattered souls in this quintessential institution of punishment. The penal colony at Devil's Island was more than punishment by ostracism, foreign exile, or hard labor. The prisoner's spirit was destroyed as well, annihilation as cruel as any crime he may have committed. Service there must have presented frightful contradictions to a caring doctor? The steward's call to dinner thankfully dispelled this heavy train of thought, an inkling of what the daemon of our trip had in store for me.

Belém, Brazil, turned out to be the next port of call. Time spent trudging about in the Amazon rainforest was followed by a day of "shopping" in the city. What impressed me most was the multihued coloring of mestizos' skin. On the afternoon of the second day, we set sail back down the mighty Amazon. While most of the passengers remained below attending the afternoon movie, I posted myself on the starboard flying bridge, a private wildlife observatory, for a wide view of the rolling Amazon, a river now so wide that from its center neither shore is visible. In particular I sought a glimpse of that rare mammal, the Amazon dolphin, a species near extinction as its opalescent eyes are collected and sold in Rio stores as an aphrodisiac.

The spectacular view from my perch echoed with discord, a sustained bickering between the captain and the river pilot. On a previous voyage, the captain had run his ship aground on a shoal in these waters. Now he and the first mate hopped and fluttered about the river pilot, questioning the pilot's every move and order, like aroused swallows harassing the flight of an unconcerned crow. Though there was little peace on the bridge, at my distance the buzz of anxious Greek and murmur of reassuring Portuguese gradually blended with the hum of the ship's engines as background music to an immense unfolding beauty.

Following a drenching shower, the setting sun unfurled a startling majestic turquoise sky outlined along the horizon by ranks of thunderheads growling and flashing their menace of yet another onslaught. There is a fascinating, elemental magic about a river preparing to surrender itself to the sea. I watched great, inexplicable upwellings of muddy water sunder roiling currents, and fish, feeling the chemistry of ocean salt mixing with fresh water, splash into the air. Dignified wrecks of shattered trees sailed by, bearing immobile, peering cranes, their pilots to undisclosed destinations. The intimidating power of primeval nature was occasionally broken by a lone fisherman, balanced erect in his fragile canoe, an insignificant apostrophe of human enterprise, afloat in the vast expanse of impatient waters.

The solitude gave time to reflect on our brief encounter with Brazil. Again, the daemon of my trip took hold. Belém had presented the physiognomy of Africa, faces more African than Native American or European. Here was evidence that Brazil had been the final destination for more Black Africans than any other port of call in the Americas.

My daemon merits explanation. Though forever alert in directing my attention, this disembodied spirit remained concealed from my conscious awareness until late in the voyage. Eventually, coincidences of travel became so clearly aligned that I was forced to reckon with the presence of this well-intentioned spirit. The first time my genie escaped his bottle, at least as I could make out, came in choosing the trip. My wife and I were looking for a North Atlantic voyage but failed to find one that met our desire until a flyer arrived in the mail advertising a once-in-a-lifetime trip across the South Atlantic to view Halley's comet. The flyer proved a shining spinner, my daemon's lure.

The night before we left I cast about my library for a book to read during lazy days at sea, but found nothing appealing. Dutifully I threw in an account of Richard Burton's travels in unexplored Africa, but my daemon would not leave it at that. Unaccountably I reached to a high shelf and pulled down an unread scholarly medical history book, Sheridan's *Doctors and Slaves*.[1] Thus my daemon set the hook that eventually drew me to her purpose.

As we crossed the wide South Atlantic, our resident oceanographer lectured on waves and weather, of vast tides of wind and current perpetually following a regular course about the earth; currents which unexpectedly matched the reading I became immersed in. He explained the Coriolis effect resulting from the rotation of the earth, giving as an example the Southeast Drift current, which passes down the coast of Europe to the African equator to become the North Equatorial current which in turn crosses the Atlantic with the westerly trade winds. Once this great Atlantic flow reaches the Caribbean it turns north and in the horse latitudes bears east, swinging back to Europe.

My book on slavery recognized these currents as well, but with different names and meanings. During the age of European exploration, like chips on the tide, fifteenth-century mariners, followed by merchants, followed the circular flow of the currents. From Europe they made their way down the coast of Africa to exchange their cargos of guns and cloth for human beings. Heavily laden with human chattel, they sailed westward, following a route that came to be known as the Middle Passage. In the West Indies, their cargo of fresh slaves was traded for another of sugar, rum, and cotton. Again at sea, they sailed north and east in the great gyres of favorable winds and currents, returning to Europe to sell their cargoes. It was profit all the way. With a little luck a single voyage could turn a fortune. Then it dawned on me that our ship was retracing, albeit east to west, the African slave trade.

Halfway across the Atlantic the weather took a nasty turn for the worse, strong winds and high waves. When I retired, I packed pillows against the bulkhead and bed rail, rocked to sleep in a cradle of sweet delight. In the morning, the sea ran high. Only by bracing myself in a corner of the cabin could I stand one-legged long enough to pull on my trousers. A particularly sharp toss of the prow gave me to understand why I read so much of the Guinea surgeon treating his slave cargo for abrasions, skin worn to the bone. Packed six hundred in a ship one-tenth the size of ours, the naked cargo, chained prone to the deck, slid back and forth with each wave, relentlessly grinding off their black skin on rough oak planks.

The common complaint of exposure and pneumonia among slaves of the Middle Passage became real when we put in for supplies at São Vicente in the Cape Verde Islands. In the evening, local musicians came aboard to serenade us. Of course my wife and I attended the aft deck concert, but only after we had bundled up against the cold night wind. Chilled to the bone, seven Creole Cape Verdians, with horns, flutes, and accordion of unusual design accompanied a soft tenor in the melancholy songs known locally as "morna." The music is a plaintive blend of Portuguese, Arabian, and African melodies, a sorrowful sigh of despairing resignation echoing voodoo incantations, which haunt those wind-chilled, bone-dry islands. While listening and sipping hot coffee on the aft deck in a wind of eight knots at a temperature of 59 degrees Fahrenheit, I came to appreciate what it might have been like for naked human beings shivering aboard the slave ships. How it could, and often did, prove fatal.

My daemon-directed education continued once we were ashore in West Africa. Dakar, Senegal, is an interesting landfall. Though I spent most of the time ashore visiting hospitals, learning from local colleagues what I could of medical practice in that part of the world, my wife and I set aside an afternoon to casually explore Gorée Island, a speck of land five miles off the westernmost tip of Africa.

After boarding a small motor ferry, we found a bench near the gangplank which promised shade from the equatorial sun. Quickening to the tempo that inevitably accompanies casting off lines, the dockhands began dragging aboard the lines securing the gangplank, when a large military truck drove on to the wharf, backed about, and disgorged a load of prisoners. Four guards marched up the swaying gangplank, rifles at the ready, and with a guttural command sent the prisoners, rough and tumble, scrambling, straight off the dock, over the railing, all but into our laps. Once aboard, the gang, short, tall, thin, and wide, talking and silent, had two qualities which immediately set them apart from the other passengers: shoddy blue-denim uniforms and mean faces. One brute of a prisoner stationed himself with his back to the railing, staring at us with eyes that seemed permanently focused on revenge.

With a shared glance, my wife and I slid under the rifle barrel of the nearest guard and scurried to a more distant part of the ship. Later we learned that the captain, in taking prisoners to Senegal's largest prison on Gorée Island, like Charon, the ferry man of the Styx, made no distinction among passengers. For just a moment, we had more adventure than we had bargained for. My daemon was at work giving us a brief taste of intimate commonalty with prisoners. Momentarily, we had been enrolled in a contemporary slave gang.

Gorée Island, all eighty-eight acres of it, is a museum aspiring to be a resort. Those Senegalese who have the means retreat to the island to enjoy its "fever free" breeze, an escape from malaria, the curse of the Guinea doctor. The president of Senegal has his summer home there, and a simple French hotel can put up a traveler for the weekend. However, we were drawn to a warren of buildings clustered below the ruin of Fort Saint Michael. Over the last four hundred years, the fort had been occupied in turn by the Dutch, Portuguese, British, and French, each intent on protecting their interest in the slavery business.

Ambling down a sandy byway, we came upon what was once the world's largest slave mart. Pushing open its shuttered gate, we passed through a dark passageway into a large, round, sun-drenched courtyard with ascending stairways circling the walls to the balcony above. The stairs afforded bidders opportunity to choose their position, distant or close enough to handle the merchandise paraded below them. Off the courtyard and beneath the balcony are the remains of holding pens; airy ones for salable grades, dismal pits for the sick and untamable culls.

Despite an array of frayed whips and rusty leg irons, the foreground horror of human suffering gave way to an appreciation of the wholly commercial nature of the enterprise. With less consideration for pain and suffering than a Chicago stockyard, Gorée Island processed untold millions of Black Africans for sale.

Like one of the three Fates spinning out the thread of human destiny, the "weighing" man decided the future of all males. Sixty kilo or more and life was assured as a salable product; for those not meeting the mark there was a month of grace to fatten up. Women slaves were graded by breast size and fertility. Failure to meet wholesale specifications was fatal. Unmarketable slaves, like any factory waste, were discarded. Regularly they were marched or dragged down a forbidding cobblestone corridor running under the building, through a series of gates, out onto a long dock, then pushed off its end. Sharks did the rest.

Not that casting slaves into the sea was uncommon. The seamen did what the mate ordered, the mate what the captain ordered, the captain what the owners ordered, and the merchant owners ordered profit. Therefore, the crews of slave ships routinely cast sick slaves over the side, since cargo insurance ruled that cargo lost as flotsam and jetsam was indemnified while cargo spoiled in transit was the merchant's loss. Nor was this a "business" secret. In 1840, J.M.W. Turner caused a minor stir in England with his graphic painting "Slavers Throwing Overboard the Dead and Dying."

The slave trade's denial of humanity found startling counterpoint that evening on Gorée Island. The inner courtyard of a crumbling building had been converted into a small amphitheater with seats fashioned from rubble. The age-worn facade of a house served both as a proscenium and dressing room for local artists who danced on the large, packed-dirt orchestra, much as choruses once danced in ancient Greece. Here a troupe of bare-breasted maidens and lithe young men stamped out pandemonium to the penetrating beat of three African drums.

No plaintive morna here. Instead, a crescendo of whirling, throbbing protest, the defiant cry of those who saw, knew, and lived to tell the tale. Rarely does classical ballet convey such direct and intense emotion. Descendants of slaves acting as chained slaves dragged from their wailing families, with separation and enslavement decreed by an imperious, white-masked captain on the balcony above; drums beating, voices wailing, and bodies writhing beneath the scourge of the press-gang boss. Then, with a great roar of jubilation, a stilt-dancing monster, certainly the God of the Congo, exploded onto the stage to scatter the slavers and set the people free. Though the Bible proclaims the sins of the father shall live unto the seventh generation, here in the fifteenth generation the sins are alive in the African dance; sins burned into the consciousness of a living multitude.

Up the coast of Africa, off Mauritania, our voyage was at its roughest, for we ran into a force 9 gale with thirty-five-foot waves. The twisting pitch and labored roll of the ship sent more than half the passengers and a quarter of the crew to their bunks, while the few who still had appetites shared a nearly empty dining salon, complete with sliding plates, broken glasses, and passengers pitched from their chairs. Smashed wristwatches and a broken wrist certified that climbing about the open decks was dangerous. I sought refuge in the upper lounge where, with my legs hooked about the fixed pedestal of a cocktail table, I could continue my daemon's assignment, reading on about the medical profession and African slave trade.

In addition to the Guinea surgeon who served the African branch of the slave industry, the British West Indies produced the plantation doctor who played an indispensable role in sugar production. Understanding his role demands a close look at the system.

Plantation sugar technology centered on the slave field gang. Much as with the ancient galley slave, the field gang did not depend on individual motivation. Despite the actuality of the whip-snapping task master, the galley slave was driven more by fear of his fellow slaves than his master's scourge. If the galley slave "pulled a crab," caught his oar in the water on the return stroke, he threw off his bank of rowers, placing all in jeopardy of punishment. Consequently, his fellow galley slaves proved swifter to punish and slower to forgive than any task master. So it was with the sugar plantation field gang. Hoes raised and fell in unison. It was machine production. Should one slave fall behind the tempo of planting, hoeing, or slashing, the whole gang suffered. The field master was paid a percentage of the production extracted by exploitation of available labor, that is, the gang. He meted out rewards and punishments to the gang, unconcerned with any individual member.

The plantation line gang was run at minimal cost of maintenance, determined by the value of a work unit, the going price of an African human being. Under usual field conditions of malnutrition, punishment, and relentless labor, the average life expectancy of a unit was seven years, paralleling today's expected useful life of an automobile. A single Caribbean island, Barbados, needed five thousand replacement units a year to maintain the island's sugar production. As units wore out, economic prudence dictated that it was better to discard rather than maintain the inefficient part. One overseer observed of sick slaves that they were "tools to be mended only if they could be available again; if not, to be flung by as useless, without further expense of money, time or trouble."[1]

For three centuries, young British doctors contracted for two or more years of "duty" on sugar plantations. They entered the "medical marketplace" of the British West Indies much as debt-ridden, hungry-for-cash, contemporary medical graduates enter the present-day medical marketplace. An entrepreneur among entrepreneurs, the new doctor joined the fiercely competitive bidding for plantation capitation contracts. Consequently, he was continually tempted to lower his bid by reducing overhead to minimal equipment and medicines while overextending his clinical range. It was not uncommon for plantation doctors to "care" for four to five thousand slaves as well as the plantations' staffs. Records exist of physicians with ten thousand slaves on their lists apparently acting more as busy maintenance engineers than healers.

Though it took time to assemble the facts and impressions into an understandable whole, I now could make out what my daemon was pointing me towards. Gradually there appeared in my mind's eye a man-made machine extending across a quarter of the globe, centered on the Caribbean, reaching from the upper Congo to the cotton fields of the Carolinas, from the depths of the Amazon jungle to offices on Harley Street, London.

Such an amazing mechanism. It was constructed by a happenstance of entrepreneurs, a wheel in a wheel, with the immense gyre of Atlantic currents serving as the flywheel, spinning lesser wheels of congregated lords, merchants, farmers, sailors, doctors, tribal chiefs, and purveyors, with compound gears of charter companies, all well oiled by governments, fueled by fifteen million bits of energy, African human beings, focused on the production of wealth. The manual of operation for this monstrous dynamo was written to ensure efficiency and certified with the motive of greed.

Two days later, the gale blew itself out and the passengers returned to the dining room, but the table conversation never broadened to accommodate my growing curiosity in the parallels between our voyage and the slave trade route. Any attempt to raise kindred interest was abandoned after my first sally went aground on an icy response, "They sold their own kind into slavery, didn't they? How could anyone care about such people?" There seemed little purpose in pointing out that Britons were once prone to sell their own people into Roman slavery or that Joseph was sold into Egyptian slavery by his brothers. Obviously, pursuing the possibility of human values in the antiquated yet profitable business of slavery did not sit well with my dinner companions. For some, perhaps, the cost of a larger sense of humanity comes too high to even examine its price tag.

The remainder of the voyage to Nice was filled with musing over two niggling questions. Why, in four hundred years, had organized medicine never taken a stand against slavery? Why did, and perhaps do, physicians tolerate slavery, depersonalizing a fellow human being into a thing, an object?

As I struggled with my daemon, African slavery generated strong emotions in my mind. It sometimes filled me with indignation and blind prejudice. Lest I complete the voyage with a heavy burden of unresolved feelings, I turned my mind to finding a workable understanding of the dynamics of the medical profession's four-hundred-year involvement in the evil of African slavery.

As I leaned against the ship's railing with thoughts directed beyond the horizon, my confusion over the evil of slavery grew. For example, to dispassionately consider that the African native simply represented a natural energy resource, much as the Arabian oil fields do today, and that fifteen million units were pumped through the Middle Passage conduit did little to reveal the logic of the traditional, generic acceptance of slavery by physicians. Yet a practical view emerged when comparing my reasoning with the logic of a Guinea surgeon or plantation doctor.

By applying higher magnification on the predominant values of slavery's service personnel, including the beliefs of physicians, my mental microscope revealed possibilities. The plantation owner pursued material gain, following his goal by risking personal capital for a possible return against the chance of losing both his wealth and position. Apparently, managers, supervisors, merchants, and physicians as well, chose to risk their skills and lives in pursuit of personal fortune in a morally ambiguous enterprise. Enabled by social consensus, they redefined the race of man, the better to deal with their difficult moral issues. For slavery's entrepreneurs, all men may have been created equal, but the African, by definition, was not a man, simply a beast of burden.

With the African defined as an animal, slaves were no more recognizable as participating in a moral system than machines are. The rights of man, the laws of government, the beliefs of morality, and the doctrines of religion did not apply to animals or slaves except as property. The exploiters' assumptions thus eliminated consideration of any encompassing morality. The universality of this thinking is perversely demonstrated in a few cases in which slaves were given their freedom, only then to establish themselves as slave owners within the plantation system by buying their own slaves.

Consequently, it was not the African's ignorance, his hopeless lack of reimbursement for his labor, nor even his helplessness before the marauding slave traders that determined the evil of slavery. The evil of African slavery rests on a single point, technology in which the slave, as beast of burden, was deprived of voice in the "moral" society that sustained slavery. Here is true north of a moral compass when navigating a voyage along the Middle Passage.

My first landmark on this route to corruption was establishing whether medical practitioners in those days were capable of protesting against slavery's denial of human values. This did not prove difficult to establish. In 1844, the Medical Society of Virginia took a strong stand against the plantation doctor/capitation system because it jeopardized their fee-for-service system of reimbursement.[1] This and other documented protests, all based on economic issues, make clear that organized medicine was capable of protest. However, rather than considering the rights of human beings, organized doctors focused their protest on *their* right to pursue profit. Slavery paid dividends, and doctors, like many others, used their organizational strength to ensure their share of technology's bounty.

Apparently, few physicians as individuals voiced protest against the generic evil of slavery. The cruelty of beating a slave to death could be, and was, attributed to the idiosyncratic brutality of an unscrupulous owner, much as some present-day physicians view cruelty to animals; animal experimentation is a moral issue for some, but not for others.

Nor was protest a simple matter of personal inclination. Society actively suppressed individual protest against slavery. One such tragic tale, complete with the modern threat of malpractice, began when a spiteful Jamaican master punished a slave he considered malingering with an overdose of tartar emetic. When the slave died of vomiting, an outraged physician noted the full facts in the public register. Incensed that anyone might question his right to do as he pleased with his property, the master demanded a public inquest, predictably made up of other plantation owners, and secured a verdict of "died by a visitation of God." Not content with rebuking the doctor, the plantation owner sued the physician for defamation of character and secured a judgment of one thousand pounds, large enough to bankrupt the physician and send him to an early grave.[1] Clearly, a slave was never to be more than a commodity.

A view of physicians acting as carriers of a virus of the moral plague of slavery was, in those times, unthinkable. Physicians, like everyone else, focused their thinking and skills on the economics of maintaining work units, to the exclusion of any contextual moral issues. There simply was little shared inclination for anyone to protest the source of their livelihood. Devoid of significant record of protest, for hundreds of years the slavery doctor went about treatment as a commercial enterprise, a technological skill independent of a patient's being.

By this time, the stewards were acquainted with my tastes, so a nod from my place at the aft rail sufficed to refill my glass. However, what I needed most was enough time before we docked to think out the contemporary parallel of the second question, do individual physicians tolerate slavery—today?

The pleasant click of the wooden discs of the shuffleboard players was not so much a distraction as a clue to finding an available doctor to put the question to. As I looked about, who should my eye light upon but the ship's doctor, in his immaculate white uniform, at the buffet table chatting with a cluster of attentive passengers, selecting among the freshly baked cookies and scones for his afternoon tea. Was it possible that he had an ancestor, a physician who had shipped out of Edinburgh with beliefs subsequently handed down to our ship's earnest doctor? But, of course I could not ask straight out if he was a little soft on slavery. He would consider me balmy. Rather the question must be put in a context that would have meaning to him as a physician.

This called for a bit of mental legerdemain, a simple thought experiment to be put to our ship's doctor. Not about sugar technology, in which his great-great-great-grandfather may have participated, but about modern medical technology where the ship's doctor might see some latter-day form of slavery.

The aft deck was littered with sunbathers about the pool, and convivial parties of nibblers and sippers clustered beneath bright striped umbrellas. Too public for "doctor talk." I invited the ship's doctor to the privacy of my wildlife observatory, the starboard flying bridge.

Passing between the two promontories known as the Pillars of Hercules, accompanied by flights of dolphins, flipping and frolicking as they once did beneath the bows of Roman galleys, the ship was entering the Strait of Gibraltar. Now perched high above the wide rolling sea I moved time ahead to summon a question which might capture our ship's doctor's attention.

Unfortunately, we failed to achieve a respectable intellectual exchange. My less-than-balmy question, "In your experience, have you encountered any difficulties with medicine's burgeoning high technology?" prompted a return volley of questions, "What do you mean? Are you against the British National Health System? Against medical science?"

"Why no," I replied, "I am not against any health delivery system as such. Just that I see so many systems which increasingly appear to treat patients in a technical and bureaucratic manner."

Obviously, he was not satisfied that I might not harbor some angst against "his" system. To mollify him, I continued, "In my experience, technologies—chemical, mechanical, or bureaucratic—so easily dehumanize those involved that I wonder about medical technology, particularly hi tech medicine."

His eyes sparkled in the Mediterranean sunlight. "Oh, that may be true for some systems, but not ours. In the U.K. we take better care of our patients than elsewhere in the world."

Though tempted to respond that he sounded like a long-gone British surgeon on a slave ship, "Oh, other nations may abuse slaves but British ships have the best record for caring for slaves," I refrained. Common sense dictates never confront a physician declaring his brand of medicine superior to another's, since so often the proof comes down to "We treat our slaves better than you treat yours."

Concentrating hard on remaining openly curious, I continued, "Well as I see technology, dehumanizing technology, it has a way of binding weak, dependent people to a system. Consider the problem of prescribed drugs. By estimates, 20 percent of the people in my city are on some form of tranquilizers, antidepressants, mood elevators, or other mind-altering drugs. We know 10 percent of physicians prescribe 90 percent of medications. It sounds a bit like medical bondage to me."

I knew I had lost him when he replied, "Ah, but that is your system," and then observed, "I say, look at that school of dolphins. What a remarkable display." He then politely excused himself with, "I must check the sick bay."

With my preaching I had lost my token doctor. To little effect, I resumed contemplating the sea. Actually, watching ocean waves can become depressing. Unlike a river or a stream, which has been somewhere and is intent upon going someplace else, once the eye is fixed on the sea's undulating plain of water, the mind dulls. Gradually, waves transform themselves into a vast, defeated army. A few officers in white caps perhaps, but most, head and shoulders, climbing over each other in a retreat from some rumor of a distant storm hastening them to flee they know not where. Waves may have a past but they lack a future so eventually the lookout must search the liquid desert for some spark of life, a flying fish, a sporting dolphin, lest the grim, unbroken universe of the sea drag him down through boredom to despair.

With my eyes fixed on the bow, I summoned the only available physician, the one I profess to be, to answer the question of modern-day medical attitudes towards slavery. Am I a technician regulating patients? What does it mean that I, as a psychiatrist, prescribe mind-altering drugs? Do I raise or lower the patient's full quality of life? Have I made an iatrogenic addict, a pharmacological slave, of the patient? Medically prescribed bondage accords with the society and science that I am immersed in. Yet for humane, if not moral reasons, I should offer the patient his or her choice of a full life and dignified death, including a pharmacologically fashioned persona. Certainly the path to healing includes the patient's choice of the amount of pain and suffering inseparable from their full life.

With my eyes still fixed on the bow, an even more ominous modern "slavery" issue surfaced. The patient's choice to "rebel," to kill the physician. Remembering that homicide is reported as the sixth major cause of physician death in the United States, I pondered deeply the implications of facing this fierce side effect of medical care gone awry.

Science has looked at homicidal reactions in slaves. The Black psychiatrist Frantz Fanon used his medical experience in nearby North Africa to carefully document the various forms of homicidal reaction colonized people displayed toward their exploiters. The syndrome is described in his book *Black Skin, White Masks*, where "doctor" may be substituted for "White man." "Face to face with the White man, the Negro has a past to legitimate, a vengeance to exact."[2]

The heavy thought of a patient choosing to murder his white-coated physician, who "first means no harm," proved oppressive, particularly as I thought of the two psychiatrists who in the last six months had been murdered in my home state of Oregon and of obstetricians across the nation murdered for performing abortions. Fortunately, the memory of the words of a Black doctor I had talked with in South Africa sustained me. In reflecting on politically active Black medical students who look to the day of their "vengeance," the doctor said, "I see them from time to time and I tell them, 'We will have no part of inequality. If they [the Whites] come in wounded, we will heal them even if it means they go back to man the guns that are pointed at us.'" He made it clear that for him there is no alternative in being an ethical doctor.

In a most unusual way the memory of this wise doctor opened my eyes to my own slave owning. He had talked of apartheid and I asked him what we, in my country, should do for him to remove the evil of apartheid. He did not ask for money, sanctions, or arms but paused just a moment to reluctantly confide, "Please do not ask me to suffer for your political beliefs." In my cultural ignorance I had stumbled again, asking him to shoulder this White man's "burden." Tactfully, he suggested I take responsibility for my own choice.

With this memory my daemon's message fell into place. Now I could see that quality of care, medical or otherwise, is not determined by my social, economic, or political value of the patient; those are but circumstances, albeit powerful circumstances, which confuse understanding of fulfilled caring. Caring turns out not to be a concept but an experience, a shared choice of one with another. Only by choosing to recognize each and every man, woman, and child that I encounter as a unique fellow human being, do I free my slaves.

That evening, after the Last-Night-Aboard party, my wife returned with me to the bow for a breath of light Mediterranean air. In the darkness she asked me, "With the storm and all the time at sea, are you disappointed with the cruise?"

Unhesitatingly, I replied, "No, not disappointed, grateful."

Endnotes

1. R. Sheridan, *Doctors and Slaves* (Cambridge: Cambridge University Press, 1985).
2. F. Fanon, *Black Skin, White Masks* (New York: Grove Press, 1967), 225.

Shoah
A Film Review

>...thou has sore broken us in the place of dragons, and covered us with the shadow of death.
>—Psalms 44:19

Shoah is remarkable for its goal as well as its path to the goal. Many if not most children are reared in the United States with the admonition that they should eat all the food on their plates because "children are starving in Ethiopia, Biafra..." Thus an incomprehensible truth is used in a way that will never make it comprehensible. Director Claude Lanzmann devoted ten years of life to make the incomprehensible fact comprehensible that "millions of Jews were slaughtered at the hands of the Nazis." His technique is superb; rather than patching together old documentary films and newsreels, he asks survivors to describe as best they can what they saw and felt from within the Nazi death machine as it annihilated millions of Jews.

Some criticize the film for its length (nine and one-half hours), others for stirring guilt, despair, and revulsion. Neither criticism is valid. In nine and a half hours Lanzmann did not say enough; and the past, replete as it is with mindless destruction, offers a foundation of meaning to an individual or a culture. The fact is, you cannot know the role of human nature in Western culture if you have not read Homer's *The Odyssey* nor seen (or read) Lanzmann's *Shoah*[1]—not that either are easy on the reader/viewer, but then moral growth, the expanding appreciation of mankind in the full, is never easy, drawn as so often it is from human sacrifice.

Shoah trods the path to the Final Solution, mapped out that fateful January 20, 1942, when Reinhard Heydrich assembled a pack of Nazi state officials at 56/58 Grossen Wannsee, Berlin, to implement the German national policy for complete destruction of the Jews.[2] The parts of the destruction machine were available, waiting to be assembled as a gigantic, military bureaucracy. What remains to be filmed of this ultimate disassembly line is the still-existing ghetto of Corfu, the cattle cars used as transports, the railroad tracks winding over Europe to the death camps, the snow-covered ruins of the Auschwitz crematorium, the summer trees flourishing over Treblinka, the monument where the Warsaw ghetto once stood, and the faces of the survivors.

What you hear is account after account of survivors: the account of the Nazi assistant commandant of the Warsaw ghetto, a Polish peasant's account, the Brooklyn housewife's account, a Vermont historian's account, an Israeli barber's account, a Polish stationmaster's account, so painful in the hearing that the first time I saw the film my body tensed enough to force me out of my seat, to pace the lobby of the theater for relief.

As survivor Abraham Bomba cuts hair in a Tel Aviv barbershop, the voice behind the camera questions, "How did it happen?" and he details in a dispassionate but tense voice how he cut the hair of still-living victims in the Treblinka gas chamber, hair the Nazis "salvaged" for use in Germany. He explains the need for speed; sixteen barbers worked two to five minutes with each group. Then they stepped back, the doors closed, and the women and children "showered" with Zyklon gas. The bodies were removed out a back door. Then another group of sixty or seventy naked women and children were herded in for a quick barbering, and so on, again and again, for years. When asked what he felt about this he stumbles, hesitating. "I felt that accordingly I got to do what they told me."

Softly but implacably the camera voice asks again, "What did you feel?"

"It was very hard to feel anything....Your feeling disappeared."

Then reluctantly he begins to describe how it was when a transport arrived from his home town with neighbors, friends, the wife and sister of one of the other barbers among them. He wipes his face on a towel; tears fill his eyes; he looks out the window, licks his lips, swallows, clamps his jaws, pauses interminably.

"I can't. It's too horrible. Please."

"We have to do it. You know it."

Wiping his face again with a towel, "I won't be able to do it." But he does.

Armando Aaron, president of the Jewish community of Corfu, stands in the square of Kerkira relating what it was like June 9, 1944, when the local Greek officials collaborated with the Gestapo in rounding up the 1,650 Jewish inhabitants of the island. Sick from the hospitals, retarded from the institutions, children and the elderly, together with all others jammed aboard ferries, which in turn delivered them to trains. They were packed in too tightly for anyone to sit until the dying relieved them by slumping dead underfoot.

Aaron tells what it was like to travel in the cars from June 11 till they arrived at Treblinka on June 29, eighteen days and nights without food, water, or sanitation. He describes children crying for water, women slashing their wrists, dead bodies completing the journey in quicklime. Then, not knowing where they were, the half-crazed refugees were disgorged onto the Treblinka arrival ramp, to be driven by the whips and dogs of the Ukrainian guards to the crematorium. All but 119 were incinerated the night of arrival. As Armando Aaron speaks, the camera follows the wake of boats, the tracks of the train, into the camp to finally move down the steps into what is left of the crematorium.

The camera switches to a surviving Nazi assistant commandant at Treblinka, SS Unterscharführer Franz Suchomel, explaining his revulsion at the pervasive smell when he arrived at the death camp. He apologizes for his rendition of the "prisoners song," learned by the slave gangs in one day or they died, but his pride in the efficiency of the camp remains undisguised. He helped in reorganizing the camp when the load began overwhelming the system. He points out how necessary it was for the Jews to arrive exhausted, without food or water, consumed with overwhelming thirst, so they would believe and do anything in response for a promised drink of water.

The assistant commandant's detailed technical description of the smoothly running machinery of death is matched by ex-Nazi Walter Stier, former head of Reich Railways Department 33 of the Nazi Party, who, with a train dispatcher's informed memory, recounts the specific routes and financing of the transport trains (the Jews were treated as passengers and forced to pay for the transport).

The camera asks, "Did you know Treblinka meant extermination?"

"Of course not!....How could we know? I never went to Treblinka."

One brief respite comes at the end of Filip Müller's account. A Czech Jew, he survived five liquidations of his "special detail" and over the years came to know every detail of the four giant Auschwitz crematoriums, each of which killed two thousand people at a time. At one point, overcome with the horror he was part of, he tried to remain with neighbors and friends in the gas chamber, only to be driven out by a woman. "Your death won't give us back our lives....You must get out of here alive, you must bear witness to our suffering."

Looking back he reflects, "The situation taught us fully what the possibility of survival meant. For we could gauge the infinite value of life....That's why we struggled through our lives of hardship, day after day, week after week, month after month, year after year, hoping against hope to survive, to escape that hell."

In place by 1942, the death technology ran with oiled precision until the end of the war. An estimated eighteen million to twenty-six million human beings—prisoners of war, political prisoners, nationals of invaded and occupied countries—were put to death by starvation, cold, pestilence, torture, medical experimentation, firing squads, and the gas chambers of the German concentration camps.[3] To understand better how this process was implemented in increments small enough to avoid placing responsibility for the lives extinguished, or its agents, its source must be traced to events prior to the Wannsee Conference.[2]

The minutes Adolf Eichmann kept of the conference are all generalities without specifics. "The 'final solution' of the European Jewish problem would involve about eleven million 'practicing Jews,' including significantly those in England, Ireland, and Turkey."[2] Ironically, the committee members shared a deep concern that they "should disarm [their] critics from outside" by differential treatment of "well-known" Jews and those over sixty-five. The aged were "not to be evacuated [that is to say, killed], but to be *transferred* to an Old Peoples' ghetto," thus avoiding the possibility of international "atrocity propaganda."[2]

They wasted their concern, for once the Allied leaders learned of the Final Solution they proved to be much like the Polish peasants portrayed in *Shoah,* living and going about their business in the shadow of the death camps. Never a word of protest. The only occupied country that defied Nazis and their Final Solution was Denmark, largely as a result of the display of moral strength by its king.

A significant clue to why the Final Solution was possible is found in the extensive medical experimentation carried out at Buchenwald: the zealous collaboration of "ethical" German doctors in establishing and maintaining the death camps. The Nazis built on the German medical profession's previous use of death as a solution of social "problems." At the Wannsee Conference, the Nazis used a "medical model," a model that had been in place well before the war, as the "euthanasia" project.[4]

In 1939 hundreds of doctors with "positive" attitudes towards the Nazis cooperated in a secret classification of retarded children, psychiatric patients, bedridden elderly, and patients suspected of hereditary disease. Once classified as unfit, patients were transferred to "Children's Specialty Institutions" and "Therapeutic Convalescent Institutions," where they were killed. By depersonalizing and dividing the clinical decision to kill a child into disjointed bureaucratic bits, the "euthanasia" project "protected" all participating doctors from confronting their ethical responsibility.

When word of the killing program leaked out in 1941, clergymen protested, and Adolf Hitler officially terminated the project. However, the project was secretly enlarged and moved further from public view with the new name of Reich Work Group of Sanitoriums and Nursing Homes, "T4." By 1945 "T4" went on to kill an estimated five thousand children together with an unknown number of adults. The role of the medical profession is epitomized in the career of Dr. Irmfried Eberl. At the age of twenty-nine, he joined the "euthanasia" project as a specialist in lethal techniques for children. Later, he was rewarded for his outstanding scientific work by appointment as commandant of Treblinka.[4] Obviously, Lanzmann's nine-and-a-half-hour film merely scrapes the surface of man's inhumanity to man under the Nazis.

Why did doctors participate in research and "treatment" directed towards human annihilation? Perhaps the question should be framed in the present tense. Why do doctors participate in torture and murder of human beings? The answer of the Nazis in *Shoah*, is "I was only carrying out orders." Some doctors refused to join killing programs, but they were insignificant in number and effect when compared with those interested in good pay, social approval, and "duty" as defined by higher authority. There is no record of the Nazi regime ever having trouble enlisting doctors into their programs of extermination. The doctors participated because they wished to succeed and were morally "adaptable."

Without a moral basis, the medical profession becomes a menace to mankind. Not too surprisingly, German doctors contributed to their own moral "adaptability." Whether through reluctance to acknowledge the moral basis of medicine in the political climate of the 1930s or other reasons, German doctors delayed or avoided critical moral decisions. As one of the Nazis in *Shoah* says about recognizing the existence of the death camps, "Then, there were things best not mentioned." He and thousands of doctors did not "know" that a physician's failure to make a moral decision is a moral decision.

When should the German medical profession have made its moral position clear? *Shoah* takes up the question of timing, pointing out that it is too late to make a moral decision as you walk down the steps of a crematorium, too late as you ride in a transport, too late when you are rounded up for "transfer." It is too late when the homeless settle down to freeze to death on a sidewalk grate.

By inference and the experience of those few who successfully fought back, the right time to make a moral decision is now, today, in the present tense. Today, when there are significant others who will hear. Today, before a social, economic, or electronic technology begins uniformly to regulate physicians' behaviors. Today, as we face critical life-and-death decisions. Today, doctors, still rich and powerful, should make explicit and open moral decisions about the right for all people on this planet to live in dignity.

Does this sound like a jeremiad? See *Shoah,* and then decide when is the right time for you to "gauge the infinite value of life."

Endnotes

Reprinted from *The Pharos* 50(Fall 1972): 24-32, with permission.
1. C. Lanzmann, *Shoah: An Oral History of the Holocaust* (New York: Pantheon Books, 1985).
2. H. Krausnik, H. Buchheim, M. Broszat, et al., *An Anatomy of the SS State*, trans. R. Barry, M. Jackson, D. Long (New York: Walker & Co., 1968).
3. *Encyclopedia Britannica, Micropaedia*, v.3, p.61 (Chicago: University of Chicago, 1973).
4. R.J. Lifton, *The Nazi Doctors: Medical Killing and Psychology of Genocide* (New York: Basic Books, 1986).

An Epidemic of Suicide among Physicians on Probation

Some in fury, but most in despair, sorrow, fear and out of anguish and vexation of their souls, offer violence to themselves: for their life is unhappy and miserable. They can take no rest in the night, nor sleep, or, if they do slumber, fearful dreams astonish them.
—Robert Burton (1577-1640)
The Anatomy of Melancholy

In 1976, the members of the Oregon Board of Medical Examiners grew uneasy with the incidence of suicide among the physicians they had placed under close examination and probation. Since its inception in 1889 the board has acted through its power of licensure as the primary force regulating the medical profession in the state of Oregon. The board is composed of eight members who represent a cross section of the geographic distribution of physicians in the state. Board members are generally appointed by the governor from a list, proposed by the Oregon Medical Association, of physicians who are recognized and respected in their communities.

The disciplinary mode of the board is expressed in its powers of probation. When a physician in Oregon is found culpable of professional misconduct of sufficient weight to merit probation, his license to practice is suspended and immediately reinstated, generally for a probationary period of ten years.

In the spring of 1977, the board had approximately forty physicians on probation or under investigation for probation. Most unusual, however, was the disturbing fact that during the preceding thirteen months eight of these physicians had committed suicide, and two were recovering from serious suicidal attempts. The impact on the board members was understandably great.

While it is recognized that the present sample is too limited for statistical analysis, the suicide rate for the general population is about 15 per 100,000, and that of physicians in general is considered to be about 77 per 100,000. The Oregon rate for our sample of probationers, however, if it could be extrapolated to a larger population, would approximate 20,000 per 100,000. In any case, in the eyes of the Board of Medical Examiners, the situation with the probationers appeared to be reaching alarming proportions. As one means of action, the board encouraged the authors to examine the phenomenon and asked for suggestions concerning steps to avoid recurrence.

Ideally, two avenues of investigation are necessary for the phenomenon to be understood in-depth—a study of the social dynamics of the board's processes and structure and the psychosocial circumstances and dynamics of the victims. Because of limited resources, the study has been limited to the latter. The board cooperated in this venture, opening its full records—under appropriate professional constraints—for the investigation of the life history of the victims, with particular emphasis on the period immediately prior to their deaths.

The study was undertaken by a group of six professionals (one psychiatrist, two clinical psychologists, one sociologist, one psychiatric resident, and one medical student) who were brought together by the senior author (R. Crawshaw) out of consideration for their interest, compassion, and professional competence. The investigators named themselves the Blachly Group as a means of honoring a distinguished psychiatrist, Paul Blachly, M.D., who had recently met an accidental death by drowning and who had devoted much of his professional life to the study of physician suicide.

Methods

In the spring of 1978, the Blachly Group made arrangements to interview the closest available surviving member of each deceased physician's family. Of the eight cases, six relatives agreed to the interview. Of the two surviving wives who would not agree to a discussion of the husbands' suicides, one had moved to the Midwest and did not want discussion by telephone or letters. The other refused to talk to any physicians, blaming them for her husband's death. The interviews were performed in the survivors' homes, except for one that took place in an interviewer's office. Of the survivors, four were wives and two were daughters. In the latter group, information was not as detailed as that of the wives.

A fifteen-page protocol, which had been devised by the American Psychiatric Association Task Force on Suicide, was the guide for compiling data in the interviews. Factual information, such as colleges attended, medical school, internship, and residency, was obtained from the files of the Oregon Board of Medical Examiners. The remainder of the form consisted of questions under the following headings: Details of the Suicide, Communication of Suicidal Intent, Response to Suicidal Communication, Previous Suicidal Attempts, Intention and Motivation, Background Information, Psychiatric Information, Psychiatric Symptoms Checklist, Sexuality, Interpersonal-Social Information, Financial Information, Residential Information, Interpersonal-Familial Information, Religious Information, Developmental History, Professional Background and Activities, and Survivors.

To protect survivors, case histories will not be published. Eighty percent of the interviews took place in Oregon and, for the most part, in the Portland metropolitan area and suburbs. One interview was conducted in Eugene, Oregon, and one in California. The sessions lasted approximately two to four hours. Each session was tape-recorded. Five of the interviews were conducted with two study group members present, the other with only one interviewer. One interviewer was present for five of the interviews. Funds for travel expenses were obtained from the Community Psychiatry Program at the University of Oregon Health Sciences Center Department of Psychiatry. The remainder of the expenses were borne by the Blachly Group interviewers.

Two of the physicians were undergoing psychotherapy at the time of their deaths. Subsequently, one of the treating psychiatrists met with the study group and gave a helpful and detailed history of the patient; the other psychiatrist declined.

The Blachly Group met regularly to review transcripts and to discuss various approaches to the growing mass of data. The summary of the interviews may be explained from at least two perspectives: the first is a quantitative presentation of selected dimensions of the material contained in the answers to the protocols, while the second is a narrative generalization that is contained in the following profile.

Physician Suicide—A Profile

This profile will attempt to characterize six physicians who took their own lives in Oregon during 1976 and 1977. All were in probation status with the Oregon Board of Medical Examiners. All were men.

In age, the men fit in two groups: four were early middle-aged, from thirty-six to forty-three years of age. Two were in their late sixties. All had a history of serious, formally diagnosed psychiatric disturbance before probation status. Depression was present to some extent in all of them. The two older men appeared to suffer from reactive depression caused by loss—in one case, of spouse, in the other, of physical health. The younger group appeared to have serious endogenous emotional problems associated with instability early in their lives. Most were described as introverted and sensitive, with anxiety and depression. Under stress, they frequently showed serious psychopathological conditions, including paranoid thinking or manic-depressive behavior. Five of the six abused drugs (amphetamines or meperidine hydrochloride), and four of the six abused alcohol; all abused at least one of these mind-altering drugs.

None of the men was a native of Oregon (as is true of about 52 percent of the total population of the state). Most were transient, having held a variety of medical positions in different areas of the country. Four of the six were divorced at least once. They were unlikely to have community or religious attachments. They tended to be socially isolated persons and, perhaps even more important, professionally isolated. Several had failed to reach important goals that they had set for themselves (for example, specialty status), and several had been rejected by professional colleagues by terminating cooperative practices, dismissal from positions, withholding social contact. Four of the men had blue-collar craftsman fathers and appear to have had an upwardly mobile work ethic. None had a family history of suicide, although four of the six had attempted suicide before their final act of self-destruction.

Comment and Conclusions

The most important single element in the data appears to be the high degree of serious diagnosed psychopathological conditions demonstrated before contact with the board by the probationers who completed suicide. For most of these physicians, an overt psychopathological condition was manifest early in their careers and recurred throughout their professional lives. Also of great importance and interrelated with the psychopathology is their abuse of alcohol and other mind-altering drugs.

Case histories disclose that professional status was of singular importance to these men. This goal was embodied by professional achievement (for example, specialty boards and professional ambitions) and personal acceptance by their physician peers. These goals were of such importance that they were frequently pursued at the expense of positive family relationships and community networks. While some of these probationers experienced financial difficulties that probably contributed to their stress, financial problems were not perceived by the survivors or by the study group as having a directly causal relationship with their deaths. All of these physicians were migrants to Oregon, and in most cases their domestic and social lives were characterized by a severe sense of isolation.

Among other things, the findings speak to the importance of medical school screening of future physicians for emotional stability and for guidance of those aspirants with early, serious psychiatric disturbance into less stressful vocations. Furthermore, medical educators should seriously address the destructive side of professional competition, namely, those characteristics of the medical profession that exaggerate independence to the degree that a physician fears to admit that he needs personal help and consequently fails to seek it out or accept it.

Examining boards face a sobering task when supervising the ethical conduct of medical practitioners, especially as they bring sharp public scrutiny to focus on errant physicians. Such exposure and consequent disciplinary action itself will—and probably should—increase the probationer's stress. Social disapproval remains a powerful and necessary deterrent to antisocial behavior in all professions. At the same time, close attention must be paid to the possibility of causing even more deviant behavior, including self-destruction. Granted that boards must pursue their duty, it must be carried out in a perceptive and supportive fashion, without diminishing firmness of standards or actions. No one should underestimate the difficulty and complexity of such a task.

The following conclusions and suggestions are submitted for the consideration of medical (and other professional) examining boards.

1. When a physician demonstrates questionable practices, the earlier in the person's career that candid recognition and corrective action occurs, the more likely that there will be a constructive response.
2. Corrective action at times might be more effective if it were stronger, more clearly delineated, and closely time-limited. A few months of absolute professional suspension might be more effective in changing behavior, and ultimately easier for the

person to handle, than ten years' probation. Probation itself should probably be limited to a few years, to modify the endless (and hopeless) prospect.

3. Comprehensive mental health services (psychiatry, clinical psychology, and psychiatric social work) should be regularly used by all medical licensing boards.
4. There should be a psychosocial evaluation of all probationers at critical points in the preprobation and probation processes.
5. A board should make direct contact with and make itself accessible to close relatives of probationers.
6. A board should carry out its own psychological autopsies of deceased probationers and should maintain detailed records on these cases for a period of years.

In addition to the aforementioned suggestions to examining boards, a few general recommendations may be made.

1. The medical (and especially psychiatric) community should take steps to make access to mental health treatment for physicians easier and more socially acceptable.
2. A physician's widow interviewed during this study strongly urges that laws prohibiting self-prescription of drugs be rigorously enforced.
3. Medical societies should cease the practice of destroying the records of physicians' suicides.
4. To facilitate the study of physician impairment at a national level, it is recommended that a national clearinghouse be established under the aegis of the American Medical Association for the maintenance of statistics regarding all physicians' suicides.
5. It is recommended that the American Psychiatric Association institute a national program of psychological autopsies of physicians' suicides by volunteer psychiatrists and that the resulting data be stored in the AMA clearinghouse.
6. Given the Blachly Group's findings that domestic and especially community isolation, as well as anxiety over professional loss of face, were prominent aspects of most of the suicides in question, the medical profession and others who share this concern should foster groups who can offer support of a regular social (not psychiatric or therapeutic) nature to physicians in

need and their families. Awareness of and ability to refer to resources of school, church, recreation, and other community activity should be clearly in the minds of those who seek not only to discipline but also to help the physician-probationer and his family.

Endnotes

Reprinted from the *Journal of the American Medical Association* 243(1980): 1915-1917, with permission. Copyrighted 1980, American Medical Association. Coauthors: J. Bruce, P. Eraker, M. Greenbaum, J. Lindemann, D. Schmidt.

Stalinization of Health Care

When you live with wolves you must howl like wolves.
—Russian proverb

In 1994, the British Foreign Office sponsored a visit for me to study the United Kingdom's National Health System (NHS). I was surprised to hear "Stalinization" used by British health care professionals to describe a pervasive attitude of fear among doctors, nurses, and patients. The British Medical Journal defines Stalinization as the fear of severe organizational and economic retaliation for telling the truth about their system's shortcoming.[1] The Journal documents thirty cases of Stalinization, including doctors suspended for complaining about inadequate staffing levels in pediatric units. The question for this visitor is, Does Stalinization occur in Oregon?

Nor is Stalinization difficult for an alert visitor to discover. An acquaintance acting as an ombudsman volunteered that increasing pressure came from above not to pursue complaints about inadequate care of elderly patients. Nurses shared their despair at being shifted from bedside care to management assignments. Doctors voiced profound concern about "gagging clauses" in new contracts with the NHS.

When the NHS is not sidestepping critical questions with "the information is not held centrally," it discourages curiosity about its activities, such as auditor's reports, by charging a transmittal fee of $130 a

Xeroxed page. Censorship of publications occurs when outspoken dissent is arbitrarily eliminated. Frequently, meetings are scheduled at inconvenient times or abruptly rescheduled to discourage public attendance while findings are distributed only to a select few. If pushed hard, the British Department of Health declares information unavailable because it is held in one of their 413 "secret files" which can not be examined for "reasons of state."

The personal cost of whistle blowing in Great Britain is high. Whistle-blowers risk more than their job. Charging that misconduct has occurred can bring a libel suit against them. Ironically, the libel suit immediately closes investigation of the complaint while forcing the whistle-blower into court to defend him/herself against charges of libeling the malefactor. Understandably, the out-of-pocket cost and personal suffering of a possible libel suit is more than most wish to undertake.

Rumbles of similar developments have been heard in Oregon. Some managed care concerns have dropped panel doctors for disclosing "business secrets" by telling patients of company malfeasance. Some patients have proved reluctant to report errant doctors, voicing fears of a medical conspiracy and retaliation. However, Oregonians have a protection that British patients lack, the First Amendment to the Constitution backed by our Freedom of Information Act. When push comes to shove we can not be denied the right to publish the truth.

If Stalinization is present in Oregon it needs immediate exposure, and a remarkable proposal is expected to do just that. Our state government is seeking practical feedback from patients using the Oregon Health Plan. The Oregon Consumer Scorecard, developed collaboratively by HMOs, Oregon Health Decisions, and the Oregon Health Policy Institute, asks how patients experience the Oregon Health Plan.[2]

As planned, patients will score their reactions to health care services. They will report how well they have been informed about what is happening, staff attitudes, as well as the efficiency, dignity, and effectiveness of their care. This information will be a unique window on what the public receives and values, information open to the public at considerably less than $130 a page.

By helping Oregonians make informed choices among health care providers, the Oregon Consumer Scorecard has a healthy future keeping the emphasis of the delivery of health care where it should be—on caring, rather than protecting the position of a bureaucracy or the profits of a corporation. The use of the Card may expand to include all Oregon patients, a proper antidote to Stalinization.

The Card is a tool of democracy against Stalinization. Yet democracy's enemies, cynicism, apathy, and special interests, are not defeated simply by governmental openness. Much as with democratic government, democratic health delivery calls for citizen action. Like the vote, the Card only works if used by thinking, committed people. Oregonians must have the courage to say it as it is for quality health care. Together, and only together, can we build a healthier community.

Endnotes

Reprinted from *The Scribe*, Portland, Oregon, op-ed, May 15, 1996, with permission.
1. R. Smith, "The Rise of Stalinization In the NHS," *British Medical Journal* 309(1994): 1640.
2. The Oregon Consumer Scorecard process is repeated biannually for use by consumers and providers of health care.

Academic Sanction

It is a fine thing to face machine guns for immortality and a medal, but isn't it a fine thing, too, to face calumny, injustice, and loneliness for the truth which makes men free?

H.L. Mencken (1880-1956)
in *The Portable Curmudgeon*

The horror of apartheid was slow to break into consciousness, finally driven into "responsible" thinking by a need to take a public stand for or against my psychiatric brethren in South Africa. Were they or were they not moral pariahs? To decide, I visited them, first in 1987 and, later, twice more to make my best judgment. Returning, I affirmed my final judgment of them and of colleagues condemning them, in the following paper published in JAMA.

Medical scientists should be aware of a real and present threat to science, the practice of academic sanctions for political reasons against South African scientists.[1] Clearly, this is no apology for any of the political policies by which oppressive governments, in the name of party, creed, color, nationality, or race, deny human rights to some or all people. Such policies are abhorrent to most medical scientists.

Through the activities of the National Academy of Sciences/Institute of Medicine Committee on Health and Human Rights, and other concerned organizations worldwide, attention has been directed to the persecution of scientists in politically oppressive countries—persecution that includes loss of academic position; limited access to research, teaching, and clinical facilities; detention; torture; and death.[2,3] However, it may not be clear how some scientists in the free world and their professional organizations contribute to the hardship of persecuted scientists by the use of academic sanction as an expression of personal political beliefs.[4]

The experience of Professor Philip Tobias, professor of anatomy and former dean of Witwatersrand Medical School, Johannesburg, South Africa, serves as an example. Professor Tobias is a strong opponent to South African racist policy. At his own expense and personal risk, he appealed to the South African Supreme Court for an open inquiry into the findings of the South African Medical and Dental Council regarding the "suspicious" death of detainee Stephen Biko. Public reevaluation uncovered the gross professional incompetency and injustice of the original investigation. Subsequently, in September 1985, Professor Tobias received notice from the national secretary of the XI World Archeology Congress, Southampton, England, that all scientists working in South Africa, irrespective of nationality, would not be permitted to attend because "the policy of numerous organizations call for a boycott of South Africa."[5] Professor Tobias, noted for his original research in anthropology and, ironically, a founder of the World Congress, was barred from the congress. Here academic sanction patently limits the universality and freedom of science.

Definition

The World Medical Association defines *academic sanction* as "discriminatory restrictions on academic, professional and scientific freedoms which deny or exclude physicians and others from educational, cultural and scientific meetings and other opportunities for the exchange of information and knowledge, the purpose of such restrictions being to protest the social and political policies of governments."[6] As with so many human rights issues, the fact of academic sanction has little direct impact on the vast majority of health professionals. Until experienced, academic sanction seems a remote, even irrelevant, legalistic gesture. Upon personal encounter, however, scientists and medical practitioners become acutely aware of the threat that politicization of science presents to the free exchange of scientific information.

Academic sanction is any attempt to use law, custom, or agreement to withhold information by restricting scholarly exchange. *Boycott* is a specialized form of sanction focused on ostracizing "offending" colleagues. Both are forms of psychological violence. In contrast, a *strike* by scientists is a direct confrontation with authorities that temporarily withholds science services and information as protest against a concept or social condition and may be accompanied by physical violence. A dramatic example of a science strike can be found in the resistance during World War II of the Dutch medical profession to the Nazi invaders' attempts to draw them into the German medical profession. Unanimously, the Dutch physicians turned in their medical licenses and, despite the Nazis' retaliation of sending one hundred Dutch physicians to their death in concentration camps, the Dutch medical profession never faltered in its stand.[7] A strike calls for direct confrontation, academic sanction does not.

Heuristically, academic sanctions can be classified as governmental, organizational, or personal, and at each level a sanction may be actively pursued or passively followed.

Government Sanction Against Academics

Since its inception, modern science has remained vulnerable to sanction by government. During the Anglo-Dutch War in 1673, Henry Oldenberg, the organizer of the British Royal Society, received a letter in London from the Dutch anatomist, Reinier de Graaf, which began, "That it may be the more evident to you that the humanities and science are not yet banished from among us by the clash of arms." De Graaf then went on to introduce British scientists to the work of Leeuwenhoek and the discovery of the microscope.[8] Later, while the Napoleonic Wars raged, communication remained open between the French and English scientists, and Edward Jenner wrote his colleagues at the Académie des Sciences in Paris, "The sciences are never at war."[9]

However, with the First World War, political leaders discovered science to be a potent weapon in a nation's armory, and the laissez-faire attitude of governments toward international science changed to an attitude of increased control. Today, the U.S. Department of Defense can declare particular science meetings as classified and subsequently seek to deny visas to scientists from potentially hostile nations.[10] The most extreme example of government sanction against academics is found in the People's Republic of China's cultural revolution (1969 to 1976), when medical schools were closed and scientists sent to the countryside by the government for ideological reasons.[11]

Strictly speaking, academic sanction by governments is outside the scientist's domain. For example, when the South African government refused in 1988 to grant visas to a delegation sponsored by the American Association for the Advancement of Science including the National Academy of Sciences/Institute of Medicine Committee on Health and Human Rights, the American Psychiatric Association, and the American Public Health Association, South African scientists objected to this action but were powerless to intercede. Similarly, the Soviet Union's denial of visas to fifty-four South African geologists seeking to attend the 1984 International Geological Congress in Moscow can not be attributed to Soviet geologists. Patently, the Soviet scientists lacked direct political power.

However, the passive role of scientists in accepting these political strictures came into question with reports that "Japan, for example, has been virtually out-of-bounds, issuing visas to South Africans traveling for business purposes, but not to tourists; conferences appear in the eyes of consulates to fall vaguely in between."[12] This was substantiated by personal communication with South African physicians. Rather than passively accepting an all-inclusive stricture on Japanese science, Japanese scientists might have reconsidered their role as citizens of a country that increased its economic trade with South Africa by supplying goods economically sanctioned by other nations, yet imposed academic sanctions on the open exchange of science information.

Far from a self-serving policy, such as the South African government's action against the University of Cape Town's antiapartheid monthly, *New Era* (*The Oregonian,* January 12, 1989:A3), the punctilious interpretation of economic sanctions by the Danish government inadvertently led to academic sanction. Professor S. Benatar, professor of medicine at University of Cape Town, South Africa, reported as follows (written communication, April 16, 1988):

> In January 1987, one of the professors in my department was informed by the Munksgaard International Publishers Ltd. in Copenhagen that as

the Danish government had passed a law forbidding trade with South Africa, they would not be able to provide him with off-prints of a paper he had written which was due to be published in *Clinical Genetics*.

In the United States, use of academic sanction by the government frequently originated at the local level with selective purchasing agreements by municipalities requiring that U.S. publishers have no contact with South Africa. Consequently, many U.S. publishers refused to supply textbooks and journals to South African medical schools for fear of losing their U.S. markets. This action had a curious rebound effect of censoring U.S. municipal libraries, which were deprived of publications from "nonaffirming" publishers. For example, the *Readers Guide to Periodic Literature* and the *Wall Street Journal*, a newspaper that maintains a correspondent in South Africa, were banned from many local U.S. libraries. Even more curious was the endorsement the American Library Association gave this book banning (*Village Voice*, February 15, 1988).

Clearly, governments impose academic sanctions for different reasons, including support from politically subservient scientists. An enlightening reaction to such pressure occurred in 1967 at the Sixth Pan-African Congress of Prehistory, in Dakar, Senegal, when President Léopold Senghor refused to comply with local demands to exclude South African scientists, as he would have nothing to do with restricting any meeting of scientists. He refused to interfere with the free exchange of scientific knowledge.[5]

Sanction By Professional Organizations

A few science organizations pursue academic sanctions explicitly. The editor of the *Zoological Journal of the Linnean Society*, Professor C.H. Schally, stated clearly, "I am not accepting manuscripts from South Africa."[12] Less blatant is the exclusion of a Black South African professor of medicine by the director of a conference on hypertension in Blacks held in Atlanta, Georgia, in December 1986. The conference committee had unanimously voted to exclude from consideration any presentation of papers from South Africa. A letter from the director of the conference to the professor stated that, "This policy was formulated on the basis that there are many documented reports of unethical practices by certain doctors in South Africa without appropriate government action." Without appeal, the Black teacher of Blacks was barred, though the director subsequently apologized to the professor for this action.[13]

A few universities, such as Trinity and University of Dublin, Ireland, severed all ties with South African educational institutions.[14] Until retired, faculty at Trinity University were forbidden to collaborate with South African peers under risk of censure and/or dismissal.

While much reported academic sanction is directed toward South African scientists, there is no apparent geographic pattern to the practice, for academic sanction originates in such disparate countries as the United States, Soviet Union, Sweden, Denmark, and Japan. For example, Professor Benatar of the University of Cape Town anticipates such an experience in Australia (written communication, April 16, 1988):

> I shall be attending the 1988 Meeting of the Presidents of Colleges of Physicians [of the English-speaking world] in Sydney, Australia, as an invited representative of the College of Medicine of South Africa. All College representatives at the meeting, with the exception of myself, have been invited in their official capacity to attend the Golden Jubilee Celebrations of the Royal Australian College of Physicians during the week immediately following the Meeting of Presidents. The Royal Australian College of Physicians have decided against inviting any official representative of the South African College to this scientific meeting. An invitation has been extended to me to attend in my personal capacity.

On the other side of the world in Portland, Oregon, Portland State University proposed a brief course in Afrikaans as one of twenty-four "exotic" languages for a special 1987 summer session. When the African Student Association at the university heard of the proposal, they raised such vehement protest, seconded by some faculty members, that the administration suggested to the invited professor from Stellenbosch University, South Africa, that she withdraw from her contract to teach the course as they "could not insure her safety." Consequently, she did not attend the summer session (*The Oregonian,* May 24, 1987:D4).

More destructive than one-time sanction by a committee is the established policy of academic sanction adopted by some science organizations. In January 1987, the Royal College of Psychiatrists adopted the Commonwealth Nassau Accord of 1985, placing their members on notice that, "Any member considering a visit to South Africa should therefore carefully consider the wording of the Nassau Accord and the Resolution expressing the College views." The Accord is a political statement by Commonwealth governments sanctioning the shipping of computer equipment, oil, and arms to South Africa as well as "discouragement of all cultural and scientific events except where these contribute towards the ending of apartheid or have no possible role in promoting it" (J.L.T. Birley, M.D., written communication, June 27, 1988).

Seemingly a worthy denunciation of despicable racist policy, the pronouncement of the Royal College of Psychiatrists, which included a denial of any intention of academic sanction, was experienced differently by practitioners in South Africa. According to R.E. Hempill, M.D., a member of the Royal College who lives in South Africa, in addition to focusing science, cultural, and educational support entirely on the racist issue in a way that denied all South Africans, regardless of their race and creed, members were forced to follow College policy if they visited South Africa or incur the displeasure of the College, which "savors of intimidation."[15] The College's action was taken despite the fact that 121 members of the Society of Psychiatrists of South Africa were on record as unanimously deploring "potentially harmful psychological effects on the people of South Africa as a result of any form of discrimination based on race, color, gender, or creed. The South African Society does and will strive for elimination of all forms of discrimination that adversely affect mental life."[16] It is difficult to see in the Royal College's official pronouncement any collegial support or scientific understanding of the struggle of South African psychiatrists against racism.

In contrast, Britain's Association for the Study of Animal Behavior, after considering a proposal to exclude South Africans from membership and their papers from publication, responded to the Zoological Society of South Africa, changing its constitution to specify a nonracist policy. Referring to the South African zoologists, Association for the Study of Animal Behavior president Peter Slater announced, "We have consulted our membership, and in view of the new clause, decided that this particular group of academics deserves encouragement."[17]

The complex nature of academic sanction by science organizations can be found in the U.S. National Academy of Sciences' position on science exchanges with the Soviet Union. In 1980, with political tension between the United States and the Soviet Union over Afghanistan, the U.S. Academy decided to sanction Soviet scientists for their government's political policy of banishing a foreign associate of the Academy, Andrey Sakharov, from Moscow to Gorki, in effect depriving him of his rightful pursuit of science. Specifically, the Academy suspended bilateral symposia, seminars, workshops, and new invitations and did not negotiate a new international exchange agreement. However, it did not terminate all contacts, for each year the individual exchange program was renewed on a de facto basis. The Academy reasoned that individual scientific visits were best left to the consciences of the participating individuals, who should not be bound by the organization's position. The Academy also went to great pains to exempt their Committee on International Security and Arms Control from the sanctions, ensuring continued discussions on the arms control issue.[18] In 1984, before the release of Sakharov from Gorki, the Academy reevaluated its position and decided that its efforts to ameliorate human rights violations in the Soviet Union were greatly hampered. As a result, negotiations for organizational exchanges with the Soviet Union were resumed.[19]

Personal Sanctions

Even though personal sanctioning of colleagues exists, tracking down the facts is difficult, for reports seldom come with documentation. Tying down the details that lie behind a reported conversation in which Scandinavian medical editors acknowledge a gentlemen's agreement to "harmonize their attitudes"[12] and not publish any material originating in South Africa is next to impossible. On the other hand, to judge fairly the file of a long and generally strongly supportive correspondence between a South African research scientist and a U.S. medical editor calls for judgment beyond my ability in deciding if the editor's precipitous switch from support to complete rejection was, as the editor states, a final decision about the quality of the author's work or, as the scientist states, academic sanction.

Some medical scientists, when not concealing contacts with South African science organizations, downgraded contacts out of fear of academic reprisal. Students in the West had reported being advised to avoid academic appointments in South Africa, which would unfavorably prejudice a future curriculum vitae. Some physicians maintained two separate editions of their curriculum vitae, one complete, the other for "sensitive" circumstances, devoid of any reference to training in South Africa.

Understandably, these subterfuges were reported to me by scientists who wished to remain anonymous rather than have such activity documented in the medical education literature.

The most valid evaluation of personal sanction comes with the experience. Prof. J.C. de Villiers, chairman of neurosurgery at the University of Cape Town, wrote (written communication, June 17, 1988):

> The academic boycott is something which people outside this country [South Africa] must also speak about. We are condemned and damned even before we open our mouths and some sense has to come from elsewhere. I find it difficult to see how submitting us to academic boycott, as far as medical information and know how goes, could possibly do any good for the Black patient who has no other recourse to doctors with better information than we have. Ninety-five percent of my practice is Black, by that I mean other than White. If I go down, they go down with me.

Dr. Anthony Barker, practicing in the Alexandra Health Center, a Black township clinic outside of Johannesburg, stated: "Alas, those who suffer for our Puritanism are not the government and not the stuffy Medical Association of South Africa, but people like ourselves here in Alexandra. By withholding our help we commit the error—which Martin Luther King warned us of—of punishing the victims of oppression for the results of their oppression."[20] Perhaps the most heartfelt response was expressed by a Black professor in a South African medical school. When asked what academic sanctions meant to him, he replied, "Please do not ask me to suffer for your political ideals."

Reasons For Academic Sanction

The most common reason given for enacting an academic sanction is abhorrence of a political or social policy of a foreign country. The intent is that ostracization of a foreign scientist will encourage the scientist to change his or her country's "offending" policy. A small number of scientists in Senegal, Guatemala, South Africa, the German Democratic Republic (East Germany), the Soviet Union, and the United States who have experienced political oppression point out in personal discussion that they encourage academic sanctions for the following reasons:

1. Free international scientific interaction tends to enhance the position of the established regime through passive international acceptance, bringing valuable foreign exchange to the "offending" country.
2. Without academic sanction, the predominant philosophy, race, and political configuration of the scientific establishment in the "offending" country is reinforced.
3. The "offending" government can use international travel to reward politically subservient scientists, while in turn the "open" country may selectively give or withhold visas, with a bias toward recognized scientists but withholding visas from worthy "unknowns."
4. The advanced, high-technology institutes in "offending" countries are the most likely to benefit by academic exchange, ensuring immediate returns for the most advantaged in the "offending" country, while leaving local institutes and clinics to practice 1940s science in 1990.

Reasons Against Academic Sanction

Other scientists offer the following reasons for renouncing academic sanction:

1. Academic sanction denies the history and belief that the sole criterion for participation in science is a proved ability to observe objectively and reason independently in the service of untrammeled curiosity.
2. Severing ties denies the sanctioning organization access to information and position for ongoing influence on the course of human rights in the "offending" country.
3. Academic sanction works the greatest hardship on the most active and independent scientists in "offending" countries.
4. Punishing scientists for their country's behavior has little or no effect on national policy, since the political arm is seldom aware or even cares that one or more of their scientists might be excluded from international academic exchange.[5]
5. Politically destabilizing a country does more harm than good to the majority, particularly to the least advantaged, while the stabilizing effect of academic exchange offers implicit support for political growth.

6. Academic exchange offers scientists the opportunity to visit "offending" countries to experience oppressive circumstances firsthand.

The third point, the isolation and intellectual handicap forced on scientists in the offending country because their scientific organizations have failed to assert political power, is malignant. Tragically, the political heroism of scientists in politically repressive countries, who must practice in a gray area between what is politically acceptable and what is not, is more often ignored than recognized by judgmental foreigners. They may be working with secretarial staff who, if not covert government informers, may be political ideologists who refuse to type or transmit scientific information that does not conform with their political beliefs. Consequently, free-thinking scientists remain in constant peril of official censure. In fact, these scientists must continually balance their public thoughts and academic actions between the threat of remorseless government persecution and, on the other hand, reprisal from an opposing, militant underground prepared to burn their homes to the ground for cooperating with the existing regime.

An anonymous Central American physician described his experience in medical clinics and hospitals in which a patient, once healed, might kill the patient in the next bed, as well as the physician, for treating someone of a different political philosophy. No better example of this can be found than the death of Dr. Abu Baker Asvat, recognized in Soweto as "The Star of the Community" for his dedicated medical care of the poor and homeless, yet gunned down in his surgery on January 27, 1989, by two unknown assassins posing as patients (*The Oregonian,* February 13, 1989:A8). The reality of medical practice in an oppressive society seems lost on the judgmental physician, practicing thousands of miles from the struggle. Inadvertently, that zealot punishes frontline practitioners for being compassionate physicians, not political activists.

Author's Recommendations

Though some might expect individual science exchange to be a lever for increased human rights in "offending" countries, my experience fails to reinforce that conclusion. In attempts to discuss psychiatric patients surreptitiously held for political reasons, the treatment of children in detention, the release of dissident citizens, or a more open exchange of information on physician impairment with professors of psychiatry and officials, including ministers of health, in the Soviet Union, the Republic of South Africa, and Fiji, I have experienced a variety of disquieting behaviors including frank denial, vehement attacks on U.S. policy, cold withdrawal, and a serious abbreviation of the exchange visit. In one case, a dissident who was targeted was permitted subsequently to leave the country of his discontent, yet it is difficult to believe that one encounter by a visiting scholar accounted for his release. While abstaining from an activist role and passively, yet objectively, accumulating data from as many scientists in the "offending" country as possible, the visitor may best serve the cause of human rights by securing reasonably balanced information for subsequent publication in "open" countries.

Individual scientists of all nations should carefully review the outcome as much as the motive of their pursuit of a policy of academic sanction. Rather than a blanket condemnation for political reasons, responsible scientists and the scientific establishment of an "offended country" should judge the moral and ethical context of each case by carefully investigating all available facts. This point is made by Professor Colin Gardiner of the University of Natal, Pietermaritzburg, South Africa. Responding to the barring of three South African sociologists from a conference in New Delhi, India, Professor Gardiner said, "What we are trying to say to those abroad is that while we understand the reason for the boycott, we believe they should distinguish between opponents of apartheid and others."[13] Then, if condemnation is indeed called for, first let the judgment focus on the individual "offending" case.

Science organizations might well consider the strong stand taken by the World Medical Association[6] to which the American Medical Association adheres:

> [The WMA is] unalterably opposed to such restrictions [academic sanctions] and calls for all national medical associations to resist the imposition of such restrictions by every means at their disposal and to heed the WMA's Declaration of Human Rights and Individual Freedom of Medical Practitioners and WMA statement on Freedom to Attend Medical Meetings.

Through careful documentation, organized bodies of science may focus on actual offenders, who by word or deed subvert science's goals of unfettered thought and freedom of communication. An extended, dispassionate dialogue with scientists in an "offending" country is a constructive initial step towards judgment. In turn, science organizations of "offending" countries are best judged by their stated aims and ostracized from international collegial exchange only as it is documented that the science organization condones political repression with its consequent human suffering.

An essential requirement for effective declarations of sanction should clearly state the reason, nature, exceptions, and expected duration of the sanction, while fully delineating specific actions expected for rescinding the sanction. Such judgments can wisely contain a measure of humility, remembering the social and ethical difficulties encountered in crossing cultural barriers. Finally, effective condemnation of a scientist or scientific organization should offer unconditionally ongoing negotiation among scientists in their mutual pursuit of truth.

Unlike Jenner, we can no longer say the sciences never are at war, albeit psychological warfare. By invoking academic sanctions for ideological reasons, scientists and science organizations threaten the open exchange of science. Though reasons are advanced for applying academic sanction against fellow scientists, using science as a tool in international politics has little or no documented effectiveness. Scientific establishments of all nations would be wise to carefully examine, and regularly reexamine, their involvement in the process of sanctioning and boycotting colleagues or professional organizations for political reasons. The basic rule of medical practice, *primum non nocere*, first do no harm, applies to all aspects of science and scientific exchange.

Endnotes

Reprinted from the *Journal of the American Medical Association* 262(1989): 1499-1503, with permission. Copyrighted 1989, American Medical Association. Original title: "Academic Sanction, Targeting South African Science."

1. Data concerning academic sanction placed some physicians and their programs at risk. Hence no material was quoted without the express permission of those involved.
2. R.P. Claude, P.C. Stover, and J.R. Lopez, *Health Professionals and Human Rights in the Philippines—Reports on Medicine and the Prevention of Torture* (Washington, D.C.: American Association for the Advancement of Science Committee on Scientific Freedom and Responsibility, 1986).
3. M. Rayer, *Turning a Blind Eye? Medical Accountability and the Prevention of Torture in South Africa* (Washington, D.C.: American Association for the

Advancement of Science, 1987).
4. M. McGregor, "Apartheid and the Academic Boycott of South Africa," *New England Journal of Medicine* 316(1987): 1022-1023.
5. P.V. Tobias, "Prehistory and Political Discrimination," *Suid-Afrikaanse Tydsknf vir Wetenskap* 18(1985): 667-671.
6. World Medical Association, *Statement on Academic Sanctions or Boycotts,* Document 20, 2/88 (Ferney-Voltaire, France: World Medical Association, September 1988).
7. L. Alexander, "Medical Science Under Dictatorship," *New England Journal of Medicine* 24(1949): 39-47.
8. D.J. Boorstin, *The Discoverers* (New York: Random House, 1983), 329.
9. G.R. de Beer, ed., *The Sciences Were Never at War* (Surrey, England: Nelson & Sons, 1960).
10. Presentation of Department of Defense-related scientific and technical papers at meetings (32 CFR 249). *Federal Register.* October 30, 1987; 11707.
11. K.G. Diamond, "The Breaking of a Profession," *Journal of the American Medical Association* 252(1984): 3160-3164.
12. Science in Apartheid. *Nature* 327(1987): 272-273.
13. J. Hanlon and R. Ormond, *The Sanctions Handbook* (New York: Viking, 1987), 118, 121.
14. N.E. Davies, Letter to the Editor, *New England Journal of Medicine* 317(1987):.1161-1162.
15. R.E. Hemphill, "The Royal College of Psychiatrists and Medical Sanctions Against South Africa," *African Journal of Medicine* 72(1987): 659-660.
16. Society of South African Psychiatrists, *Position Statement,* 31 January 1985.
17. Scientists in South Africa Condemn Apartheid, *New Scientist* 119(1988): 34.
18. C. Corillon, ed., *Science and Human Rights* (Washington, D.C.: National Academy Press, 1988), 14.
19. R. Schweitzer, "Who Wins in US-Soviet Science Ventures?" *Bulletin of Atomic Scientists* 44(1988): 31.
20. A. Barker, Letter to the Editor, *British Medical Journal* 294(1987): 244.

The New Custodians

Like the bee, we distill poison from honey for our own self-defense—what happens to the bee if it uses its sting is well known.
—Dag Hammarskjöld (1905-1961)
Markings

When a medical student at Bellevue Hospital in the 1940s, my curiosity was piqued by the recurrent rumor among charity patients that the staff had a black bottle of poison for unwanted patients. One day my curiosity got the better of me and I brashly asked a patient about the black bottle. The patient was a slight, Irish man, one of those rare, bright souls who are able with cheerful wit to make light of the terrifying burden of imminent death. He suffered from advanced tuberculosis with a large fistula draining his chest. Each day we "met" at his bedside and while I flushed warm saline into the hole, catching the fetid return in a kidney basin, we would chat. He seldom failed to have a word of encouragement for my clumsy work, the faltering Brooklyn Dodgers, or the dirty weather. He winked at nurses and smiled at life.

Bluntly, I asked him, "You do not believe in this Black Bottle stuff, do you?"

He was surprised, his smile faltered, and he turned strangely grim—"Sure'n I do."

"You can't," I joshed.

He paused and flicked his head to the left—"You see that bed—the empty one—that was Dominic's. He got the Bottle."

I grew uneasy as he left his usual bantering style and turned coldly serious. "Go on—you don't mean it—"

"Oh don't I—a week ago Dominic was alive in that bed—" he coughed— "He was sick, with what I always tried not to know, and two of your smart-aleck medical students came and spent an hour examining him—Him lying like putty. When they were done they stood there at the foot of his bed." He paused—caught his breath, "Twenty feet from me—and one says 'it's his kidneys' and the other says 'it's his heart' and as they get heated up, Dominic is all eyes and ears until he hears the last of them when one pops out, 'Well he will come to autopsy before we are off this service next month—and I bet you a dollar it's his kidneys'—That's how Dominic got the black bottle—"

I did not say anything—I finished, replaced the dressing, pulled off my gloves, and shook hands with that brave man—He showed me what I would not see—there are black bottles all about—.

As the years have passed, my interest has centered not on the black bottles, which come in such a variety of sizes, shapes, and packages, but on the people who hand them out. It is how I discovered the New Custodians—the medical students, the lawyers, the social workers, the psychiatrists, all those helpers of mankind who do such a fine job but so often after a successful operation report that the patient died.

With the phenomenal growth of scientific knowledge, particularly in the behavioral sciences, and the vast increase of population, a distinct class of behavioral technicians is emerging, the New Custodians. Unwittingly perhaps, they are charged, in the interest of public tranquility, with the custody of the minds of their wards. They are the dispensers of deadly poison carried in modern black bottles, a poison intended to dissolve deviant thought, to ensure the compliant recipient.

However, they are but one of a species, for there have been Custodians as long as there has been civilization. First there were the Ancient Custodians, then the Old Custodians, and recently the new. They guard, respectively, the human's soul, body, and mind.

The Ancient Custodian rejoiced in guarding the soul—but as the interest in souls has diminished, the trade is so reduced that there is little call for Ancient Custodians. Savonarola and the inquisition might fill a movie house for the spectacle, but it would never be more than a historical pageant—black bottles being handed out by black-hooded specters. Souls no longer invite custody, for there is little economic reward or social power in collecting and controlling souls.

The Old Custodians guard the body and are still in demand. They are the first sergeants of a peacetime world—not employed to reason why but to maintain control over a unit—whether a hospital ward, cell block, or a ghetto. They are easy to pick out—they know the rules and they know how to fit people to the rules. Drawing on his experience as a physician, Chekhov eloquently described the Old Custodian, an aide on a ward in a mental hospital:

> Nikita the keeper, an old retired soldier with
> service stripes, which have turned rusty from time,

lolls upon odds and ends with his eternal pipe clenched between his teeth. His face is morose, drink ravaged; his eyebrows are beetling, bestowing on his face the look of a steppe sheep dog, and his nose is red; he is not tall, rather spare to look at, and sinewy, but his bearing is impressive and his fists are huge and hard. He belongs to the number of those simple hearted, positive, reliable, and stolid persons who love order above all things on earth, and are therefore convinced that people must be beaten. When he beats somebody he beats him about the face and chest, the back—wherever his blows may fall—and he is convinced that without this there would be no order in this place.[1]

The bodies were, or are, neatly arranged in bed, or rocking chairs, or at desks with thin smiles on their faces and their bruises covered. For the Old Custodians, human activity is a mechanical interaction which they have mastered with efficiency.

Hospitals have moved from custodial care to active therapy, no "dying" wards, no snake pits—no black bottles now, no sadistic "bughousers" loose in mental hospitals. But the Old Custodians who were displaced by modern technicians are by no means extinct. They have simply shifted to foster homes, nursing homes, correctional institutions, and all those other depositories where the simple formula of control through physical means holds sway. There remains a large, though conservative, market in warm bodies, "in human junk." This market will remain until society either directly eliminates the physically inept, as the Eskimo and Nazi have, or genuinely offers adequate rehabilitation to *all* the disabled.

The New Custodian, though of a different era, shares many traits with his predecessors. However, before examining the modern dispensers of black-bottled poison, examples are in order. Here are three—a physician, social worker, and attorney administering to an anonymous man.

John Smith was a 35-year-old waiter in one of the community's better restaurants. One evening two policemen appeared at his place of work with an order to place him in custody pending psychiatric examination. He was brought to a locked ward in a general hospital. He was not permitted access to a telephone and when he objected vigorously was given an injection to quiet him down. Late that night, his wife called his place of employment to find out why he wasn't at home. One of his co-workers told her what had happened and she called the police. After several calls to them, they finally revealed his whereabouts. She immediately went down to the hospital. There she was not permitted to see her husband but rather was told to make an appointment to see a social worker. It was too late now to make such an appointment but she should call the next day. No physician, psychologist, nurse, or social worker was available at that time to speak to her.

The following day she called both the social service office of the hospital and a lawyer. The latter told her to meet him at the hospital immediately although the social worker told her not to come until the hospital called her. On arrival at the hospital, the attorney's and wife's request to see the patient was initially denied. After the lawyer raised the possibility of immediate legal action against the hospital administrator, a resident physician was called who simply informed them that the patient had been admitted because of a petition for psychiatric examination. The physician knew little else as the patient had not been seen by the medical staff. After further discussion, reluctant permission was granted to see the patient. The meeting provided no additional information as to why he had been abducted.

The attorney then went to the county probate court to examine recent records regarding petitions. Here he found a petition signed by a social worker from the county welfare office. The petition alleged that the petitioner had reason to believe that Mr. Smith was mentally ill because he "demonstrated poor judgment in financial matters, neglected his children, was a disturbing influence in the community, and had threatened little children with bodily harm."

A telephone call to the petitioning social worker was responded to by a curt refusal to discuss her actions toward Mr. Smith. A call to the director of the welfare department also produced no information. The attorney obtained a court order transferring Mr. Smith from the hospital to the county jail. At least in jail, he would not be forced to incriminate himself, would be available for consultation, could make telephone calls, and could not be forced to undergo medical treatment against his will. He could also have a physician of his own choice, something not permitted in the hospital.[2]

For the next several days, Mr. Smith remained in jail awaiting a hearing. During this time, no court-appointed examiners appeared. No social welfare agent asked whether he wanted help. Rather, against a stone wall of hostility, Mr. Smith's attorney attempted to find out the basis of the petition from the welfare agency. Everyone there, including three social workers and a psychologist, refused to give any information. Feeling a bit like the attorney of the hero in Franz Kafka's *The Trial*, he undertook a heroic effort to get to know Mr. Smith, his life, his family, and his neighbors. Not knowing what his client was being accused of, the attorney directed his efforts at being prepared for almost any accusation, the implication being that in this state, as in probably most states, there are some mental health workers and physicians who will sign commitment papers rather freely.[3]

At this point, at the request of the county attorney and the welfare agency, two such men were assigned to be Mr. Smith's examiners. After a 120-minute examination a hearing was held. The social worker who had signed the petition admitted under cross-examination that she had never seen the patient nor his family prior to the day of the hearing. She had signed the petition because another worker had requested her to do so. This person was not at the hearing, having been "assigned" to visit another county that day. The worker now on the stand reported that it was her understanding that the other worker had found Mr. Smith an "uncooperative informant" and had therefore felt that he was mentally ill. A man appeared at the hearing who claimed to be the court-appointed attorney for Mr. Smith. However, he didn't seem to know who Mr. Smith was but promptly sat down near Mr. Smith's other attorney and in a few minutes was asleep. The same lawyer had previously been appointed by the court to help indigents. In each previous case, he had never seen his presumed client until the day of the hearing and had never been observed by others to speak on behalf of his clients.[4]

So there they are: the resident physician, certain of his position and dispensing knowledge only when it is scheduled by the staff to be dispensed—a black bottle administered by his "professional behavior."

There is the social worker—committing someone whom she has never seen as a favor to another colleague—again a black bottle.

There is the attorney never speaking to his client—sure of his fee, with the knowledge that all is right with his world, complete down to his black bottle of legal neglect.

Here are three New Custodians—pseudoprofessional professionals; they are well educated, acceptable in appearance, and most important—all three are certain of their goals. Their eyes are on their positions, their roles, and they know where they are going—they are about to secure "the greatest good for the greatest number," despite the needs of the patient. To them, human activity is a sociopsychological interaction which they intend to control efficiently.

Do not be misled into thinking that these pseudoprofessionals are either apathetic or exceptional. They are neither.

Rather than apathetic they are all actively carrying out their legitimized roles. They are caring for the helpless as our institutions have trained them to care. They are highly selected people, often tested under severely competitive conditions, and then appointed to their positions after years of study. In two cases (the physician and social worker), they remain under strict and continual supervision to insure that they act as they do. No apathy here, unless it is the judge who tolerates a sleeping attorney.

Secondly, they are not unusual. Though there are no ready statistics, simple reflection reveals that New Custodians are all about, teaching, cajoling, and sometimes ordering that all conform to their "greatest good." These are the yeomen of the modern Watch and Ward societies—intent upon removing sickness, poverty, and crime from our society, "if only everyone cooperates."

Yet another possible error in considering the New Custodians is thinking that their field of operation is limited to the Dominics and John Smiths of our world. The Old Custodians are limited to the physically helpless, while the Ancient Custodians held sway over the morally inept. For the New Custodians there are no limits on the horizon; the whole world is their oyster. For example, who is consulted about determining the route of a new freeway, or the policy for school counseling? Oh, there are public hearings but they nearly always follow the fact. The public is on the defensive, reacting to the determinations of the New Custodians who know, on the basis of their population projections, "expert" attitudinal surveys, or personality test studies, what is the greatest good. Woe to those who question their scientific findings. As the servant of the people, they lead.

When the eye is sharpened, recognizing the New Custodians is not difficult. They are the product of their class. The Ancient Custodian came from the upper classes, the Old from the lower, and the New comes from the middle class. The New Custodians are generally a little overweight, wear a slightly out-of-press business suit, and always have near at hand a briefcase, clipboard, or a bundle of papers. They carry themselves with a hurried certainty, a brusk officiousness that belies they know where they are going. Actually, the New Custodians generally oscillate about the center of their local government or agency.

The New Custodians' manner with patients is distinctive. Invariably their initial response on contact is, "What is your eligibility?" Questions concerning human needs are subordinated to, "To whom do you belong?" or "On what wheel are you a cog?" The opening establishes a style which pervades the continuing relationship.

Physically the attitude is manifest in the monumental amounts of paper that flow out and around them. Paperwork represents a permanent barrier between the New Custodian and the recipient. Even after the recipient has proven eligibility and compliance with the demands of the system, is a willing cog, a recognizable number, a compliant cipher, the paperwork remains a barrier. "If only I had the time to get to know my clients," is the New Custodian's plaintive refrain. Humanness remains at best an incidental note, characteristically touched on with, "I had an interesting case this afternoon of homelessness [incest, glomerular nephritis]".

In relating, the New Custodian is trained to first have a pen at the ready and to close with all the t's crossed and the i's dotted. Involvement is tightly defined by regulations while certainty of goals arises out of the ubiquitous briefcase.

The New Custodians' sense of identity is revealing. They are pseudoprofessionals. A profession is a group bound by ethical standards to protect those whom they serve. A union is a group bound by work standards to protect its members. A pseudoprofession combines the qualities of both to its own advantage. Thus, the question may be asked, is the local Bar Association interested in attorneys' malfeasance or in establishing tax-sheltered retirement programs for its members? It is the motive, of the individual and the organization, which identifies the pseudoprofessional, not the venerability of the profession.

Lastly, the New Custodian is recognized by her/his philosophy of social change. The New Custodian hungers for the greatest good for the greatest number, which means a highly personal interpretation of government regulations to alter the client's life. Whether it is to assign children to ethnically correct foster parents, establish high school programs for teaching family interaction, or forcing welfare recipients to work on the county roads, the greatest good is "just around the corner" and social problems are solved by bringing government power to bear.

What can be done to help the Dominics, the John Smiths, and others like ourselves who may fall under the influence of the New Custodians? The formula is simple—recognition, commitment, and exposition. The New Custodians must be recognized for what they are. Then considered thought and feeling should be welded into commitment by those willing to speak out forthrightly against the "efficient" determination of the "greatest good."

Recognizing the New Custodians is a beginning. The second and third steps, commitment and forthright speech necessary to render the New Custodians accountable, are more difficult. Together these three processes protect social service from becoming camouflaged custodial care. There are no alternatives, for, ultimately, social problems become social solutions through attentive listening and shared understanding, not power plays. Affluence and power may change the appearance of social problems, but only human understanding fashions solutions.

Custodial care will be with us until the servants of the weak and helpless know whom they serve. The Dominics, John Smiths, the young, the sick, the poor, disenfranchised, prisoner, elderly, all teach us that true service is the considered sharing of power. As understanding replaces control so care replaces custody. Should we fail to learn these truths and carry them out we are simply sophisticated dispensers of black bottles, possibly helping bodies, yet certainly poisoning minds and spirit.

Endnotes

Reprinted from *Medical Opinion & Review* 4(1968): 63-67.
1. A. Chekhov, "Ward Six," *Great Russian Short Novels* (New York: Dial Press, 1951).
2. F.T. Lindman, D.M. McIntyre, eds, *The Mentally Disabled and the Law: The Report on the Right of the Mentally Ill* (Chicago: University of Chicago Press, 1961).
3. T. Szasz, *The Ethics of Psychoanalysis* (New York: Dell Publishing Co., 1965).
4. E.S. Sulzer, "Individual Freedom, Law, and Social Welfare," *Community Mental Health Journal* 3(Spring 1967): 50.

Is There a Doctor in the Nation?

And the more ignorant, reckless and thoughtless a doctor is, the higher his reputation soars even amongst powerful princes. In fact now that medicine is practiced by so many, it is really only one form of flattery, just as rhetoric is.

—Erasmus (1465-1536)
In Praise of Folly

London is a long way from Oregon for a week's journey, but if the prize is great, the travel is worth it. At least, so I thought in 1971, when the announcement of The Anglo-American Conference on Medical Care crossed my desk. The roster was impressive: the Presidents of the American Medical Association (AMA) and the British Medical Association (BMA); the Surgeon General of the U.S. Public Health Service and his United Kingdom counterpart; the Secretary of the Department of Health, Education, and Welfare (HEW) and his British counterpart; two former British Ministers of Health, Kenneth Robinson, and the sometimes notorious Enoch Powell; Wilbur Cohen, former Secretary of HEW; John Knowles; and other luminaries. All were listed on a three-day program of papers and discussions, and the audience was to be limited to three hundred members of the Royal Society of Medicine. It was irresistible.

On April Fool's Day, I finished up my work at the office, caught the evening plane to New York and, after a thorough frisking for guns and dynamite, went on to London. The meeting began Sunday evening with a reception at Chandos House. There I heard my name loudly announced by the footman as I made my way up the long carpeted stairs. At the head of the stairs, came the immediate and lasting pleasure of meeting the host and his lady, Sir John and Lady Richardson. As president of the Royal Society of Medicine, he proved unfailingly hospitable throughout the conference, quietly concerned that the proceedings should move with the measured tempo of a symphony. Noble is the word for that gentleman, for what a combination of antitheses, reticent openness, forbearing directness, urbane naivete, and disciplined ease, a man among men, the kind of men you wished all your medical school teachers had been. Then, with a splash of champagne, the hurly-burly of meeting people and exchanging ideas began.

The first session on Monday morning started with a brief address by the Minister of State for Social Service, the Right Honorable, Lord Aberdare. He seemed uncomfortable, like a hall porter who has been asked to account for the tarnish on the brass door knocker. Nevertheless, he did a competent job of describing certain aspects of the British Health System. He focused on the tripartite confusion, the three separate services—hospital, public health, and general practice—and he did it with a begrudging air that added nuance to Sir John's thanks that he had not spoken in Welsh.

Next came what appeared to be a team out of the early nineteenth century. The pair, who would have been fair game for Dickens, were Sir George Godber, Chief Medical Officer for the British, and our Surgeon General, Dr. Jesse L. Steinfeld. First, Sir George charged the podium and, with fixed monocle and the dash and bluster worthy of Waterloo, announced that all was right with the British medical world. Where previously only a few regions had supplied service with equality and fairness, now all were doing so. The new towns were glowing examples of the growing team spirit. The general practitioners (GPs) had all been upgraded. Nurses and midwives were on the increase, and the greatest advance of medicine in the United Kingdom in the last twenty years had been its organization by the General Public Health Officer. He finished with a plea for greater communication both within and without the profession: "Cooperate we must. If we do not, we will be managed from the outside." He sat down with the applause of most of the Americans and some of the British ringing in his ears.

His U.S. counterpart sidled up with a self-demeaning air. "I am neither a surgeon nor a general," he announced, and seemed, with his soft sell of the Nixon Health Doctrine of increasing quantity without limiting quality, the very epitome of a modern major-medical general. His list of problems was explicit: (1) How do we reduce organizational rigidity and cost by giving increased emphasis to cultural and social problems? (2) How do we recognize that health is a birthright of all? (3) How can science be restrained from overriding social considerations? (4) How can the federal role be established? (5) How can we recruit and retain sufficient manpower?

The Surgeon General then went on to expound the emerging national health strategy, which should include equal access to all; reconciling supply and demand (presumably by central planning); better organization of health care with emphasis on cost/benefit ratio; building the present system upon a focus on health, not health care; and fostering responsibility of the individual. On the last point, he emphasized the need to identify responsibility for health care among the private, state, federal, and personal interests involved. His delivery was unrelieved by even the faintest suggestion of humor until, when discussing planning, he laughed at the inclusion of politicians. I never did get the precise significance.

Sir John started the discussion period by pointing out that no smoking was permitted and should he have his way smoking would be limited solely to consenting adults in private. The most impressive part of the discussion was how the masterful Sir George impaled dissenters. One chap, obviously doubting the facts, asked from the floor how, in calculating the use of consultants' time, had Sir George arrived at the figure 9/11ths. Sir George gobbled him up. "You, sir, can use your methods as you wish. But I, sir, I use arithmetic." It seemed like a mighty non sequitur to me, but it was carried off with such style that the questioner shrank into his seat, crushed by the ring of laughter in the hall. Later in the sessions, I mentioned to a member of Parliament what a masterful politician Sir George appeared to be and was informed, "That, sir, is precisely the very thing you should never tell him!"

The questioning continued with one indomitable surgeon asking Sir George if he did not anticipate that "short commons" were here to stay for national medicine. Sir George bridled, responding with a spray of statistics that, though there were some shortcomings, there were not nor would there be "short commons."

Later, in private, I asked the questioner about "short commons" and found it to be the fare of a poor boy at Oxford or Cambridge, bare subsistence diet. He also described the nursing service in his orthopedic wards as going under with the flood of demands and the loss of teachers. "We have a 40 percent dropout rate among our student nurses. The waiting list for cold surgery is three thousand and it's two to three years to get in. Of course, national health is good in places but with damnable patches."

The afternoon session on Monday started with the paper of President Bornemeier of the AMA on "American Medicine: The Good Revolution." He touched on the maldistribution of doctors in "disorganized" medicine and of the need for the federal government to increase the number and versatility of doctors, particularly family doctors and groups. His "revolution" sounded as though it had been plotted at a soda fountain over servings of apple pie and ice cream. It was as doctrinaire as a Sears Roebuck catalogue and carried a muted theme of tardy expedience. Dr. Bornemeier's delivery was eloquent American; I could almost hear the members of the Cairo (Illinois) Medical Society giving him a standing ovation for his "revolutionary" proposals. However, no such response came from the audience at the Royal Society for, as always, decent civility prevailed.

Next came Dr. Ronald Gibson, Chairman of Council, British Medical Association, whose position I never quite understood but whose anguish I never doubted. He traced "The Origin and Progress of Organized Medicine in Britain" and that is the story of the GP. Apparently, long ago the peerage system slipped over into the medical profession, for historically the specialist has had the hospital appointments, the academic positions, the rich patients, and ultimate control of the profession through the Royal College of Physicians, while the GP has had his front room "surgery," the poor, and the tag-along British Medical Association.

Describing the frustration, overwork, and desertion of GPs by the country, Dr. Gibson did not tell a pretty tale. In 1948, most GPs lost their hospital appointments, though they could still, as friendly visitors, come in out of the rain and see their patients after first obtaining clearance from the hospital staff. The flood of patients with the inception of the National Health Service was overwhelming. "They were children at a Christmas party and the GP was Father Christmas." Whatever gradual improvements have been made have come by voluntary moves from within the profession; there have been no statutory reforms.

In his closing words, the ring of bitterness sounded sharply as he explained that for two decades the BMA has worked to overcome the tripartite system with all its divided responsibility and grim duplication of bureaucracy, only to have within the last few months another political division of care originate in Parliament with the passage of the "Green Paper," establishing community social concerns completely independent of medicine. The social worker has arrived in force. Even civility was strained to applaud this suffering man.

Dr. Ernest Saward, associate dean at the University of Rochester School of Medicine, came next with "Some Values Inherent in an Organized System of Medical Care." He described the Kaiser Foundation Medical Care Program with the ingratiating smugness of a Jack Horner who had stuck in his thumb and pulled out an "HMO" (health maintenance organization). He showed how his former HMO, through planning made possible by capitation payments, utilized beds and resources better than other local services, and cost the government nothing. It sounded like the answer to a Republican politician's dream and was certain to be the darling of the conference. Since the program operates in my home town, I took the opportunity to set the record straight on one point, for the government *is* participating. The local establishment has a million dollar auxiliary service, the delivery research department of thirty-four carried by federal funds.

After the discussion, I stopped Dr. Saward to say that, though I was not in a position to judge the quality of care delivered by the local Kaiser organization in the field of mental health I was impressed by the relatively high out-of-pocket cost to the patient. The patient seemed to derive little advantage from his capitation. He replied that this was more an illusion than a fact since the cost problem stemmed from contractual arrangements. I did not understand, but went on to say that there were two facets of the local organization that impressed me greatly: (a) their physician who had volunteered for two civilian tours in Viet Nam, a living hero; and (b) the fact that I was unable to ever get the administrative staff to return a phone call. The research staff was always ready to talk or join one for lunch, but the medical administrative staff remained inaccessible, either because of their concentration on patient care or because of chaos.

Dr. Saward laughed lightly. "Oh, that is easy to explain. You see, we train our secretaries never to relay a phone call to a doctor until they can put the patient's chart in his hand at the same time. They probably think when you call that you are a patient and are still looking for your chart." It struck me that I was consciously listening to medical newspeak for the first time, but before I could clarify anything further, Dr. Saward was swept away in a crowd of questioners. Exhausted, I wandered back to my hotel to ready myself for the evening reception at Lancaster House, St. James Palace, given by Her Majesty's Government.

Tuesday morning started with zing. Dr. John H. Knowles spoke on medical manpower. He came on like the white knight with a smiling, sharp delivery, giving life to statistics (there is not enough of everything, and what we have is poorly distributed). As I heard it, he came closest of all the speakers to the larger issues. He was the first to use the word "immoral." He considers filling 25 percent of the staff positions in U.S. hospitals with graduates from foreign medical schools as immoral. What a handsome idea! At long last, I had heard a physician step beyond the safe, impersonal, supravirtuous position of "objectivity" to say that his soul could smell a stink. We, the most affluent people of all time, drain away from the underdeveloped and overdeprived nations of the world a goodly percent of their doctors to care for our needs. All the "blah" about training foreign doctors and sending them home again is, in my opinion, blah. What do we do to insure that whenever a young doctor comes to our shores for "training" we send someone to fill the gap he left? Bravo, brave white knight!

The exposition was brilliant and when he came to discuss the grave cost of governmental confusion, I was right with him. He explained that as a people we need to improve economically and politically as much as medically if we are to gain by the changes we seek. One flaw struck me harshly, when in closing he advocated, admittedly as an example, the use of television as an adjunct and cost saver in medicine. Please, must there always be ritual kowtowing to technology as the ultimate in man's world? But such a tiny flaw merely spiced the taste.

Dr. Henry Yellowlees, Deputy Chief Medical Officer of the United Kingdom, plodded over the ground Knowles had vaulted. I guess every knight must have his squire. He touched on some means of redistribution but said nothing conclusive.

Then Professor Herman M. Somers of Princeton spoke on the role of the private sector in the United States. He had a shaggy appearance, with bushy eyebrows and tweedy coat, and seemed woolly in everything but his thinking, which turned out to be direct, surprising, forceful, and challenging. He spoke of the problems of affluence which cause more demand, of universally spiralling costs (with Sweden the worst off), of irrational delivery systems, of deep discontent with all institutions, of the danger of success which encourages expectation faster than supply, of the mistakes the insurance companies have made, of the government's repetition of the same mistakes, of the government's failure to follow through on statutes, of the seeds of stagnation inherent in monolithic organizations, and how the cutting edge in social-economic improvement must be the small organization.

He finished with some general observations. The American way when setting up a new plan is never to look to the past. As for the continental systems, he doubted whether they have the managerial competence to progress, inasmuch as no political system can withstand chronic complaining or make constructive use of the ancient human trait of "complimentary abrasiveness."

Mr. E.D. Roberts, governor of the British United Provident Association, spoke on the contribution of the private sector in the United Kingdom, and the easy conclusion from his talk was that there just is not much contribution at all. Industry does the most, and that by offering some special care to its own employees. In effect, there is little familiarity with the concept in the United Kingdom comparable to our group practice in the states.

My frustration with the conference was growing as I saw so many participants playing Eric Berne's game of "Ain't It Awful." I had had enough of statistics and moans, so after the tea break I asked the panel: "I wonder if there is a lack of candor in the conference in respect to what I perceive to be the hidden agenda of the political role of medicine and the physician? The speakers center on available resources. Actually little is new—more money, more teachers. Can we not do better? What I want to know is, can we talk about the 'politicization' of medicine? For example, Dr. Knowles has received some nasty public bumps as the result of being intelligently outspoken. According to published reports, Dr. Egeberg, Dr. Steinfeld's immediate superior, does not know from day to day whether he will continue to hold his position. Dr. Bornemeier has completely evaded any mention of the intended "revolutionary" effects of the American Medical Political Action Committee (AMPAC). Are we as a conference capable of facing the politics of modern medicine?" After I sat down, a benevolent surgeon from the Salvation Army Mission Hospitals murmured in my ear, "Ah, now you have set the cat amongst the pigeons."

Knowles responded immediately. "As Harry Truman once said, 'If it is too hot in the kitchen, get out' and it is not too hot. You know that the definition of a liberal is the ability to tolerate ambiguity. I can see the far right and the far left and they are both wrong. I have learned a lot and would not want to have missed any of it. If only we had more doctors in politics."

Wilbur Cohen was next on his feet, "Doctors are political ignoramuses! More power to AMPAC or any other device to get doctors to learn something about the reality of political life." He went on, "If we can only get them to listen, to talk with, to understand the consumer. It is not too hard to understand the doctor. I could get nearly every doctor in the United States to back a form of national health insurance tomorrow if I could guarantee two things. First, a one-page reporting form and no more for each patient; and second, government-financed malpractice insurance. But to get them into politics. Ah! there is where they should be." From the floor came a cry: "Oh, I only wish I could get AMPAC to oppose my program. It helps so, politically."

Later at lunch, Dr. Bornemeier asked, "What do you think I should have said about AMPAC?" I answered quickly, "What you know of how it is an influence on medicine." "Ah," said he, "I know nothing about that. They are an entirely independent organization." "Oh," said I, wondering if it was not time for the president of the American Medical Association to look about.

In the afternoon, Dr. Walsh McDermott, chairman of the Department of Public Health at the Cornell University Medical College, spoke on "Do Medical Schools Have to Restructure?" In brief, they do, and his recommendation is to eliminate duplication in undergraduate and postgraduate studies. He recommended facing the fact that only one in twenty students wishes to be a scientist and condensing the time required for the M.D., somewhat similar to Britain's system, with a five- to six-year "lower" and one year obligatory general practice. I imagine there may be a bit of faculty resistance to this innovation, but then that gets into another political problem.

Dr. John Hunt, immediate past president of the Royal College of General Practitioners, rose to express the place and training of the general practitioner. He looked more German than English, with his youthful white-blonde hair brushed back, and eyeglasses bent out of parallel, with different planes of reflection producing an eerie death's head illusion. He explained how matters had improved for the GP and how they were continuing to improve. He used as an example his treatment of one of his patients, Sir Thomas Beecham, and with that name something began to rankle. Later I learned, quite incidentally, that his practice includes some of London's wealthiest. Anyway, as he ground on explaining the fifty services available for the GP to use in referral, a groan behind me signaled the uncontainable frustration of a man from beyond The City. "God, doesn't he know that there is a whole generation of men missing from the profession? I am the only man under sixty who operates in my district; the rest have left." When asked during the discussion period, by a Virginia anesthesiologist, about the misconceptions of British medicine from which American doctors suffer, Dr. Hunt assured him that the British GP was not overworked, that those who had emigrated would have left anyway, and that financially the GP is better off than he has ever been. I had the urge to settle down immediately in the U.K., but in time it passed.

Dr. Lloyd Elam, president of Meharry Medical College, gave a fine paper on the changing patterns of health care for Afro-Americans in America. He spoke in detail of his local program; later I was able to ascertain that its success rests on the shoulders of one man who has literally gone into the neighborhood and established community cooperation in a direct, viable way. Calmly and clearly, Dr. Elam explained the problems of involving the White neighbors in the community health center, their original suspicion, and their eventual cooperation and gratitude. My own experience had not been as pleasant; I had been asked to leave an Afro-American clinic in the planning stage, "since no White psychiatrist could ever hope to understand a Black mind." Moreover, I understand that at the Charles Drew Postgraduate Medical School in Watts the whole drive is toward total segregation: staff, administration, and board. Dr. Elam understood it that way, too, and explained it as a development of politics, not medicine—politics again. My envy of his program is profound.

Following the afternoon tea break there was to be a paper on "Is Excellence Possible in a National Health Center?" Since I had no wish to see a man stand on his head and talk backwards, I left for my hotel bed and an hour's nap before the banquet at the hall of the Worshipful Society of Apothecaries of London.

Rushing to the banquet late, heavy with residual sleepiness from the enforced nap, I gave the cabbie the address but placed the accent on the first syllable, "A-pothecary Hall." "Indeed, Sir. And would you please tell me how you can be a member and not pronounce its name? Too much wine and cheese?" Rather than explain the havoc that a nine-hour time change wreaks on tongue and mind, I summoned up my best imitation of a Texas drawl and "'lowed as how thut wur righ."

Ah, and what a hall, what a banquet, what a company! The hall's foundation, laid in 1221, was part of the Black Friars monastery, but of course it was not the 1671 stained glass windows, nor the handhewen beams of Oregon pine, nor the adjacent site of Shakespeare's Blackfriars Theatre, nor Reynolds's sketch of Hunter that made the difference. It was the people: The Grand Warden, limping on one leg since he had lost the other to the Germans in '41 saving the building from a five-hundred-pound bomb. It was the gracious physician on my right prepared to talk of the role of humility in medicine. It was the delightful lady on my left who could maintain without hesitancy that Soames, of *The Forsythe Saga,* was not a good man though he led a good life. But here as always there are limits and when I went on to suggest that Irene was a scheming, beautiful wretch, the air suddenly became turgid, and with an unbelievably deft touch, I was womanhandled into line: "A man's thought. So like a man, but, of course, you are right." She won by losing and I was left to muse, "Soames, will you never learn?"....

The final day started with Dr. John Brotherston, Chief Medical Officer for Scotland, asking, "The Ideal Health Service—Does It Exist?" Well, we all guessed the answer to that one. It does not, but we are trying "in what seems to be a twenty-five-year cycle of seismic spasms of improvement." He neatly phrased the differing attitudes of the American and the British at the conference: "The North Americans act with ardor as they go with the bride whereas the U.K. people view twenty-three years of marriage with mixed pessimism and optimism."

Next, Dean Wilbur Cohen of the University of Michigan gave what he thought were the essential provisions of an American national health insurance program. He came on as a warm and bouncy *enfant terrible* to capture the imagination of the British, possibly by harking back to their history of court jesters. However, the Honorable Wilbur J. Cohen is anything but a court jester, as was revealed by one slip of the tongue that came late in a late discussion. He was before the audience referring back to the days when he had been "Secretary of State." Such a slip would have easily cost an authentic jester not only his job but his head.

Mr. Cohen knew his goals better than anyone else, and did not hesitate to point to the tomfoolery should anyone at the conference be deluded into thinking that the professionals, the president of the U.S., or the people were going to have much to say about the forthcoming U.S. National Health Program. That decision would belong to Mr. Wilbur Mills, chairman of the House Ways and Means Committee. He went on to point out that our meeting would have been impossible in the United States, and that we had to come to England to regain freedom of speech on medical problems. His points concerning a national medical strategy followed clearly.

1. Although it would save two billion dollars to eliminate Blue Cross Blue Shield and to collect funds through social security, this will not be possible.
2. Eligibility for service must be federal (not Blue Cross) with appeal to the federal courts where necessary.

3. New innovative systems of delivery must be developed. (This is not just to put the emphasis on cost efficiency, since the patient is more important than the system.)
4. Preventive medicine must be greatly expanded.
5. Manpower must be increased, remembering that the possibility is infinite since new positions create new demands in spiral fashion.
6. Do not expect perfection; even the best man at bat seldom hits .400.
7. Many should be involved in decisions (unions, consumers).
8. Growth and advance should be reasonably fast, taking into account that not everybody is interested in social idealism.
9. Cooperation with the professions must be sought to help them focus on the patient.
10. The pluralistic system must be maintained.
11. Administrative reality must be recognized; there is a limit to administrative competence.

And then there was a tea break.

As I stirred my cup, I paused a moment to catch my breath then drifted to a corner. Here a kindly, gray-haired man was sipping his tea and flexing the fingers of his open hand. I could not help noticing his open notebook resting on a ledge beside him. Thinking that he was another participant, I mentioned my envy that he could take notes in shorthand.

"Oh, these are not notes. I take down the discussion and, unfortunately, it is not too easy since I have rheumatism crabbing my fingers."

"Spasm," said I, knowing now I could safely play doctor and not be caught by an expert.

"Yes, it's spasm and is a little worse since I retired."

"Retired?" I asked.

"Yes, for twenty-five years I worked in Parliament and now I travel all over the world doing much of the same thing. I just returned from three months at the U.N. Did some of Nixon."

I was intrigued. "Why, twenty-five years in Parliament means you took down Churchill's speeches!"

"Oh, yes, I actually go back to Baldwin, Chamberlain, and Ramsay MacDonald, though of course he was not PM then."

"Churchill must have been an easy one to take down with his ponderous tempo?"

"Heavens, on the contrary! Those cursed pauses! You never knew where he was going next: such phrases and references; you worked all the way. But then when he made a joke, he always did a little dance step [which he demonstrated] and we could catch up. The easy ones are the repeaters, you know. 'There is one thing I wish to say' or 'There is one thing I want to make perfectly clear.' So easy, and, of course, since you know there is only one thing they hope to make clear, the rest is bound to be pretty much of a muddle anyway." The tea break was over.

The rest of the morning was dramatic. First, Kenneth Robinson, Minister of Health from 1964 to 1968, then Enoch Powell, Minister of Health from 1960 to 1963, and finally Elliot Richardson, our Secretary of HEW. Kenneth Robinson came on as predicted, the good guy. Almost out of a British Western, if there is such a thing, in an affable, "white hat" style, he was prepared to see everything working out for the best, and to predict that meanwhile, back at the ranch there were going to be enough beds for the thousands on the waiting lists. And as the sun slowly set in the west, he called upon all to recognize the need for conscious and deliberate organization and distribution: "Service born in idealism—to each according to his need." It left you wanting to see the reruns.

The Rt. Hon. Enoch Powell came on as the "black hat," a good old-fashioned hissable villain: "though what you hear about me may label me as a cynic, I simply report it as it is." And report he did, for he spoke in such a clearly logical fashion that he left me wondering if I were listening to a wise man among fools or a fool among sages, for certainly he wished to think, not expound. It was beautiful to follow a mind honed in Greek, sharp as a medieval scholar's, crowding one "angel" after another off the head of a pin. The demon of rationing and governmental control was thoroughly exposed. When there is a disequilibrium of supply and demand, other forces inexorably come into play, and it is unlikely that they are man's love for his fellow. Rather, the devil will be rationing at the ministerial end of politics through irrational acts. He went on, gloomily predicting that some social processes, such as national health programs, are made irreversible by their destruction of alternatives. Beware, beware. Perhaps Mr. Powell has delineated a new syndrome—Institutional Pollution. He left the audience in such a state of despair that Kenneth Robinson, the good guy, could not contain himself, but burst out with, "I've known

Enoch from years in Parliament and he has always been our Cassandra." To which Powell replied, "And Cassandra was right!"

Then in rushed Elliot Richardson to discuss the strength and shortcomings of the U.S. system of health care and its future development under proposed legislation. There he was, a real live, up-to-date Boston Brahmin, sporting a Jack Armstrong smile above a flaming red tie and passing out artful yet distracting waves to friends and relatives in the audience. I had trouble placing him until he stood up to speak. He was the living image of Clark Kent, and I momentarily expected him to strip down to his Superman outfit before our very eyes. Apparently lacking the necessary phone booth he stuck to mufti and a Clark Kent personality.

Carefully he made it clear that he had nothing to add to the proceedings and proved his point magnificently. He started with a supposedly humorous but an unalluring tale of his great-grandfather, a Yankee surgeon, who had been cheated in some preoperative fee bargaining by a patient and had in turn cheated the patient. It was additional evidence of mutual suspicion between patient and doctor and inadvertently made the point that in other times doctors must have seemed a greedy lot. Probably his clearest points were the need to keep open as many options as possible, and to look to HMOs to lead the way. As he said, there were volumes he could say but would not and did not. No Emerson here, firing the minds of men with thoughts of dedication and transcendental self-fulfillment.

The discussion period that followed was instructive. Dr. Knowles was on his feet immediately, directing a question about capitation to the president of the AMA. However, before he released the floor to Dr. Bornemeier, he turned it over to "Elliot," who added some further twists to the question, and then turned the floor over to "Wilbur" for even more twists. It was "from Tinker to Evers to Chance," and though Dr. Bornemeier may give a good speech, he is no floor debater, so the question flashed by him like a fastball over the center of the plate. He did manage to state the position of the AMA. He survived, but it was doubtful that much was done by anyone for U.S. patients. So it went, three ganging up on one, the great American tradition of personal violence. Enoch Powell remarked from the panel, "This is very much like watching a man being eaten by a boa constrictor." After that, a little too nauseated for lunch, I went back to my room and took a shower.

COMPASSION'S CRUEL COMPANIONS 433

The last afternoon session was anticlimactic. One paper went like a Robert Benchley satire—misplaced pages and the slides permanently out of focus, a bit of comic relief. One paper was so poor that a gentleman in front of me turned and remarked, "I thought it was we Englishmen who were the bores."

The closing ceremonies were brief, with Sir John graciously thanking his staff, the speakers, and the audience for the combined effort. Dr. Bornemeier closed with a plea to reduce tensions, to see each other as working for a common goal, and a proposal that Wilbur Cohen be made an honorary member of the AMA. The latter suggestion set Mr. Cohen to clapping and stamping like a latter-day Rumpelstiltskin, and the conference closed with loud applause.

As I moved to leave, a pleasant, slight man came up to me and asked if I would talk with him "since you seemed militant." I did not know what he meant but was intrigued, so despite my fatigue I settled in a back row with this South African physician turned reporter. He was six months out of medical residence and was now full time with a wire service. His question was persistent: "But what were the U.S. doctors so tense about? I could feel it but I could not understand it." I explained I did not know, for a number of reasons: my ignorance, a provincial outlook, and the confusion of too much input. In my opinion the meeting was a success, but the kind of success twenty blind men have in describing an elephant. However, I was willing to speculate on the tension and hazarded that the cause was not economic, even though an eloquent case could be made for the economic pressures, particularly when one considers that by 1980 approximately 10 percent of the gross national product was spent on health (in 1998 it had reached 17 percent). With those unbelievably gigantic sums involved, IBM begins to look like a cottage industry.

I added that professional identity seemed closer to being the crux of the matter. The U.S. doctor, assailed by forces that he does not understand, resists change and unwittingly becomes the proponent of the status quo. These forces, like the problems of race, politics, education, and yes, even of religion, are difficult to comprehend. They are complex and complicated. When I asked if he were following me, he replied with an unconvincing, "Yes, I guess so."

"Well, look at it from the British view: What are the U.K. doctors so tense about? I will tell you one thing that has them tense but that never appeared on the agenda: race. Informally, three different physicians spoke to me of the race problems, one sharing his dismay that his wife had been spit upon and told to 'just wait till we take over.' Or maybe you watched that sea of coal-black heads surrounded by communistic flags in Trafalgar Square last Sunday and perhaps you heard them roar 'Kill the Bill.' Race tension is in both our worlds and affects everyone. We Americans are more explicit than the British, but that may be just a matter of timing. What is happening are deep shifts of power; those who have power are anxious and those who do not are anxious, too. It is as though the ship of state has cargo rolling free in the hold. Irrespective of responsibility, if the violence is not made fast the hull will go and we all sink.

"It all sounds irrational but not entirely so, if you take a broad enough view. Look, it may sound outrageous, but even Henry the Eighth is in the act. When he drove the Pope and the priests out of England, no 'legal' doctors remained, since the priests had controlled the medical delivery system of that time. He got around this by directly giving a royal charter to the profession, forming the Royal College of Physicians. In his wisdom, Henry made them independent, with the written proviso that they would never use their power to harm the state. This is where part of today's tension originates for the British, since now the state wants back some of that power.

"It is not money, it is not position, but it is threat to the very identity of the profession that makes for the tension. How else could a next-to-nobody like Dr. E.V. Delphey in the 1920s have successfully used sleazy tactics, screaming Bolshevism, to permanently derail the AMA's program of social leadership. I understand that Sir Henry Brackenbury was a little less obvious but just as successful about the same time in permanently defusing the BMA as a progressive social force. If you doubt what I say, take a look at why Lord Russell Brain, an illustrious president of the Royal College of Physicians, was dumped by the BMA, or so I have been told. Certainly medicine has its corridors of power worthy of a C.P. Snow, but it is not in power nor in money, but in identity that the real tension lies in the form of chronic, pernicious, professional paranoia. In the individual or the group the dynamics are the same: 'Who am I? I am the person against…!'

"But you still do not understand? Let me try once more. It is the content of what is happening that is so difficult to understand. I do not mean the content of what is being said, but the historical content. Again, I may not be clear, but it is structure versus content. Structure is what everyone seems to be coming up with: how to build the world's mightiest, all-American, low-cost, self-service health industry. Again and again it is approached as an engineering problem. 'Systems' is the 'in' word but the word could just as well be 'statics'. They all seem to be engineers, hardly an architect in the group. The social engineers are prone to jurisdictional disputes because they fear the real challenge—the content. What we should look for is the most human institutional structure for the health of man, his whole health, mind as well as body. It makes as much sense to have Philistines plan universities, or atheists build cathedrals as it does to have social engineers design health strategies. Oh, all the government building codes will be met, and the roof won't leak, but what goes on under the roof?

"All the talk of medical assistants, nurse practitioners, and the like is an illusion. It is an illusion because most patients, especially blue-collar workers, know or at least sense that doctor substitutes lack perspective, content if you will. Perhaps doctor substitutes do something cheaper or faster like drawing blood, checking a diabetic patient's diet, or screening for immunizations. But when things get serious, touch-and-go, the man you want when your child has a temperature of 104° or your wife has a lump in her breast is someone who knows alternatives, not just the next person along a line of referrals. You want a man or woman who knows alternatives and has had experience with and in them. The only way he or she can be replaced is with another thoughtful, well-trained, compassionate physician. And don't think I am invoking a holy caduceus before you. I am talking about the crying need, largely unconscious, that the plain people have for content in their life and in the lives of those on whom they depend.

"But it is not just the people who need content. It is the profession as well. It takes a philosopher, historian, scientist to supply content. In a few words, it takes the ancient ideal of the complete physician—a man of character. But where is he or she? Where is the man who will listen to a distant discipline? Where can we find someone who is not intimidated by a computer readout? Who will compassionately live with the fact that every man, woman, and child is prejudiced? Where is the physician who is not intimidated by a government program, or worse, seduced by a government grant? A physician unafraid of the clamor of three hundred thousand organized doctors? There is the problem. Find such a physician, and you can start with the real challenge, human content, not institutional form." I slumped in my chair; clearly I had said too much. My listener murmured his thanks and left me alone in the hall.

Weary and hoping for rest, I wandered from the Royal Society and into the underground. Down I went, surprised when I came out on the platform to find but two people waiting. One was a Black man, with the face of an aged Aborigine. He was sitting on a bench, shouting and pleading in a guttural tongue across the tracks to a poster of a handsome White man who proclaimed in bold letters that baldness was unnecessary. The other waiting man was a wren-like, worn clerk, in fitted coat and pointed shoes restlessly dancing the quick step of the courting consenting adult. Time dragged on and nothing happened. Then, remembering the threatened railway strike, I left the two of them waiting for Godot or the Great National Medical Express, or whatever. As I started back up the escalator, a train roared in from the opposite direction sending a blast of noise and dust up the shaft after me. Suddenly, with all the commotion came the recollection of the last scene of *The Bridge on the River Kwai*. After the whistling was over, every plan and scheme destroyed, the bridge blown, the train wrecked, and the principals dead, only the frontline medical officer remained to sum it all up. He looks out over the carnage to repeat: "Madness. Sheer madness."

I hastened to the street and made for a small elegant restaurant, the Ivy, where, with the help of gnocci, a tenderloin of venison sauteed in wine with truffles, an eloquent hollandaise on the broccoli, a bottle of St. Emilion (Chateau Pavie Decesse-62), Sicilian *cassata,* coffee, and a panatela of pure Havana, lit with a flourish by the wine steward, I recovered what I was looking for: the sense that though every life has more pain than is necessary, all need not be suffering.

And so the next day home by the polar route, hours of flying over Greenland's glaciers, the Arctic ice pack, Canada's lifeless tundra, a vast white frozen world awaiting a distant spring. Then the final deplaning, in a rush of joy, in my beautiful green Oregon home. Ah, Paradise regained!

Endnotes

Reprinted from *The Pharos* 35(Winter 1972): 2-9, with permission.

A Modest Policy Proposal: The National Health Selective Disservice

I profess, in sincerity, that I have not the least personal interest in endeavoring to promote this necessary work, having no other motive than the public good of my country.

—Jonathan Swift (1667-1745)
A Modest Proposal

Early on a raw February morning, I discovered how close upon us is George Orwell's prophecy. A bright colleague, thought by some to be a loudmouth, by others a renegade, opened my sleepy eyes to strange possibilities when he sat down beside me at breakfast exclaiming, "I've got it all worked out. To hell with HMOs and PPOs; it is NHSD, the National Health Selective Disservice all the way!"

It was 6:45 A.M. and we were at the counter of the Central Cafe, a hole-in-the-wall beanery, a block and a half from the local hospital. It's the kind of place that tries to live down its honest working man's heritage of red plastic upholstered chrome-plated stools and formica countertop by piping in classical music and labeling hash-brown potatoes on the menu as "cottage fries." My friend, or more precisely, my acquaintance, was still in his jogging clothes as he went on unbidden, "I have been working it out in my head every morning for the last three weeks."

"Not another of your plans to reform the medical profession," I groaned, over my bacon and eggs.

"Reform, nothing! This is a genuine development. A born-again ecdysis for the world of health care delivery, as inevitable as the sun rising in the east. The only wonder is that the truth of the NHSD has not dawned earlier."

"Please, Jonathan, it is too early in the morning for rhetoric. In plain words, what are you talking about?" Then, to the background music of Vivaldi and with his regular bowl of bran flakes before him, Jonathan began, "Look how the health strategy of the country has shifted; voluntary sharing in the 1940s, sometimes called charity, then the period of health entitlement starting in the 1960s with its great cry, 'Health is a right.' Well, it did not take Powell's law long to prove that unlimited access to health care would mean unlimited demand. So, here we are with our present marketplace strategy, which will not work unless we eliminate emotionalism from the system. The NHSD is the next natural development."

"Everyone knows the system is out of control and has to be cut back, but who is to do it? The politicians won't, for the simple reason they would be out of office the day after they did. Consequently, the uproar focuses on you, me, and every doctor and hospital in the nation to cut the cost of health care. On a dollar basis, the medical profession is expected to decide who shall be excluded from hospital beds and emergency rooms, forego neonatal intensive care, or have their expensive life-support systems disconnected. We fumble, trying to accommodate the public both ways, by applying 'brakes' through cost controls and, since braking friction always generates heat, simultaneously attempting to keep the political situation cool by concealing gross injustice in health services. The NHSD is the answer, technically, economically, and politically."

"Please, Jonathan, stick with the facts," I threw into his accelerating chatter.

"Facts, I will give you facts. In 1940, the nation decided that, for the greater good of the greatest number, a particular class of people, men between the ages of eighteen and twenty-six, would be placed at a remarkably high risk of life. With the National Selective Service Act, citizens were screened for physical and mental status; the appropriate ones were drafted and sent to war. Predictably some died, some were injured, and some escaped physical and mental harm, but all took their chances according to the will of the people. Selective Service served the nation well and today stands as a clear precedent for the NHSD. Why not use this historically proven social mechanism to solve our present health crisis?

"For the good of the nation, boards of local citizens would convene across the nation to judge a class of citizens, health care utilizers. Everyone would register with their local board for a health care classification. Each board would have a yearly quota of private and public health resources, much as with any scarce resource during times of war. The necessary data base was established in 1974 by Public Law 96-641, which suggested the Secretary of Health and Human Services establish guidelines for the supply, distribution, and organization of health services. The local board would then determine a citizen's expected health expenditure compared with their value to the community. Lest you think this an unfounded or presumptuous enterprise, determining individual worth in dollars and cents is a frequent practice in today's courts and legislatures."

Rapping my cup to interrupt his torrent of words, I broke in with, "Perhaps that is true for lawyers and judges, but doctors would never go along with placing a dollar-and-cents value on patients."

"But, you know such judging is even more common in the daily practice of medicine, where it is referred to as 'valuing the quality of life.' Take, for example, the judgment of a family practitioner comparing a forty-year-old male president of a manufacturing firm suffering from acute appendicitis with a six-year-old foster child suffering from Down's syndrome complicated by spine bifida. Frankly, which one will have prompt, easy access to quality health care? You do know physicians participate in a selective health delivery system based on the patient's financial worth.

"Granted, these practiced values of individual worth are not drawn up clearly and published the way physicians' judgments of fees are in the California Comparative Value Scale, yet they exist. The only things needed to codify patient worthiness for health care is candor and a computer. With the assistance of receptionists, business managers, and hospital administrators, we regularly turn people away from necessary medical care through a host of commonly accepted conventions. By referring the economically disadvantaged to overloaded clinics, by giving diabetics a prescription for insulin they cannot afford, to say nothing of the considered neglect of the infirm elderly in the backwaters of custodial care, we protect hospitals from the "cost shift" while reducing the burden of health care costs on the general public. There is little difficulty seeing that a calculus of patient worth exists, ranging from 'crocks' through VIPs. Although these values presently lack the imprimatur of the government, which is now busy with the relative values of Therapy and Diagnostic Reimbursement Groups, the relative value of patients will be part of the NHSD.

"The NHSD is the logical extension of medical marketplace strategy, finally establishing the sought-for rational mechanism to protect the medical marketplace from overutilization which is presently leading to bankruptcy. With a direct health worth appraisal, similar to a credit rating by which a computer validates the purchase of a refrigerator, an immediate determination will be available to control access to health care. At present, health care eligibility, sometimes referred to as need, is a muddle of secondary measures of productivity, media coverage, accumulated wealth, and insurance. This jumble is used to determine eligibility, rather than a clear measure of the prospective patient's productivity. A personal evaluation of productivity (PEP) is readily determined by subtracting a citizen's expected productive life span from his expected biological life span. For example, a hardworking fifteen-year-old boy with an anticipated productive life span to sixty-five years has a PEP of 50. However, if he became a paraplegic as a result of an automobile accident, his PEP would, of course, be adjusted downward. In fact, many, say an eighty-five-year-old unemployed woman, would have a negative PEP. The PEP becomes essential in deciding which of two patients should use a limited resource such as an intensive care unit bed. Neither the hospital staff, the physician, nor the family will be faced with complex judgments, as the computer prints out both patients' PEPs, with the bed going to the patient with the highest PEP."

"How about the elderly patient with the money to pay for long-term care?" I asked.

"For those who have the financial resources, registration with their local board could be handled like the original draft law in 1863, which allowed draftees to buy out of the system. However, in the modern instance, the person could buy in. The PEP ratings would be issued as vouchers good for stated periods, during which health care could be redeemed by the voucher. The vouchers would be openly negotiable in the marketplace, and Merrill Lynch could trade in vouchers much as they do in futures for wheat or soybeans. You would have an inalienable right to give, trade, or sell your health rights, much as you have if you wish to sell a pint of your blood, or a woman renting out her uterus for insemination.

"As you might expect with social change, difficulties can arise during the transition. Weeks, perhaps months, may pass before attorneys adapt their present preoccupation with malpractice to PEP arbitration. Some old-fashioned physicians, those dependent on fees from patients, will object to limiting their hospital admission privileges, but these doctors can be handily dealt with by stuffing their throats with gold, much as the English did with their old-timers when establishing the National Health Service. They would be paid not to practice, much as farmers are paid not to raise cotton or wheat. For salaried academicians, the emphasis shifts hard dollars to social reform, the greater good for the greater number, which concept should suffice when accompanied by assurances of tenure. HMO doctors will understand intuitively how well the NHSD fits with their present economic incentive to keep patients out of the hospital. For those physicians employed by the corporations of the medical/industrial complex, personal reimbursement incentives plus stock options can be expected to clarify their thinking. As always, government doctors can be handled by fiat.

"No opposition should be expected from business and labor, since the NHSD will eliminate the present hospital cost shift, which places a considerable burden on the employers, forcing them to bear ever increasing health insurance premiums. In fact, the medical corporations will undoubtedly contribute a strong lobbying effort to ensure quick NHSD enactment since it eliminates most of the present unprofitable hospital services for the aged and chronically disabled. The NHSD will clear obligatory losses from health corporations' accounts while promising higher profit margins."

As Marie, the waitress, topped off our coffee cups, I interrupted, "Wait a minute. People are going to object. Priests and ministers will be up in arms."

Jonathan pounced on my idea, "I thought of that. Religionists will see the NHSD as a way of returning patients to the hands of God. Granted, some objections may arise from those moralists maligning the NHSD as reminiscent of the Nazis and their racist policies. Blinded by dogma and prejudice, that lunatic fringe will miss the point; no one will be secretly denied life; there will be no secret about it. All activities will be legal and above board, pursued in open meetings with the record published in the newspapers. This is no policy of dictatorship, but a people's policy arrived at democratically. If any historical example is appropriate, it is the Greek city-state and that gloriously militant democracy, Sparta, which exposed infants deviating from accepted standards. Neither infant, Oedipus or Moses, would have survived Nazi Germany's gross use of political subterfuge, but with the NHSD's policy of scientific natural selection, any latter-day Oedipus or Moses would be afforded the same opportunities that the original infants had, survived, and were actually better for the experience.

"In the case of those protesting that the NHSD is equivalent to Jonestown, hysterical genocide, a calm explanation that no one will be encouraged to commit suicide should suffice. The basic strategy remains: the 'national lifeboat' is full, and as a triage measure, some of the passengers are encouraged to swim, rather than sail, to shore. In fact, there are many who will welcome the therapeutic value of the NHSD as a way of deinstitutionalizing the sick, offering them an alternative, holistic, self-actualizing way to health through exercise, diet, and education. Now, what do you think of it?"

"I think it is time for me to start rounds and for you to take a shower." Obviously disappointed, he pleaded, "But what of NHSD?"

Without another word I took my raincoat from the bent hook behind me, and squeezed down the narrow aisle to the cash register. Marie took my money and, with a nod of her head toward the far end of the counter where Jonathan was finishing his bowl of flakes, returned my change with an added, unexpected comment, "He might be the best in town, but I wouldn't take my sick dog to that Dr. Swift. Not me!"

Endnotes

Reprinted from the *Journal of the American Medical Association* 252(1984): 261-262, with permission. Copyrighted 1984, American Medical Association.

Nurturing Hate in Psychotherapy
Address, Children in Distress Conference, New York City, 1987

The tigers of wrath are wiser than the horses of instruction.
—William Blake (1757-1827)

At a board meeting of a charitable enterprise, or rather, sitting at the table before the meeting began, in informal talk the member next to me inquired about my recent trip to the Republic of South Africa. The visit to that benighted land had given me an opportunity to observe their health delivery system about as close as anyone can get in a month. My friend was not so interested in the state of heart transplants or the value of the Krugerrand as he was in what I had seen and learned about the care of children. I laid out the abysmal social conditions for many Black families. The problems of children held in detention, the self-righteous but mindless policy of the United States, professionals and lay people alike, with our academic sanctions, our utterly destructive policy of disinvestment, our encouragement of strife and reinforced disregard for those, under the burden of apartheid, striving for some semblance of human dignity and concern. I showed him a newspaper clipping from a Cape Town paper that I carried in my wallet, and then I all but exploded that we in this country were in a conspiracy of destruction, nurturing hate and fostering terrorism worldwide. His response was, "You are an expert in outrage." Indeed, I have become an expert in outrage at the way the richest country in the world fails in its duty to children, worldwide, while it fosters the very hate it deplores.

Remaining dispassionate is not easy once you have seen the killing fields in Guatemala, talked with clinic directors in the third world who despair of training indigenous health workers, recognizing they are only training bright, caring peasants for death as their clinical teams are slaughtered twice over by the government and guerillas intent on eliminating any form of impartial local leadership. It is difficult to remain calm once you have walked through the slums of Bombay surrounded by crowds of penniless children, begging for the price of a dose of dapsone to treat their leprosy. This, when you know that the dose for a year costs but fifty U.S. cents, but might as well be fifty thousand dollars for the children's lack of resources. Becoming an expert in outrage may seem easy but remaining one is not; you are in danger of having your spirit crushed by the sheer mass of childhood suffering. I try not to be overwhelmed.

Nor do I have to go to Sri Lanka to find immense, immoral discontinuities in the care of children. Simply getting up from my psychotherapist chair and descending from my ivory tower with its spectacular view of the snowcapped peaks of the Cascades affords contact with more than enough outrage for a lifetime. I find myself in a great and beautiful American city, Portland, Oregon. A city which supports three hundred full-time child prostitutes. Here, let me read you a recent headline from my local paper, "13-year-old guilty of ruthless murder." The newspaper filler goes on, "The young killer could be confined until he is 21 for the coldblooded rifle slaying of a Bend fisherman." What horrendous weight of hate has crushed this child's soul and what unimaginable abominations of rage will be added?

What can my outrage mean to you? I ask you as I have asked myself, and the answer, as plain as the face of George Washington on a dollar bill, is that we, as a nation, are busily nurturing hate. You and I and the rest of the citizenry of the nation that has 40 percent of the world's wealth are industriously going about the business of trashing a significant portion of the youth of the world. I hope you are squirming, for I need company as I squirm at reading that we are "forced" to cut the budgets of most if not all child programs. Is there anyone who even remembers the blessing of Medicheck, the erstwhile federal program to identify and diagnose the sick children of the U.S.A.? As a people we have eliminated not the thought, ahh how we love to trumpet noble sentiments, but the obligatory action that gives meaning to the word "charity," the ancient word for love. "Sacrifice" is our least spoken public word. You will not hear it mentioned by the media, nor from our leaders, by our colleagues. Ours is a world of progress and progress has come to be spelled, "M" "E". If you doubt what I say, squirm harder as you listen to the latest television report on how we must accommodate to reduced resources, the phrase is "cut to the bone," in order to avoid new taxes, the prime resource for deprived children.

But outrage is brash emotion which at best only inflames not enlightens. Offending you with the label of unconcerned serves no purpose. The fact is, you are concerned, otherwise why would you be reading this. Nor is my outrage unique. You share it. But what are we to do with your unasked-for passion? Luckily, you, like me, at least profess to be reasonable. So like reasonable men and women, let us look at how we hate our children and consequently nurture hate in our children. Thus we can struggle to understand what is possible; how we may use what strength we have, not to attack and destroy, for, lo, that is the path which has brought us to such a parlous state, but to act out of reason with the highest emotion, courageous compassion, considered active charity, action for the inarticulate and deprived children of our world.

As men and women of good will we, the professed concerned, find it difficult to even consider that in our daily lives we might nurture hate in those dependant on us. Yet I fear we do. A terrible truth lies in the ethical dilemma which the psychotherapeutic relationship reveals, for it always bears acknowledging with the patient the profound artificiality of the security and freedom simulated by the relationship. The question is, How do we remain "therapeutically neutral," free of hateful actions when the frail ship of therapy floats on a sea of exploitation and destruction? Society grants a protected space for the exploration of the inner person, the patient's soul, and with that privilege comes the temptation to believe the thin illusion that the implacable demands and crass values of public life are barred by the office door. But consider how much time with the patient is used to mitigate, rather than identify and work with, the hate which leaks in at every crack and crevice?

Should you consider this issue purely academic, let me ask where you stand on the great federal program of the 1960s, the deinstitutionalization of the mentally ill by the establishment of nationwide mental health centers? Was it a good idea to eliminate child guidance clinics by converting them into multipurpose community centers? Was it a good idea to dilute the emphasis on child care, deemphasizing the need for beds for children in psychiatric hospitals? I was a zealot in that misbegotten cause, until I discovered that the child guidance clinic I had founded was being turned into a mental health sedation center and left in disgust. For me, the advent of the psychotropic drugs seemed a scientific achievement, until I discovered that what the public wanted was "not to know" of the suffering in children. The public proved grateful for the money saved by chemical restraints and made it clear through their elected representatives that the public demands even more "scientific pills," technological breakthroughs, to remove the problems of children from public view. Today we view the disaster of this "therapeutic triumph" in the blank faces of those children, now grown to adulthood, who wander the streets of every city, the homeless.

Specifically, how much is psychotropic medication used to genuinely "make the patient amenable to therapy" as contrasted to how much are chemicals used to screen from our eyes and the eyes of relatives and the public the horrendous suffering of a sick child? Teenagers suffering from schizophrenia plead with me to reduce or eliminate their mind-numbing Prolixin and, I acknowledge with mixed feelings, if not shame, I continue to control their symptoms at a level society will tolerate, since our society denied, at reasonable cost and accessibility, the safety and freedom of inpatient care, the necessary therapeutic space to address the teenagers' suffering openly. I temporize with hate, cover it while acting as an agent of society to avoid it.

Do not hear me as a zealot against the use of psychotropic medications, though I remain a zealot against lobotomy, that medical device patently intended to permanently seal hate into a damaged mind.

The ethical dilemma of the psychotherapist in using medications is profound and must be considered by any therapist with each and every pill prescribed. I am not against psychotherapists using these drugs, but I know from personal experience how easily drugs contribute to nurturing chronic hate.

Most of my present practice focuses on adults. However, I do see children as sometimes the patient arrives in the waiting room with a child. Should the receptionist be turned into a babysitter? Is the child, as therapists have been trained to consider, a defense against the intended intimacy of therapy, a distraction to dilute or distort the treatment? Or is the presence of the child a clue to something else? Unfortunately, I missed the parent's plea for help in dealing with his hate of his child. I ineptly fudged the issue by suggesting family therapy with another therapist, to completely miss the human drama unfolding before me.

One insidious way of reinforcing the patient's hate lies in the therapist's reaction to the patient's global complaints about money. What to do with the "poverty" lament of the middle-class patient? What to say when they present the cost of therapy, added to a hundred other bills, as an unbearable burden? How frequently do therapists remind the patient that as members of the economically top 5 percent of the world they have choices? Even in treating our underclass, how often do therapists remind them they are above 50 percent of the world's population when it comes to quality of life? It may sound hateful to point out broad advantages to a narrowly disadvantaged patient, but again it is an approach to hate in the form of greed generated by a culture which leaves nearly all hungry with a pervasive sense of deprivation. Such explorations of hate can open patients to appreciating sacrifice, paradoxically, sacrifice for their own benefit.

Another dodge therapists use, and I know because I am guilty of using it, is to dilute the language of therapy, to tacitly agree to avoid naming elemental feelings. This semantic trickery is analogous to the nefarious family obfuscation, the defense against feelings which has one family member saying to another, "Of course I love you. I do not need to tell you so, since you know I do." How difficult it is to remind the patient, "Yes you do hate your child's behavior and you must measure it against your love."

Consider the physically abused wife of a physician who describes her reaction to her husband's blows as an example of "how disappointed she is in him." Is the therapist's job to explore this "disappointment" or to discuss the fact of hate, real, straight-out, undiluted hate? Is the abused child, like the abused wife, too sensitive to know what she really feels when "Daddy does those things to me"? Now I am not suggesting concerned therapists play the surgeon's game of citing statistics, "Your complaint is statistically significant, for recent studies by a Georgia clinic show 19.2 percent of prepubertal girls and 8 percent of boys have been sexually abused." It is our job, not the patient's, to know that in our country a child is killed through abuse once every twenty minutes. But I ask, does the therapist label the emotion for what it is, abject hate, or join in the national pursuit of euphemisms, a game which has us talking mechanically about "stress," a technological condition, when what is experienced is "suffering," the ancient and inevitable price of witnessing to the human condition?

We openly nurture hate in psychotherapy when we shrink from our personal experience of hate. We nurture hate in the patient as we distance ourselves from the patient by language and position. We are hateful, like it or not, when the emotions of the patient reincarnate personal dreads. The daily, up-front experience of hate in practice is either explicated in our minds or further buried in the patient's illness. There is no middle ground, no safe neutrality in this. We have a choice which is fatefully limited to either/or. As therapists, we either help the patient by identifying their elemental feeling in order to work with the sufferer or foster the disease by covering and concealing hate. Jeremiah that I may be, I fear the latter predominates.

Why do I judge the profession of psychotherapy so harshly? My eyes are jaundiced for the sight of the natural product of integrated and personally worked-through mature hate in my colleagues. If the psychotherapist has remained enough in touch with his or her personal hate to discipline it into a workable therapeutic tool, hate, that tool must appear in other parts of professional life. It follows, at least for me, that the complete therapist must experience outrage. We know there is a legion of dragons loose in our society, but where are the St. Georges? I have seen some but, frankly, they are too few to dignify the profession as a latter-day order of the Knights Templar.

Please bear with me, for I am much like the bemused Mr. Dick in *David Copperfield* whose every conversation invariably ends up discussing King Charles's head. My King Charles head is outrage at the lack of caring for the deprived children of our world.

The health professions of the world must learn to speak, to plead, to demand, to command that "The children of this world are suffering and we, one and all, must recognize their suffering." It is not enough to treat in a clinic, to lobby for a budget, to inveigle an endowment. Please, no more public relations sedation. No more cheap-shot, satellite television extravaganzas for the starving children of Ethiopia, no more collection boxes for abused children in Somalia, no more committees to decide what the needs of children may be. Please, no more self- effacing professional do-gooding. Let our hate mature over time. Our outrage drives the citizenry to action for deprived children.

What professionals should do with necessary, healthy, heartfelt, spirit-sustaining outrage is to let out a tremendous, sustained, yes, an ever-strengthening roar, an arresting chorus of protest. Both the people and the leaders of this nation need to hear that the bottom line is not dollars, the bottom line for us to survive as a moral nation is the bonding of every living child to a loving/hating adult who cares. Every idea espoused, professional association endorsed, clinic supported, yes, every policy our nation proposes, for ourselves and for others across the world, from highway taxes to Star Wars, should answer to an inevitable, elemental question, "What will this do for children?"

Part 9

Manifest Tragedy

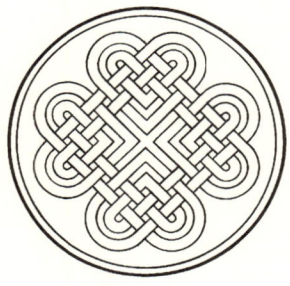

Through me lies the road to the City of Grief.

—Dante (1265-1321)
The Divine Comedy
The Inferno, Canto 3, line 1

Overview to Part 9

Experienced compassion not only recognizes its possible absence but also absence of hope for compassion as well. A brief venture into fantasy, a thought experiment, should make the indispensable presence of compassion's companion, hope, undeniable. Have you ever wished to have sufficient wealth to send your personal benefactions rippling wide in every direction? If so, on whom would you bestow your generosity, friends, relatives, the uneducated, the worthy poor, those close at hand, those far away?

Predictably, in deciding how to distribute any newfound wealth, the only certain response comes as a band of sorcerer's apprentices suggesting their favorite charity, helpers who, ironically, swiftly dispel goodwill. Aggravated by stereotyped pleas and financial advice, the momentum of unbounded wealth should eventually carry you to the edge of the abyss of bottomless needs of the poor, ignorant, and sick of this world, needs beyond hope of satisfaction.

Recognizing the grim fact of finite means is neither a scandal of festering corporate exploitation nor an indictment of charity's claim on respect. Rather, the fact of limits reinforces authentic fellow feeling, perforce as a personal experience rather than an institutional program. Compassion is never "given at the office." Great or small, the complete gift brings with it an ultimate beneficence, albeit often anonymous, the donor's considered position on the edge of another's need. Without the imprimatur of free choice, any gift, no matter how fancy the wrapping, withers as mindless welfare.

Our troubling thought experiment teaches that despite the best of intentions, no one has the power to alter the course of mankind's fate, which is enforced by the Eumenides, as they measure out our destiny. In considered detail the movie review *3 Women* weaves fate's unalterable course through the lives of three modern women. Nor should there be doubt that our ever present fear of the unknown future draws its strength from mankind's universal dread of death, the knowledge that the time will come when the Eumenides cut us off from the thread of life.

When peering into the pit of mankind's limitless poverty of means, our limited ability to discern the true significance of shared feeling becomes starkly real. What can an individual's wealth avail in filling that ghastly maw? What hope of compassion flickers even briefly in that abyss? Assailed by the fact of finitude, we reach out for infinity in the form of problematic immortality offered by institutions. Despite any inspiring rhetoric to the contrary, fear of the oblivion of death binds us, by way of unrequited hope, to bear allegiance to our religious, governmental, educational, and charitable organizations. The tyranny of fear of death turns even mindful men and women into agents of institutional ideologies, fired with the desire to live through some illusion of eternity.

Like it or not, ours is a corporate destiny determined by theology of religion, politics of nation, policy of economics, and lately, faith in medical science's chimerical promise of ever extended life span. Our institutions program us and reprogram us again, to serve their corporate immortality. Once as slave, then serf, now as citizen, common man supports "necessary" institutions. Today we have a new designation: as consumers we tithe our health insurance premiums, signifying obeisance to health care services. **Technological Zeal or Therapeutic Purpose?** examines the unpalatable fact of enforced servitude occurring at the bedside.

St. Paul and Medical Technology, originally given as an address to a religious congregation, examines the patient's helpless condition as a dialogue between what is done and what families wish to be done for their endangered members. **My Brother and His Keepers** asks who among the medical profession bring care to hopeless, impaired physicians.

Failing to save a terminal patient's life need not be a tragedy; failing to respect the needs of a dying patient is always a tragedy. To place a human face on the tragedy of compassion forsaken, **Requiem for an Unknown Leper** explores the withering of humanity in a man's heart numbed by disease and by the treatment of disease.

3 Women
A Film Review

When shall we three meet again?
—William Shakespeare (1564-1616)
Macbeth Act 1, 1, 1

Ah, here is a worthy film! Here is a film that is beautiful and speaks of honor. Here is a film in which the hero is destroyed for his shortcomings, not pickled in sentiment. Here is an elemental tragedy. See *3 Women*!

But, why is the film complete? It seems a thin tale of a farm girl, Pinky (Sissy Spacek), who runs away from her Texas home with nothing more than a sewing machine and a few dollars in her purse, searching for a larger life in California. She finds a job at a rehabilitation center on the desert where she meets Millie (Shelley Duvall), a young woman and fellow worker who is also searching. Together they frequent a bar owned, in part, by Willie (Janice Rule), an older, pregnant woman. All three seek personal meaning, and gradually, as their earnest wish to grow is savagely destroyed, they fall into a strange, yet logical, relationship by offering a meaning of life to each other. It is high drama, because every last chance of escape from their narrow lives is explored only to be found wanting. Their fate inexorably unwinds and captures them and us in a web of human suffering that overwhelms, as tragedy must, leaving only the memory of what might have been.

The slow pace of the film is deceptive; in the initial scenes Pinky is introduced to the rules and regulations of the rehabilitation center, and action drags with the boredom of a child's experience, expectations far beyond fulfillment. Pinky, perhaps seventeen, finds Millie the only staff member willing to help and consequently develops an adolescent crush on her. Through an obvious subterfuge Pinky manages to move in with Millie, who at about twenty-seven years of age is a Mary Hartman trying to become a Martha Stewart. She has the personality of a character in a television commercial—blathering mouth and shallow mind coupled with unchecked compulsive behavior. Millie keeps her apartment in *Good-Housekeeping*–Gold-Medal style, astounding Pinky with its orderliness and cleanliness. Millie's compulsiveness is all-consuming ("Clean is sexy").

She approaches men with a direct by-the-numbers friendliness that may be accepted by Mickey Mouse Club members but has no place among swingers. "Hello, Tom, how is your cold?" gets a passing cough for a response from her neighbor at the Purple Sage singles apartment complex.

Millie and Pinky frequent the Dodge City Bar, a hokey miniature Disneyland, a worn-out Western movie set where Millie hangs out with Edgar and the boys. Edgar (Robert Fortier) is landlord of both the Purple Sage apartment and the Dodge City Bar. He is a pathetic stud, a broken-down ex-Western-movie stunt man. In the sandlot behind the Dodge City Bar, Edgar's faceless male buddies cavort on motorcycles ("dirt racks"), when they are not displaying their machismo at the shooting range. Willie, the third woman, is Edgar's strange, silent, pregnant wife, who decorates all the available concrete walks, walls, and swimming pools with painted murals.

So far I have told you absolutely nothing of the ambiance of the film, which strikes you immediately, within the first moment of the film. As the titles flow by, the background is filled with the strange creatures Willie paints. There she is, completely covered in a flowing gown, sunscreening floppy hat, brush in hand, slowly painting in the colors and outlines of horrid, violently struggling, hominoid figures. These bestial, tailed creatures slither over the pavement, across the walks, under the water; and as you watch, gradually they run into the lives of the three women.

To begin with, life flows along smoothly for Pinky and Millie at the rehabilitation center and with their social life. The swinging singles at the Purple Sage, however, have nothing to do with these "innocents." As the girls prepare a dinner party, Pinky slavishly imitates Millie in the hopes of becoming a look-alike copy but predictably fails. Consistently, Pinky is clumsy, spilling sauce, making messes, and actually bearing bad news. When Pinky inadvertently remarks that their party is a bust, Millie for the first and only time rejects her. The rejection is violent, for Millie wants to prove she is a woman where Pinky is a child. Millie gets drunk with Edgar and returns to the apartment with him to scornfully force Pinky out of the bedroom. Pinky is so devastated by the blow that she attempts suicide, jumping from the balcony of the apartment into the swimming pool. She suffers a fractured skull and nearly drowns but is saved by Willie who rushes her to a hospital where she remains in a coma for weeks.

The hospital scenes are probably as authentic as any the movies can produce, more real than most documentaries. The patient in coma, Pinky, does nothing, as a person in coma would do nothing. There are no intrusive "to-pac-ata" sounds, and the portrayal of the physician is the most sympathetic that the film world has shot since the long-gone days of Dr. Christian. He cares as he can care. The officious nurse as well as the understanding nurse are as believable as nurses in real hospitals.

Millie is shaken by Pinky's near suicide and summons Pinky's parents from Texas. They prove to be liabilities. Nor is there any other help, as the staff at the rehabilitation center simply does not care. As Pinky recovers, Millie takes her home, but Pinky is a changed person with a severe post-concussion amnesia. Severed from her past by the amnesia, Pinky resumes the fantasy that had originally so enthralled her; to become Millie, and she does. The women's personalities merge, with Pinky coming out on the other side of the relationship as Millie. She takes over Millie's apartment and her personality, but unlike Millie she is a loose female on the make. The transfers of personality were facilitated by Millie's diary. Pinky broke into it to learn her friend's secrets while beginning her own diary. The exchange of personalities can be followed in the excerpts they read from each other's diaries, ending when Pinky commandeers both diaries and relegates Millie to a nonperson.

Pinky's precipitous jump into hedonistic living is interrupted by a series of dreams, which, again, are handled like dreams and not as an excuse for the director to fill the screen with well-labeled symbols. The dreams are chaotic, terrifying, and end Pinky's flight to phony sophistication by reviving the forgotten past and returning her to her original search, for what she wanted from her Millie, not competition but mothering.

The fact of mothering then explodes into the lives of these two women when the drunken Edgar surreptitiously sneaks into the apartment late at night for "a little fun." He intends to celebrate his impending fatherhood, abandoning Willie at home to have her baby unattended. Millie immediately recognizes Willie's danger and, with Pinky, rushes to the house behind the Dodge City Bar, where Willie's in labor.

The birth scene transfixes the audience. Millie screams for Pinky to go for the doctor, rushes into the house, and intuitively becomes midwife for Willie. Like Pinky, the audience remains outside, watching the whole gruesome event through an open door. The baby is born dead. As Willie cuddles the stillborn, Millie staggers out in shock, a bit mad, blood dripping from her fingers, and confronts the paralyzed Pinky with the wild anger of despair, for Pinky had failed to go for help. A blow to Pinky's face ends the scene.

Time passes, conveyed by an unbelievably long shot of a Coca-Cola truck approaching the Dodge City Bar, straight on, down an endless road. The rewoven shreds of the three women's lives are now revealed as Pinky explains to the delivery man that her "mother" will have to sign for the Coke, and Millie appears, now a matron. After Millie agrees with the delivery man that Edgar's sudden death was unfortunate, the two women return to the house behind the bar, where the silent Willie sits on the porch swing. With a few grandmotherly nods she reports she has had "a most wonderful dream," which she cannot remember, and affectionately she welcomes Pinky to the swing "while supper is getting ready." The women have become each other's need and reason for existence, they are now a family.

If you are simply interested to learn the plot in order to decide whether or not you wish to see the film, I have done my duty, and you need read no further. The critic, like the physician, may offer a report, an opinion, a diagnosis, and leave it at that. Neither critic nor physician can be sued or run out of his organization for such "professional" behavior. But then there is the physician who has a hankering to see more, to understand more deeply, to relate more completely to his world; such becomes the art of medicine, an art that is not restricted to the patient-doctor relationship, but is also part of the doctor-self relationship. Perhaps any of us with a hankering to know more may discover a bit about ourselves in this film.

I left the theater possessed. Robert Altman's daimon had captured not only my imagination but my very spirit as well. What was this business of these three women, so vaguely familiar, so impossible, yet so believable. Altman is reported to have written the story from a dream, but whose dream and of what? Getting through to the heart of any artistic dilemma, much as diagnosing a disease, takes engaging with the dissonance, the abnormal signs.

Some of the film's signs and symptoms—the talk of tomatoes as love apples and the spilling tomato sauce—are obvious for the blood and menses they represent. The strange creatures that Willie is forever painting seem in place as expressions of unconscious drives and desires, together with their violence. Such hominoid figures often appear in schizophrenic art, exaggerated symmetry and compulsive design posed in extremes of destruction, as the psychotic artist projects his internal violence onto the canvas. Nor is the use of water shots in the pools and through the aquarium too difficult to understand. They illustrate the chaotic dissolution of the culture the three women are immersed in.

The sign that caught and held my curiosity was Pinky's sewing machine. Was Pinky's preoccupation with sewing symptomatic of something more? Why did Willie prop an advertisement for a computerized sewing machine on the bedside table next to the comatose Pinky? It seemed incongruous, and when I asked someone in a position to judge fairly if a girl might run away from home with her sewing machine, the answer was affirmative. A suitcase full of clothes, yes, a doll, maybe, or, like Dorothy in the Wizard of Oz or Little Orphan Annie, a pet dog, but a sewing machine? It still did not fit and like an otherwise "normal" sign that intuitively catches your attention in a physical examination, the sewing machine remained in the back of my mind, complete with its question mark.

Another sign that did not fit was Willie's silence. What was the oppressive message in her implacable gaze? It was not the wild-eyed hostile stare of the severely depressed, nor a look of unspoken reproach, nor dark curiosity. It was a piercing eye of knowledge. What did she know but would not say? In contrast, Millie, a froth of a woman, a flotsam in a social world, posed no questions, simply talked about herself.

Still another sign led me deeper into the mystery of the film's artistry— color. Pinky, all reds; Millie, all yellows; and Willie, blues. Pinky Rose's name proclaims "her" color. Pinky's reds are light, youthful, with a dainty tentativeness, while Millie's yellows are saturated, heavy, and intentional. Millie discourses at length about her car's particular shade of yellow, carefully differentiating the hue as "mustard yellow, not English dry, but French, mustard." Then there is the shaded, smoky, perhaps muddy, chiaroscuro of Willie's blues. Ah, here is a series of signs that add up. Here are the primary colors, red, yellow, and blue. The women must have some elemental relationship. Three women, three women, and then, it dawned—the Three Fates, the working sisters of the Muses. Here you are, Robert Altman's daimon, I have caught you by the tail.

So, we have Clotho, the spinner of life (Pinky's sewing machine is revealed for what it is), Lachesis, the measurer (Millie, literally the name means one thousand, with your thousand values), and Atropos, the inflexible executioner (I know now what you are looking for, Willie, my final day, and, Willie, we both know who did in Edgar).

It becomes possible to return to see some scenes again, for more than their flickering shadows; for example, the initial introduction to the spa. It is the river Styx, the same metaphor Fellini used in *8 1/2*. Old people are being helped into the waters, knee deep, by the first two of the Fates, who are continually alert for death. Pinky grows sleepy in the tub room and is derelict in her duty as a custodian of the dying, just as the "beginning" Fate might be expected to be. Pinky's experiment of completely dunking herself in the hot waters, her baptism in the river of life and death, presages her later trip to an underworld after she jumps into the Purple Sage swimming pool and nearly dies. Even Charon is there worrying about collecting the toll. In the person of Dr. Mass, the medical director, he is overly preoccupied with cost, bills, and malpractice insurance. Cerberus, the mad three-headed dog guarding the gates of hell, might easily be the doctor's assistant, fawning before her master, the growling, snooping physical therapist who bites any who get out of line. In classical mythology, Cerberus devoured time, past, present, and future, and the physical therapist acts out the ancient role when she catches Pinky making a mistake punching out at the center's time clock. Finally, the girls have no personal relationship with their patients, who come and leave at appointed times which none can question or even comprehend. The Fates mark out the path of human destiny. They are not the authors of what is "written in the stars."

But then the question of the girls' clothes at the spa is interesting. Why so ill-fitting a tank suit for Pinky, and why purple? In this death house, the new girl never finds clothes that fit. Clotho is a spinner of her own clothes as well as the initial pattern of life. The purple is the color of royalty. Millie's favorite flower is the iris, the purple flower named for the male messenger of the gods. They, Pinky and Millie, are forced into the employment of the gods, at a task they can never fulfill, literally or mythologically, since the Fates' allegiance goes beyond the Gods—even beyond mighty Zeus.

But the significance of the "royal" purple continues to spin out through a strange internal story, for they try to make a home for themselves at the Purple Sage Apartments. The apartment name is an obvious reference to Western movies, and Zane Grey's *Riders of the Purple Sage* is a clear example of this name designating the cowboy Valhalla. The Purple Sage is the place of heroes and gods. For the Greeks, it was Mount Olympus, and how like a modern Mount Olympus this swinging singles apartment is. Apparently no one works; the swingers sit around the pool, as the gods once sat around the heights of Olympus, indulging themselves in feasting and petty games, impervious to the cares and suffering of mortals.

Who then is the king, the Zeus, in this latter-day celestial abode? Why Edgar, of course. The sound track literally thunders when he first appears. He lusts and drinks like a Greek god, indiscriminately letchering after any woman who strikes his fancy. Edgar, who boasts he once was the stand-in, "stunt double," for a real movie star, Hugh O'Brien, is a virtual hero-god stand-in for Zeus as well. Here the mythologies of Hollywood and Olympus merge. Both are bankrupt, unconcerned with the human condition and liable to dissolution. Altman's daimon reveals our gods as dead or dying.

But men cannot live without gods. The three Fates know this. In the end Pinky, Millie, and Willie retreat from a life that is deadly to find shelter in the house behind the set of the Dodge City Bar. They live on as destiny does, awaiting a new culture, new gods. Fate does not cease with the loss of a mythology, only a culture does.

The historical insight of Altman's daimon is fully valid. Centuries before their "glory," the Greeks of classical antiquity had their mythology synthesized for them by Homer. Whether Homer ever existed as an individual is unimportant, much as the question of who wrote Shakespeare's plays. What is important is that about 800 B.C. the remnants of a tattered Mycenaean culture, which had flourished four hundred years before, were spun out as tales that bestowed gods on a Greek culture of 400 B.C. The poet founded a "new race of men" by investing them with new gods, and as a nation, the Greeks flourished until they lost belief in their gods. Later, the less imaginative Romans appropriated the pantheon of Greek gods and by simply changing the names made use of cultural retreads for nearly a thousand years. Little wonder the Romans were short on creative originality. Christianity attacked these pagan tales only to reassemble them as saints and sinners in a mythology that found its apotheosis in Dante's *Divine Comedy*. The Renaissance re-reassembled the tales in a style that, mixing the old with the older, initiated and supported a vast rebirth of European culture. So on down through the ages the recurrent cycle goes of poetic genius, gods, cultures, growth, dissolution, and again genius, down to our most modern, and unfortunately bankrupt dream factory,

Hollywood. The gods (stars) of Hollywood are tangible, and in drama, if not their lives, Hollywood, until recently, has been able to preach the ideals and honor of our people, epitomized in our latter-day miracle play, the Western.

But to understand fully the genius of *3 Women*, we must recognize it as a complete tale and not simply another debunking of our contemporary worship of mass media. Simultaneously, the story moves two ways in time, anticipating the future while revealing the past. As we are willing to suspend immediate judgment of the film, *3 Women* reveals the origins of culture itself.

Historically, the Greeks derived their religion from the Mycenaeans who took their mythology from the Aegean-Minoan culture of Crete, which with the help of wandering Phoenicians, had seized upon both the gods of Egypt and Mesopotamia for its mythology. This moves us back through 1800 B.C. to 3000 B.C. and the origin of writing. Curiously, a consistent theme running through all these mythologies is that writing is a gift of the Three Fates. In the film, Pinky and Millie are forever struggling with their diaries. Both of them are intent upon chronicling their lives, Pinky in imitation of Millie, both attempting histories of themselves. The fundamental gift of writing is the magical power to suspend time, hold it in abeyance. With writing, mankind stands against the ephemeral moment with a record that can last longer than an individual's memory. Writing does more than communicate, it frees man in time.

The archeologist's observation that writing began as a commercial need to record the exchange of goods does not invalidate the magic of stopping time. Archaeologists are only too aware that the early Assyrian tablets that have been recovered are long on the number of sheep some man exchanged for jugs of wine and short on personal reflections about the cosmos. Bookkeeping is where writing began, with the measurers such as Millie. Millie-the-measurer was there first when it came to writing the earliest pictographs and hieroglyphics, clocking off the housekeeping realities that nurture culture.

So Altman's daimon leads us back to prehistoric times, which we intuitively knew when looking at Willie's paintings. Her figures, painted over the surface of the grounds and pool, will last. Here are the earliest forms of records, and they have lasted the longest. They reverberate to pictures on cave walls, the hunters of Lascaux, and Font-de-Gaume, the barbarian killers of old, recording their lethal history. In contrast, the paintings Willie does on canvas are so transitory that she peppers them with bullet holes. The primordial, animal/man figures in the film, which grossly represent the three women and Edgar, go on eternally, underground, underwater, under consciousness, in the "Land Beneath the Waves." They are forces in mankind, more bestial than humane, that culture unsuccessfully strives to tame. The humanoid beasts are legion; all folklore has them—the griffin, the gorgon, the chimaera (an Etruscan chimaera in the Piazza della Signoria of Florence is so weirdly contrived it can make the spectator's skin crawl as the price of a glance), the sphinx, the dragon, the catoblepas, the vodyanoy, the Wyrd (which a true hero, Beowulf, went to meet—"His heart was sad, uneasy and deathready: wyrd immediately nigh" [*Beowulf*, lines 2419-2420]), the manticore, the kekeko. The list is endless, for these strange half-human creatures are more than ghosts of our distant past; they are the past alive within us, teeth, claws, and insatiable appetites, always there. They are what mankind was and may become again. Willie can never conquer them, these immortal demons. Death does not kill mankind's wish to kill.

Within the film *3 Women* the mechanism of culture lies revealed. To rise above a barbaric past, men must believe in something beyond the moment, something beyond the immediate urge, something beyond themselves. Man's inventive mind has seldom been at a loss in suggesting form for these monsters, evidence of the belief in the Devil, and then some genius, in turn, through song, epic, and religion dresses up the delusions as reality. Thus, the belief made common, becomes a shared reality, a commonality of thought and action, a cultural tie. These geniuses, spiritual artists, are always busy making glue of culture, fashioning honor, tradition, the countless checks and balances that hold Willie's demons in bondage, harnessing the individual's bestial instincts to the community's need.

Nonetheless, this same mind of man has curiosity and the possibility of free imagination that simultaneously challenges and questions the accepted belief of the culture into which he/she is born. At times, thought inspired with curiosity leads to stronger beliefs, newer and more effective mythologies. Then these "doubters" on the edge of culture reinforce the artist's bonds about the demons. At other times, particularly when changes brought by war, religion, or technology within the culture outstrip belief's ability to adjust to new circumstances, the imaginative mind may "fall off the edge." Then, either through madness or willful self-destruction, the artist contributes to the culture's destruction. Picture Adolf Hitler enthralled with visions of new worlds to destroy inspired by Richard Wagner's "Götterdämmerung," an old world torn asunder. Without belief in "gods," the people fall away from their commonality and seek distraction, hedonistic amusement in the moment, typified by the Dodge City Bar. Then the common man, naked to his emptiness, despairs of values beyond self-indulgence. The Circus Maximus, the burning of Christians, the rendering of gladiators, reinforces for the audience the culture *they* live. They embrace the demons of Willie's art, only to become one with the demons.

But does the film say something even deeper than this, the revolution of epochs? In focusing on the women, the point is made that in chaos and destruction, the hub of cycle, the ineluctable center is human love, that the fundamental and irreducible component of culture is mother love, Pinky, Millie, Willie become daughter, mother, grandmother. The treasure of culture is the madonna. Archeology agrees, for despite the fact that Greeks had Zeus as the father of gods, the Fates actually flourished long before there was a language within which Zeus could exist. Fates are handmaidens of the god of the first men, the ancient earth-mother. She has been worshipped since the time when primitive men diminished their elemental fear of other animals with the belief that the earth was a protecting, superhuman being, Mother Nature. With mythology arrives a system of moral order, the source of protection and strength. Like the three primary colors—whether Pinky, Millie, and Willie; or Urth, Verthandi, and Skuld of the old Norse; or the Weird Sisters of Macbeth; or Clotho, Lachesis, and Atropos of the Greeks—in each triad, each entity is part of the whole, the essential earth mother. They manifest the primary elements of life, birth, marriage, and death; becoming, being, and became. They are the fullness of truth beyond mythology.

Psychology, too, in an ultimate sense, joins with Altman's daimon by asserting that there is a predestined fate for each of us, a fate that measures all our day-to-day mythology. Our destiny is determined for us with our birth. We are prisoners not only of the moment, time, but of language as well. Any thoughts we have about man or god are thought in personal language, which we learned as our mother tongue. We may worship the gods of measurement (science), of pleasure (culture), of power (politics), or mythology (religion), but worship we must in a predetermined way.

As has been observed, the Buddhist monk transfixed in ecstasy of spiritual otherness sees Buddha, not Christ, while the Christian saint lost in his religious revery sees Christ, not Buddha.

Philosophy, too, following an immeasurably great arc, returns to study language as the ultimate meaning of man. Semantics and grammar are the first causes that today's philosopher sorts and sifts in search of elemental particles. And though the philosopher speaks an eloquent language of his own, his broad path is yet another form of Millie's diary, an attempt to find meaning beyond the moment.

So there we have a film that is a film. The possible meanings of *3 Women* are barely scratched by this review. Consider the questions remaining; for example, Is this film but clever artifice or is it the work of authentic genius? More particularly, lest you claim I have wired the film by explaining not only that "the butler did it" but "how," let me ask you, should you see the film, Why is Willie's baby born cold? Millie exclaims over it repeatedly. The stillborn, like any tissue or fluid issuing from a living body, must have the temperature of the body it is leaving, yet Millie repeatedly exclaims, "It is so cold." What lies behind her scream?

Like life, and any other profound mystery, there is never a solution, only a partial solution. Science is always at a frontier of "just about to discover"; health is a state that is continually pursued by the wise yet never held; knowledge proves as relative as any other belief, yet man's fate is to know he is human only as he tolerates reality's ambiguity. Most need tight structure; some few constructively bear the agony of mutable beliefs; still fewer can move from one belief structure to another, experiencing the terrible void between, yet making of both beliefs something better for themselves and for their fellow man. These very few are the heroes, the geniuses, the inspired leaders who set the redeeming course of culture, but always within the limits imposed by Pinky, Millie, and Willie.

Endnotes

Reprinted from *The Pharos* 40(Fall 1977): 40-44, with permission.

Technological Zeal or Therapeutic Purpose?

The incessant concentration of thought upon one subject, however interesting, tethers a man's mind in a narrow field.
   —William Osler, M.D. (1849-1919)

The anxious voice on the other end of the telephone queried, "Ralph, this is Eugene Medford. I would like to talk to you soon, today if possible." I immediately placed him as a colleague I knew for his reputation as an excellent surgeon. Pausing, I looked at my schedule and located a canceled patient at 4 P.M. "I will be there at four," came his immediate reply, and as it turned out, he was precisely on time, burdened with a tragic tale of medical care out of control, the tyranny of medical technology.

Although retired, Gene came through the door as if entering an operating room, disciplined, concentrating on the problem at hand, determined to see it through to a proper resolution. His erect carriage and trim body belied his silver-haired, seventy-three years, and once seated squarely in the center of the patient's chair, he wasted no time. "No, it is not malpractice, but a matter of ethics. I have been to the Medical Society and they suggested I lodge a formal complaint. Perhaps I should." Then, as though working with a scalpel, he coolly began incising through the layers of the problem. "It concerns my brother Tim. He was eight years older than me and always there to be depended upon. His marriage was childless, and as it turned out, he was more than just an uncle to my children. I guess the two of us thought we would go on forever. That is, until last year when he turned up a bit anemic.

"My wife and I now live in Florida, settled in a condominium, but we get back for summers, and when I saw him in July, I insisted on a checkup. Well, the anemia was not serious, part of chronic renal failure which had been going on for years. However, the hematologist discovered rapidly developing multiple myeloma.

"Tim was a rock, always taking care of someone, and for the last five years it had been Betty, his wife, who is going downhill with Alzheimer's disease. If he could help, he wanted to be around. If he could not, he wanted to be on with it. He questioned whether the myeloma should be treated, and we talked about it for a long while. Finally he decided to go ahead with the chemotherapy, but from the beginning, the treatment was doubtful. His BUN was 60, and in anticipation of the chemotherapy load, he checked into the hospital for three days of supportive dialysis.

"Well, his stay was a lot longer than three days. His calcium level proved extremely difficult to control, he became lethargic, developed a bacteremia, pneumonia, and in two weeks was in coma in Intensive Care.

"I had not flown here after he decided on treatment, but when I sensed things were not going well, I began calling his nephrologist, who turned out to be impossible to get through to. I was told he was away for the weekend and could not be reached. I called again on Monday, and after reaching him, he said he would like to see Tim before he talked with me. I stuck by the telephone, I waited all day, but he never called back. Concerned, I got on a plane.

"Back in Oregon, I still could not get him on the telephone, so I just stayed by Tim's bed and waited. Tim had come out of coma, and though he seemed drowsy most of the time, he could talk. He had fallen out of bed the night before, and when the doctor did come, he immediately ordered a flat film. I followed the doctor to the nursing station and waited until he was done with charts. The hallway was the only place I ever got to talk with him. He volunteered that Tim's calcium level was difficult to titrate. Then I asked why he ordered a flat film. You know flat films tell nothing in multiple myeloma. He said it was to see if there was a fracture. I asked him what he would do if there was a fracture, and he said he would tell Tim that he had a fracture and that there was nothing he could do about it. I remarked it would have saved $43 to tell him that in the first place. The bill was now at $47,000. The doctor just walked away.

"As the nephrologist never returned my calls, I turned to Rex Stayton, who had been his supervisor in training. Rex volunteered the fact that he had originally questioned Tim being placed on dialysis, but did not want to get involved.

"Tim lacked appetite from the first so I brought in special dishes I knew he liked. Now they were hyperalimenting him through a cutdown on the subclavian. I consulted Rex again, and this time Rex admitted that when he talked with Tim he got the strong impression that Tim wanted to give up the machines. Do you know what those things cost? A run of dialysis is $604; one day in Intensive Care is $760, while hyperalimentation is $123 a liter, $10,000 a month. It sounds gross talking of money when your brother is dying, and I know Medicare pays for most of it, but to what purpose?

"Later I caught the nephrologist while making rounds, and we had a shouting match in the hall. I guess in fairness I should say it was a harsh discussion. I asked how much longer this was going on, and he answered, 'As long as the patient says he wants to live.'

"I told him Tim did not say he wanted to live, explaining I asked the nursing supervisor to take me to every floor nurse and orderly who had any contact with him, and none of them reported he had ever said he wanted to live. I cannot remember precisely what he said, but when I suggested a second opinion, he came back with, 'No second opinion can be satisfactory, since no one has had the experience I have had with the patient.' Although the encounter was most unpleasant, I persevered, reminding the doctor he could be dismissed. His reply was, 'Not until he indicates he wants to die.' Then I proposed that we talk with Tim together, to which he replied, 'I will not talk with him if you are present.' He had made it a point to ask everyone to leave the room, even the attendings, when he was with Tim. When I asked Tim about this, he said, yes, the doctor talked with him; he climbed onto the bed to talk; in fact, he never stopped talking long enough for Tim to say anything, so he supposed he was not much for listening.

"Finally, with the help of the other attendings, we stopped the machines. Tim grew brighter each day, and we talked of old times. Tim lived five days and then died in his sleep. He was my brother."

Gene had arched forward and now, on the edge of the chair, was crying as surgeons do, not with tears, but with full eyes, face frozen, still in command of his emotions, but just barely.

"You were right to come and talk with me," I said as he began to pull himself together.

We both paused, and he sighed, "I feel unburdened."

Knowing he wanted some answers, I went on. "It seems to me little can come of a committee calling in the nephrologist now. I know you came to see me because I sometimes write about such things. May I share this experience with our profession?"

"Yes, please; do as you think best. Not a man or woman my age I have talked with wants to get caught on the life support machines, but how can we stop them?"

"I do not know how they can be stopped. I have not thought it out." I was tempted to go on exploring possibilities, but plainly he was exhausted. "Suppose we think about what you have been through and keep in touch."

He rose, grasping my hand. "Thank you. You will hear from me. What has happened should never happen again," and he was out the door.

Grateful that catharsis had lessened his grief and anger, but most aware how his bright mind sought more than solace, I stared out the window at the winter dusk beyond and let my inchoate thoughts stumble one upon the other. What to do?

His frank, doctor-to-doctor talk could be passed along, but that might stir more concern than closure. Certainly this problem of a zealous physician preempting medical decisions by way of a fancied, Hippocratic right to preserve life must be happening in other hospitals. Hippocrates elevated the goals of all physicians by writing down our humanistic tradition, but did he dream of such a thing as a medical machine?

Obviously, physicians need a broader ethic that understands, informs, and accounts for the degree and reason for each technological barrier introduced between patient and doctor. In Tim's case, the nephrologist had unlimited power to use a machine without accountability for cost, iatrogenic suffering, or patient dissent. Although most physicians, including most nephrologists,[1] are compassionately aware of their mortal limits, the machine allows some physicians to assume priestly powers unto the patient's last breath and beyond, powers rivaling a demigod's.

Although correct, the limited logic that the physician, not his machine, is responsible for aggravating human suffering does not address the broader truth that machines foster poor medical judgment through intellectual entropy. "Since it (the machine, technology, or test) is there, we will use it" typifies such short-circuited thinking. Nor is intellectual entropy limited to a particular machine, for it can happen with a stethoscope, kidney dialysis machine, or a computer. "It can do no harm to have blood gasses (CAT scan, angiography)" leads to such scandals as a pediatric patient undergoing six separate bloodlettings in one day.

In the name of objective science, we can become integrated into the machine rather than the machine integrated into patient care. Although machines are defined as slaves, they have a way of becoming masters of clinical judgment through dependence, diffusion, distraction, and, most important, through fixation, experiencing the machine as an extension of self. Why else did Tim have a flat film of the abdomen?

Two elemental problems of the medical profession are revealed through the suffering of Gene and Tim. The first, an ancient one, is physician judgment, but with a new twist, the "too ept" physician. We have peer review committees in medical societies and hospitals, committees prepared to uncover and correct inept physicians. We now need a broader charge to those committees that will judge the too ept, the medical zealots. Such a change will take a definitive national educational program within the medical profession. To be implemented properly, the zealots must be leashed, not punished, by their peers.

The second problem, the medical machine, is of a higher order of complexity, so much so that it has become imperative to rethink the physician-machine relationship. The machine of itself can become an agent of unwanted change, and although some angry reformers may wish to do away with all medical technology, we need no medical Luddites smashing our superb medical technology in a burst of anti-intellectualism.

However, this problem of the machine dictating the treatment, which is as old as the stethoscope, goes largely unrecognized and unchecked by physicians. Physicians appear blind to how much the machine intervenes between the patient and doctor, crowds into their relationship while profoundly complicating physicians' ethical behavior. We are unconsciously integrated into our medical machines, with both physicians and patients becoming their unsuspecting agents.

Lest some scoff, remember Gene; despite his superior intelligence, his economic independence, his clear articulation, his unique position of respect within the profession, his friends on the hospital staff, despite all the power of his spirit, Gene was powerless against the zealot with the machine. This problem calls for much more than educating doctors, since we lack clear knowledge of the forces involved or even how to conceptualize them properly.

We need a new order of understanding of medical technology developed out of the suffering of patients and their families, which will lead to a better evaluation of every medical technique within the context of its use with every patient. We need an expanded Hippocratic tradition in all hospitals that deals constructively with the implicit counterproductive cost, pain, and arrogance of medical technology. To begin with, every hospital in the nation should treat such "ethical" problems as medical emergencies just as critical as diabetic coma or a myocardial infarction and equally unresponsive to "cookbook" solutions. Every hospital should have an appeal mechanism for patients, families, and physicians suffering from uncontrolled medical technology. Again the medical profession needs to return to the bedside to study a new disease, in this case the syndrome of the technological fix.

By a curious inversion of human values, scientific therapeutic zeal has generated this new, iatrogenic disease. The technological fix is the extension of the machine into the psyche of the physician, an invasive malignancy capable of becoming a plague. To avoid mechanical distortion of our humanity, we need to witness to our purpose as physicians who value life as a quality, not blindly worship it as a quantity. The ancient tradition, *primum non nocere,* calls for focus on new developments, *primum non nocere cum machineae.* Let us first do no harm with our machines.

Night had fallen. My office was dark. Time for home and dinner, and as I locked up, I resolved to better discipline my thoughts, although I knew that Gene would have intuitively followed where they led. We must decide, not the machines.

Endnotes

Reprinted from the *Journal of the American Medical Association,* 250(1983): 1857-1859 with permission. Copyrighted 1983, American Medical Association. Original title: "Technical Zeal or Therapeutic Purpose—How to Decide?"

1. N. Kurtzman, "The Ultimate Problem," *Seminars in Nephrology* 3(1983): 75-76.

St. Paul and Medical Technology
Chadwick Memorial Lecture
Good Samaritan Hospital, Corvallis, Oregon, 1985

Now as touching things offered unto idols, we know that we all have knowledge. Knowledge puffeth up, but charity edifieth.
—I Corinthians 8:1

A commonly accepted truth holds that the wisdom of the past should be reinterpreted into the unique language and experience of each new era. Yet in our times of instantaneous communication, where wisdom is replaced by knowledge only to have knowledge buried under information, the task of being wise grows ever more difficult. Interpretation of greater values into the daily lives of our people becomes the task of the minister preaching, the lawyer pleading, the politician speaking and, in my case, the physician advising. To do this, I will reach a long way back, to move properly a deep way down into our beliefs, by asking, in this case of St. Paul, "Are Faith, Hope, and Charity enough for our world of medical technology?"

The question may seem far-fetched, archaic, since faith, hope, and charity are presently generally conceived of as historical concepts rather than actual behaviors. We best begin with a translation so our question makes sense to both ourselves and the beloved Apostle.

A modern medical translation of "faith" is "science." Science is a faith, a belief system, whose adherents are convinced they can abolish human suffering if not defeat death. The number of scientists who have sacrificed their lives to this belief are legion. I hold that the true believers of Science maintain that with enough time and money their system of thinking, their faith, will so improve the lot of mankind that we can expect heaven on Earth.

The modern equivalent of "hope" is "progress," a ubiquitous social persuasion that mankind is perfectible through assisted evolution of the human species from unlettered monkey to overarching enlightenment. Progressive self-monitoring of the arrangement of our genes, chemistry, and psyches will eventually produce a universally benevolent animal called future man, perhaps superman.

When pronounced, the ancient word "charity" may evoke a vague, uneasy sense of demeaning servitude together with images of poorhouses or long, hard benches in a clinic. More the pity that such a rich word should fall on hard times, and we are left with the word "welfare," a legislated form of sharing, primarily intended to force the electorate into apportioning some of the community's wealth to a group, the poor, disabled, or as some maintain, the unworthy.

Thus, when we translate the words of St. Paul into present-day language, the modern virtues become "Science, Progress, and Welfare, and of these Welfare is the greatest." Granted, a certain sense of humanity is lost in the translation but who would deny that for many, perhaps the majority, "Science, Progress, and Welfare" says it as it should be said. In any case, I pursue our question of St. Paul's words since, with your indulgence and no disrespect, I intend to take up the matter of medical technology with him. Such is possible by invoking his memory, his presence, to chat with him, about his original judgment that "love" is the greatest of these.

Before we do this we should first make clear the meaning of medical technology. However, not as an entomologist or scientist might, but as St. Paul would be most likely to understand, in terms of human beings, in terms of you and me.

To do this, I propose a simple thought experiment. I would like each and every reader to think of the one you love the most. Bring that person into central consciousness. Now imagine that a stranger quietly enters the room, looks about, marks where you sit, and comes over to whisper in your ear, "Would you please come to the Emergency Department? There has been an accident and you are needed." You immediately get up and leave. In the Emergency Department a man in a green scrub suit, presumably the doctor in charge, confronts you, explaining that a drunken driver has run up on the sidewalk and pinned your loved one against the wall. Your loved one, unconscious with a ruptured spleen, is behind the curtains at the end of the room. He asks your permission to surgically remove the spleen.

Would you agree to the surgery?

Twelve hours later, after you have spent the night pacing a hospital corridor, a neurosurgeon appears and explains that your loved one is doing as well as might be expected, but that intracranial pressure has developed from the head injury and he wishes to do a shunt to decompress the brain.

Would you agree to the procedure?

Twelve hours later an anesthesiologist appears to explain that there is a blockage of your loved one's airways causing respiratory distress. He would like permission to place your loved one on a respirator.

Would you agree?

The next day, an internist takes you aside to explain that the intravenous feedings are not going well and he would like permission to have a venous shunt established to facilitate hyperalimentation necessary to maintain hydration and nutrition.

Would you agree?

The same day, a nephrologist seeks you out to report that for unclear reasons your loved one's kidneys have begun to fail and kidney dialysis is needed. Your consent is necessary.

Would you consent?

That evening, a cardiologist asks you to step away from your loved one's bed in intensive care, escorts you to a quiet place in the corridor, and explains that acute myocarditis with signs of congestive failure has developed and though it is possible to save your loved one's life you must agree to the installation of an artificial heart.

Would you agree?

At this point, your here-and-now feelings are predictable, but you might pause to consider your reaction to such intense stress.

A common reaction to our thought experiment has been reported as a sense of confusion, anger, hopelessness, and abandonment. However, the point is not to stir your emotions, but to define medical technology in a way which both you and St. Paul would understand.

Not surprisingly, the consequent definition is inhuman, devoid of the spirit of humane medical care. Medical technology is the use of tools, machines, which have at best little relationship to the spirit of a human being. Medical technology, lacking values of good and evil, does not generate moral values. Quite the contrary, machines can erode the user's values to the point where the technician is a valueless person. Tools have a way of distancing people, one from another, while corroding faith into ritual, hope into a lottery, and charity into economics. That is, the medical specialists (technologists) who put the question to you "Do you agree?" are not asking for your values of human life but agreement with their belief in the preeminence of science, progress, and welfare. Should you doubt me, ask them.

Enough with definitions. Now let us seek out St. Paul. Another thought experiment should do this nicely. Let us travel to his world, to his time: Corinth in the year 48 A.D. It is a boisterous city with its grand acropolis to the east, but we will make for the marketplace, the Stoa, where St. Paul has been speaking and once was called before the Roman consul for judgment of his professed beliefs. He knows the city and the people well. There he is, wrapped in a simple wool toga, bundled up against a cold October north wind, blowing down from lofty Mount Parnassus beyond the Gulf of Corinth. To speak with him, we must shoulder our way through throngs of merchants and prostitutes, for which the city is so famous. His features are not commanding, for his face has a soft, questioning look, not foreboding but serious. Hearing out our question about faith, hope, and charity in a technological world, he nods for us to follow him to a secluded spot behind a marble column, out of the traffic and wind, to ponder our question.

However, as he thinks long over our question of faith, hope, and charity in a technological world, impatiently I ask him a more pointed one. "You have omitted the matter of judgment when you say charity is the greatest of these. How are we to judge in these matters?"

His answer is direct, "When I was a child I used to speak as a child, reason as a child. When I became a man I did away with childish things. For now we see in a mirror darkly. But then face-to-face, now I know in part."

"St. Paul, if I may paraphrase your answer in the speech of my time, judgment is a mature activity which at best is unclear, in that things never seem as they are, and prove most difficult to see as a whole."

Even though a saint, he shows a bit of irritation at my impudence and asks me what I am driving at, to which I explain that I am a physician seeking the power of good judgment. Much as a humble minister of the Lord might seek grace, I seek to share prudent judgment with patients and colleagues.

Then, increasingly insecure in such a sacred presence, I involuntarily shift to doctor talk. "St. Paul, here is a modern case of caring for the sick in which I know not what to do." To catch his interest while putting myself at ease, I continue, "Recently I was asked by an EMT if she should have done other than she did."

With his focused interest, St. Paul interrupted me with, "Though I am graced with heavenly omniscience when it comes to things of the spirit, as well as the knowledge of many tongues, would you please tell me what an EMT is?"

"Oh, excuse me. An EMT is an Emergency Medical Technician. Someone who rides in an ambulance. I mean, a woman who goes about the city helping the sick and injured." To this he might nod knowingly.

"She was called to a small room in the worst part of our city with the report that there was a sick woman there. The EMT, I mean, good woman, entered the room to find an elderly woman unconscious on a bed. Later it was determined she was eighty-six and suffering from an invasive Grade IV adenocarcinoma of the pelvis and abdomen."

"Again, please speak in the language of human beings, not machines."

"Excuse me, she had a great tumor which was killing her. A note was pinned to her chest which said, 'I have little food, no money nor friends, my dog died last week, my pain is unbearable. The pills do not help. Let me sleep.' An empty pill bottle was at her bedside. The good lady considered staying with the unconscious woman until the spirit left the body, but instead called the hospital, related the situation, and asked if she might not simply leave the elderly woman as she was. The hospital doctors told her she must start all available machines immediately. Then the woman should be carried to the hospital as soon as possible. The good woman did as she was told and the sons of Aesculapius at the hospital pumped out the woman's stomach, placed her on more machines for two weeks, and when they revived her body enough for her to walk, sent the ancient woman back to the room where she had been found. Later the EMT asked me what *I* judged best, and I could not say. Now, I ask you, St. Paul."

Leaning back and looking towards the heavens, St. Paul might say, "To paraphrase what you have told me, your soul is tried as you suffer from the news that the good handmaiden acted as though she was loving, but without love, and you fear you have failed her for not saying so to her. But why did you not share with her your soul's belief?"

"I hesitated because the good woman had explained to me that she lives in a world where she may exercise judgment only at great risk. She is trained to render unto Caesar that which is Caesar's, and in her world *science, progress,* and *welfare* belong to Caesar. She said, she feared to do as her soul wished since Satan in the form of the demon Malpractice, demanded that she leave judgment to the owners of machines."

Now St. Paul was alert to the problem. "You are sore tried indeed. I feel your soul smarting."

"But what am I to tell the EMT, as she is certain to ask again?"

"Is she strong of soul?"

"Yes, but not saintly. She wishes no martyrdom."

The saint responded, "Then there would be little sense in advising her to sacrifice herself. Certainly, the suffering of her experience suffices unto her need. I see your problem clearer. Neither you nor she sees love as real enough to illuminate faith and hope, or as you might say, science and progress."

"Now, I do not understand."

"Well, the two of you need to make clear the place of faith (or as you say, a belief in machines) and hope (that is, 'progress') in being charitable. Forgive me, I simply can not use your word 'welfare.'"

"Precisely, but our mirrors are dark."

"Please, I accept that. It goes with the sting of suffering. But take heart. You and she have taken the first step in seeing charity as it is. You have recognized singularly and together the fact of your suffering."

"But does not everyone?"

"Ah, no. If they did, your problem with machines would not exist."

"How so?"

"Whenever compassion is reduced from an experience to concept, the ability to know suffering is first weakened, then lost. A toothache remembered is not the same as a toothache, and the memory of someone else's toothache is even further removed.

"The fact that children starve in the land of the upper Nile is but a fact to most of the people of Corinth. Even when the procouncil rules that wheat shall be sent to these children and the people agree, yet they agree without compassion. There is no shared fellow feeling with the children's hunger, only thoughts of the head without power of the heart that nurtures the soul. So when decree moves men to give food, there is no recognized awareness of the humanness of the children who are hungry. The words of the decree form a void in the hearts of people; to be filled by other machines. The cymbals of the musicians, the circuses of the gladiators, are machines to distract and entertain, attempting to fill the void between what people are and what they might be. Compassion lives only with full discovery through suffering shared with those who suffer."

"I understand, but what has that to do with my friend and me?"

"You both seek to be loving in a system without heart. No one faults the reasons of your people when they wish to save the sick lady. They intend to be charitable, but charitable as a machine, as you say, welfare: knowledge without wisdom, head without heart. They act in good faith, but their faith is machine faith. The faith of science is a faith of reason, a contradiction in terms. It is similar to a congregation of true believers who form a church in which the pursuit of faith becomes the faith, empty theology. Then the worship of God makes them ungodly as the revelation of faith is lost in the study of ritual. I believe Hippocrates remarked on the operation that was a success but the patient's spirit died, or something like that. Mind you I speak not against the word of God, but *for* the word of God, as it contains living spirit."

"But what am I to tell the good woman?"

"Ah, how dark is your mirror. What you tell your handmaiden, first, last, and always, is that you suffer together, not alone. Together you can find the strength to listen to your own souls."

"Yes, but then what?

Then with the patience of a saint, Paul would repeat and repeat again, "Then tell others."

"But what has that to do with the judgment that charity is the greatest of these?"

In measured tones Saint Paul replied, "Judgment, seeing things as they are, is the distillation of experience wrought from suffering. This is the moment when we approach highest human fulfillment, for thus are the secrets of the heart disclosed. As you share more and more of your judgment of suffering it can be shared in charity and grow in charity."

"Then I should organize people to hear of this suffering and my judgment of it."

"Hardly, for if you do, you will end up with a congregation, not a judgment. What you do is share. Sharing is the ultimate of love; share in words about your suffering, for your words give words to the suffering of others, who in turn may feed on the words and become full-souled. Together, and only together, can you ask the people of your time what place their present faith in science has in their soul caring of the sick lady."

"But they may not understand nor wish to understand her plight."

"Only if you have failed to love your listener enough to know that they too have thought of being abandoned like the sick lady, of being pain wracked by the dying of their body; only if you fail to believe they have feared the loneliness unto death, as you do, only then your words will sound without understanding. Should you share the loneliness of the sick lady with them as you experienced her loneliness, their souls will hear."

Confused and deeply disturbed, I blurted out, "But should I not do something. All you say is talk and talk again. I live in a world where talk is cheap. We have money and we have many charitable societies among the men and women of good will. Should I not do something, so that this will never happen again to some other old woman?"

"Oh, how dark your mirror. Render unto congregations that which belongs to congregations, yet know in your mind if not your soul, that though you bestow all your goods on the poor and give your body to be burned it profiteth you nothing. Where there be tongues, they shall cease; where there is knowledge, it shall vanish away. I fault not your science and all its good deeds, but if it is without charity, the sharing of one to another in the spirit of love, your science is a prophecy of nothing, not even evil."

"You do mean I should simply say what my soul says when it is moved to speak."

"Now you begin to see over and beyond that vast mountain of congregations and machines which apparently blocks your view of truth. But remember: it is for you to speak so that others may speak with you. You are not in a wilderness, but in a community with suffering all about. You and the good woman are not alone, nor is there but one sick lady who wishes to give up the ghost with grace and dignity."

"But I fear that I have not the courage that goes with such a task."

With a beneficent smile, the good saint confided, "I must be on my way. It is late. The marketplace is nearly empty. See, beyond the pagan temple, friends beckon me. If my words have confused you, simply remember my behavior, how I live my life in sharing. Then your fear will become a strength to remind you to rejoice in a truthful sharing which beareth all things. There is no world made of man, not even yours with its wealth and power, where charity is not the greatest of human virtues."

The dark night was upon us, and with those words the good St. Paul drew his cloak closely about himself and made off, leaving us to ponder.

Perhaps you read to learn of modern medicine and its dilemmas, of the wonder of MRIs or the dangers of AIDS. Hopefully, this flight of fancy has left you neither disappointed nor bored. What I have to say is a weak echo of the words of St. Paul, who lifted my thinking and showed a way to grow in wisdom. We all know that there are many elderly ladies and gentlemen, many children and adults who now ask that their spirits be heard by those who minister to them. It is our responsibility not to look to others, but to remind all who minister to the sick that each spirit can be listened to in love. Into our nursing homes, our hospitals, our offices, our foster homes we must carry our personal meaning of suffering. Like the shadow of St. Paul, whom I have evoked for you, let us lead our lives compassionately, expressing the suffering which is forever a part of us and of our world.

My Brother and His Keepers

"But I am not guilty," said K., "it's a mistake.
And, if it comes to that, how can any man be called guilty?
We are all simply men here, one as much as the other."
"That is true," said the priest, "but that's how all guilty men talk."
—Franz Kafka (1883-1924)
The Trial

A reverberation that Abraham Flexner set in motion in 1908, when he established national standards for medical education and consequently standards of practice, was the revelation of how many impaired physicians practice within our profession. Since then physicians, medical school hospitals, state boards of medical licensure, and specialty organizations have struggled with the thorny problem of what to do with wayward colleagues, disabled through ineptitude, ignorance, unethical behavior, alcohol, drug dependency, and/or mental illness.

Despite the continual and unfounded gossip that physicians do not discipline their own but maintain a conspiracy of silence, the American Medical Association has been in the forefront, prodding members to protect the patient from failings of impaired physicians. The Second National Conference on Disabled Doctors, sponsored by the AMA in Atlanta, Georgia, some twenty years ago, is an example of the association's push for answers to a tough problem.

The meeting was held in a fancy new hotel, complete with an immense atrium and a gallery of balconies reaching up to the twenty-first floor. Despite the posh chandeliers and windowed elevators, the modern "open" hotel leaves an unfortunate impression of a cell block from a 1930 prison movie, for it would be no surprise to find James Cagney leaning over the thirteenth balcony to shout down to the lobby, "Okay, warden, I ain't gonna eat no more of this slop. I'm breaking out!" Well, there was no "breaking out" of this meeting, since it quickly caught the interest of the participants.

Through happenstance I was anchor man on the opening panel and had a chance to listen to the introductory dialogue. Perhaps I am getting old and hard-of-hearing, but what filtered through to my brain was a harsh order to meet the public's demand for professional accountability, to detect and control the disabled doctor through "constructive coercion," and to hurry on the business of getting the rascals out of the profession. Unfortunately, with age my verbal stability has decreased; consequently, my turn to speak was described by a member of the media as an "outburst." Seems to me I but gently hinted that the disabled doctor was not an adversary whom we should legislate out of existence. Touching softly on the necessary balance of justice and compassion, I asked if anyone might be interested in compassion, since I had missed mention of the subject to date. But then I am hung up on the prejudice that coercion is a last resort for physicians and patients both, while persuasion through example comes first. It seemed to me that the audience agreed, for thankfully no one ran me off the platform.

No matter how many times I hear the statistics concerning doctors in difficulty, I feel the same disheartening wrench at my innards, and this meeting was no exception. The profession loses the equivalent number of a medical school class each year to suicide, while the equivalent of three medical school classes are incapacitated by alcohol and drug dependency. Behind these patent statistics are the enumerable tales of broken homes, broken hearts, broken minds, and broken lives. Some tales are startling in their brash disregard for common sense and humanity. Take the case of a doctor who makes a business of selling prescriptions. At twenty dollars a prescription for any drug taken in the city, he grossed three or four thousand dollars a day. He is difficult to detect and when apprehended he hires lawyers to defend his "treatment methods." Alone, he has enough moral blindness to cloud the vision of an army. Then there are the tales of men and women of intractable self-destructiveness, such as the physician who believes that alcohol is an innocuous pleasure, until he has run down a pedestrian during a drunken joyride. His long slow travail back to practice is redeeming, though ever so painful to hear.

The conference moved through a series of workshops, with the 350 participants arranging their participation as they judged worthwhile. Confrontation techniques, the subject of the first workshop, dealt with the resistance the profession and the professional have in recognizing illness among doctors. There are many different kinds of "confronters," but generally the best available one is either an old friend who, whether a member of the immediate family or of the professional family, can with sincerity and in a nonpunitive way point to the terrible cost of the wayward physician's destructive behavior. Even better is a physician who has successfully confronted his impairment. "It takes one to convince one." More formal confrontation exists in some states, such as Ohio, Georgia, and New York, where, upon verification of a complaint against a physician, physician committees can send a delegation of board members to the impaired physician as a beginning of a difficult dialogue.

A second workshop focused on the physician and his family. Here the group worked through many of the deep-seated and hidden problems that occur in the physician's family life. The taxing demands and conflicting roles of the physician frequently generate hostile feelings towards him from within his own family. The particular problems physicians' children have with an "unattainable" father who often loads them with overwhelming academic and social pressures were discussed in detail. The physician son of a physician was explicit in outlining his anger and resentment toward his father for drinking and how only with outside help was he able to reestablish contact with his father. The structure of the doctor's family is changing with new problems appearing as more physicians are women and their spouses are men. Problems seem to multiply.

Three workshops considered treatment techniques, centering on the terrible difficulty some doctors have in seeing themselves as patients, leading to the special problems that the physician/patient has in being treated as a patient. The plethora of possible treatment modalities often proves confusing to a physician/patient, while the threats of license revocation, loss of hospital privileges, loss of confidentiality, and loss of practice all conspire to lead physicians to deny recognition and postpone treatment of their problems. Particular emphasis was placed on the drug-dependent physician/patient's unique opportunities to indulge his illness behind a cloud of professional immunity. The group concluded that anyone who treats physician/patients must have a unique adaptability to meet the special needs, and that the highly structured, extremely demanding therapies that isolate the patient from the reality of family and professional life are generally of little help. More successful treatments are those in which the therapist acts as a team leader, adapting the therapeutic situation to the changing needs of the physician/patient.

One workshop tackled legislation related to the sick doctor. The Florida Sick Doctor Act was recognized as historic, and the AMA model Sick Doctor Act has been used as the basis of legislation in nearly thirty states. But that enactment must serve the needs not only of the doctor and patient but also of the legislators and community. Successful passage of laws protecting patients demand consistent, well-thought-through teamwork within a community.

A workshop on challenges to enforcing the law brought forth many of the immediate difficulties that presently confound attempts to reach the disabled doctor. The styles of state medical licensure boards, as seen in the statistics, vary from strict to casual. Different levels of intervention, whether a friend working with the physician, through a medical society, through a Professional Standards Review Organization, hospital, or public denunciation, leave the situation confused with no clear recommendation for any one approach. The dangers of false accusation were outlined; also the ability of some physicians to use their legal rights for perpetual appeal, while maintaining a destructive practice, even known as charlatans.

One former head of a state board of medical licensure related his unhappy plight. In the course of a hearing, a member of the board made remarks that offended the physician under scrutiny, and subsequently, after the head of the board had left the board, the angry doctor sued the members of the board for slander. Now the former head has to retain an attorney at his own expense to protect himself in court against the charges of bias and slander. The wicket is a sticky one for any member of a licensing board these days. The whole question of who should do the licensing is unresolved and without clear direction while consumer advocates decry "turning the chicken coop over to the foxes."

Another workshop dealt with the economic and readjustment problems of the recovering physician. Probably the two most powerful difficulties a physician meets are an acute economic one (it is amazing how few physicians carry adequate disability insurance) and the horrid problem of professional scorn. Once the mighty have fallen it is a long climb back into an accepted practice. Any minor slip becomes a potential disaster for the recovering physician. The most important fact remains that it is possible to recover.

Still another workshop dealt with the medical student. Here, we heard the old cliche that it's too late to deal with doctors by the time they are in practice, and that only noble men and women, of unquestioned moral strength, should be chosen to enter medical school. If there is a good way of screening the characters of one thousand applicants to find the one hundred without flaw, please let your local medical school selection committee know. In my experience, there are two central measures—the individual's actual past record and the hunch of the examiner. Both can prove wrong as there is no infallible selection process, but it is possible to change prevailing attitudes towards doctor illness in the first years of medical school. Some schools have instituted programs, formal and informal, that permit medical students and their spouses to explore the fears, ambitions, competitions, angers, and overload that so powerfully shape their lives. The emotional side of professional life begins well before the medical degree is granted, a fact that should be incorporated into every medical school curriculum.

The last workshop was on the inept and unethical physician. Here we have the charlatan, the scoundrel hanging to the edge of the profession, dealing in soft drugs, rainbow pills, exotic massage (inflating balloons in the nasal sinuses to relieve mental deficiency), and those other strange rituals that the public so enjoys. How to hold the attention of these illicit, if not illegal, members of the profession long enough to change their behavior is a difficult problem. Concern for and about the aging physician was expressed. How necessary it is for the aging physician to find a continuing meaning in life, reassurance that his or her contribution to mankind has been appreciated and will continue to be appreciated. How difficult it is to guide gently the shaking hand of an aging surgeon away from the scalpel and toward some other rewarding work. The National Association of Retired Physicians has a vital role in capitalizing on a manpower resource that too often is wasted.

A luncheon program was devoted to reviewing the Georgia Medical Association's program for alcohol- and drug-dependent physicians. A self-motivated group of physicians, the Caduceus Club, are boot-strapping their way out of alcoholism. At present there are about forty members, all of whom have had serious problems with stimulant and depressant drugs. The program in Georgia runs approximately four months for a candidate, including hospitalization, supervised reentry into practice, and continuing rehabilitation with heavy reliance upon Alcoholics Anonymous, AlAnon, and Alateen. An important aspect of this group is that it is doctor controlled, eliminating problems of notoriety. By remaining anonymous yet within the profession, problems are avoided such as the physician, following resumption of sobriety, who confessed his years of alcoholism in a lay group only to be slapped with a nasty malpractice suit. An unscrupulous attorney in the audience of the self-confessed alcoholic surreptitiously searched the physician's past hospital files until he uncovered a likely case for malpractice and prompted the otherwise satisfied former patient to sue. The sober physician was successfully sued for a quarter of a million dollars for a history of alcoholism. By doctors helping doctors start a new and constructive life, the Georgia program has a great deal to commend itself to other state organizations.

When judged against other conferences this was a success. It was so successful, and I am serious, that another national meeting on the impaired physician is unnecessary. The problems are open and solutions possible. The next move is for regional meetings to carry the word closer to the physician in need.

Reflecting on the plight of the impaired physician brings to mind his keepers as well. The helper is as much to be judged as the helped, and as keepers I judge physicians as barely passing. Oh, if there is a continuing medical education course on the errant physician, probably most practicing physicians will muster a respectable score on the final test, with most coming in with a blazing 90 or 95. They would be able to define the inept, the unethical, and the sick physician, together with a cogent differential diagnosis. That is how we were trained in medical school, "by the numbers." Statistically, programmatically, and legally the median grade for physicians as keepers is above 90, but for me there are still doubts about our ability to act humanely as our brothers' keepers.

Am I harsh? You judge. With the medical profession up for pass or fail, this conference would lead us to believe that we are progressing famously. However, the actuality appears more governmental than human, more coercive than cooperative. This point was made indelibly the evening the meeting closed. While I was riding up to my room on the elevator, another physician turned and looked me in the eye saying, "I am grateful for what you said about compassion. It needed to be said. I'm an impaired physician. I'm a severely impaired physician, but I have come back, and let me tell you that it's been coercion all the way. No, we need to learn a great deal more about compassion." You see, I judge our profession by our brothers' words and not by what our keepers say. Harsh as this may be, the facts are there.

Endnotes

Reprinted from *The Pharos* 40(Summer 1977): 23-25, with permission.

Requiem for an Unknown Leper

> *You wish me to renew ...*
> *that grief incurable, which breaks my heart,*
> *Even at the thought, before I speak it.*
> —Dante (1265-1321)
> *The Divine Comedy*
> *The Inferno,* Canto 33, line 4

A winter attack of the 'flu accompanied by a persistent, hacking cough pointed me toward a warmer climate to convalesce on a sandy beach, mindlessly listening to lapping waves argue with rustling palm trees. Molokai proved the place, out of the heavy tourist track, and after a few days of rest I stirred enough to take one of the few tours offered, a visit to the leper colony at Kalaupapa.

Getting to Kalaupapa is an experience in itself, as there are but two ways for the tourist, by mule down the cliffs or by airplane over them. Choosing the less strenuous way, my wife and I climbed aboard an ancient six-passenger Beechcraft, flown by a very unscheduled pilot who proclaimed his plane more mule than bird. Presently, we arrived at the Kalaupapa air terminal, an open shed at the end of the airstrip marked off from a sun-bleached, crushed coral parking lot by a row of simple benches.

Deplaning, we met our guide, Ida, a woman of medium height whose more than medium width was draped in a brightly flowered dress. She may have been fifty or she may have been seventy; her age went undeclared by her presence. Nor was her leonine face, shaded by a broad-brimmed palm leaf hat, easy to read. Her complexion was mottled by indiscriminate dark pigmentation. She lacked eyebrows, and her broad Polynesian features were peppered with small swellings extending to clustered nodules on her ears. Her smile ended at the corners of her mouth. In greeting she did not offer to shake hands, perhaps because the distal phalanges of many of her fingers were missing. With the rolling gait of a restless sailor, she led our party of six to her open van and began a line of matter-of-fact patter that, though similar to that of countless other tour guides, directed our attention away from the obvious: she was a leprous patient.

Not that Ida concealed her condition. On the way to pick up the remainder of the party, who had spent the morning coming down the cliffs on mules, she readily acknowledged her disease, reassuring us that she no longer was infectious but also tying this disclosure to the row upon row of graves we were passing. "I was scared as hell by those graves when I first was sent here as a girl in 1939." As though continuing with an as-yet-unannounced agenda, she handed some pamphlets on Hansen's disease back over her shoulder to be passed among the passengers. "Hold your questions. I will answer them later."

Once the full party had assembled, we made our way in two vans over a dusty, rutted road tracing the base of the cliffs of Kalaupapa. In the 1860s, King Kamehameha of Hawaii decreed all island lepers were to be quarantined for life on Kalaupapa, an isolated peninsula of land bound on the south by sheer mountains and otherwise guarded by the relentless Pacific Ocean. Once brought to Kalawao, Father Damien's parish, the lepers were left to fend for themselves.

The road ended high above the surf at the door of Father Damien's church, St. Philomena. The building is well preserved. Though no longer sanctified by the Catholic Church since Father Damien's body has been returned to his native Belgium, the church and nearby grave site remain forever sacred ground.

We entered the immaculate 30-by-100-foot miniature cathedral while Ida moved to a place before the altar. Quietly our party settled in the front pews to hear a most moving sermon.

Now a different woman stood before us. The tour guide had disappeared and before us appeared a concerned shepherdess—scanning her flock. She spoke in the rasping voice of a leprous patient, devoid of timbre but with inflection all the stronger. "This is Father Damien's church and he was one of us. He had his troubles with the authorities, but he never gave up." The involuntary congregation quickened to her words. "We are what remain of the colony. There will be no more coming here. It was closed to new patients in 1969. Now leprous patients are treated at home.

"You do not know about leprosy. I know because over the years I have talked with thousands of visitors and few know about this disease. Caucasians have little experience with leprosy though fifteen million people in the world suffer from it. The number is growing. Leprosy still comes to the islands, now from the Philippines. You have it in the States with the Vietnam refugees. It is a disease that is hard to know about since there are so many wrong ideas." For emphasis she repeated, "So many wrong ideas."

"Even the government knows little about leprosy. Until 1970 all the mail leaving Kalaupapa had to be fumigated with formaldehyde for eight hours. Madness!" She drew the word out to a clear hiss.

"Until 1959 I had to have all my clothes fumigated before I could talk with visitors, and I am not infectious. Leprosy is a disease of poor nutrition and ignorance. It is spreading over the world where the people are poor and uneducated." Her voice softened. "But we still die of it. We lost a good lad today. He was young, fifty-four. Just this morning he put his head down on the steering wheel of his jeep and died. Perhaps it was hypertension? Not that we do not have medical services. There is a staff of forty-five, three doctors, twenty-five nurses, a fourteen-bed infirmary with three dialysis machines. We have better medical service than the other side of the island." With a wry smile and a glint to her red-rimmed eyes she added, "You know, just the other day we had a ninety-nine-year-old leprous patient transferred to the hospital in Honolulu for a double inguinal hernia operation. He died three days later of pneumonia. More madness?"

Moving forward, close enough to touch those in the front row, she confided, "But let me tell you about myself. I was born on the island of Maui. We were poor. My father was Japanese, my mother Hawaiian, and I was the seventh of nine children. They all amounted to something. I wanted to be something myself, a schoolteacher, but on my way to the fifth grade I was suddenly taken to the hospital in Honolulu. I never had a bit of schooling since, but I run my business, work seven days a week, learned everything on my own.

"I spent five years in the hospital and they used me like a guinea pig. Oh, I agreed to their experiments. If I didn't, it was Molokai."

She half-twisted her torso and slapping her back sides exclaimed, "Did you ever have someone draw your blood and then inject it right here? Day after day. They were looking for something to stop the disease. But nothing much happened. Then I got this letter from the government with that second paragraph, 'Since you have shown no improvement, it has been decided you will be transferred to the colony at Kalaupapa.' I was seventeen years old and came with twenty-one others. Eight of us were children. The shock of those graves, the corpse I saw buried that first night, the advanced cases everywhere. I cried for two months and the doctors thought there might be something wrong with me. That I might be depressed. Madness!" Again with a hiss.

Her stance shifted. "Let me tell you something of the spirit of our people. We never despair. No suicide here. We always try to make it better. We grow bitter at times, but we must think positively, even though we tell ourselves, 'Once a leper—always a leper.'"

Her voice grew more intense, with a ring of anger. "I am a positive-thinking woman." Then she added what at the time seemed a curious observation, "I do not believe in shock treatment for those who get upset."

Our guard and guardian paused to collect herself, then went on. "Let me tell you what the disease is like. For some there is fever; 105 degrees can make you think you are going mad. Your forearms swell so you cannot...." She flexed her extended arms. "You cannot make a fist for the swelling of your fingers," and she shook her clenched, disfigured fist at the congregation, proving that what remained of her fingers could close. "And then there are the ice tubs to keep the fever down. Do you know that the disease only attacks those parts of the body that are cool? Leprosy grows in the skin. The hair about your eyes falls out but not under your arms where it is warm.

"Your body changes with the disease. You see my red eyes? My eyelids turned in so much they rubbed my eyeballs and for six years my eyes hurt and tears ran. Finally, I had an operation in Honolulu that turned the eyelids out again. You die in bits and pieces, but you do not feel anything. That is the danger. You have to watch all the time for any scratch. It can be bad but you never feel it." The tattered Band-Aid clinging to the stump of what remained of the finger she pointed at us made the point indelible.

"When I came over there were 21 in our group. Four are still alive. No more come, 102 are left. I should say 101. A good lad died today. There he was slumped with his head on his steering wheel and the doctors did nothing. They did not even give him a shot. You know what I mean." She pointed at her breast, appealing to the congregation. "A shot of…you know." Someone responded, "Adrenaline." "Yes, that's it, adrenaline. Nothing was done. He just died."

As Ida paused again, sudden presentiment filled my mind. This must have been how Father Damien spoke. He was fashioned from the same simple clay, believing in "our people." Proud of his humble origins, natively wise, dogged in his faith, forthright yet wary, self-taught in the school of human suffering, he too was a positive thinker about the human condition in its dark hours.

Sighing, Ida offered us her closing benediction. "Do not think I am ungrateful. I am grateful, grateful for the care we have now and the sulfones. I take three pills a day and the disease is stopped. Oh, if only it had come sooner.

"I am grateful for all the money you taxpayers spend on me and the others here. When I go to Honolulu to have H & R Block make out my income tax, I am happy to pay. Yes, happy, for money can stop this disease everywhere. Poor people in countries run by dictators need treatment. They can be helped. I thank you for paying your taxes." Abruptly she broke off. "Are there any questions?"

A few tourist questions surfaced, but most of us were silent. After a few perfunctory answers, Ida sent us off with a nod and her abbreviated smile.

On the way back to the airstrip we drove past the Catholic church. Some cars clustered about it, and Ida explained. "We bury our people the same day they die. This is where his funeral is being held." Though she never said so, Ida had wished to attend that funeral. Frustrated by circumstances, her duty to us, she had presided at a surrogate funeral service for this lad of "our people," for all who had died of the dread disease and for the impending death of the colony.

As it turned out, a resident had urgent need to leave Kalaupapa, and as our plane held but six, the seventh, the resident, was odd man out. My wife and I volunteered our seats. Ida saw what had happened and determined to wait out the return of the plane that would take us out of Kalaupapa.

As we loitered beneath an ohia tree, I was free to draw her out. "If there is one thing you would say to all the doctors in the world, what would it be?" Immediately she removed her palm leaf hat, raised her clublike right hand, and drew it across the top of her head. "I would have chiseled here on the top of every doctor's head that when a patient comes in complaining of numbness to immediately take some skin scrapings and send them off to a pathologist. That is what I would say!" We talked about the need of doctors to be knowledgeable and, as she put it, "to have human feelings." In no time the Beechcraft returned and with as firm a handshake as possible, we bade farewell.

As the plane cleared the cliffs, I found myself thinking of Ida's advice, and most particularly of her cryptic remark about shock treatment. Why had she singled out that treatment, controversial as it might be, when talking of leprosy? It was probably the tip of some personal experience with psychiatrists. I will never know. But then, suddenly, I thought I understood. Electroshock treatment is iatrogenic numbness. Born of her physician- and society-imposed isolation, Ida was an enemy of numbness of the mind as well as body. Her message was "Beware of Numbness."

As tourist rather than physician, involuntarily I relearned a lesson all compassionate physicians should hold in mind, if not chiseled on their brows: "Be aware of human feelings." Like compassion, the practice of medicine should nurture active feeling, not passive numbing. First do no harm with our mind-numbing tests, procedures, and deadening pharmacopeia. Do not diminish the patient while diminishing his or her pain. As I have come to believe, Ida would have patient and physician strive for full feeling in body, mind, and spirit, together, becoming children of promise, sharing all suffering, enduring all things, alive to all life.

Endnotes

Reprinted from the *Journal of the American Medical Association* 266(1991): 3411-3412, with permission. Copyrighted 1991, American Medical Association.

Part 10

Compassion's Challenge

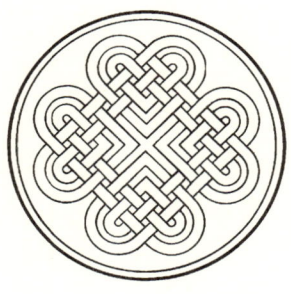

Beware of social efficiency bereft of reflection that treats compassion as an optional benefit rather than an essential need.

—Ralph Crawshaw

Overview to Part 10

The experience of compassion is more complex than an unbidden sense of grace received. That momentary epiphany has a way of bundling many elements into a new and welcome higher understanding of yourself while quickly dissolving into immediate circumstance. Even the experienced, empathetic therapist who offers an interpretation of the patient's suffering, which blossoms into accepted insight, must work at examining the feelings of relief and reward that accompany the patient's enlightened access to a previous black corner of his or her life. Compassion has an ineluctable way of shimmering away into the recesses of the mind leaving but the finest traces of memory. But then those traces are the substance of enhanced maturity and there lies compassion's challenge.

Reflection does more than simply weave the recollection of compassion into personal recognition of how the experience of shared feeling changes us. Gentle yet sustained consideration of what shared feelings have done gradually informs the ancient saw that the giver receives in giving. Bestowing insight serendipitously bestows on the thoughtful increasing capacity for insight. As the vast horizon of compassion emerges along the edges of a tested life, reflection is transformed into the commonsense pursuit of increasing insight and understanding. As each responds to compassion's power, unconsciously we become more responsible for the world we share with others.

One focused aspect of the phenomenon of compassion's challenge is found in how professionals of the caring professions who live their vocation are drawn to social action. **Civic Medicine**, while speaking to physicians' loss of autonomy, encourages if not challenges them to lay aside their white coats long enough to help the community understand dimensions of social suffering. Curiously, **Mini-Internships** does just the reverse as it suggests ways for caring physicians to take concerned citizens under the aegis of those same white coats and come close to the heart of shared suffering.

The Better Health Business Bureau takes a wider view as it reveals, with its gentle antidote to compassion's ancient opponent, prevalent apathy, a possible way for both citizens and physicians to enhance a culture of compassion, considered reflection, and action. **Breaking Out of Gridlock** offers voice for physicians in the toils of system suffering, the enforced, blind ignorance of political institutions blocking the natural flow of vocation.

A guide for community outreach, **Grass Roots Participation in Health Care Reform**, offers an unusual roadway to commonalty in caring. The popular concept of an "invisible hand" of the marketplace brokering health care through gatekeeping doctors is set aside. In place of patients, as consumers, pitted against physicians, as providers, an inclusive approach calls upon citizens, hospital administrators, nurses, and physicians to work together in establishing life and death community priorities in health care.

Lest failure to meet compassion's challenge go unremarked, **Lying** outlines many ways vocation is corrupted. As a broad view of intentional misrepresentation, this essay suggests a bestiary of liars.

Perhaps the most insidious form of opportunity aborted appears when "experts," dedicated to eliminating human suffering, use the challenge of caring to fashion words that never connect to action. **Intellectual Nemesis** discloses how the poor and ignorant can stand unnoticed at the door of a mansion of the wise.

Though unfilled or ignored, the challenge of compassion will never disappear, but the capacity to respond, the ability to be a caring profession, a caring people, may. Unbelievable as it may seem, the collective capacity for dedicated vocation is fragile to the point of vanishing. Our culture capital of caring erodes insidiously under the power of forces beyond the control, if not the ken, of those intent upon vocation. **Medicine, A Challenged Profession** looks back on an organization for collective caring forever destroyed, knighthood, drawing attention to similarities with today's profession of medicine. The bleak conclusion that physicians can wither down into a band of well-paid technicians in the service of an economic system may be impossible to accept, much as it was impossible for the Knights Templar to think their noble profession could be dismantled before their eyes, but it was. We are well advised to consider in our reflections that a time may come when response to compassion's challenge will have neither collective force nor shared meaning. Beware of social efficiency bereft of reflection that treats compassion as an optional benefit rather than an essential need. As history reminds us, ignoring the daily challenge of shared feelings is fatal to shared vocation.

Civic Medicine

> *Medical education does not exist to provide individuals with an opportunity to make a living, but in order to make possible the protection of the public.*
>
> —Rudolf Virchow (1821-1902)
> Address to medical students
> at Pathological Institute, Berlin

A fundamental issue preoccupying practicing doctors is our loss of professional autonomy. Whether rooted in inflexible government regulations, strident consumer demands, economic exigencies, technological complexity, paraprofessional competition, managed care, or malpractice threats, a pervasive concern haunts American doctors that they are losing control of their practices while becoming provider technicians. Civic medicine is a countermeasure that historically has proved a mainstay for public trust in physicians.

Many doctors consider any enterprise which is not immediately and directly clinical as inconsequential or irrelevant. Extraoffice work, such as volunteering medical service at a Salvation Army clinic or training a mountain search-and-rescue team, is frequently seen as peripheral to practice, while running for public office is frankly irrelevant. Similarly, physicians may deny their satisfactions in civic service since they cannot be computed in cash terms. However, great value exists in this essential part of medical practice.

Definition

Civic medicine is medically insightful action by physicians for the commonweal from which they derive a sense of participation in citizenship rather than patients' gratitude, money, or scientific knowledge. It is the study, development, and use by physicians of the social power which mediates between the medical profession and the community within which a physician considers her/himself to be a citizen. For some, perhaps too many, physicians, community is circumscribed by a medical institution such as a school, health maintenance organization, or hospital.

Social power, as used by physicians, is defined by enlarging on Bertrand Russell's[1] definition of power as "the production of intended results" to include that mixture of scientific knowledge, moral rectitude, spiritual conscience, psychological insight, economic facility, and social position which a physician may use to affect public issues.

Civic medicine is not public health medicine, which entails a paid career under the aegis of a government. Nor is it political medicine which, though generally unpaid, seeks the aggrandizement of an individual or the profession.

Dynamics of Civic Medicine

Civic medicine has a reciprocal in direct service medicine, the care of patients for financial reward. Clearly the practitioner of medicine, no matter what his specialty or institutional setting, must balance these two conflicting elemental motivations: self-interest and interest for others.[2]

The balance between self-interest and others' interest has some physicians coming down hard on one side or the other, voicing a rationalization for either extreme. "I am out for all I can get before government takes over." Or, in a distant echo of Virchow's injunction that physicians are trained for the protection of the public, "My colleagues are so miserably mercenary I am considering joining the Peace Corps." For the practitioner of civic medicine, this ambiguity is not resolved by taking sides. Rather, there is a conscious search for social/ethical homeostasis to maximize the best of both forces.

Development of Civic Medicine

Civic medicine is not and probably cannot be taught; it is learned through personal reflection and experience. The ideals of service that frequently bring young people to study medicine are seldom strongly reinforced during their student years. They hibernate while the student slaves to please many masters. However, when the long-delayed autonomy of medical practice arrives, these dormant humanitarian ideals may reawaken, to be burnished by the ethical dilemmas of patient care in the community. Then the practitioner learns civic medicine firsthand.

Historically doctors have dreaded government, for until modern times governments accorded them little power and less respect. The execution of Servetus and the persecution of Paracelsus are examples of irrational public acts that made physicians favorites of kings or the scapegoats of mobs. However, with the advent of quarantine as a control of plague, governments grudgingly developed rudimentary health policies based on medical skills and with them a recognized interrelationship with the medical profession which slowly grew in the nineteenth century until scientific medicine cemented it with proven ability to protect the public's health. Today, the complex dynamic between government and the medical profession floods legislatures with innumerable issues, from funding research to legislating specific medical therapies.

Heroes of civic medicine, physicians without prospect of personal gain, prepared to apply social power to civic problems, appeared in the eighteenth century as the interface between government and medical science grew more complex.

Benjamin Rush (1746-1813) risked his life and fortune by signing the Declaration of Independence and spent considerable professional energy on unpopular public causes such as the abolition of slavery, the development of public schools and colleges, the higher education of women, and hospitals for alcoholics. The unquestioned Solon of civic medicine is Rudolf Virchow (1821-1902), who founded modern cellular pathology, was a member of the Berlin Anthropological Society, served in the German Reichstag, and by his forceful integration of medical science with municipal politics made Berlin the first example of a healthy, modern city despite its high-density population.

Practice

The practice of civic medicine is largely the everyday work of thoughtful application and diligent follow-through in response to mundane civic needs. Countless examples exist, ranging from helping with charity fundraising to running for the legislature, all of which contain the possibility of applying medical insights to the community's advantage.

As in general medicine so in civic medicine: practice should aim at quality, seeking an appreciable positive influence on the community by preparation, deliberation, and action. For the young doctor under the pressures of practice and family responsibilities, time and energy for civic medicine are understandably limited. Yet even a beginner can make provision for community service, anticipating fuller expression in later years. The complete physician continually seeks increasing maturity through civic expression to complement direct service and broaden perspective as a human being.

Probably the most important, and yet most difficult, element in civic medicine is consciously sharing a civic gift. Curiously, both discipline and courage are necessary to recognize a self-chosen civic duty. Feelings of frustration and resentment over the thicket of irritating governmental regulations invading medical practice must be faced and overcome. It is easier to make a gift of time and effort to a deserving patient or to donate money to a worthy cause than to share medical insight with a government official. Yet, without this concept of medical sharing, the essence of the gift is weakened and that most worthy of ideals, constructive patriotism, is denied the physician. Only as the physician consciously and independently contributes to government does he or she become a free professional, the complete practitioner of civic medicine.

One of the best areas for developing skills in civic medicine is the government of medicine itself, organized medicine. Here, skills of communication, awareness of interacting networks, thinking through opposing ideas, and developing practical judgment of colleagues' motives and potentials are sharpened. Civic medicine is not for the shy or timid, nor for the social climber. Yet participation leads to larger arenas where parochial attitudes and limited professional identification can give way to broader concepts and genuine leadership.

Wisely, the goals of civic medicine should be pursued with caution by avoiding the waste of fruitless committee meetings, useless work, importuning of zealots, and unreasonable goals. Since no doctor has unlimited resources, each contribution should be carefully balanced against its real return to the physician as personal satisfaction. Then, the concept of medical practice in the largest sense, as the art of serving the community, naturally evolves.

Rewards

Though no calculus of physicians' contribution to the public weal exists, a 10 percent donation of time and thought by all doctors to community service would undoubtedly enhance public trust as nothing else could. Physicians bring a unique and constructive leaven to civic problems, for without medicalizing politics but rather offering broad alternatives so often lacking in public deliberations, physicians can become concerned leaders of their community.

For the physician the rewards of civic medicine may seem intangible, yet a lifetime of service to the sick is richer in meaning when devoted to the world of the sick as well as their bodies. The common frustration of facing patients' finite limitations is relieved for the doctor who sees his community healthier and wiser for a greater contribution. Specifically, when charged with accumulating money at the expense of the sick, guilt need not color the thoughts and fear of retaliation need not threaten a physician's autonomy. The rewards bestowed on the practitioner are balanced by a voluntary gift of service to the community. Civic medicine reinforces the community and the physician through an interrelationship of mutual benefit.

As the medical profession loses autonomy with fractionating specialties, redundant manpower, technological obsolescence, manipulative reimbursement, and intervention by third parties, many doctors are preoccupied with professional survival. Yet there is opportunity for them consciously to use medical insight for the commonweal. Civic medicine is a bulwark against significant social and economic forces presently eroding the medical profession's autonomy.

Endnotes

Reprinted from *South African Medical Journal* 72(1987): 735-736, with permission.
1. B. Russell, *Power* (New York: W.W. Norton, 1966), 35.
2. A.R. Jonsen, "Watching the Doctor," *New England Journal of Medicine* 308(1983): 1531-1535.

Mini-Internships: An Experience in Health Care Delivery for Community Leaders

There are many truths of which the full meaning cannot be realized until personal experience has brought it home.
—John Stuart Mill (1806-1873)

A number of lay leaders, including legislators, public officials, administrators, business executives, judges, reporters, and the trustees of philanthropic foundations, substantially influence health policy decisions. Although a few lay leaders have had coincidental involvement with clinical medicine, most experience medical service only as patients or relatives of patients. Concerned with the lack of clinical perspective displayed by lay leaders in the determination of city and state health policies, while president of the Multnomah County Medical Society in Portland, Oregon, I initiated a series of integrated "white-coat" experiences, called the Mini-Internship Program, for recognized civic leaders in the community.

Lay people who are curious about the delivery of medical care are frequently exposed to the technical side of medical science rather than encouraged to develop insight into the healing arts. Consequently, an afternoon may be spent touring surgical suites rather than appreciating the dynamics of a surgical team with its implicit focus on personalized patient care. Though the mini-internship exposes lay people to medical techniques and technology, surgical operations, CAT scans, and obstetrical deliveries, throughout the program these techniques are interpreted as extensions of the patient-doctor relationship—a perspective emphasized by encouraging lay students to examine the treatment of human illness and suffering through the eyes and ears of their host physicians.

The lay students are largely self-referred, having heard of the program by word of mouth. Former lay students include businessmen serving on hospital and foundation boards, state legislators interested in health legislation, school superintendents concerned with health education, city officials interested in developing innovative health programs, insurance executives perplexed about health care costs, and reporters seeking greater understanding of the local delivery of medical care. Lay students are screened for involvement with health care policy by the Mini-Intern Committee, which is made up of four members of the Multnomah County Medical Society and one staff executive, backed by a faculty of approximately forty volunteer physicians. A few applicants with demanding personal agendas or obvious voyeuristic motives have been refused. Quarterly, eight selected guests are invited to dinner at the Medical Society, where they meet six host physicians for an initial evening of informal discussion and preparation. The cost to the Medical Society each quarter for the entire program is about twenty-five dinners, twelve hours of coordinating work by one executive, and the efforts of approximately six volunteer host physicians and two coordinating staff physicians.

The initial dinner meeting is directed toward both intellectual and emotional orientation. Each lay student receives a personal, detailed schedule of activities, a map with directions for every location for the next two days, and a central telephone number to call in case of any confusion. At least one of the lay student's host physicians is present at the dinner to ensure continuity from the start. The dialogue focuses on two essential points: patient confidentiality and the lay student's anxiety. The host physicians emphasize that though the patients have been or will be asked for permission to have the lay student present during consultations, everything the student sees and hears remains confidential. When either the physician thinks it unwise or the patient declines to have a third person present, the lay student is excluded. For example, lay students are not present for any counseling of an intimate nature, during pelvic examinations, or if the lay student is personally acquainted with the patient. To the best of our understanding, the legal implications are precisely those that apply to any medical education circumstances to which the patient has given informed consent.

In eight years of program experience, the only untoward problem of confidentiality occurred when a lay student who was a city official was photographed watching a mastectomy, and the photograph appeared in the next day's newspaper. The unidentified patient and her family had been fully informed before the operation that this person would be present and had voluntarily agreed, yet there were protests that the patient was exploited by being put on exhibit. No other public complaint about the program has been heard.

The range of physicians who volunteer as faculty is as wide as the practice of medicine: family physicians, internists, psychiatrists, surgeons, emergency-room physicians, and representatives of all the medical specialties have participated. The lay student has some preliminary choice, so that, for example, a Medicare administrator can be matched with a family physician serving geriatric patients. Sometimes the match proves serendipitous, and it is generally educational; only rarely is there a mismatch, with a serious difference of opinion on the delivery of medical care.

Occasionally, the host physician is called from the dinner meeting, and the clinical phase of the mini-internship begins immediately with the lay student accompanying the physician to a delivery or emergency surgery. Usually, however, the work begins the next morning when the lay student joins the host physician on early hospital rounds. During the ensuing two days, each lay student accompanies an internist or family doctor, witnesses an operation, sees an emergency room in action, and learns something about one of the medical specialties. Invariably, these hours are intense, and they are shared with a candor that surprises most lay students, overwhelming some. After retiring from the bedside, lay student and physician discuss questions of cost, technique, life, death, and taxes with the intellectual vigor that characterizes the best in medicine and with the openness that is found in successful patient-doctor relationships. These spirited exchanges in themselves reveal a new dimension of medical care to the lay student.

Process

The lay student appears to pass through three attitudes of mind. As documented by staff notes and tape recordings, the initial attitude at the introductory dinner is frequently denial parading as skepticism. Lay students have said, "Oh, I know about doctors and hospitals—I had an appendectomy fifteen years ago," or "I'm not put off by the sight of blood. It never bothers me." Denial gives way to unreserved enthusiasm during the actual clinical interaction: "It's just marvelous the way he sutured blood vessels with those tiny curved needles." The final attitude, an understanding of the human interaction, is expressed during the debriefing dinner in statements such as, "I'll never know how she makes rounds among those dying patients day in and day out," and "I have come to see that the medical profession is made up of individuals and that patients are individuals as well. I must never forget this." Invariably, the lay students' preexisting ideas have been seriously reexamined after their clinical experiences.

Debriefing Dinner

To ensure understanding and closure, a debriefing dinner is held on the evening of the second day, which the host physicians do not attend. Invariably, the lay students have many ideas and questions. Candid remarks and insights are shared late into the evening.

The most common immediate observations reported by lay students are, "I expected this was going to be some kind of a political hard-sell by the doctors, but it never happened," followed by, "I never had any idea doctors worked so hard." For many lay students the most amazing experience is to witness the rapid and respectful intimacy between patient and physician. Each lay student is given ample opportunity to recount what the two days have meant. Cases are recalled, alternative procedures considered, suggestions made, positive and negative feelings examined, and conclusions drawn in the light of the group's experience. No holds are barred as the profession stands exposed. Questions about physicians' styles, etiquette, techniques, and failures and successes with patients are discussed in detail. Here are some remarks that have been made by lay students: "Six hours standing in one spot! How come all surgeons don't end up with varicose veins?" and "Only one of the doctors washed his hands after every patient." A string of observations may be stimulated by the remark, "I never knew it took so much energy to listen," but lay students consistently return to expressions of awe at the power of the patient-doctor relationship. "He changes the minute he is with patients; instead of orders and rush, he is all ears for the patient." Thus, two goals of the program are achieved: educating the public to many of the intangibles of high-quality medicine and developing an ongoing, constructive dialogue with civic leaders.

Though it has not been formally measured, the rapport between the medical profession and the community is reported by both lay leaders and physicians to have improved perceptibly as a result of this program. Legislators in need of health policy advice use a personal consulting service, born of mutual experience and respect. When writing regulations, government officials have informal yet functional access to practicing physicians. Business and labor leaders gain practical experience with health care costs and cost avoidance, and they involve their former host physician in health cost coalitions. Reporters who have gone through the program subsequently check with their former host physicians when in doubt about the facts of a story on local health care.

One unresolved problem with the Mini-Internship Program is the lack of adequate formal feedback from the faculty. Particular problems that arise at the debriefing dinner are carried back to the host physicians through informal channels, along with the committee's thanks for adding another task to their busy schedules. Frequently, lay students write or call their host physicians to express gratitude. To date, we have not had the time necessary to assemble the faculty—all busy practitioners—and assess their reactions against those of the lay students. However, there has never been a lack of volunteer physicians prepared to take the lay students along with them on their days' rounds.

The practical payoff of the program can be seen in the development and maintenance of communications. One labor leader, who was an administrator of a large health trust, participated in the program and subsequently became a board member of the local professional standards review organization. Another labor leader, who later became president of the Statewide Health Coordinating Council, invited his host physician to a labor organizer's tour of the city's factories. We are aware of other county medical societies that have initiated similar programs and report sustained positive results. Hospital executives have developed similar programs within their institutions for their boards of trustees. We have been repeatedly asked for "mini-residencies" by former lay students interested in pursuing a particular interest in medical care delivery. There is no lack of public interest in the program, though a formal evaluation of the public reaction has not been attempted.

Conclusions

This program has introduced community lay leaders to the patient-doctor experience. It has increased the quantity and quality of dialogue between local physicians and civic leaders. For a very modest exposure and about 150 hours of volunteer physician time, a medical society can appreciably raise the level of public sophistication in the determination of local health policy.

Endnotes

Reprinted from the *New England Journal of Medicine* 309(1983): 992-994, with permission. Copyright ©1983 Massachusetts Medical Society. All rights reserved. Coauthored by William Zieverink, M.D., and Collette Wright.

The Better Health Business Bureau

It's me and you against the world—when do we attack?
—Graffiti, New York City wall

Medical practitioners are learning firsthand how significantly the business of medicine has changed during the 1990s.[1] With the entrance of the American corporation into the health care marketplace, many of the transformations Paul Starr predicted in his 1982 study of American medicine have come true, leading to a "new" business of medicine—the medical-industrial complex.[2,3] The operational philosophy of the "new" business of medicine—maximizing profit—is at odds with the traditional standard of practitioners—putting the patient's interest first.[4-7] There is a fundamental contradiction of goals between marketplace corporations and their first-line practitioners. A Better Health Business Bureau (BHBB) offers an approach for participants seeking sustained, shared, ethical solutions to the marketplace's elemental contradiction.

Definitions

Defining roles and how marketplace participants perceive them is essential for understanding the function of the proposed Better Health Business Bureau. Marketplace participants may be thought of as members of one of three groups, each with a clear role: service recipients, healers, and stewards.

The service recipient group consists of patients and their families and, as the scope of health services has grown to include disease prevention and health promotion, an increasing number of healthy citizens. This group's actual level of health, considered along with their satisfaction in how that health is maintained, is the ultimate marketplace measure of health care quality.

Healers comprise those hands-on practitioners in the marketplace who are reimbursed under a benefit plan. They include primary care and specialist physicians, nurses, nurse practitioners, physical therapists, psychologists, and social workers. Through their scientific skills and considered art, they seek to relieve patients' suffering. In return, healers expect reimbursement commensurate with a reasonable standard of living.

The steward group is made up of private corporations and public organizations. Stewards are entrusted with funds, premiums, or taxes to protect service recipients from the burden of the costs of health care. The stewards, public and private, have a contractual responsibility to insure that funds are prudently expended on necessary service, not wasted on inefficient or fraudulent treatments. In addition to covering the cost of care and administration, private stewards expect to make a profit in the competitive marketplace.

To insure maximized efficiency and utility, stewards carry out or contract for managed care. Managed care is defined as "intended to direct patients to efficient providers who are responsible for giving appropriate medical care in cost-effective treatment settings. It seeks to maximize value to health care purchasers...in health maintenance organizations (HMOs), preferred provider organizations (PPOs), or other 'point-of-purchase' arrangements."[8, p.3] Managed care companies are agents of stewards.

Clinical Examples of the Marketplace Contradictions

Case histories give focus to vastly different perspectives held by various participants in the health care marketplace. The following example was offered by a managed care staff member.

> An eight-year-old girl exhibiting severe night phobias was referred to a clinical psychologist who saw the child in individual psychotherapy for eight sessions covered by insurance. He then discharged the child as untreatable, referring her to a psychiatrist for medication. At no time did the psychologist interview the parents, secure a family history, or consider the role their divorce and its legal-custody battle had on the child's condition.

The managed care staff member saw the funds for the eight sessions as wasted, observing that had the insurance coverage continued, the psychologist would still be ineffectually treating the patient.

From such experiences a number of managed care companies derive three corollaries for correcting the marketplace contradictions as expressed by healers:

1. Economic discipline to reduce ineffectual treatment that appears as overutilization and overcharging for healing services.[9]
2. Methodological discipline for healers to act and communicate in a manner that is understandable to significant other marketplace participants.
3. Expectation that healers produce a warranted product capable of uniform production that is interchangeable among healers.

Approaching the delivery of health care as a mercantile enterprise, health industry organizations commonly use standard economic methodology for judging production, that is, measuring the number of patients seen per hour (income) against the fee per hour of the medical practitioner (cost). Focused as they are, they seek not quality of care but a dominant position in a competitive marketplace.

In contrast, a healer's perspective was offered by a psychiatrist.

An eight-year-old boy who acknowledged intense suicidal thoughts and auditory hallucinations was admitted on an emergency basis to a psychiatric hospital following his attempt to strangle his baby brother. The patient openly expressed suicidal ideas, while reporting auditory hallucinations. Upon the boy's admission, the hospital's utilization review nurse notified the family's managed care company. The company agent ruled the admission unnecessary and requested to talk with the treating doctor. The agent told the doctor that the patient should be treated as an outpatient, a recommendation backed up with six-weeks authorization for outpatient treatment but none for inpatient care.

The doctor spent a considerable part of two days attempting to reach the managed care medical director to plea for three days of inpatient care. These were granted and, as the child's condition warranted continued hospitalization, four more days were negotiated. Beyond that, the company spokesperson denied any further inpatient care for fear of "institutionalization," a circumstance left undefined.

The doctor informed the parents that payment for medical care was about to become their responsibility, as the managed care company refused further coverage for inpatient care. The father took this problem to his employer, who in turn asked the company's insurance carrier for an accounting. Upon learning of this feedback, the managed care agent promptly informed the doctor that she was dropped from the company's medical panel for "splitting," jargon for disclosing confidential business procedures. The doctor was told she might appeal the discharge but that neither she nor the hospital could expect any reimbursement during the company's appeal process.

As the family was unable to bear the financial burden of the child's medical care, he was transferred to a state institution. Legal "charity" regulations required that the child become a ward of the state; consequently, the family relinquished custody of their son.

Some healers, building on similar experiences, define stewards as merchandising sharpers investing minimal services into patient care while passing the savings on to shareholders.

The distance and hostility implied by these informal, yet ubiquitous, definitions generates destructive stereotypes, which in turn threaten quality care of patients. Unless these attitudes are understood and dispelled, the health care marketplace becomes an arena of hostile confrontation rather than collaborative effort.

Where to Begin

Resolution of the balance between quality and cost, central to the conflict between stewards and healers, is ultimately determined by what patients seek. It little matters what quality review committees say, how managed care companies rule, or even what profit corporations achieve, the patient and the patient's family are the ultimate judges of the quality of care they receive. Common sense appreciation of the patient as the end user of health care should bring the other participants together in a shared goal of serving the patient. Therefore, prime consideration should focus on the patient and the patient's family, the least well-informed yet most important participants in the health care marketplace. Stewards and healers must insure protection of patients through a prudent, therapeutic consensus on their respective application of professional and economic power.

The working proposition that stewards and healers are capable of building therapeutic consensus comes with the expectation that they share a goal. It can be assumed that there are well-motivated and poorly motivated participants in the marketplace. Experience teaches that there are good and bad physicians, good and bad managed care companies, good and bad third-party payers, and good and bad employers, when good or bad is measured by coherence between what is professed as service goals and what is produced.

Establishing the shared goal calls for "good" healers and "good" stewards to examine, through a mutual dialogue, deeply held professional values and beliefs. Since such dialogue has little precedence, meager language, and insufficient conceptualization, it must be considered as pioneering.

As the proposed dialogue enters new territory, it should adhere closely to actual circumstances. Thus, discussion should, in the main, focus on relevant cases to facilitate communication among marketplace participants towards improved, prudent care for patients. New ethical principles for the marketplace could well emerge from the discussions.

The first site to consider for such a dialogue might be the managed care companies themselves. Experience teaches, however, that negotiating with powerful corporations on their terms is unsatisfactory. Some managed care companies offer appeal mechanisms that upon close inspection appear to function much as chicken coops designed by foxes, with ultimate authority for medical decisions retained by the company.

Some might suggest that such a dialogue is best pursued in courts of law. Expecting that health law will resolve marketplace contradictions is a faint hope for a number of reasons. The law is costly. Courts generate rulings rather than recognized standards of moral behavior sustained by a shared ethic. Lawyers are in the business of establishing rights rather than clarifying process. It is highly unlikely that complex ethical problems present in local health care marketplaces can find resolution in the courts. Courts are best left for final appeal in the event nothing else succeeds.[10, 11]

Another approach to marketplace consensus might be through government legislation and regulation. Previous attempts through the National Health Planning Act of 1974 came to naught, however. That attempt at community consensus by pitting consumer against provider was abandoned in 1981.

A suggestion for professional regulation has come from the American Medical Peer Review Association, with quality monitoring at the state level.[12-14] It naturally follows that national health professional organizations such as the American Medical Association, American Nurses Association, and the Health Insurance Association of America would join in fostering local consensus in the marketplace.[15] One-on-one consideration, however, of local, nitty-gritty, clinical/ethical issues, those intended for the proposed forum of the BHBB, do not lend themselves to national agendas. Though local clinical/business conciliation may have national impact, it is more likely to filter from the grass roots up rather than from the boardroom down.

Local citizen health reform organizations, such as the Health Decisions movement,[16] might offer the BHBB a home. It would be a possible but difficult match since none, including the League of Women Voters, focus on the marketplace of health care. This leaves the American Association of Retired Persons, with its expressed interest in HMO practice, as a slim possibility for nurturing a BHBB.[17]

In any case, concerned participants in marketplace contradictions should call local gatherings to explore ways of better serving patients and their families. Then, the Better Business Bureau (BBB) could be examined as a template for the proposed forums. The Better Business Bureau has been resolving marketplace contradictions through discussion of good and bad business practices, the ethics of the general marketplace, for seventy-five years.

The Better Business Bureau operates directly and consistently in a surprisingly unsophisticated manner, worthy of emulation by the proposed BHBB. Membership is open to all local companies that agree to twelve stipulations, the most important of which are (1) participation in an open BBB file of complaints against the member with disclosure of responses; and (2) response to customer complaints within a reasonable time as well as demonstrated willingness to enter into mediation or arbitration when informal BBB action fails to resolve disagreements.

Such an open, voluntary process may prompt the question as to where the muscle is found to produce functional results. The answer is that the public is hungry for reliable facts and that an informed public will respond intelligently. Each working day, BBB's telephones are busy with potential buyers reviewing the customer history of members from whom they are considering purchasing.

Citizens with complaints are expected to comply with BBB rules as well. The complaint must be written out, with as full documentation as possible. An actual transaction, a contract, must have been entered into. The average complaint is responded to in ten days, and most complaints are resolved in thirty.

The Initiators

Only two members of the health care marketplace are necessary to initiate a functional Better Health Business Bureau, a respected leader of the stewards plus a respected leader of the healers. They can begin by deciding that "something has to be done" and drawing together some kindred souls to brainstorm a new approach to ethical problems of the health care marketplace.

Consider the history of hospital bioethics committees, a development of the last twenty years, which lends credence to the idea that new ethical standards for physicians can evolve at the local level. Bioethics organizations, initiated as study groups investigating a felt need, have become necessary and powerful instruments of quality medical care.

A similar development can be anticipated in the health care marketplace as some healers develop reciprocal trust with some stewards, both groups motivated towards promoting prudent patient healing. A new *modus operandi* for the health care marketplace evolves, complete with institutional memory, as a sustained mutual dialogue focuses on serving patients with the best prudent care possible. In addition, as the need for ethical solutions in the marketplace is shared and understood, the possibilities for funding the BHBB follow.

Results

An organization with a mission similar to the Better Business Bureau can be expected to address and clarify the following:

- Promoting the highest ethics of prudent care through the integrity of the health care marketplace.
- Protecting the public from fraudulent and uncaring practices.
- Providing factual reports to consumers and providers concerning local and national provider organizations (presently, in part, being done nationally by the National Association for Quality Assurance).
- Mediating and arbitrating "health delivery" disputes among stewards, healers, and patients.
- Monitoring and arbitrating advertising and marketing practices.
- Investigating and publicizing unfair and unethical contractual and professional practices through education and referral to appropriate governing bodies.
- Promoting and distributing useful information aimed at both academic and consumer education related to the complex process of securing appropriate health care security.
- Promoting research into the most efficient and prudent means to serve the public through the health care marketplace.

Conclusion

With a Better Health Business Bureau healers can enhance their mission. Organizational needs, community credibility, clinical experience, and professional angst demand a new and broader conceptualization of the health care marketplace. Healers can mobilize, plan, muster resources, rally colleagues, and act. A civic organization along the lines of a Better Health Business Bureau presents a significant opportunity for stewards and healers to serve patients and their families better.

Endnotes

Reprinted, with permission, from *Portland Physician* 33(1976): 16-17, and from *The Pharos* 59(Summer 1996): 39-42. Original title: "The Better

Health Business Bureau: a modest suggestion for leveling the health care marketplace."
1. T. Cooper, "Who Manages the Managers?" *Journal of Neurosurgery* 71(1989): 311-315.
2. P. Starr, *The Social Transformation of American Medicine* (New York: Basic Books, 1982).
3. L.H. Lapham, "Notebook: Devout Observances," *Harper Magazine*, Oct. 1994, 8-11.
4. D. Burda, "The Two (Quality) Faces of HCHP," *Modern Healthcare* 21(11): 28-31.
5. G. Lundberg, "Countdown to Millennium—Balancing the Professionalism and Business of Medicine," *Journal of the American Medical Association* 263(1990): 86-87.
6. D.M. Eddy, "The Individual vs. Society: Resolving the Conflict," *Journal of the American Medical Association* 265(1991): 2399-2406.
7. M. Rodwin, *Medicine, Money, and Morals: Physicians' Conflicts of Interest* (New York: Oxford University Press, 1991), 1-8.
8. P. Boland, "Market Overview and Delivery System Dynamics," in *Making Managed Healthcare Work: A Practical Guide to Strategies and Solutions*, ed. P. Boland (New York: McGraw-Hill, 1991), 3-24.
9. J.J. Saalwaechter, "Hiding Your Criteria Will Never Work," *Physician Exec* 18(1): 48-49.
10 J.S. Todd, "Must the Law Assure Ethical Behavior?" *Journal of the American Medical Association* 268(1992): 98.
11. D.M. Levitt, "Examining Exclusionary Conduct of HMOs and PPOs: A Case Comment on Northwest Medical Laboratories v. Blue Cross and Blue Shield of Oregon," *American Journal of Law and Medicine* 17(1991): 271-288.
12. A. Webber, "Health Reform and the Quality Assurance Imperative," *Quality Letter for Healthcare Leaders* 5(1993): 15-18.
13. P.M. Romano, "Managed Care Accreditation: The Process and Early Findings," *Journal of Healthcare Quality* 15(6): 12-16.
14. C.W. Clanton, "What Managed-care Doctors Can Do to Contain Costs, Do We Really Need Uncle Sam's Help?" *Postgraduate Medicine* 95(3): 38, 44-45.
15. C.J. Schramm, "Healthcare Industry Problems Call for Cooperative Solutions," *Healthcare Financial Management* 44(1): 54-61.
16. R. Crawshaw, "Grassroots Participation in Health Care Reform," *Annals of Internal Medicine* 120(1994): 677-681. The essay appears in part 10 of *Compassion's Way*.
17. R. Maxwell, "The AARP [American Association of Retired Persons] Perspective," *HMO Practice* 4(1): 12-14.

Breaking Out of Gridlock

We are confronted with insurmountable opportunities.
—Pogo (1949-1973)

After years of expert research and months of public debate, forty million Americans are still without health insurance and prudent access to health care. Millions more are threatened by marginal insurance coverage and/or loss of coverage should they change employers. All this, while our national health care costs approach a trillion dollars a year.

Americans and their physicians want the health care system to improve. However, tightly focused groups as well as narrow-minded partisan politics combine to gridlock movement towards effective reform.

The Clinton Task Force Goal of Reform

Caught in a riptide of conflicting forces, the Clinton Health Plan merits reevaluation. The Clinton Health Care Task Force worked from the premise that health insurance guarantees access to health care and consequently the health of the nation. Its recommendations clearly stated its objective as securing necessary health care insurance for every American.

It turns out that neither assumption, health insurance for individuals or increased level of national health through insurance, are valid under existing circumstances. The government health care "insurance" programs of Medicare and Medicaid find increasing numbers of practitioners declining participation. Any reform plan that offers Americans a form of insurance that is unacceptable to large numbers of physicians can not be expected to solve the present crisis.

In addition, the availability of insurance is only part of the solution. Health care is a complex issue that inevitably includes elements of housing, employment, education, commerce, and law enforcement. A workable solution must take these additional factors into practical consideration.[1]

Gridlock

The national health insurance debate that President Clinton courageously initiated ground down to a feckless squabble among special interest groups. At the same time, developments in the health care industry of managed care, merger, and acquisition add severe complications in understanding the underlying dynamics of a nation seeking reform. Too often, groups with special interests have used their financial and political power to confront each other rather than address the tough issues that assail patients, citizens, and physicians.

A Renewed Goal for Reform

It is time to shift the paradigm of the national health care debate. Health care leaders can set a renewed goal—determining what it takes to prudently assure health for all Americans. This goal is fully consonant with the universal wish for a healthy life as long as humanly possible.

By sharing their vision of a healthy America, pace-setting thinkers can challenge the American people to find the means for fulfilling our universal wish. Much as President John F. Kennedy set the goal for going to the moon without telling scientists how, and President Dwight D. Eisenhower set the nation to building the greatest interstate road system in history without detailing the kind of concrete to use, so future presidents can stir the imagination and productivity of the American people by voicing the determination to achieve a healthy America—the renewed goal for health care reform.

A Strategy for Consensus from the Grass Roots Up

After renewing the goal, the leaders can challenge the public to speak up through broad-based, nonpartisan, not-for-profit, community-based groups. American Health Decisions (AHD) serves as an example of this opportunity for consensus building.[2] It is a confederation of twenty-one state citizen groups who have held thousands of community and focus group meetings to educate Americans about the policy implications of health reform including the need for trade-offs. Simultaneously, AHD has been eliciting the public's values in considering health care issues.

The need, according to AHD, is first to shift the national debate from a facts-based agenda, though facts should never be ignored, to a civic clarification of values underlying successful health care reform. Now is the time for Americans to engage in discussing what they value in health care at a national level. For example, the relative values they hold for preventive versus curative services. To do this, citizens must debate broad issues confronting society as a whole. Only after accepted values are in place can we, as a nation, effectively discuss how much of our wealth we wish to devote to health care.

Out of such national "research" a blueprint of the critical values will emerge to encompass and direct the subsequent debate based on facts. Thus our leaders can set the goal of reform leaving to the people the determination of the extent and nature of reform implementation. Nor will these values turn out to be a list of clichés, sound bites, to be ignored in the heat of debate. They will stand before all groups and legislators as national parameters for change.

A National Health Care Community Meeting

As a means for initiating consensus, the President can convene a National Health Care Community Meeting to challenge citizens to decide about a series of tough health care issues. The first, and prototype of the other meetings, can include a broad representation, certainly representation from all concerned organizations. The goal of the meeting will be to ascertain the values dimensions that health reform demands. Only with broad participation at the meeting can representatives be expected to "own" its findings. Openness of the meeting can be insured by national television coverage of the full proceedings and debates.

By addressing particular cases, the needs and wishes of participants will quickly reveal implicit trade-offs that health care reform must embrace. As these trade-offs are discussed, the implicit values for health care reform will surface to be captured by the staff for subsequent debate and agreement. This is the path to national consensus, the blueprint for acceptable change.

The values findings will then be referred to the nation in general for grass roots clarification, rejection, or validation. The findings will also go to each of the participating organizations for their constituents to discuss, reject, or validate. The findings will not be referred to national and state legislative bodies, for the source of citizens' health values lies with the people, not with their representatives. After the findings are confirmed at the grass roots level, legislators can use them in determining the interplay between citizens' values and health care facts and funding. The legislators are expected to use the values in building government programs that the people will accept.

A Model For Achieving Consensus

A model exists for this form of consensus building. The Oregon Health Plan was crafted in this manner, resulting in working consensus of special interest groups, public interest groups, and partisan political leaders.

The agreed upon goal was access to basic health care for all Oregonians. In determining Oregon's values for state health reform, Oregon Health Decisions was rewarded with twenty-five thousand hours of voluntary citizen input. Physicians volunteered another seven thousand hours to insure the plan would be workable at the bedside.[3]

Despite national clamor raised against the Oregon Health Plan, Oregonians took a calm and deliberate look at policy developments. When national special interest organizations for specific illnesses or disabilities entered the debate to "protect their interests," their local counterparts carefully outlined the real gains under the plan for their constituents. As one member of the AARP (American Association of Retired Persons) testified about the plan, "We want no additional health care benefits that come at the expense of our grandchildren."

The results of the value/fact approach had dramatic effect on the legislature. Bipartisan legislative support for the plan, SB 27, emerged. The bill was approved by 57 to 3 votes in the Assembly and by 24 to 2 votes in the Senate. Legislative success can be attributed, in part, to the way legislators were armed with an explicit statement of their constituents' values about the issue. Legislators made a tough decision knowing they would not be savaged by their constituents. They listened to the voice of the grass roots.

Oregonians' acceptance of the plan can be measured in the fact that eighteen thousand citizens signed up in the first three days the plan came on line, four times the expected number. At the six-month mark 84,253 people had signed up—24,083 more than anticipated.[4] The need is there, confirming the concerns and consequent values of citizens.

The Role of Physicians

It is important for physicians to take a broad view as well as a personal position towards implementing health care reform. Complacency and despair have no place in advocating health care reform. American Health Decisions and comparable grass roots organizations offer physicians a vastly enhanced power for effective patient advocacy in facing our complex and difficult health care issues. The process is as American as Thomas Jefferson, for the strength of our nation does not lie in the privilege to vote but in the responsibility to vote intelligently. Let the people do more than speak, help them experience their community. Gathering together they talk out their beliefs and values with each other. Physicians have an indispensable contribution to make to these community discussions. They are the spokespeople for humane patient-doctor relationships, the goal of every sick patient and caring doctor.

Traditionally, physicians have been respected leaders in society. By demonstrating their commitment, locating the nonpartisan activists in their community, offering advice, donating time and resources, physicians can influence change to the benefit of patients and the nation.

Endnotes

1. W. Gaylin, "The Health Plan Misses the Point," *New York Times*, 15 Sept. 1993, A27.
2. R. Crawshaw, "Grass Roots Participation in Health Care Reform," *Annals of Internal Medicine* 120(1994): 67-81. This essay appears in its entirety in this part of *Compassion's Way*.
3. R. Crawshaw, M. Garland, B. Hines, and C. Lobitz, "Oregon Health Decisions—An Experiment with Informed Community Consent," *Journal of the American Medical Association* 254(1985): 361-363.
4. The Oregon Health Plan, *Oregon Health Forum* 4(Aug. 1994), 6.

Grass Roots Participation in Health Care Reform

To escape from imposed systems, the yoke of habit, family maxims, class prejudices, and to a certain extent national prejudices as well; to treat tradition as valuable for information only and to accept existing facts as no more than a useful sketch to show how things could be done differently and better; to seek by themselves and in themselves for only the reason for things, looking to results without getting entangled in the means toward them and looking through forms to the basis of things—such are the principal characteristics of what I would call the American philosophical method.
—Alexis de Tocqueville (1805-1859)
Democracy in America

Traveling from Alaska to Florida representing American Health Decisions, a citizens' organization for grass roots health policy, I confirmed that the nation seeks effective health care reform, often in the form of state initiatives, the direct result of the health decisions movement, which, since its founding in 1990, has developed into seventeen active state chapters.

American Health Decisions (AHD), a nongovernmental organization, is dedicated to fostering state-based citizen initiatives.[1,2] AHD's work offers insight into the dynamic of the grass roots participation of citizens and physicians in shared commitment to broad, nonpartisan reform.

Frequently, health care reform is presented as a prescribed plan; for example, the Pepper Plan, the plans of the American Medical Association, the American College of Physicians, the California Medical Association, the American Association of Retired Persons, and the granddaddy of them all, the Clinton Health Reform package. Each of these programs is a top-down approach, representing vast collections of data sifted by provider, academic, and government experts under the direction of special groups, vested interests, or both.[3] Frequently, plans are presented with the cachet of citizen-based discussion through staged, public relations town hall meetings or through proponents' appearances on television talk shows. The thrust is for Congress or a state legislature to turn the proposals into law and thereby solve the nation's health care crisis. Thus far, these wholesale approaches from the top down have come to naught.

In contrast, the bottom-up, grass roots approach does not thrive on special interest turf. American Health Decisions, a proponent of the grass roots approach, is a national consortium of state organizations sponsoring grass roots discussion networks among citizens committed to education and consensus development on the ethical issues of health care. The goals are informed community consent and the assured public understanding of the personal, institutional, and societal implications of health policy decisions (medical, legal, and economic). Although citizen response efforts have been organized in many parts of the country, most can be characterized as program-specific efforts, such as citizens for a one-payer system or for increased mental health services. American Health Decisions' strategy of bottom-up, grass roots, broad, civic enlightenment has a common pattern of development that could prove helpful to reformers, citizens, and providers of health care services.

Rationale

The desire of citizens for participation in policy-making has been pointed out by the President's Commission for the Study of Ethical Problems in Medicine and Behavioral Research:

> Since the early 1960s there has been an extraordinary emphasis on the rights of citizens to direct the course of

their own lives, from voters' rights to consumer rights. This stress on the individual has been coupled with a skepticism towards the claims of specialized expertise and a suspicion of powerful institutions and the 'establishment." Health care has not escaped its share of criticism in the process.[4]

Fueling this desire for participation is a palpable, public angst about the cost and complexity of modern medicine. This surfaces as a deep concern of an aging population about personal health care choices associated with chronic rather than acute disease: a shift from factual questions of health and illness to value questions of quality of well-being in the face of competing needs.

These two forces seek voices in the public realm, a role formerly discharged by articulate political leaders. However, in these days of complex issues that do not respond to political rhetoric or traditional values, politics as usual often ends up in legislative deadlock. A functional alternative enables people to speak for themselves, the health decisions movement. The most powerful rationale for the health decisions movement lies with the certain fact that health reform calls for many sacrifices. Should the government expect citizens to buy into sacrifices of services and money, the buy-in will only follow wide public participation in determining the nature and extent of those sacrifices. The political science of the health decisions movement follows the work of Benjamin Barber[5] and his participatory politics of "Strong Democracy." Where Thomas Jefferson saw independent farmers as the support of American democracy, the modern counterpart for this human potential now lies with concerned, independent citizens pursuing their beliefs in political freedom.[5]

National Perspective of State Health Reform Processes

Minnesota, Florida, and Hawaii have initiated innovative state health reform, yet have not followed the grass roots route that Oregon and Vermont pioneered. Although Minnesota has been exposed to the health decisions movement, its reform program grew out of the "Gang of Seven." Four Democratic and three Republican legislators were so frustrated by the powerful state senate health committee blocking a single-payer bill that they quietly built a legislative consensus for broad-based reform. They then involved special interest groups while developing a strong positive relationship with the press in a successful pursuit of public approval.[7]

Florida, with a large population slanted towards the elderly, followed the commission route favoring top-down legislative leadership with their dedicated governor leading them to comprehensive reform. Using the commission, task forces, and policy "clubs," the Floridians' prime involvement comes down to a formal, one-time statement at a hearing. Consequently, their commission's approach to grass roots input lacks group discussion, the forging of values through argument, which the health decisions movement considers imperative in developing functional policy.[7]

Hawaii, a state with an enviable health record to begin with, had a health decisions organization founded in 1985, long after the passage in 1974 of their unique bill mandating employment-based health insurance offering access to most Hawaiians. Although Hawaii was first to grant broad access to its citizens, complex health issues followed as diverse ethnic groups sought widely disparate forms of delivery. The Hawaii decisions process targeted community consensus on health values through workshops in neighborhood centers, churches, temples, senior clubs, union halls, and cultural centers. The untimely death of the initiator of the Hawaii Health Care, Culture and Social Values Project precipitated the demise of this health decisions organization.[8]

Health decisions organizations in Vermont and Oregon pioneered the broad grass roots approach to health policy. California, the largest state organization with five chapters, and Georgia experimented with variations of community meetings to fit their state needs in specific ways. In all cases, the health decisions organizations have followed a broad yet similar pattern of development.

Stages of Development

Citizen-based, grass roots health care reform has five stages of development: initiation, mobilization, implementation, acceptance, and affirmation. Each stage appears to generate a seemingly unrelated configuration of thinking and leadership. How the stages build on each other is a fascinating self-empowering civic process as yet dimly understood. The result is not a constituted team but a league of improvised or shadow teams made up of people working together. Rather than having clear roles the improvised teams display impressive flexibility in exchanging and using volunteers and community power. The resulting civic dynamo of political will seems applicable to other complex social issues. Citizens in Oregon, for example, are presently exploring applying this interaction of team with team, accompanied by informal, fluid adoption of mission goals and organizational authority to the perplexing ecological dilemma of allocating water resources.

Initiators

State health reform does not begin, although it may die, as an expert's abstract concept for fine-tuning the existing system. Reform starts with real-life experiences of people injured by the system. For these people, the initiators, complaining is not enough as they resolve to correct a counterproductive system of health care that neglects or abuses patients. Efforts to improve states' delivery of health care uniformly begin as responses to local calamities involving any of the three key elements of health delivery: equity in access, containment of cost, and maintenance of acceptable quality of care. Invariably, some concerned individual experiences an egregious failure of the health delivery system and reacts by determining to "do something about it."

The initiator may be a state legislator whose belief in a reasonable civic basis for the delivery of health care is shattered by the arrogance of an importuning turf-manager. The initiator may be a provider whose eyes are opened by the inhumane care received by a sick relative.[9] A pediatrician treating a seriously ill child whose treatment is "disallowed" by a third-party payer may turn his concern into action by becoming an initiator. A small business owner with a sharp eye for cost accountability who carefully reviews the complete, itemized computer printout of the hospital bill for an injured employee can go public in calling a halt to accounting nonsense.

The initiator may be a lay person whose experience of illness has led to seeking ways of avoiding unintended complications. Mary Strong, a former president of American Health Decisions, founder of the New Jersey chapter, the Citizens Committee on Biomedical Ethics, stated it this way:

> My interest in this topic [personal choice in the use of advanced high technology] stems from an event in my life when I was 17. Three of my friends got polio. One died, one was crippled, and one was put in an iron lung. Most troubling to me was, if I got polio and was put in an iron lung did I have a choice? It was the first mechanical technology that could change your way of

life. My concern over this issue has grown as the technology has grown.[10]

Most initiators go without recognition, for what follows in the health reform process has a way of taking on a life of its own. The anonymous initiators, like latter-day Johnny Appleseeds, sow the seed of grass roots reform. The critical point for the initiator is "reporting it as it is" clearly, repeatedly, emphatically. The initiator's message is generally presented as a special case until it reverberates for others as a shared disregard of an essential community value. As a member of the North Carolina Bioethics Resource Group put it, "When I saw my father die the way he did [on unsolicited and unwanted high-technology life support systems], I swore at his bedside this should never happen to another human being." Undaunted, the initiators frequently confront both profound public lethargy and intimidation by experts for criticizing the "best health delivery system in the world." Initiators are the first and most important heroes and heroines of a healthy and health-promoting democracy.

Mobilizers

The next step of grass roots health reform is the mobilization of others with similar points of view and experiences. The case must be made, and made repeatedly, that the dysfunction of the system is general and not a one-time happenstance. It is not enough to cry out in protest. To be heard, the voice for change must echo with the cries of many suffering souls. Mobilizers tune the initial outrage to the public's ears through broadening appeal and civic relevance.

Oregon Health Decisions offers an example of civic mobilization. It was founded in 1982 as a spin-off from a grass roots conference of concerned citizens, providers, and government officials who recognized that Oregon, as a state, had to decide some tough basic health care issues. "Society must decide" became the organizing motive behind sustained efforts to "harmonize" issues to the public's ear.[11] The critical point for mobilizers is developing a constituency with a message that is broader than the grim facts of a particular system dysfunction. Fact-oriented organizations quickly devolve into special interest groups. Worthy as Citizens for a Single Payor Health Plan or American Heart Association may be, they do not aim at explicating fundamental community values needed to support the full spectrum of basic health care.

Mobilizers act through community forums to assist citizens in clarifying and ranking health priorities. Mobilizers may respond to different initiatives: a community leader's call to change an unacceptable condition, a task force recommendation for public reinforcement, an initiator's personal plea for help. In each case, armed with relevant information, mobilizers bring the issues to public forums for citizens to discuss, recognize, and prioritize. Mobilizers understand that only by articulating and bringing issues to the public will the public "own" the issues. Sometimes a dramatic clinical case, such as that of Cobey Howard, an Oregon child needing an organ transplant that the state decided not to fund, arouses the media's interest, lending urgency to deciding tough issues about funding for expensive, high medical technology.[13] It is the mobilizer's task to bring the public's outrage into a responsible, responding arena.

To secure infrastructure support, the money for hiring halls, printing flyers, postage, and telephone expenses, mobilizers in different states face different problems with grass roots communication and funding. Mobilizers need a keen appreciation of local attitudes, resources, and possibilities for political will. Georgia Health Decisions raised sufficient funds to pioneer a focus group approach for residents of Georgia. Mobilizers know the practical limits of volunteerism, its need for sustaining funding.

At the leaner end of the funding spectrum, New Mexico Health Decisions is largely volunteer. The mobilizer, an ordained minister, found it expeditious to join twenty-six different ethnic community boards to give New Mexico Health Decisions community credibility. Whatever the resources available to the mobilizer, validity for the mobilizer's work flows from public appreciation that a substantial number of citizens wish to actively express their personal health care values. Then can mobilizers' findings make a difference that permits a new level of development.

Implementors

Building on public momentum for reform, the implementors receive citizens' "raw" values from the mobilizers. The next step in functional reform is transferring citizens' values to implementors. In Oregon, the implementation team, though it was never called that, was led by Dr. John Kitzhaber, a respected emergency room physician, then serving as president of the state Senate. By using the findings of Oregon Health Decisions in working with staff, experts, and fellow legislators, a health reform bill

(Senate Bill 27) was passed creating the Oregon Health Plan. The bill was based on citizens' expressed health care values, a fact every legislator could easily check with his or her hometown constituency. Dr. Kitzhaber's legislative experience and critical contacts as an implementor ensured a fair hearing for the bill, which passed without major opposition. In fact, only two of the sixty members of the House voted against it, while the Senate passed it with a healthy margin.

The importance of mobilizers is apparent in Oregon Senate Bill 27, as it mandates Oregon Health Decisions' return to the public with the legislative findings to assist in integrating health values into the administration of the Health Plan. A similar relationship of public and legislators informs Vermont's health reform effort. Through an act of the Vermont legislature, the grass roots Vermont Ethics Network is mandated to conduct a series of public forums ensuring that Vermont's health reform laws are in concordance with values expressed by Vermonters. Integrating the work of mobilizers and implementors calls for a refined understanding of the complex relationship of what is possible, what is desirable, and the scope of operant political power.

Acceptors

The next informal team in effective health reform is made up of acceptors. Acceptance by substantial community leaders signals to the people of the state that a workable consensus has been reached. Acceptors establish a statewide ambience of tolerance and hope. As leaders they validate that the cost of reform—social, economic, and possible human suffering—is worth the sacrifice.

Acceptance begins with the titular heads of state and local government who are solicited for their approval of fundamental change. Then pertinent private and public organizations throughout the state, including the presidents of health associations (state medical, nursing, hospital, and ancillary), leaders of academic medicine, citizen groups, health insurance companies, philanthropists, and key industrialists. As leaders recognize and in some cases strongly approve reform, programs cease to appear as special interest manipulations and become accepted policies! Endorsement of the Oregon Health Plan came from Oregon's congressional delegation, from the governor, and from nursing, hospital, and medical associations, with the latter taking the plan to the House of Delegates of the American

Medical Association for AMA endorsement of Oregon's request for a necessary federal Medicaid waiver, a necessity in implementing the plan.

Failure to link political leadership with expressed public values, as when the president of the United States refused to grant Oregon a Medicaid waiver, results in more than a barrier to health reform. Governmental action counter to the expressed will of the people diminishes trust in government, retarding national as well as state efforts for health care reform. Subsequent rulings by the federal administration granted the Medicaid waiver, returning the issue of funding their reform to the people of Oregon—those that must sacrifice.

Dissenters and Affirmers

Experience teaches that health care reform is a never-ending quest to constructively influence vast governmental and private bureaucracies. The quest has its dissenters. Dissatisfaction with the health decisions process takes several forms, ranging from "just another hot air session," to "civics 101," to "it can not authentically represent the diverse public." Pointed criticism is directed at health decisions organizations for not representing ethnic and disabled minorities. Though 85 percent of the membership of health decisions organizations is made up of white, middle-class, professionally oriented citizens, the health decisions process actively strives to reach those deprived of easy, or any, access to political power. Meetings are scheduled in ethnic neighborhoods at times when working people can attend, with babysitting provided for working mothers. Discussions are held in the language of the neighborhood people (for example, Spanish and Russian). In addition, American Health Decisions conducted research in ethnic outreach in three states (California, New Mexico, and Georgia) to learn what people in targeted ethnic groups believe makes community meetings worth the investment of their severely limited time and resources.

Nor does the all but hidden fact of implicit health care rationing in our nation lessen protest against the grass roots approach to health care allocation. To the critics, the attempt to explicitly ration health care in Oregon was construed as burdening "the most vulnerable and defenseless patients" with the cost of reform.[13] Despite the uproar of protest a significant number of citizens acknowledge that the resulting basic package might well give Medicaid recipients and otherwise uninsured persons improved health care compared to what might otherwise be available.

Although it gained faint praise, the Oregon grass roots effort did bring the state, if not the nation, to openly recognize that "everyone cannot have everything" and that equity must be considered in health care allocation.

In contrast to dissenters, those who affirm reform enhance citizen contributions of expressed values, trust, and political will. Citizens must hear, in a cause-and-effect manner, that their help made a constructive difference in reforming social institutions. At every step in the grass roots process, the principal actors need to publicly affirm that the ultimate judgment rests with the public.

Members of the extended grass roots reform team naturally develop talent as two-way communicators. Each player communicates with and listens to other team members, when successful. Back and forth, up and down, this patchwork communication net buzzes with belief in the worth, endowment, and dedication of fellow participants.

Success and Failure

When presented with a clear goal and adequate resources, health decisions organizations prosper. However, a vulnerable aspect of health decisions work is its episodic nature, highs of focused activity in political seasons followed by lows of inactivity while participants are distracted by other issues. Nor do the abstract elements of health policy goals promote continuity. Complex health care issues, such as advanced high medical technology, legal alternatives in making personal and family health decisions, the ethical dilemmas of genetic medicine, and individual responsibility in promoting health, call for continual public education. However, raising public awareness is an elusive undertaking. Each issue quickly accumulates political implications as increased understanding translates into a call for reform. Hence, the bumpy road of highs and lows, the waxing and waning that go with grass roots initiatives for prudent, accessible health care.

Examples of organizational waning are not hard to find. In 1985, Colorado Speaks Out on Health, the Colorado health decisions chapter, pioneered a community education program under the leadership of Dr. Fred Abrams, a practicing obstetrics-gynecology specialist. The initiators found no mobilizers to move the grass roots awareness to civic action. Consequently, with its immediate goal accomplished, the chapter became dormant, with only a volunteer secretary answering the mail. This has happened in Arizona and Hawaii where the momentum petered out in the absence of a carry-through mobilizer. Sustained success calls for the mobilizers to continue building on the cadre of dedicated members the initiators have organized. Teamwork holds the health decisions organization together during the lean times between high visibility activist programs.

"Citizen" includes physicians, and the health decision movement represents a window of opportunity for medical practitioners and teachers to foster health policy from the grass roots up. Physicians can help initiate, mobilize, implement, and affirm the political will necessary to reform health care. The process is little less than the extension of the patient-doctor relationship directly into the community with the intent of civic healing. Augmented by direct support of physicians, the evolving grass roots health decisions movement demonstrates its ability to enhance the equity and quality of health care throughout the nation.

Endnotes

Reprinted from *Annals of Internal Medicine* 120 (1994): 677-681, with permission.

1. The States That Could Not Wait—Lessons for Health Reform from Florida, Hawaii, Minnesota, Oregon and Vermont. Milbank Memorial Fund. 1993.
2. B. Jennings, "A Grassroots Movement in Bioethics," *Hastings Center Report* 18(Suppl): 1-16.
3. P.E. Dans, "Perverse Incentives, Statesmanship, and the Ghosts of Reforms Past," *Annals of Internal Medicine* 118(1993): 227-229.
4. United States. President's Commission for the Study of Ethical Problems in Medicine and Biomedical and Behavioral Research. Making Health Care Decisions: A Report on the Ethical and Legal Implications of Informed Consent in the Patient-Practitioner Relationship. Vol. 1: Library of Congress Card Number 600637. Washington, D.C. 1982; 34.
5. B. Barber, *Strong Democracy* (Berkeley: University of California Press, 1984).
6. H. Leichter, "State Model: Minnesota, The Trip from Acrimony to Accommodation," *Health Affairs* 12(1993): 48-58.
7. L.D. Brown, "Commissions, Clubs, and Consensus: Florida Reorganizes for Health Reform," *Health Affairs* 12(1993): 7-26.
8. D. Neubauer, "Hawaii: A Pioneer in Health System Reform," *Health Affairs* 12(1993): 31-39.
9. R. Crawshaw, "Technological Zeal or Therapeutic Purpose—How to Decide?" *Journal of the American Medical Association* 250(1983): 1857-1859. This essay appears in part 9 of *Compassion's Way*.
10. S. Blakeslee, "Health Care Choices: Letting the People Decide," *New York Times,* 14 Jun 1990, B7.

11. R. Crawshaw, M.J. Garland, B. Hines, and C. Lobitz "Oregon Health Decisions: An Experiment with Informed Community Consent," *Journal of the American Medical Association* 254(1985): 3213-3216.
12. R. Crawshaw, M.J. Garland, and B. Hines, "Organ Transplants: A Search for Health Policy at the State Level," *Western Journal of Medicine* 150(1989): 361-363.
13. D.D. Hadorn, "Setting Health Care Priorities in Oregon: Cost-effectiveness Meets the Rule of Rescue," *Journal of the American Medical Association* 265(1991): 2218-2225.

Lying

The cruelest lies are often told in silence.
—Robert Louis Stevenson (1850-1894)

To tell the truth, physicians lie. But can you believe they lie when you hear it from a physician, who therefore is an acknowledged liar? A pretty paradox this, which since ancient times has haunted the most trusted of professions made up of men and women who have always told most of the truth and sometimes more than the truth. To begin with, why would physicians be so willing to swear a Hippocratic oath if we were not aware of a wish to lie and conceal? Certainly patients are aware in their hearts of our moral flaw, for who among them would want to hear, let alone bear, the truth, the whole unvarnished truth about their human condition. The doctor and the patient are joined in a tacit understanding that they should approach the truth, should nurture the truth, but need not worship the truth to the exclusion of the patient's well-being. As I say, what a pretty paradox, perplexing physicians as their lying extends through patients' lives, all the way from birth to death, from the profession's distant past into the foreseeable future.

But the tale to spin is not about a passel of well-paid liars pandering to the hypochondriacal whims of the public nor of a coterie of corrupt priests of science building a comfortable niche for themselves by hoodwinking society into believing there will be a cure for cancer tomorrow. What we are about is an attempt at understanding both sides of lying. One side is an intentionally misleading act or statement. The other side is truth saying, intentional, full disclosure in word and deed. By understanding them together we may better develop that essential to healing, trust, for without trust no therapy prospers. Only by understanding the care and nurturance of truth will our journey through the dark side of the patient-doctor relationship become worthwhile.

Henry Thoreau observed, "It takes two to speak the truth, one to speak and another to hear,"[1] which illuminates that patients lie as well as doctors. Physicians, particularly psychiatrists, are keenly aware how patients lie, for it is a truism of psychotherapy that this week's interpretation (truth) is next week's resistance (lie). This phenomenon of converting a truth into a lie, one of the wonders of transference, works for both the patient and the doctor. Take, for example, the specialist who concluded the diagnostic workup of a young man with carcinoma by answering the patient's question of how much longer he had to live with, "Not long enough for us to ever become friends," a "truth" intended to maliciously mislead with confounding rejection. Experience teaches how easily both patient and doctor can become enemies of trust.

To make absolutely clear how few wish to know the whole truth and nothing but the truth, simply imagine a remarkably sophisticated computer capable of predicting the time of your death. It would model your life by tracing out your lifestyle, calibrating your genes, measuring the accumulation of sclerotic plaques per square millimeter of your blood vessels' surface, judging the risks connected with the form, extent, and destination of your travels, the degree to which you are exposed to violence including nuclear holocausts and report that you will cease to exist at 4:21 A.M., October 21, 2044, or, perhaps, tomorrow afternoon. Would you jump at the chance to get a copy of that computer readout?

Some people, in a burst of overwhelming curiosity, would rush to discover their fate; some would hesitate; others, burdened with soul-freezing dread, would attack the machine and destroy it. What would you do? Though the question of the whole truth becomes uppermost in your mind, it can take a different form in the mind of your physician. What the caring physician considers, since he is simultaneously an analogue for the computer and your ally, is, should you be forced to know the truth? Should the computer readout be mandatory reading for you or should you know what you want to know and no more?

Nor does it take an imaginary computer to put our common wish to be lied to into personal perspective. There is a high probability that each of us someday will be a patient, stretched out in a hospital bed, when a caring physician will enter our room knowing that he can offer some comfort but no hope. His question will be how much of the truth do you wish to know and how do you wish to go about hearing it. As the wise man says, it takes two to tell the truth, and we are back to our paradox that the most trusting of professions is sometimes trusted not to tell the truth.

Bestiary of Lies

Agreeing that the quest for the holy grail of medical truth has more directions than a compass has points, we can, with a measure of humility, look closer at medical lying, its forms and processes. The taxonomy is daunting, for there are colored lies, white, yellow, and black, anatomical lies, barefaced and tall. There are protective lies, malicious lies, habitual lies, unconscious lies, fibs, perjury, deceits, exaggerations, evasions, excuses, myths, fictions, falsehoods, self-deceptions, quibbles, omissions, as well as ignorant, expected, social, institutional, scientific, and statistical lies, to name but a few. They are intended to mislead and together make a veritable zoo of corrupt practices.

An excellent classification of lying can be found in Sissla Bok's book on the subject.[2] She starts with white lies and moves through excuses, lies in crisis, lying to liars and enemies, lying for the public good, protective and paternalistic lies including the lies of science and medicine, all of which makes a start at an inclusive outline of the possibilities for lying in our culture. However, for our purposes we do best focusing on purposeful misleading by physicians and how they act as toxins to trust.

Given the size of our zoo of liars, we cannot expect to make a complete survey of all the animals, neither time nor inclination permits such a scholarly approach. However, we can select a few beasts for close examination and hope they represent a broad enough sample to identify most species when encountered in the wild. I propose we look at white lies (rabbits), institutional lies (wildebeests), and self-deception (hyenas). Knowing these three inhabitants of our bestiary of prevarication will not make experts of us but will permit a workable cross section of our zoo and, for the curious social naturalist, open a way to identify other creatures when encountered in their native habitat.

Physician's White Lies

A white lie is one that is considered by the liar as trivial and harmless, much as those cute, long-eared, burrowing creatures, the rabbits, are considered as incidental to the great scheme of things. "So nice to see you," murmured as greeting to the patient by a harried physician, or the salutation of some pediatricians, "What a beautiful baby," seem less than worth the time to think about when considered as lubrication intended to smooth the way for an involved and difficult encounter, the patient-doctor relationship. Who ever heard of anyone hurt by a rabbit?

Take, for example, the white lie to the sick and weary filling a waiting room, announced albeit by the physician's surrogate, the receptionist, "Sorry the doctor will be a little late as he is delayed by an emergency at the hospital." Occasionally this may be true but too often it is a white lie to cover the physician's dallying at lunch, or a quick trip to the local marina to check the battery of his cabin cruiser.

My authority in judging this rabbit as a rabbit rests on the public's report. As president of the local medical society, some years back I let it be known through the media that I would be available Monday afternoons at society headquarters to hear the public's complaints, praise, and questions of the medical profession. All they had to do was call and make an appointment and I would listen. Each week four or five worthy citizens stopped by and over 50 percent of their complaints were of doctors wasting their time. There were, and presumably are, too many times that physicians were late to attribute it to emergencies. There appeared to be as many emergencies as there are rabbits, white lies.

One man did not leave it at complaining to me. He wrote his physician pointing out that the three hours he lost in the waiting room was time away from his job and money out of his pocket. He enclosed a bill for forty-five dollars, his lost time. The doctor, with a playful arrogance sometimes attributed to all the medical profession, wrote across the patient's bill that indeed he may have wasted the patient's time but the patient was going to have a hard time collecting anything. How wrong the doctor was. The patient took the bill with the doctor's acknowledged lapse to small claims court and collected.

The prospect of all the patients in the nation collecting on such a prolific hutch of white liars is daunting to the imagination and should be frightening to the profession, yet this is but a minor incidence compared with those who live, day-in, night-out, with physician white lies, medical answering service operators. They report the prevalence of white lies too high for comfort.

Here are some examples of this cute beast gamboling innocently across the medical landscape. The doctor who asks the operator to page him at a certain time so he can get out of a meeting at a medical society or church. The operator gives the doctor a call that he does not wish to take so he says, "Just tell them you cannot find me." The doctor who has been paged many times by several operators and calls in to say that it must be operator error; when the operator requests a test call, the pager works fine. A call to the doctor's residence, the wife says he is out of town and she does not know who is on call. Checking with his associates, they insist the information is incorrect. Upon calling back to the residence the doctor answers and takes the call. Or a call to the doctor's residence and a child answers. The child drops the phone and calls out, "Daddy, are you home?" The child returns to the phone and says, "He is not home." These white rabbits have an incredible ability to multiply.

At this point I feel a little uneasy, like the magician who having pulled a rabbit from a hat, goes on pulling more and more, unable to stop though the stage is alive with bunnies. By simply moving to a different medical area and quizzing others—nurses, hospital administrators, emergency medical technicians, nursing home operators—how many physician's white lies would appear? But then if asked, what would patients report, since the physician's white lies are so purposefully screened from them? However, there are those physicians who believe white lies are good for the patient and give therapeutic reasons for deception. The process is dignified with a name, placebo, translated from the Latin "I please," and what we are observing are the March hares of medical white lies, placebos.

Placebos are medications not intended to have any therapeutic value beyond deceiving a patient into believing he or she is being treated. Placebos are the official, established, fully licensed white lies of the medical profession.

Dr. Howard Spiro dealt with the question in detail,[3] citing his own experience as a gastroenterologist where he estimated that placebos relieved the pain of peptic ulcer in approximately 60 percent of the cases. He recommended the use of placebos if the physician keeps in mind that they "(1) Delude (physicians) into thinking their patient has no significant organic disease since they relieve the patient's pain, (2) find placebos as a first step to more major deceit or diagnostic ennui; or (3) mistakenly, believe that the placebo response indicates that the complaint is feigned." A sizeable list of warnings to add to the label of this therapeutic dose even when it fails to include the dangers of introducing a foreign substance into a sick person's metabolism as well as a foreign concept into their psyche.

On the positive side, Dr. Spiro suggested that the placebo acts as a symbol signifying that someone cares and is doing something in the patient's behest. This questionable icon at best is simply pleasing, at worst is lying about possibilities for a relationship. If talking with patients helps, and it does for a number of reasons, it is enough to take the time to listen and reply, rather than surmise and escort the patient out the door with a promissory symbol of what may happen.

Not that the physician is alone in suggesting placebos. Again the patient is prone to use the questionable credibility of symbols when seeking a cure for what ails. A patient I saw insisted that she could not sleep without phenobarbital. Our sessions revolved about the wonders of that drug in taking her to an oblivion beyond the insomnia and suffering of her daily life. For me it was a placebo devoid of the ability of relieving her condition, while keeping her depressed and dependent on magic. What she needed was help in overcoming her lowered self-esteem by constructively facing her reality, not fleeing from it. We were stuck at loggerheads, back and forth, with her demanding and me denying.

Finally, I succumbed to her pleas and wrote her a prescription for one phenobarbital capsule with the instructions that it was to be used only when necessary and she was fully accountable to me for that necessity should she wish a refill. The psychotherapy prospered as she explored her fears, now with her talisman that if things got "too bad" she could resort to the magic pill. I altered the original condition and renewed the prescription about every six months not because she ever took the capsule but because she carried it in her change purse where the rough and tumble of coins and keys wore it out. If the lady wished to lie to herself I was not going to zealously preach her out of her misbeliefs; however, neither was I interested in complicating her psychic or physiological defenses. She had enough troubles without adding my ignorance to them. We talked about troubles, in and out of the relationship, with a minimum of iatrogenic symbolizing.

But then what cost can we lay to these little white lies of medical practice? It is a little like asking what harm rabbits do. Harmless Easter bunnies hopping around a springtime pasture cannot be of much concern. That is, unless you own the pasture and the prevalence of rabbits is enough to preclude other species. But in our profligate country the price of white lies may not seem as exorbitant since the complaint is seldom raised to any significant degree. When we look at prescribed drugs, not including any surgical, manipulative procedures or any over-the-counter drugs, it is estimated that between 35 and 45 percent of all prescriptions are for substances that are incapable of having an effect on the condition for which they are prescribed,[4] we have a sizable cost. The lower estimate, 35 percent, of the 28.75 billion dollars spent in 1982 for prescription drugs[5] yields a dollar cost of ten billions for but a portion of one form of medical lying, some rabbit patch that. (The rabbit patch has only gotten proportionally larger in the intervening years.)

Should there be immediate concern about either the harmless rabbits or the white lies of doctors? Ask an Australian who can, with alarm, relate how rabbits have all but stripped the grazing lands of that continent, crowding out other species through starvation in the competition. Ask a nurse, receptionist, or answering service operator about the white lies of doctors, the plague of mistruths, that disrupt communication about patient care and erode medical teamwork. Only an experienced concern which replaces the indifference of indifferent physicians can contain the pernicious plague of "harmless" creatures.

Physicians' Institutional Lies

Few realize, including physicians, how seldom medical cultures encourage candor in dealing with the dying patient. Informing a patient suffering from a fatal disease of the diagnosis is difficult for both the patient and the doctor, so difficult that many believe the issue should be avoided, and physicians are sometimes trained to avoid this difficulty by lying. In fact, some medical teachers, particularly in other cultures, teach deceit for dying patients, which brings us to the institutional lie, another inhabitant of our zoo of prevarication. The institutional lie is a beast that goes where the herd goes and does what the herd does for the simple reason, "everyone does it." It is not lack of brains but "mass think" that makes the "dumb ox." For without the herd, the ox knows not what to do but eat and work.

We can best see the universal nature of such deceptions at a distance and as foreign. Wildebeests, for example, live in large herds upon the African veldt close to water holes and when disturbed they dash away for a short distance, then wheel around to confront what has frightened them with a toss of the head, a wild prance, concluding with a meaningless buck and resumption of grazing.

The largest medical culture on earth in the former Soviet Union may have been just such a herd where the institutional lie flourishes, "because everyone does it." The Soviet medical culture mandated the denial of a fatal diagnosis for any patient, a practice common in other countries. Denial is almost a law in countries such as Japan, where systematic denial by doctors passes as simple custom, the instinct of the wildebeests.

A clinical example, from the experience of Dr. James Muller, a Harvard cardiologist, illustrates both the disruptive power of candor as well as the magnitude of expected medical deception in the name of the patient's well-being.[6] In the course of collaborative cardiological research in Moscow, Dr. Muller worked on a small cardiac ward where a patient suddenly suffered a cardiac arrest. With immediate resuscitation, Dr. Muller saved the sixty-three-year-old engineer but was called away from the scene before he could follow up with more than emergency care. Later the convalescing patient asked him if his heart had actually stopped. The way he put it was, "Was I dead?" Dr. Muller was amazed that the patient had not been told about his condition and of the steps taken to save his life. He explained, "No, you were not dead. Your heart stopped beating briefly during the first minutes of the attack, but we were able to supply blood to your brain by pumping on your chest." He then went on to explain in detail what had happened, only to have the patient hug and kiss him on the cheeks for his help. Dr. Muller was unaware that the encounter had been reported in detail to the director of the hospital who called him into the office the next day to admonish him, "Jim, in the Soviet Union we do not generally tell patients when a cardiac arrest has occurred. We feel such knowledge is often harmful to the patient's psychology, and in rare cases may lead to reflex cardiac arrest." There was no confusion in Dr. Muller's mind about what he should tell or not tell the next Soviet patient he might treat for severe cardiac disease.

My personal Soviet experience was to have the head of Public Health in Leningrad, a creditable source, assure me that a Russian physician never acknowledges a fatal diagnosis to a patient. At times he may confide the deadly prognosis to the family but always on the condition that the patient is not informed. Dying was not a shared experience in that country since all patients in Soviet hospitals had an "optimistic" diagnosis.

Such deception was part of the regular training of Russian physicians. Their ethical education falls under the rubric of deontology, the philosophical study of duty where ethics is the study of choice. The outstanding Soviet academician and research physician N.N. Blokhin has written at length on the need to conceal unfavorable prognoses, emphasizing that "Informing a patient in the last stages of a disease about the impossibility of aiding him is the equivalent of a death sentence and cannot be justified."[7]

This kind of medical lying is not as obvious as the white lie, for it is hidden in the regular behavior of the herd that recognizes the lie as a universal good rather than an individual evil. The fear of patient and doctor together, largely unconscious, is institutionalized into a mutual denial as they shrink from the dreadful news that life is ending. Much the easier path is to play on the survival instinct of the patient with the unfounded hope "that surely something can be done." There is no placebo, pleasure or pleasing, for the judge who renders a fatal prognosis. By the very nature of physicians' training we are placed at odds with such a verdict. Only as the physician is prepared to share courageously with the patient can such news be conveyed honestly and compassionately. The truth of our mortality is ever present whether or not it is denied; the essential question is, "Do we have the strength to recognize it?"

Self-deception, Physicians' Lies to Themselves

Undoubtedly the most difficult lies physicians have to deal with are the unconscious distortions of reality we manufacture to make our lives seem, though not actually become, more tolerable. In childhood we all lie, the peak is between the ages of five and six, and boys seem more profligate with the deception than girls. We lie as children for a number of reasons ranging from simple playful imagination, "I killed a monster from outer space last night," to vanity, "My father is the strongest man in town," to fear, "I did not do it. Johnny did." As we mature in the natural order of things, we attempt to put lies behind us. It is part of the training a functional family imparts to their children. Yet a pattern of lying once established does not go away but retreats into a deeper part of the mind to wait and pounce on the truth when least we expect it, even into our professional life.

In our bestiary, these lies of self-deception are more than rabbits. They are hyenas, stinking, skulking scavengers, active day or night, in packs or alone, omnivorous to the point of devouring their own young, yet an integral part of the world. Because hyenas are retiring and characteristically flee with the least confrontation, like the unconscious lies of physicians, they are difficult to observe and understand.

In fact, physicians' unconscious lies are so elusive I must cite a personal example. Late one night while on duty during my psychiatric training, I was awakened by a telephone call from the duty nurse exclaiming that one of the patients in the hospital had just been cut down after a suicide attempt at hanging. The nurse was distraught recounting how the patient had gone to the toilet, strung a belt around her neck and over a shower stall, and hung herself—only luckily to be discovered by an alert aide. Would I come quickly as the patient was unconscious? I listened, asked if the patient was breathing, and ascertaining that yes, the patient was breathing, explained to the nurse that since she was not my patient, having a "strange" doctor whom she did not know would only disturb the patient once she regained consciousness. With that I hung up, turned over, and started back to sleep. It took a full thirty seconds for me to recognize that my instantaneous, intellectual explanation of why the patient was not my problem was a bald-faced lie. As I pulled on my trousers, I called back, saying I would be there pronto. Ever since then I have remained alert to the "laughing" hyena which exists within me.

Unconscious lies plague the practitioner because their very nature is so deeply entwined with the wish to seem "complete," to have the proper answer quickly and at minimum emotional cost. These lies live on the carrion of our ignorance, so often wrapped in empty medical language. One such lie is that given by the narcissistic surgeon to the recovering patient, "We got it just in time." What a miraculous figure the surgeon appears to be in the eyes of the patient, a savior of science, omniscient and omnipotent, that is, until the surgeon is asked to define "just in time." Does his fancied knowledge of the chronology of the patient's illness permit our omniscient surgeon equal glibness with the other side of his lie? Does he announce to the patient with equal certainty, "We just missed getting it out on time." I doubt it, since it is no longer a preening lie which feeds the physician's unconscious sense of omnipotence. We can safely assume the latter lie will never be heard at a patient's bedside.

But the most common form of this unconscious juggling of the truth occurs in assuring the physician he "knows" because he has made a diagnosis. During the early part of the 1900s, Osler spent a good part of his professional life attacking the diagnosis of "typhoid fever," a diagnosis which had replaced "ague" only to be abused in his day the way the diagnoses "virus," "allergy," and "stress" are abused today. The patient's vague symptoms are tidily wrapped up in deceitful packages to reassure the physician that he knows when he does not know. It is a strange process in which the unconscious lie of "a lot of that is going around these days" is not abandoned until a treatment is found for the lot-of-this-has-been-going-around disease.

The wish to be seen as knowing is so strong among physicians that we often shrink from our ignorance, relying on the fact that the vast majority of illnesses patients present us with are self-limiting. Listening, as a psychiatrist, to a gastroenterologist decry family practitioners for treating gastric ulcers when they should refer the patients to him, the specialist, does little to increase my trust in the man. The distrust becomes intense when he proclaims he knows that 40 percent of these ulcers are caused by "stress" and he is best equipped to treat "stress" with antidepressants. His solipsistic belief does more than stimulate any rivalry I may have in garnering a fuller practice. It exposes to my view, if not his, the unconscious lie of believing he knows.

The great problem with the physician's unconscious lie is how easily it is reinforced by a "scientific" knowledge of the symptom, coupled with an immense and growing armamentarium of symptom-relieving drugs. These anodynes should never be denigrated, sometimes they are a blessing. However, these seductive drugs should always be viewed with a jaundiced eye as potential sources of dependency and interpersonal avoidance. So much so there is a need for a latter-day Homer to proclaim that one and all should beware of physicians bearing drugs.

In my practice the lie is uncovered when patients come asking, "Please no drugs. I have been all through the Valium, codeine, Elavil, and Prozac routines with too many doctors. I want to know why I shake and cry so much." The patient seeks a truth which lies beyond physiology and pharmacology in an area where no physician "knows." Nor does the patient wish to learn my jargon of "identification," "countertransference," and "neurosis," ways in which I might scavenge off the patient's canker of symptoms. To help, I must acknowledge that I do not know the source of the tears and tremors but will share in searching for their true cause. A process of truth-finding that thoughtful physicians learn through grim experience. I know because I have a hyena within me ready to explain why I should not be intimately involved in the patient's struggle with illness.

What to make of physicians' lying? It is an acknowledged, perhaps necessary, ingredient of the practice of medicine. Yet it comes with a fearful price, for whether a white lie, an institutional lie, or self-deception, the alteration of the truth will in the long run lessen the effectiveness of the physician and consequently hurt the patient.

Simple as it may seem, no treatment prospers without trust. Treatment can exist without trust but only to the degree that it is mechanical and thus fails to reinforce the complete healing process which includes the patient's mind having peace as well as the body having strength.

When a patient loses confidence, trust, in a physician there is a dreadful and destructive force set loose which finds expression in more than malpractice suits. Too often the loss is expressed as the patient's diminished self-confidence. There is a dreadful loneliness which goes with disillusionment in those we love and depend upon and ultimately we hold ourselves responsible with, "I shall never trust again." Such disillusionment corrodes all that is healthy in a person or a people.

It is easy to deplore the times, claiming medical lying is an evil on the increase. Certainly the plethora of malpractice suits which rive today's medical profession is evidence that trust is suffering in the practice of medicine. But it is not enough to cry havoc.

Though finding the cause of this loss of trust is more unyielding than simply decrying it, the cause can be uncovered. What it takes is a close and continuing appraisal of belief systems of the physician, the patient, and the society. We must be honest about our dishonesty. This is an initial premise to be clearly stated over and over.

Despite our animalness we need not despair. With all the faults and weaknesses which are so clearly part of present-day medical practice, still the physician can be looked to as a leader in standing firm for integrity. First, because his strength has grown through a science which openly examines facts. Second, because he has a traditional alliance and vast experience with the human condition. Third, and most important, the physician knows, no matter how difficult it may be, he serves his patient best by serving honestly.

The elemental reason why truth telling is indispensable for the physician is that for care to flourish there must be that special form of love called trust. Lies are poison to love and in large enough doses kill. The search for truth is eternal. Together in a bond of trust, patient and doctor have made much progress seeking that truth. We are more open with each other than ever before. Despite the complications of a vast technology and a complex delivery system, we grow in spirit, fulfilling, ever more completely, our capacity as human beings. So it is I share my true belief.

Endnotes

Reprinted from *In Search of the Modern Hippocrates*, ed., Roger J. Bulger, Iowa City: University of Iowa Press, 1987, pp 183-197, with permission.
1. H.D. Thoreau, "Wednesday" in *A Week on the Merrimack and Concord Rivers*.
2. S. Bok, *Lying* (New York: Pantheon Books, 1978).
3. H. Spiro, "Placebos, Patients and Physicians," *The Pharos* 47(Spring 1984): 2-7.
4. S. Bok, "The Ethics of Giving Placebos," in *Ethics in Medicine*, eds. S. Reiser, A. Dyck, and W. Curran (Cambridge: MIT Press, 1977), 251.
5. U.S. Bureau of Census, *Statistical Abstract of the United States-1984*.
6. J. Muller, "Experiment in Moscow," *Notre Dame Magazine* 6(4): 10-20.
7. N.N. Blokhin, "Deontology in Oncology," in *The Practical Physician's Library—Malignant Neoplasms*, trans. through a grant from the American Cancer Society (Moscow: Medisina, 1977).

Intellectual Nemesis

I am done with great things and big things...I am for those tiny, invisible, molecular moral forces that work through the crannies of the world...which, if you give them time, will rend the hardest monuments of man's pride.
—John Dewey (1859-1952)

Unfortunately, traveling in a foreign land makes a thief of me, not a customs cheating, restaurant-ashtray filching, hotel-towel stealing, mincing footpad but an authentic international jewel thief worthy of Interpol's close attention. Let me give you two examples of gems I smuggled out of Mexico, one a rough cut diamond, undoubtedly of great value, and the other a dark opal, dusky, aglow with smoldering, inner light.

The first gem (remember, I consider human beings the most precious of all the world's bounty) was uncovered in Mexico City, on a boulevard to the west of the Chapultepec Park as I was returning from a visit with a colleague in the University district in the south of the city. Ahead was a trolley, an old-fashioned street car, flying down the center of the boulevard with three urchins, as nondescript as cobblestones, hanging on for dear life. It took a bit of doing but my driver, full of self-righteous menace, managed to pull alongside the trolley and began haranguing the ragamuffins. It was all his idea for even if I could I would not have interfered since, unbeknown to him, he was taking me back fifty years to Brooklyn, New York, and the Fulton Street trolley, when as a slip of a lad I had watched with envy as the big kids hooked rides downtown.

The action was fierce for the juvenile freeloaders. They were wildly alive to their precarious ride on the dust-raising, hell-clanging, mechanical steed. All three had their heads below the level of the rear window as a precaution against catching the conductor's eye. In the center was a ten-year-old safely squeezed between the bell and pulley cord. Closest to us, his head pulled in like a turtle, was a nine-year-old with a white-knuckled hold on a bit of projecting wire screen. He was a rigid ball of terror, a mind full—of prayer and panic, obviously on his first ride.

Then there was the twelve-year-old, on the far side of the trolley, the leader of the gang, with the toes of one foot barely wedged on the bottom bit of wheel guard, two inches above the tracks, the other foot raised and braced with insouciance against the trolley's rickety nameplate, one hand holding a rusty bit of ornament and the other free to feel the breeze. His head was low, thrown back, with his tangle of black hair streaming behind, a boy become hero, prepared to take on all the world. The twelve-year-old was the principal target of my driver's blast of unintelligible Spanish and in return we secured a look of sheer exuberance I hope never to forget. The boy had found the last and missing element in his pursuit of paradise, an adult who could speak but not act. As he took in the situation, a resplendent smile transfixed the boy's face. Suddenly, however, our ways parted, for the taxi was forced to screech to a stop at an intersection while the trolley sped on through. In that instant of parting, the boy raised his free hand in the eternal salute of impudence and disappeared into a cloud of Mexico City dust, radiant smile and all, the incarnate, flashing, ultimate human spirit, a free, unbound, master of his fate. There he went, Huitzilopochtli, the humming bird wizard, the Aztec Apollo, riding his sun chariot across the heavens. Though the boy was a diamond in the rough, one facet was polished to incredible brilliance, and I stole it from the Mexican people for my collection.

The opal, actually a pair, I took from Cuernavaca. Late one evening as my companions and I were meandering back from the central square, we passed through some byways, twisted and ancient. I was so taken with the scene, the bare streetlight, the varied shadows, the crazed cobbles of the sidewalk, that I hesitated, allowing my companions to stray ahead. Suddenly I was alone with little to remind me I was still in the twentieth century. I gazed at the walls of the buildings across the street with their worn texture of an old man's skin, white-gray splotches bared from the rough, spalled, sepulchral green stucco, cracks wandering from a worn wooden doorstep up to the casement of a second-story window, scars of forgotten wounds. The rusted bars across the deep-socketed embrasures of the shuttered windows, like the bent spectacles of an ancient man, allowing but the least glint of warm human light to escape into the public world.

I felt uneasily alone, a spectator on the moon, for the gentle rub of my companions' huaraches on the stones had disappeared along with the murmur of their soft laughter into the darkness ahead. Pausing for one last look, I followed the crooked course of a rainspout up the face of the wall to the fringe of light at roof's edge and there made a most frightening discovery. I was more observed than observer. Two burning eyes were fixed on me. Against the muted blend of wan street light and night sky was silhouetted an immense black dog, a Doberman pinscher, clipped ears back, immobile as a gargoyle. There was not a sound. Shaken, I paused, then stole away. Keeping his two glowing eyes, shining with the opalescence of burnished Toltec basalt, fixed on me, only his head moved. Evil incarnate was watching, ever watching. I had unwittingly stepped into a canvas of Henri Rousseau, with the black animal of the night stalking me as I stalked life. Breathlessly I made off for my companions, carefully holding these two opals of priceless chatoyance I had stolen from an ancient Mexican culture. Stealing jewels is risky business.

Like all thieves I must have a cover, a respectable appearance to hide my illicit life. There is no government in the world that would knowingly issue a passport to a jewel thief—certainly never a professed jewel thief. My passport describes me as a physician and my declared reason for travel is the search for wisdom not beauty. This trip to Mexico was to attend a seminar at CIDOC (Centro Intercultural de Documentation) on the over-institutionalization of medicine, a condition Mr. Ivan Illich, the guru of CIDOC, labelled the Nemesis of Medicine.

CIDOC sits high on a mountain ridge overlooking Cuernavaca and could well be the original for a thousand California mansions. A hacienda with palatial tiled rooms, verandas opening out through the bougainvillea and jacaranda onto pools, palms, and beyond to a distant view of cathedral towers, as fine a place for a think tank as this world might afford. The group that congregated were economists, college professors, medical students, philanthropists, homemakers, physicians, social workers, engineers, sociologists, and just plain people. The format was unstructured, a lecture or general discussion, followed by small group discussion, each day for a week.

A lecture by J.P. Dupuy, a futurist from Paris, was particularly interesting, for he dealt with the dilemma of French physicians. These men devote an average of three minutes to each patient, and with the "consumption" of medical services in France increasing at an accelerating rate (pharmaceutical drugs are consumed at a 16 percent higher rate each year) the physician is further and further removed from the human needs of his patients. Monsieur Dupuy showed the coherence of this seemingly irrational condition by pointing out that the drugs are used primarily as placebos, for to remain in practice the physician is forced to give chemical talismen, magic, in place of understanding. Dupuy's book, which analyzes the phenomenon in depth, *L'Invasion Pharmaceutique*,[1] has unfortunately earned him the enmity of the French medical profession. They have declared him anathema, no treatment for him if he gets sick in France.

Dr. Quinten Young, medical director of Cook County Hospital in Chicago, one of our largest hospitals, gave an interesting account of his experiences "outlawing" the seductive drugs, sedatives, and tranquilizers, from the pharmacopeia of the hospital outpatient department. When he enforced his dictum that the staff had to be at the clinics on time and each patient was to get at least twenty minutes of the doctor's time, the interns and residents were up in arms, close to rebellion. He stuck by his belief and, lo, the doctors survived, the patients seemed no worse, and as a minor point, the hospital saved thirty thousand dollars a month. We see eye to eye, Dr. Young and I, when it comes to believing that people are more important for patients than chemicals.

For me the small group discussions did not go well; as it turned out, many participants were interested in replacing old systems with new. The systems might be economic, political, social, or educational but whenever I asked where the patient-doctor relationship, the human factor, fitted in their revised system, the talk ground to a halt. It was hard for one engineer to believe that it could be more difficult for a physician to treat a dying patient as contrasted to "just" a patient and there was no explaining the point. I suggested that when he returned home to the States he visit a local ward for leukemia patients and talk with the staff, but practical advice seems to do little to assuage the modern lust for systems.

One group came up with twenty-one alternatives to present-day medical care delivery, ranging from nationalizing the drug industry to encouraging more volunteers. To me it smacked of more and more systems but I wrote down all twenty-one alternatives hoping to find something of value for my practice. However, the groups proved subordinate to the presence of Mr. Illich, for he, with his book *Medical Nemesis*,[2] easily out-awed, if not out-thought, all other activity at CIDOC.

It is difficult to write about Mr. Illich since he has that rare quality, charisma, and for his influence to be properly evaluated would take a book on wizardry. Charisma is a magic cloud made up of an undefined amalgam of independence, beauty, sex, intellect, and physical and spiritual strength. To watch Mr. Illich, with his transcillient smile and sumptuously modulated voice, interrupt his talk with a request for a cup of water and to see the recipient of his request, a cool, collected, young, liberated, professional woman, dissolve into a simpering female chauvinistic slave is magic of the most personal kind. Perhaps personal distance is another characteristic of charisma for I was never close enough to Mr. Illich to be sure where his skepticism became cynicism. The distance left me unsure of whether I was examining a diamond or a zircon.

But, as is so often the case with travel, the informal encounters are the best. The feasts for example, Mexican green corn soup, as spicy on the lips as the first kiss of adolescence, sultry Pacific squid broiled in black butter, and Mayan chocolate cake, each slice heavy with enough sweet, opulent, degeneracy to bring down an empire.

And the great, good camaraderie which went with the feasts. The Canadian woman's account of the terror of her childhood on the winter prairie of Alberta. She was reared there in a private English school which required a formal uniform while the winter weather demanded long underwear. In the fall the costume was possible, for the fibers of the underwear cuffs had enough resilience to hold the shape of the leg. However, as the winter season advanced the fibers relaxed with each washing and since long underwear lacks stirrups, pulling long cotton stockings up neatly over the underwear became more and more taxing. No matter how careful the fold, no matter how gentle the tug, the loose underwear moved up under the stocking to bunch about the calf. By March, she claimed, her legs looked like they had been jointed to her body by a clumsy plumber. Oh, the laughter, till the tears ran. I thank whatever gods may be that warmth of the heart is yet to be computerized.

Some of the improvised side trips, impromptu adventures, proved more valuable than the sessions themselves. A few of us went higher on the mountain, to a recently abandoned Benedictine monastery, and met the former prior, Gregoire Lemercier. For me the experience was discovering a mother lode of spiritual value. This beneficent man gave us of his time freely to explain his gradual development from a strict monastic life to a loving marriage and dedication to the care of wayward youth. He converted the monastery into a home for young people; a home in the fullest sense of the word. In describing his work, he spoke of his concern for his wife. A lad had left impulsively without saying goodbye to her. "I understand his feelings, his guilt and fear, but it is so hard for her, for she takes these matters so close to heart." Who could doubt how close that lad had been to his heart too?

He explained that when he died the endeavor would die as well. No monuments for him. The last time I had heard this was from Dr. Karl Menninger reflecting on his talks with Dr. Albert Schweitzer, "But the man is not building a school. He is not surrounding himself with young men and students. All that he is doing will slip back into the jungle when he dies." Thus it is that some men look over the void into eternity and, renouncing institutional immortality, waste no time nor effort in personally addressing this world's immediate problems.

How to weave the Mexican experience into a meaning which can be more than stray memories and colored slides? Reflection makes it clear that our world is about to be filled with many more people, more rich people, more poor people, more educated people, more ignorant people, more sick people, more healthy people, more politicians, more policemen, more doctors, and more, much more, suffering. The burning question for the medical profession is not where we will fit into the crowd but whether we will, with rectitude, compassion, and personal commitment, respond to the crowd's suffering. Nor do I mean more medical systems, more charts, more pills, more oscilloscopes measuring pain thresholds—that is our intellectual nemesis. Our unique challenge as physicians lies in voicing the suffering of mankind, endowing the suffering we perceive in others and in ourselves with personal meaning. Can we respond to men as men, not masses, to women as women, not assistants, to children as children, not interesting cases?

I encourage you to join me in thievery of priceless gems which may be found for the looking in Mexico, but if it is wisdom that you are after, you need go no further than your patient's bedside. If we take heart to peer through the multiple tests, the thick charts, the rising costs, the innumerable regulations, to focus on our fellow man or woman, prone before us, we discover the patient is seeking self-meaning, meaning for self. The patient is wrestling with the ever present dilemma of finding dignity in the human condition of rising expectations and diminishing resources. Nor is this too great a prospect—a view shared by patient and doctor of the diamonds and rubies buried in the human experience. The lode is there for the mining in patient-doctor relationships. Let us be about finding and polishing them.

Endnotes

1. J.P. Dupuy and S. Karsenty, *L'Invasion pharmaceutique,* Paris: Edition "Du Seuil," Collection "Points."
2. I. Illich, *Medical Nemesis: The Expropriation of Health,* London: Marion Boyers, Inc., 1982.

Medicine, A Challenged Profession
Molly and Sidney N. Zubrow Award Lecture
Philadelphia Hospital, Philadelphia, Pennsylvania, 1997

> By the historical method alone can many problems
> in medicine be approached profitably.
> —Sir William Osler (1849-1919)

Considering one's own death may be neither a symptom of intractable depression nor stoic resignation but the reasonable acceptance by a wise soul that all must die. Nor does it take a leap of imagination for the thoughtful physician to appreciate how social organizations such as our profession could also face a finite end.[1,2] Much as endangered species lose their environmental niche to vanish from the environment so social organizations can lose their *raison d'être* to disappear into the dustbin of history. Knighthood was such a profession, replaced by more efficient social/technological means after centuries of public service that had brought with it wide acceptance and eminent renown. Comparing the organizational development of knighthood with that of the profession of medicine presents some striking parallels that may in themselves be warning signs of the demise of the medical profession as it is known today.

Considered comparison of knighthood and medicine must initially deal with and dismiss prevalent romanticizing of both. The image of "The Doctor" as a latter-day Galahad is a disservice to both professions. While avoiding the soft ground of literary fantasy, consideration can begin with the historical commonplace in Western culture that knight and doctor represent human beings with a vocation of caring for the weak, sick, and disempowered. However, proof of such an assertion rests on documented facts and seasoned scholarly interpretation. Certainly, both professions are human undertakings with self-regulatory systems based on members witnessing to a vocation. While both professions always attempted to reward merit, in fact, both bestowed, to greater and lesser degrees, position and power on greedy and cruel as well as charitable and caring members.

In assessing change within a profession, the role of professional autonomy in caring, judging the motive in personal choice, often proves a sticking point.[3] An unselfish choice to care so often brings with it unique and perplexing moral ambiguities difficult to judge; for example, the act of willfully grasping or artfully avoiding the extended hand of a stumbling leper. To merit the title of professional, a knight or doctor must freely address these ethical issues. Consequently, professionals are invested by self, client, profession, civic authorities, and the law with independent autonomous judgment. How this right to independent choice waxes and wanes for knighthood and the medical profession, particularly under the pressure of technological innovation, reveals similarities of organizational growth and dissolution.

Elements of Professional Service

Professions are callings that express dedication to the welfare of others through an arduous discipline of specialized knowledge and skills. Consequently, a profession's accepted body of fundamental knowledge, skills, and ideology makes up its ethos, which serves as conceptual center as well as a guide and support for the profession's members.[4] Since so much of what follows bears on understanding the medical profession's ethos, heuristically it is important to recognize that professional powers during interactions with patients are generated by domains of specialized knowledge, economics, civics, and art. In turn the domains of social force spawn "support" systems with parochial stewards. These fields of social force may be designated the four domains of medicine to serve as checkpoints in comparing medicine with other professions.

The domains of medicine may be designated as: the domain of knowledge, formal scientific training the physician must master; the civic domain, the legal relationship with the state; the economic domain, who pays how much for what; and the art of medicine, the psychological domain of interpersonal relationship. The latter domain serves and supports the patient's social position, personal beliefs, expressed wishes, and ethnic culture. Together the four domains constitute the ethos of medicine, a whole greater than the sum of its parts. The whole acts as an ineffable social phenomenon, sometimes characterized as the soul of medicine.[5]

A Brief History

Historical context is essential for fully understanding changes in autonomy for knighthood and medicine; perspective enlightens by focusing on how each profession addresses its domains.

Knighthood, like medicine with Hippocrates, had antecedents in ancient times such as the Batavi, chosen horsemen of Emperor Augustus's personal bodyguard.[6] However, during the sixth and seventh centuries Europe was submerged beneath a sea of barbarians who withdrew to leave the continent a vast desolate wasteland, the Dark Ages. In the eighth and ninth centuries Europe slowly recovered but yet remained a no-man's-land with savage bands of Muslims ravaging Rome and looting the treasures of St. Peter's (853 A.D.). For the populace as a whole there was little or no civil order. Only a few dared venture far afield and then seldom further than sprinting distance back to their local fortifications.[7] It was a time when adventurous wanderers with a "calling," knights-errant, emerged without documented reason. These anonymous pioneers proved yeast for the profession of knighthood. Some may have been among those who responded in 804 A.D. to Charlemagne's call to arms of those able to protect the defenseless Church.[8]

Though modern medicine did not spring from a dark age of culture in ruins, the outlook for scientific medicine in the early nineteenth century was dim, having yet to completely discard the lingering heritage of the Middle Ages with its reliance on Galen's humors. However, by the latter years of the nineteenth century, through the application of scientific principles by such medical scientists as Boerhaave, Schwann, Rokitansky, and Virchow, modern medicine emerged.[9, 10]

The Growth of Professions

In their early development, professions seldom demanded much of initiates. The original requirement for becoming a knight was little more than a "calling" to a quest, much as in the early nineteenth century an aspiring medical practitioner with a "calling" to medicine had only to hang out his shingle to be in practice. Initiation costs, start-up money for both professionals, were minimal. Knight and nineteenth-century medical practitioner supplied the meager tools of their trade out of pocket, a helmet, shield, sword, and a horse for the knight, for the doctor a few books, scalpel, a black bag containing doses of physic, and a horse and buggy.

Both professions originated without benefit of manifest ideology. Early knights, like nineteenth-century medical practitioners, found professional commonalty in a shared, albeit inchoate, body of moral beliefs, their experienced ethos. Perhaps their most pressing need at this stage of development was companionship of each other, mutual reinforcement.[11]

As training increased in quantity and quality, the professions' leaders recognized a need for standards of training and practice which led both professions to promulgate rules and regulations.[12] These in turn became not only the knights' and medical profession's operating standards but also the profession's implicit guide to further development.

Knighthood's strict rules and regulations coalesced into a canon called chivalry.[13] The twelfth-century *L'order de Chevaleri*[14] epitome of chivalry is a clear and detailed documentation of the codification of knightly behavior into a warrior's catechism without troubadours' embellishment, much as the sixteenth-century edition of the code of the Japanese samurai, the Bushido.[15] By the eleventh century knighthood's ideology of service was recognized by Europe's soldiering class.[16] Predictably, universal acceptance brought with it prominent social position and considerable political influence.[17,18] One offshoot of knighthood's growing renown was the founding of independent knightly orders such as the Templars and Hospitallers who undertook specialized missions.[19,20] Centuries later this professional development was echoed in the medical profession with the formation of medical specialty societies.[21] Both knights and medical practitioners appear to have identified with their specialty organization rather than their profession at large as their focus of "professional" organization.

In both professions unlettered practitioners gradually gave way to those trained by experienced instructors. Simultaneously, socialization of the knights with the nobility and doctors with the "carriage trade" brought a need for social skills, if not a heightened sense of gentility. The knights became advisers to their lords while the nineteenth-century medical practitioner found increasing presence in public affairs on school boards and as trusted advisors in charitable enterprises. The interpersonal domain, the art of the profession, prospered significantly at this stage of their development.

Unlike the art of the profession, the domain of professional knowledge and skills experienced steady external pressure from evolving technology. By the tenth century, increased quality of steel required that knights wishing to prevail in battle secure expensive Damascus swords. In parallel fashion, the successful nineteenth-century medial practitioner, keeping up with his times, invested first in a stethoscope, later in a microscope. With the advent of plate armor, knights needed immense, specially bred war horses capable of bearing full battle regalia.[22] This in turn necessitated a retinue of paid followers to service the knight and his increasingly sophisticated equipment.[23, 24]

As change comes with a cost, knights gradually aligned themselves with those capable of underwriting the expense of necessary equipage, a baron or bishop with the ability to tax.[25] Similarly, when physicians, unable to meet growing costs of medical technology, turn to governments and profit-minded underwriters, corporations, they mirror the earlier growing economic dependency of knights. Eventually, the knights' traffic with money, much as with physicians, led to an unexpected expansion of their economic domains. One consequence was the subtle redirection of the knight's dedication from autonomous service into preoccupation with organizational aggrandizement, allegiance to a lord rather than principle. As will be seen, this significantly altered knighthood's ethos.

By the eleventh century and the First Crusade, knighthood experienced significant political pressure from the Church. In the previous century the Church had undergone a profound internal reorganization that placed a cadre of militant priests in control of the Vatican. To accommodate their desire for expanded hegemony, the Curia revoked the previous religious ban on violence by knights to direct it against heathens and heretics.[26] By bestowing the title of "Soldiers of Christ" on knights, the Church gained in two ways.[27] Organizing knighthood as an arm of the Church reduced the threat of military action against the Church's authority. In addition, the edict invested significant military power in the Church's crusades against Muslims in Spain and Saracens in Jerusalem. By abjuring their oath of individual vocation for a new calling, a collective loyalty to a religious organization acting politically, knights altered their civic domain. The consequent political trajectory of allegiance to a religious organization irremediably eroded knighthood's original autonomous civic domain.[28]

Similarly, the medical profession experienced a gradual shift in its behaviors mirroring knighthood's shift in ethos. In the fifteenth century, governments began employing doctors to contain disease, that is, determine and enforce quarantines.[29] However, not until the late nineteenth century was legislative control of the profession vigorously pursued, especially in the United States, to establish a state-licensed monopoly on healing.[30] Historically the state remained uninterested in the medical profession as such except in wartime when manpower drafts targeted doctors.

Following the social upheavals that came with World War I, organized medicine in the United States was seized with a political wariness of "state" medicine.[31] The reaction approached hysteria with the 1920 American Medical Association (AMA) Convention resolving, "that the AMA declares its opposition to the institution of any plan embodying the system of compulsory insurance against illness…controlled or regulated by any state or the federal government."[32] Organized medicine underwent a remarkable shift of policy from a balanced ethos of service to a tendentious and at times irrational preoccupation with political action. The emphasis on political policy so unbalanced the profession's ethos that many alienated members transferred their professional allegiance to medical specialty societies, societies that stressed medicine's domain of scientific knowledge and skills over the civic domain.

However, antipathy of the medical specialists, particularly academicians, to political aggrandizement evaporated in the 1960s and 1970s with the advent of generous national health care and medical research programs. Where British politicians were reputed to have prevailed upon the civic domain of British medicine by dealing with consultants' objections by "choking their throats with gold," U.S. legislators implicitly promised to pave hospital wards with silver by federal "usual and customary" reimbursement for what had once been charity care. As American doctors found their pockets filling and hospital residents boasted salaries in place of the cold comfort of room and board, the doctors were brought over, if not bought over, to join the AMA's endorsement of a federal "war on poverty" and a "crusade against cancer." The switch of sentiments echoed the knights' pursuit of economic security under the aegis of Church and kings. Apparently both professions paid little heed to the shifts in their ethos that came as contractual loyalty diminished autonomous professional power.

Effects of Ethos Transformation

As the profession of knighthood matured, its orders increasingly cultivated their economic domain by pursuing profitable ancillary services, becoming international bankers.[33] Their hunger for capital to underwrite expensive technology, build state-of-the-art castles, and maintain an overseas presence in Jerusalem led to increasing facility in raising and distributing funds, a significant expansion of their economic domain. Inadvertently, knighthood's orders proved to be Europe's most reliable fiscal institutions for depositing and transferring funds, a diversification which brought with it great wealth and an unanticipated side effect, the envy of rulers.

In 1306 chivalry fell on hard times when Philip IV of France decided to assume the assets of knighthood's more prosperous orders. His plan was remarkably simple: cut off the heads of the beasts. With the collusion of Pope Clement V, he invited the Masters of the Templar and Hospitaller orders to Paris, ostensibly to consult about a proposed crusade. When the Masters, bright in burnished armor, arrived with their entourage and twelve packloads of gold and silver, the king promptly had the Masters thrown in prison. It appears he had suspected them of witchcraft, heresy, and greed, an assumption quickly validated by confessions exacted by the royal torturers.[34]

The event came as unexpected news to the people of the times much as the fall of the Berlin wall astounded a later generation with what seemed an utter impossibility, the collapse of a central agency of culture. After due deliberation, King Philip, in *his* wisdom, determined that the right thing to do was to burn the Masters at the stake, confiscate their ill-gotten gains, and secularize the orders of knighthood into his employment. By removing all vestiges of autonomy the King's act transformed the knight from an artisan of charity into a technician of violence, a soldier of the realm.

The Residual

As with most tales of vanquished virtue, in this case of honorable knights, the heroes do not die but live on in myth. The afterlife of knighthood's ideology took the form of a soldier's code bestowed by kings on their employees, men at arms. It was not until World War I, with the Christmas truce of 1914, when German and Allied soldiers climbed out of their trenches to wander about no-man's-land like knights at a tournament celebrating a brief respite, that the last, quixotic shadow of chivalry flickered out.[35]

While drawing conclusions from history is often problematic, there is yet a contemporary ring, a resonance of reinforced metaphor, when "Wall Street" is substituted for "Philip the IV," "inefficiency" replaces "heresy," and "regulating government" is substituted for "colluding Pope."

A creditable interpretation may be ventured. When, as the result of the demands of burgeoning technology, knighthood incrementally replaced its primary mission of service with allegiance to external organizations its professional autonomy devolved upon church and state. With the loss of vocation went the profession's sustaining constituency, the countless poor and sick.

A possible lesson to be drawn by thoughtful physicians, especially by those practicing in the United States with its high culture of entrepreneurialism, suggests developing in the forebrain a profound respect for the capacity of technology to destabilize the professional organization of medical practice. More important than the economic cost of heavy plate armor or of a sharper focusing MRI, are the accumulated costs to the culture of caring. It is a wise profession that checks every column of their accounts—knowledge, money, law, and art—for costs.

Nor is accounting for the impact of technology on a profession simple. Present-day medical technologies are significantly more complex and cloaked than knighthood's technology of warfare. Physicians are not unaware of these as ethical costs but the number and intricate combinations of trade-offs defy easy understanding and direct expression.[36] For example, the patient's immediacy for the clinician can be subtly eroded by involvement in medical technology. Technology's infringement on the relationship has been recognized and discussed by the profession since the introduction of the stethoscope in the nineteenth century. Interestingly, during my internship in 1946 one of the more senior staff members maintained that the proper manner of listening to patients' heart sounds was through a silk handkerchief. A holdout from a distant age, he refused to use a stethoscope and positioned his ear against the patient's chest.

The challenge of technology is not restricted to medicine's domain of scientific knowledge and clinical skill, but bears on the other three domains as well. The economics of medicine has become a mysterious series of esoteric accounting systems beyond the ken of any practitioner who does not hold a master's degree in business administration. The civic domain is a clutter of medical regulating agencies jealously controlling the flow of relevant data from beneath mountains of paper. Perhaps the most acute threat to autonomy by technology is to the domain of the patient-doctor relationship, the art of medicine.[37] Here confidentiality of the patient's electronic medical chart has become highly problematic. Purported safeguards are in technicians' hands, not in the hands of the patient's doctor.

Taken together these challenges prompt a deeper, personal challenge to members of the medical profession: how to respond to preserve a "caring" ambiance for patients. Nor can the response be similar to that of my mentor: we can not dismiss but must use and involve advancing medical technology in care that cares. We need accomplish what the knights could not, maintaining a vocation in the face of overbearing cultural forces. We can only accomplish this as patients trust our ability to stand firm for shared fundamental beliefs.

Countering technology's intrusion between patient and physician demands a strategy of enhanced communication. The central issue for two-way communication is, "What does this particular test, treatment, or procedure mean to both of us, doctor and patient?" It may sound ludicrous to expect a patient to judge medical technology that even the doctor may not wholly understand, but it is not if the technology is dehumanizing the patient-doctor relationship. Instead of a question of fact about technology the dialogue needs to center on values, such as, "What will it mean to you, your quality of life, to undergo this proposed course of chemotherapy?" Thus shared communication enhances autonomy for both. Additionally, this question contains within it another critical question of values for the medical profession, "What effect does this technology have on our ethos?" Beginning with this question our collegial discussion moves to how, where, and why our fundamental beliefs are being challenged by technology. Only with collegial solidarity can we act with confidence and strength to fulfill our profession's unrealized future.

History reminds us that the medical profession is encountering cultural forces remarkably similar to those that destroyed the profession of knighthood. As physicians clearly conceptualize destabilizing forces within the four domains of medicine, there need be no professional capitulation nor ethical compromise to conflicts of interest. Armed with our autonomously established goal of service to the patient, the family, and the community, physicians' constructive response to the present threat of professional diminishment remains ethical solidarity in caring for the patient.

Endnotes

1. E. Krause, *The Death of the Guilds* (New Haven: Yale University Press, 1996).
2. R.J. Maxwell and P.H. Maxwell, "Do Professions Have a Future?" *British*

Medical Journal 315(16 Aug. 97): 382.
3. E. Frerdson, *Profession of Medicine* (New York: Dodd, Mead, 1975), 137.
4. Ibid., 71.
5. R. Crawshaw, "The Soul of Medicine, A Contemporary Proposal," *Transactions of the College of Medicine South Africa* 58(1993): 58-63. "The Soul of Medicine" can be found in part 11 of *Compassion's Way*.
6. M. Spidel, *Riding for Caesar* (Cambridge: Harvard University Press, 1994), 16.
7. B. Kreutz, *Before the Normans* (Philadelphia: University of Pennsylvania Press, 1994), 16.
8. Charlemagne, *Transcript of a letter of Charlemagne to Abbot Furrad, 804-811*. In A.S. Easton and H. Wieruszowski, *The Era of Charlemagne* (Princeton: D. Van Nostrand, 1961), 140.
9. W.E. Bynum, *The Science and Practice of Medicine in the 19th Century* (New York: Cambridge University Press, 1994).
10. L. King, *The Growth of Medical Thought* (Chicago: University of Chicago Press, 1963), 175.
11. M. Keen, *Chivalry* (New Haven: Yale University Press, 1984), 243.
12. R. Shyrock, *Medical Licensing in America, 1650-1965* (Baltimore: Johns Hopkins Press, 1967), 43.
13. M. Keen, *Chivalry* (New Haven: Yale University Press, 1984), 8.
14. F. Geis, *The Knight in History* (New York: Harper Row, 1993), 80.
15. A. Saler, *The Code of the Samurai* (Tokyo: Charles E. Tuttle, 1941).
16. M. Keen, *Chivalry* (New Haven: Yale University Press, 1984), 35.
17. N. Cantor, *The Civilization of the Middle Ages* (New York: Harper Perennial, 1993), 198.
18. R. Shyrock, *Medicine in America: Historical Essays* (Baltimore: Johns Hopkins Press, 1972), 162.
19. P. Partner, *The Knights Templar and Their Myth* (Rochester, Vt.: Destiny, 1990), 59.
20. D. Seward, *The Monks of War: The Military Religious Orders* (London: Penguin Books, 1972), 211.
21. R. Stevens, *American Medicine and the Public Interest* (New Haven: Yale University Press, 1971), 115.
22. C. Ffoulks, *The Armourer and His Craft From the XIth to the XVth Century* (New York: Dover Publications, 1988), 119.
23. M. Preswich, *Armies and Warfare in the Middle Ages: The English Experience* (New Haven: Yale University Press, 1996), 18.
24. J. Keegan, *A History of Warfare* (New York: Random House, 1993), 290.
25. M. Keen, *Chivalry* (New Haven: Yale University Press, 1984), 243-245.
26. H. Lea, *The Duel and the Oath* (Philadelphia: University of Pennsylvania Press, 1988), 33.
27. P. Partner, *The Knights Templar and Their Myth* (Rochester, Vt.: Destiny,

1990), 7-9.
28. N. Cantor, *The Civilization of the Middle Ages* (New York: Harper Perennial, 1993), 468.
29. F. Lane, *Venice, A Maritime Republic* (Baltimore: Johns Hopkins University Press, 1973), 18.
30. J. Keith, *The Formation of the American Medical Profession 1780-1860* (New Haven: Yale University Press, 1968), 32.
31. R. Stevens, *American Medicine and the Public Interest* (New Haven: Yale University Press, 1971), 143.
32. P. Carter, *The Doctor's Business* (New York: Doubleday Pocket Books, 1967), 155-156.
33. P. Partner, *The Knights Templar and Their Myth* (Rochester, Vt.: Destiny, 1990), 17.
34. D. Seward, *The Monks of War: The Military Religious Orders* (London: Penguin Books, 1972), 211-232.
35. L. Macdonald, *1914 The Death of Innocence* (London: Penguin Books, 1997), 3.
36. R. Gorlin, *Codes of Professional Responsibility* (Washington, D.C.: Bureau of National Affairs, 1991), 181-246.
37. M. Edwards, "Doctors and Patients: Facing Life-threatening Illnesses," *The Pharos* 60(1997): 20-23.

Part 11

Compassion Pursued

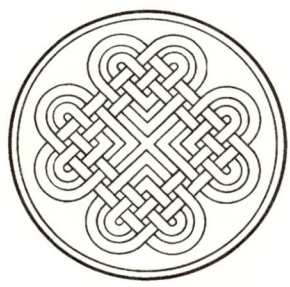

Hope
There is no such thing as idle hope....
The hopes we develop are therefore
a measure of our maturity.
Selfishness, vengefulness, hate, greed, pettiness,
bitterness, vindictiveness, ruthlessness, cruelty,
destructiveness, and even self-destructiveness—
all these are in us.
But not only those.
Invisible at first but slowly pervasive
and neutralizing
came love, and then—
perhaps because of it—
came faith, then hope.
Love, faith, hope—in that order....
...Hope, alongside its immortal sisters,
Faith and Love.
            —Karl A. Menninger, M.D.(1893-1990)

"Hope," Karl Menninger., *Perspective* magazine 3-4, 2001, courtesy of The Menninger Foundation.

Overview to Part 11

A successful pursuit of compassion brings us to a paradox, the prey capturing the hunter. Stalking compassion, like chasing a rainbow, is the quest for a pot of emotional gold. During the chase, shared suffering transmutes any acquisitive desire for social encounter into realized compassion. At that moment of transformation the human spirit bestows upon the seeker the sought-for reward, the richly woven robe of heartfelt compassion.

With profound understanding, **The Great Santini** illuminates how a father's ruthless pursuit of flag, fame, and honor turns itself inside out to become the medium of a son's compassion. As the lad seeks the best in his insensitive, dogmatic father, he discovers the worst, yet by accepting his father's mortal sacrifice, the son's quest becomes life-affirming spirit.

A humble bean may seem an unlikely symbol of lifelong affection, yet **What to Do with the Bean from the Patient's Ear** proves otherwise, underlining how substance plays servant to caring when sharing the balm of healing.

A reliable reference to the compassionate life comes with asking others where they believe their daily path leads. **Fraternizing with the Enemy** reveals a national leader's quest for compassion in health care. Senator Edward Kennedy confides, from his position near the peak of the U.S. political system, that the ancient dictum, *noblesse oblige,* is his humanitarian compass.

Answers to the question of how we become attuned to our personal voice of conscience are found in recognizing that caring, human spirit incarnate, like our sense of balance, develops from uncoordinated instinct. Beginning with a child's heedless encounter with the world, willful exploration gradually shapes what is possible for mature body, mind, and heart. How else to explain a child's desire to precariously balance along a narrow curb rather than amble down a wide sidewalk? Is there a child who reckons the cost of exuberant skipping against a docile walk? Even though reason may triumph, establishing rules for strolling sidewalks, a sense of testing the possible, preserved from childhood, regularly recharges our ability to engage with our compassionate feelings, ensuring an active and refined balance to caring.

Consider yet again the little lass so rudely shoved to the end of the school bus line. Despite the immediate blow to her self-esteem, she regains her emotional balance by treading her way through social hazards to a goal, albeit dimly formulated, of shared support with caring classmates. Thus she gradually transforms the social instincts of a child into the charm of a lady.

By overriding the preemptive social question, Who is in charge here? **Powerless Groups** stands in opposition to the operative rule of jostlers awaiting a school bus. Recognized powerlessness is an exercise in temporarily relinquishing social power and professional hierarchy for congenial relationship. By replacing duty of any kind with mutually respected powerlessness, space is provided in the mind for intimately shared thinking. Thus common consideration can open to unbidden and unexpected alternatives.

Friends of Medicine speaks to physicians' essential need for collegial compassion. Despite a wilderness of organizational neglect surrounding the impaired physician (see "An Epidemic of Suicide among Physicians on Probation" in part 8), a path of enhanced dedication is hewn to bring fellow feeling to abandoned colleagues.

In the marketplace, mercy and justice are easily displaced by the pursuit of profit. Consequently, patients, especially those forty million citizens without health insurance, are confronted with severe economic problems—the means to pay medical bills. In turn the doctor, when acting as agent of health care managed for commercial profit, is confronted with a profound ethical issue, whether to treat the patient as an individual or as a unit of organizational profit. Under marketplace stress, compassionate care for forty million Americans without health care insurance becomes as much an oxymoron as "caring for mankind," extrapolated feelings devoid of context.

The concerned physician finds ethical affirmation in civic action, community-based medicine, when the action is based on a consensus of shared values, such as in the Oregon Health Plan. Then, as a caring healer, the practitioner finds direct validation from community members in sincere thanks from grateful patients. "With coverage by the Plan, I even get coverage for drugs. That means I have money to buy food instead of most of it going for pills." **The Patient-Physician Covenant** explores how citizens and doctors may work together in holding systems accountable to felt human needs.

But then physicians, trained as we are by science to expect evidence before accepting theory, sometimes have difficulty in acknowledging the concept of the human spirit, the ethos of medicine. Aware that there are none so blind as those who can but will not see, **The Soul of Medicine** attempts to quicken physicians' full discovery of themselves as healers, as much in the patient's life as in the curing of the patient's disease. **The Humanitarian Imperative and the Practice of Medicine** weaves the physician's quickening into a global perspective.

The Great Santini
A Film Review

Semper fidelis
  —United States Marine Corps motto

The Great Santini is a fine film, no thanks to Hollywood. In fact, Hollywood wrote it off as a flop, planning to bury it in the "cans," until the producer peddled it to the airlines for in-flight entertainment. Genuine appreciation by a flying audience sent the film to neighborhood movie houses.

The Great Santini is successful for a number of reasons, including superb acting. Robert Duvall should have received an Oscar for his starring role as Lt. Colonel Wilbur "Bull" Meechum, while the supporting cast is close behind in portraying believable people. The photography of coastal Carolina is dramatically evocative; the story is the elemental oedipal conflict between an ambitious father and a loving son; while, like it or not, the issues revealed (racism, patriotism, and family survival) are close to the hearts of all.

The tale is simple. A Marine Corp fighter pilot is routinely transferred home from overseas duty, forcing his growing family to work through a new unity. After three years as a "bachelor" officer in Europe, he is ordered to the Marine Air Station at Beaufort, South Carolina, to, among other responsibilities, resume his role as a participant father in his family. It is a big jump, which Bull makes without much visible effort by applying his set solution for all problems—"by the regs." The family's reaction makes the tale worth hearing.

Bull issuing the "orders of the day" to his children, Ben, seventeen; Mary Anne, sixteen; Karen, fourteen; and Matthew, eleven, as they stand at attention on the front porch may sound like child abuse, but it is not.

"O.K., hogs. I have listened to you bellyache at moving to this new town. Said bellyaching will end at 15:50 hours and will not affect the morale of the squadron henceforth. Do I make myself clear?"

Chorus of children, "Yes, SIR!"

"I know it is tough to leave your friends and move in here. But you are Marine Corp kids and can chew nails while other kids are sucking cotton candy. You are Meechums. You are thoroughbreds, winners all the way. The best grades, the most awards, and excellence at sports. A Meechum never gives up. Now I want you hogs to let this burg know you are here. I want these crackers to wake up and wonder what the hell blew into town. O.K., by nightfall I want this camp in inspection order. Do you read me loud and clear?"

"YES, SIR," answer the children, one just a bit slow.

"I said did you read me loud and clear?"

"YES, SIR!!!" again chorus the children.

"Sergeant, dismiss the troops." He marches away and the children grumble, as Ben the oldest son (Michael O'Keefe) mumbles, "Dismissed."

Despite the noise and bluster, Bull's children unquestionably know that he loves them. What evolves as Bull renews his family life is a style of love that is both dated and questionable, namely patriotic. Set in the United States of 1962, the era of J.F.K., Bull Meechum's patriotism seems to be an anachronism, perhaps even then, certainly now. Here is pre-Vietnam War patriotism, which seems to have gone the way of the covered wagon and fly swatter. Set in the context of lived lives, however, "basic" patriotism may still be comprehended if not understood by a citizen younger than forty.

Bull first appears on screen in an idyllic passage of superb aerial photography—marines dog fighting with a squadron of navy fighters in practice maneuvers over Spain. Here he is, a knight in armor, complete, one with his steed, jousting under a serene blue sky, among immense cathedrals of billowing cumulus clouds, a knight whose honor is tightly bound to victory. Of course, Bull and his marine buddies fix their sights dead center on each and every navy jet. "Kill" after "kill" is racked up by the marines. But once the tournament is over the knights retreat to their local round table, a fancy Spanish restaurant, where Bull acts more like a buffoon than a hero as he drunkenly plays sophomoric college pranks on the patrons. Obviously, this hero lacks much appreciation of the social world that surrounds his battlefield, not because he is ignorant or short on social graces—no gorilla he, but because as a dedicated killer/hero he never sees the world at peace. In his thinking it is the "fighting" Marine Corp all the way. Like many warriors, Bull has his toughest problems dealing with peace.

Counterpoised against Bull's fierce power is the gentle love shown by his wife Lillian (Blythe Danner) and the tolerance of her respectful son, Benjamin (Michael O'Keefe). The believable development of the tender love between mother and son is one of this film's triumphs. Mother and son stand in a quiet bond of tolerance against the father's violence in all its forms. Although never examined with the depth of D.H. Lawrence, there is nothing mawkish in the acknowledged mother-son love that moves them to their mental struggle with the contradictions of family life. Their love is expressed as allegiance to the Meechum family and to a husband/father who is eventually transformed from tyrant to family member by their love.

Few war films tell the silent battle fought by servicemen's families, but *The Great Santini* does. Should Congress ever wish to do justice to the "team," which is a serviceman's family, that great American family with the undeserved reputation for churning out "army brats," they should strike a special medal for the regular serviceman's spouse. She is a long-suffering soul who follows the military's whims for twenty years or more, rebuilding the homelife every three years, living on the edge of debt, and tolerating an iron-bound social system, without so much as a single official thank-you-ma'am. The high emotional cost in shepherding Mrs. Meechum's little flock is talked about in the film but not developed. Lillian unfailingly carries on as the ever dutiful, cheerful colonel's lady. Generally she is apologizing for Bull's gross behavior, but she has her limits, particularly when her son is being taken unfair advantage of by his father.

Benjamin is the military "point" for the Meechum family plan of attack on Beaufort, South Carolina, their new home, for Benjamin is expected to become a basketball star in high school. Benjamin practices basketball with the trained ferocity that his father displays as a marine, resulting in the predictable yet unacceptable. He learns to beat his father in one-on-one basketball. The unexpected success of his son triggers an elemental contradiction in Bull's character: if you must always be a winner how do you compete with a loved one who is better than you? Bull tries changing the rules, and Lillian flashes with such self-righteous indignation over the patent injustice that husband and wife nearly come to blows. Bull then tries to degrade his opponent by teasing his son to make him cry and thus gain a macho satisfaction by humiliating the lad. Since the contradiction goes unresolved the family is left in shreds, but like most families they regroup and go on.

Bull's internal contradiction cannot be ignored, however, for it reappears as overidentification with his son. At the season's opening basketball game Bull becomes so domineering as an obnoxious sideline coach that Benjamin is goaded into breaking an opponent's arm. The disgrace only complicates the father-son conflict, which finally becomes intolerable under the duress of a predictable yet surprising racial incident. Benjamin's Black friend is threatened with a lynching, and, failing to appreciate the seriousness of the situation, Bull commands his son not to go to his friend's help. Benjamin rightly disobeys and wins his emotional independence at a frightful cost, the loss of his boyhood loyalty to family and belief in his father.

The authenticity of the film is easy for me to attest to, as I was stationed with the marines at Parris Island in South Carolina as a medical officer a decade before the Meechums arrived. The film has the full mellow atmosphere of South Carolina coastal waters, with miles of tidal sloughs woven among interlocking low-lying islands. Sandy lanes meander under arching, moss-hung oaks, hushed with the drone of insects; and wet oppressive heat holds the tacky, somnolent town suspended somewhere between the nineteenth and twentieth century. An ambience of genteel primitiveness was characterized for me by the obvious developed style with which the produce man in the local supermarket stamped the heads off mice as they scurried among baskets of vegetables. It is the land where Gullah is spoken, that strange American tongue that has all but abandoned English out of lasting respect for its African ancestry. The rich but shaded beauty of the coast country offers a full but never overwhelming background for the film's human drama.

Should you wish a penetrating look into American military history, the film proves a provocative set piece as a war story. It is almost as though *Patton* were being retold against a peacetime background. The characters of Bull Meechum and George Patton seem interchangeable, down to their overweening disgust for any sign of cowardice. Where Patton struck a psychiatric casualty, Bull, with the same overbearing irrational hubris, drives his son to disgraceful violence. To these men the code of honor is cast in concrete, never to be reconsidered nor adapted to the times. They are leaders who are prepared to win battles or die in the attempt, without the least notion of negotiation or compromise. Except as victorious hero, the movies have always had difficulty portraying this manner of military man. As peacetime men they simply do not fit in, and both George Patton and Bull Meechum perish in peacetime deaths for the lack of a "sustaining" battle.

The Caine Mutiny attempted to deal with the awesome problem of autocratic command in a democratic society—the charismatic military leader. Who can fail to remember how eloquently Humphrey Bogart led the audience down the deceptive path into believing that the leader, Captain Queeg, was mad? What relief the audience felt when at last the court-martial judges saw Queeg's steel balls restlessly rolling in his hands as a diagnostic symptom of his madness. Medicine, in the person of the physician/psychiatrist, got everyone off the hook by redefining the issue not as conflict with authority (the crew's problem) but as madness in a man (the captain's problem). That was answer enough during the fifties, for the Korean War never seems to have been rated by the nation as a war, but as a "police action," exemplified in the films *M*A*S*H* and *Pork Chop Hill*. In the latter, Gregory Peck played a thoughtful but unrealized company commander of United Nations troops fighting an unseen enemy to an exhausted draw; it was as though the problem of command and commanded was too foreign to be taken seriously. *The Caine Mutiny* and *Pork Chop Hill* represent a transition in the development of war movies as well as our national understanding of the place of war in our culture, a transition from the John Wayne shoot-em-up war hero, best portrayed by Gary Cooper in *Sergeant York,* to introspective films dealing with conflict within, within a country, within a command, and within a commander.

The sixties blew apart any remaining credibility of the shoot-em-up-and-save-the-nurse-from-the-fate-worse-than-death war film. The created void was filled by documentary genre war films, each with a "stupendous" cast of Hollywood actors playing themselves, landing on Omaha Beach, or defending a bridge at Arnheim, or flying to victory in the Battle of Britain. The size of war became the principle subject, while the command problem remained relegated to psychiatry, as in *The Bridge on the River Kwai.* As the British prisoners, renouncing their previous lack of discipline, march away to begin yet another useless project, the medical officer makes the final diagnosis of the action, "Madness, all madness."

Remarkably, the exposé films of "horror" of war, which colored the screens in the thirties, did not reappear. There were no reruns of *All Quiet on the Western Front* or any similar films. *Catch 22* along with *M*A*S*H* make a joke of horror. In contrast, a serious genre moved to sicker and sicker commanders, center stage as unrealizable heroes. *Apocalypse Now* plays up a genius gone mad in a manner that is as vague as it is large. In the end the audience leaves with the uneasy feeling that Green Beret

Colonel Walter Kurtz is somehow justified in going bonkers. If Kurtz had only been given his way and allowed to slaughter as he was trained to, the war would have ended sooner and victoriously. It is a theme pushed in *Patton*. If given the gasoline and unrestricted command Patton would have had his troops in Berlin before the Russians, and all our Iron Curtain problems would have been solved; but, alas, our frustrated generals can only die or go mad.

Predictably, the next step up is finally announcing that all military geniuses are mad and thus excused from civic or moral responsibility. This theme was central to Hitler philosophy and may be just around the corner for us at our local movie house. It is a case of not only loving the bomb but learning to love the mad bomber as well, that is, we have all gone mad. This theme is a set piece for director Stanley Kubrick and can also be seen in *The Deer Hunter*.

The difficult national problem that arose during the seventies and that the war films have ineffectually grappled with ever since is that we have lost a war. Surprisingly, *The Great Santini* implicitly comes closer to addressing our defeat in Vietnam, the reasons for it, and the proper way of dealing with our loss than any war film yet screened, a resolution that may account for its unexpected popularity.

It is not difficult to take Bull Meechum as the epitome of the military mind of the sixties, when you hear him address the troops of his new command.

> Good morning. You men have the privilege of serving under the meanest, toughest squadron commander in the Marine Corp. ME! Now, I don't want you to consider me as just your commanding officer. I want you to look on me like I was—well—God. If I say something pretend it is coming from the burning bush. We are members of the proudest, most elite group of fighting men in the history of the world. We are marines, Marine Corp fighter pilots. We have no other function. That is our mission, and you are either going to hack it or pack it. Do you read me? In thirty days I am going to lead the toughest flying sons of bitches in the world. Three Hundred Twelve Squadron will make history or die trying. Welcome aboard.

Put this man at the head of the most powerful armed force in the history of the world, against a pitiful handful of "gooks" running round in a distant jungle, and there can be no question that the "mess" will be responded to by the prescription, "We are going to clean out those miserable boondocks with a few passes of napalm and a BAR." This is the way that Bull flew his missions, uptight, precise, in the military manner. What lets Bull down in the end, however, is not the conflict with his son, nor his own judgment, but the technology. His jet fighter flames out, first in one engine and then in both, and over the populated world of South Carolina this spells disaster for a whole town if the pilot fails to crash the plane in a deserted area. Bull does not bail out, but dying as he lived, a straight-out hero, crashes his plane and himself in the boondocks.

The metaphor for the Vietnam War is clear: it is the technology that failed us, not as it failed Bull in performance with frank misfire, but in promise. The illusion of technological omnipotence led our leaders to believe our nation could run a mechanical push-button war as an all-American sideshow. What started as a skirmish much like Bull's scrub basketball game in the backyard with his son, that is, military advisors going into South Vietnam to help clean up a minor league event, gradually became the most counterproductive military effort in our entire history. The "kids" finally had to stop the war by grabbing their fathers by the back of the neck and pulling them off the enemy, even though it meant abandoning victory. Technology became a fix for our leaders and their advisors; "guns *and* butter" was the policy, when it should have been either "blood, sweat, and tears" or "peace at any price," a decision to be made by the whole family, the whole nation, not just the technical advisors. It is not now important to blame the leaders of the 1960s for their error. That is about as valuable as the state of Georgia passing a resolution condemning General Robert E. Lee for failing to win the Civil War. The important lesson is that our thinking about patriotism has changed forever.

Bull Meechum was mistaken when he saw the backyard basketball game with his son as a simple incident in which he happened to lose a game, much as Secretary of State John Foster Dulles was mistaken when he saw the Vietnam situation as a simple skirmish which twenty or thirty American military advisors could set to rights. Bull Meechum was evil when he persisted out of ignorant pride to "win" by commanding his son's unquestioning obedience rather than permitting his son to judge how to save a friend, much as President Johnson was evil to escalate the Vietnam War after he was elected on his promise to reduce it. When the leader's judgment is focused on remaining leader, and that is what Bull Meechum and President Johnson wanted, to remain unquestioned leader, the result is tyranny, not social good. Understanding how fathers and leaders move from error to tyranny is essential to healthy patriotism, and in the end Benjamin is able, with his mother's love, to sort out the difference and with a sense of loving honor fill the void left by his father's death.

When Bull Meechum realizes his egregious error in choosing to command rather than to listen to his son's need for a greater honor than obedience, Bull pulls a predictable stunt. He goes out and gets dead drunk. But in one of the most touching scenes in filmdom Bull is not abandoned to public derision. Despite Benjamin's wish that his father disappear off the face of the earth, he is told by his mother that he must go out and find his father and bring him home. The moral could not have been stronger: if we are to be patriotic we must forgive those who were unable to forgive. Reluctantly Benjamin searches the night streets of Beaufort until he finds the man he hates as no other and brings him home. Thus he regains for his father as well as for himself a sense of dignity, a necessary part of family feeling and, consequently, patriotism.

The elemental quality of necessary father feeling as part of patriotism was never made so strongly for me as by a taxi driver on a ride from the then National Airport to downtown Washington, D.C. It was in the seventies on a sultry summer evening, when the Capitol buildings seemed to glow not only with floodlights but with the chain reaction of the exploding Watergate scandal. Everyone was talking of the politically linked disasters, and we in the cab were no exception. But this gray-haired Uncle Remus of a hackman said it as no one else could, in his gentle patois, "I ain't sorry for these men. Perhaps they'll go to jail and perhaps they won't. They'll find a way like they have before! It's their kids and their grandkids I feel sorry for. For all their lives, those po' kids ain't never gonna have no father they can love and be proud of."

Our country made a mistake. We became involved in a war we should never have slid into. The mistake was compounded, some say by fighting too hard, some say by not fighting hard enough, but it was a mistaken war either way. Men and women died, and though the war was a mistake their suffering was not. They died as patriots; they died, some willingly, some unwillingly, because their nation needed them. It was a mistaken war, if not in involvement and development, certainly in final defeat, and as a nation we have yet to face up to this defeat.

The Great Santini is a step in the proper direction. We have lost a part of our national belief, namely, "My country right or wrong." But that loss is also a part of a growth process, much as Ben loses his father but simultaneously grows as a man, and this time as a man who is no less patriotic than Bull Meechum but with a considered appreciation of the horror of violence. It is easy to see Ben becoming a career marine officer in the tradition that his father has handed down to him but with a different style of command, as different as the style of General George Marshall, who won the peace after World War II, was different from that of General George Patton, who won a considerable share of the victory in Europe.

This film is superlative in revealing the terrifying ambiguity of violence residing in the human condition. Power corrupts in family life as much as in civic, but that does not mean power should be abolished; it is part of us. The film reveals how we can learn to see power for what it is. If we train to kill, and that is what a standing army is all about, we must also train to "live." Strength without balanced understanding is disaster; strength without balanced understanding of the many kinds of strength and their proper application simply makes us social dinosaurs—blundering survivors moving to final catastrophe. The process of life as Bull Meechum would see it is winning, and he is right, but the style in winning is as important as the winning. A style that permits survival of the humanness of the opponent is essential lest we simply "kill or be killed," in government, in politics, in medical practice, in family life, in all our loves. Certainly then patriotism becomes the last retreat of the scoundrel.

What we have to learn is not whether the Vietnam War was or was not a noble war. We must learn that there are no noble wars and that pride that goes with a war is ignoble. What is noble is the sacrifice that one human being makes to serve and save another, a friend, a family, a nation. That sacrifice and suffering is alone ennobling and worthy of sanctity. Ben sacrifices in trying to save his Black friend, and though he fails to save his friend's life he saves his own, even while disobeying his father. The nobleness of Ben comes not from his pride but from his humility, his sacrifice. Disobedience to his father, disobedience to a repressive "system" in the service of the love of a fellow man, is the basis of Ben's redemption and ultimately offers him reconciliation with the memory of his father. If he did kill his father, he did it as his father would have ultimately done it himself, a man who faced self-sacrifice to save the lives of others.

Difficult as it may be to see the lesson for our hidden grief as a nation, it is there as wide and high as the movie screen facing the audience. It is a fact that we lost the Vietnam War. We suffered forty thousand casualties because of a fatal national weakness—denial of reality. The war was never ours; inadvertently it became our leaders' war. We cannot turn this weakness into strength by further denial but only by relearning, as individuals and as a nation, that we can turn to violence only as we serve and sacrifice in the preservation of friend, family, nation that is emotionally real for us. We can never have an impersonal "push-button" war; technology destroys the soul of the button pusher. National action cannot be divorced from national spirit, if we are to flourish. Finally, we have been called to forgiveness as a gesture of patriotism, by a physician/patriot who sought to bind up the wounds resulting from our Revolutionary War. Listen to another Benjamin, Dr. Benjamin Rush, a physician who served in the army, speaking out after that war.

> Patriots of...1776...come forward! your country demands your services.—Philosophers and friends to mankind, come forward! your country demands your studies and your speculations! Lovers of peace and order, who declined taking part in the last war, come forward! your country forgives your timidity, and demands your influence and advice!—Hear her proclaiming in her sighs and groans, in her governments, in her finances, in her trade, in her manufactures, in her morals, and in her manners, "The revolution is not over!"[1]

So, by accepting a balanced understanding of the lesson before us, that our patriotism can be of the spirit of understanding and sacrifice, not of blind obedience, we may soften bitterness, banish scorn, and bridle pride. Our grief work continues, and Ben, by lovingly filling the void left by his father, leads the way to our understanding. See *The Great Santini* for the deeper story, the undoing of the myth of national hubris, the fear of patriotism that so hinders our continuing growth as a nation of loving patriots.

Endnotes

Reprinted from *The Pharos* 44(Winter 1981): 36-40, with permission.
1. B. Rush, *Selected Writings of Benjamin Rush*, ed. D.D. Runes (New York: Philosophical Library, 1947), 31.

What to Do with the Bean from the Patient's Ear

Every great advance in science has issued from a new audacity of imagination.

—John Dewey (1859-1952)
The Quest of Certainty

The question of what to do with a bean from a patient's ear may seem unimportant in the great scheme of present medical progress. Perhaps it is hardly worthy of attention, time, or space. However, in the coast-to-coast dialogue concerning our national health strategy there may be room to squeeze in a few minor questions among the many monumental problems of managed care, cost-benefit ratios, administration, and peer review. I hope the bean question makes it.

For the systems analyst, stalking clinic halls with slide rule and clipboard or checking medical productivity in the business office, the question of what to do with the bean is obvious: throw it away. However, any pediatrician and most physicians who have done a stint in an emergency room can point out that the bean question has ramifications, for not only beans, both dried and jellied, are removed from ears (and sometimes noses) but also pebbles, beads, lozenges, bugs, seeds, Cracker Jack prizes, marbles, ball bearings, and gems. There are a host of foreign objects which find their way into human orifices and physicians are continually extracting them, often from children. On the off chance that the systems analyst becomes interested in what to do with this myriad assortment, it is predictable he will turn to his computer, feed in the information, and expect a read-out with the precise dimensions of a proper can to dispose of all this junk.

Eventually this right-size receptacle will appear in local clinics with embossed directions for disposing its expendable contents: "When the receiver is filled to the red line, fold over the top of inner liner three times and replace with plastic disposable inner liner #X-22-99."

But how to get physicians to use the can; I mean for the beans they take out of ears? So often a new building, institution, or reform appears only to find little interest in using it. Even with the hypothetical bean receptacle there is more than may meet the systems analyst's eye. Of course I refer to the well-removed bean. Bloody mashed beans are unquestionably for the disposal can. But the intact, barely scratched, white dried bean, teased free in toto—now that is a different story. Intuitively, any physician worth his stethoscope is not going to drop that bean in the can. No, as soon as the patient sits up from the examining table the bean is shared, for mother to look at it, then the father, then the patient, then the nurse. Finally, the physician plucks it up from the pan with the careless ease of a Rotterdam gem merchant appraising a brilliant two-and-a-half-carat diamond. Briskly, confidently, yet with professional deference, he exhibits the bean to the appreciative audience. At that moment, the question clearly uppermost in everyone's mind is what to do with the bean.

Probably the last thought in any physician's mind would be to drop it, plunk, in the disposal can. No, the question becomes, "Who merits this elusive gem?" If the physician happens to be a pathologist there is no confusion, as it will go into his museum collection. Incidentally, I once knew a urologist who boasted a sizeable and frightening collection of objects removed from urethras. I most certainly would hesitate to label "friend" a proctologist with such a hobby. Happily, most physicians displace their innate acquisitiveness to more mercenary matters and consequently display beneficent freedom in bestowing the bean. Their prime consideration is, "Has the patient learned enough from the experience to be able to handle the bean without inserting it in the other ear?" The patient who passes this maturity test gets the bean back, with a short solemn sermon (complete with the tired cliché of putting nothing in the ear smaller than an elbow). While mother turns an ashen shade at the prospect of another harrowing few hours of helpless terror, the patient leaves with smiles, the trophy, and the prospect of an exciting tomorrow at "show and tell."

For those patients who do not pass the maturity test, there is the possibility that the bean will be given to mother, who can treasure the gem in the small jar on her dresser along with a lock of baby's hair as well as a tooth or two. She often also receives a gratuitous admonition about childcare from the doctor, which only sets her guilt at keener edge, leaving her little alternative but murmured gratitude.

For the systems analyst, such medical vignettes probably do no more than raise a smile of whimsy. But before he gets away, there is yet another alternative to consider. This possibility surfaced during psychotherapy, when a patient recollected his respect for his family physician, a man who had cared for him since infancy. The patient put it simply: "You know, he still keeps my pussy willow taped to the chart." In his early adventures the patient had stuck, not a bean in his ear, but a pussy willow bud in his nose, and after it was extracted this "bean" was taped to his chart where it has since remained. Now years later, on each visit to his doctor he catches a glimpse of a bit of fuzz taped to the inside of the chart. He remembers his physician with affection, trust, and respect, as manifest in the pussy willow bud taped to the chart.

Not that the bean problem is a complication in the patient-doctor relationship. That special mutuality is an amalgam of the concern of two human beings in achieving a shared goal. There is reason for guarded optimism that the relationship will make its way through the electronic maze of the future. I am concerned, however, with the doctor-systems analyst relation. They sorely need a common language and a common goal.

I suggest whenever possible that physicians take systems analysts to leisurely lunches and begin building the necessary vocabulary for a genuine exchange. Such meetings perhaps will help, particularly in developing a mutually understandable language. As the doctor shares the dynamics of the patient-doctor relationship, the systems analyst may discover that the patient is ultimately dependent for life on the patient-doctor relationship and, though this vital dependency may not be explicit in many of their contacts, it is implicit in all of them. However, if rational communication fails and the idea remains fixed that the central element of the patient-doctor relationship is whimsy, there are other means for changing the thinking of a systems engineer.

Many voices are in the wind these days exhorting physicians to irrational behavior. There are those who say physicians should run for office or form a third party. Some urge formation of medical unions complete with strikes. Other gloom-mongers maintain it is best to flee the country while there is still a chance. I am not alone in suggesting to my fellow physicians that reason may not be enough. However, I am not one for drastic medicine or radical procedures. Rather than indiscriminate purges or repeated bleeding, I believe in a personal approach which has the treatment match the illness; in this case a major systemic disease.

I do not call for saintly, medical martyrs. No need for fatal self-immolation. But there is a need to make the connection in the analyst's mind between the machine and the human—a link the Luddites made by destroying their mechanical looms.

Why not demonstrate the degree of unintended but real impairment that technology brings down upon the patient-doctor relationship by incorporating "the bean" directly in the system?

Let each physician, once he has freed the patient's bean, insert it in his own ear. Admittedly this final, desperate alternative may sound drastic or bizarre but I maintain it is not as bad as some already voiced. First of all, it gives the physician a handy way of dealing with the increasing demands by the politicians that the practitioners cure everyone at reduced cost. By turning his "beaned" ear to the political crowd each time they open their mouths, he may continue caring for patients in a relatively undisturbed manner. But most important is the long-run effect, for leaving the bean in his own ear over a period of time will certainly cause it to sprout. Just a few weeks ago there was an account in the newspaper of a lad in Chile who had a bean lodged in a sinus, a bean that germinated and grew to surgical proportions. In a physician's ear the bean would naturally flourish, winding out the ear and about the head. No surgical problem here, but a reminder to all that the modern physician has learned how to use his head in making clear to everyone that the elusive bit of synchronized cortical and myocardial symbiosis, called the patient-doctor relationship, should never go to seed.

So when it comes down to helping patients by choosing between a bean in the ear or running for Congress, few physicians would hesitate to pop the bean, even if it means they must make their rounds garlanded in fresh greenery rather than ancient laurels.

Endnote

Reprinted from *Archives of Internal Medicine* 131(1973): 278-279, with permission. Copyrighted 1973, American Medical Association. Original title: "Powerless Groups, A Vector in Mental Education."

Fraternizing with the Enemy

Leaders are the custodians of a nation's ideals, of the beliefs it cherishes, of its permanent hopes, of the faith which makes a nation out of a mere aggregation of individuals.

—Walter Lippmann (1889-1974)

As a physician, I have been tried and found guilty of sometimes saying something good about "those people in Washington." Now I am up on a second charge of consorting with the enemy. I appeal to you. Is an afternoon chat with Senator Edward Kennedy a capital crime? Here let me explain the circumstances. Then, you judge.

Frankly curious how one man could become the nemesis of American medicine and cause such extensive hypertension and insomnia among physicians, I sought an interview with the senator. My goal was not to ask him the routine questions—"What do you think about health manpower legislation?" or "Why are you wrecking American medicine?" No, I sought to ask him what he would do if he wore a white coat and made rounds—"What would you do, Senator, if you were in practice, rather than observing from the sidelines of clinical practice?" The senator proved agreeable and through his medical aide-de-camp, Dr. Phil Caper, put aside an hour on a Friday afternoon, a courtesy to cut my out-of-office time to a minimum. All went well and on a snowy January afternoon I was on deck.

It's strange how much you may learn from a man's receptionist; but I am ahead of myself. Remembering Wellington's response when asked to what he attributed his military successes, "Be Punctual!" I was more than punctual for the encounter. I arrived at the senator's crowded reception room fully twenty minutes early and was greeted by a bright young lady seated behind a crowded desk. As soon as I identified myself, she said the senator was on schedule and suggested I hang my coat behind the door.

Waiting in that room proved a bit difficult, difficult because of the crowded space and the nature of the crowd—people with folders in their arms sliding by people with cartons in their arms squeezing by people with coats on their arms expectantly waiting—and difficult for the rapid rate of flow of the crowd.

I slid into an empty wicker chair directly in front of the receptionist's desk, not out of fatigue but to occupy the least space. A door at my back, a door on my left, a tiny space in front, the high walls covered with pictures of Kennedys and a fiercely busy young lady directly on the right, just one nose above me. The receptionist was one of those clear-skinned, naturally attractive, high blonds, at the discriminating age, a bit beyond thirty, when a woman begins to feel undressed in public without eyeliner—

Suddenly there was a pause in the bustle at the desk. She picked up a paper, put it down, peered over the phones and then down into my right ear. I turned and she surprised me with, "You are here to talk with the senator about health—?" I felt in hostile territory, not quite like a bad commie in the trench about to be bayonetted by a good American nurse but more like last month's medical bill about to be spindled.

"Yes," I smiled up sickly.

"What issues do you plan to discuss?"

Before I could answer, the phones rang. How well we all know that disjointed "May I help you" language of receptionists.

"Yes, if you will please wait a moment."

"No Harry, it must be in black."

"Senator Kennedy's office—would you hold please?"

"I'm sorry she is not at her desk now."

"Yes, may I take a message?"

I will not belabor what follows with these bursts of helter-skelter messages. At times the receptionist seemed as busy as the traffic control officer at O'Hare Airport but she was a master of multiple communication and in the pauses descended to my level, where single-mindedly, as though fending off a pre-senile dementia, I clung to the thread of what I hoped it was all about.

But there were other interruptions besides the telephone—delegations of bright-eyed students, a sorrowful man seeking to get his sick mother into this country—and each individual was welcomed with dispatch, tact, warmth. I simply waited at the interface.

"Yes, what issue?" she asked, coming back to me.

"Well, I'm not that interested in issues. I am more interested in how the senator sees the feelings and spirit of practice that go into the processes of medical delivery."

She paused, clearly I was not spindling predictably.

"Manpower?" she tried tentatively, much as when a foreigner conveys he is unable to speak English and you ask, "Are you sure?"—

"No. Legislation is not my thing. It is the thinking that precedes legislation that I wonder about. I am more interested in how a person would see himself from inside the medical profession looking out. Say, for instance, what would you do with your life if you were graduating from medical school in June?"

"I would be going into something to fill some of the pressing needs—"

"Yes, but what?"

"I guess family practice."

"And what would you do?"

"I would go to one of those areas where there is a pressing need."

"Where would you go?"

"To where I was needed."

"In family practice?"

"Yes, I would work two days a week in a storefront clinic."

"As a family practitioner?"

"Yes, as a family practitioner. Making $40,000 to $50,000 a year, which I think is what a hard worker should make, I could see people free of charge, say two days a week. It should cover the need."

"You would do a general family practice if you were starting in this June and take the money from your practice to open a storefront clinic?"

"Well, women have a great need for women doctors."

"Oh—instead of family practice you would be going into OB-GYN."

"Yes, cancer in women is very important and much research is necessary."

"You would take an OB-GYN residency?"

"Yes, with emphasis on thanatology. We need more people in medicine who understand how people die. They need to die at home rather than in hospital. I would do everything I could, encourage halfway houses, like that nurse in England. We don't have people and places in this country that understand—like that place."

"St. Cicely?"

"Yes, I guess that is it."

"And you would work full time with the dying?"

"Yes."

"Do you know about the toll working with the dying takes, about the difficulties staff members face on a children's leukemia ward?"

"Yes, but I know about life and death."

Before I could ask more, and I have many, many unanswered questions about life and death, a sudden hush fell over the reception room and just above my left ear there boomed, "Doctor Crawshaw."

The senator had come partway through the door behind me, and good general that he must be, had taken me from the rear with complete surprise.

Now, I did not have a myocardial infarction, at least there was no chest pain, but as you might expect from a psychiatrist, my response was psychological, *déjà vu*. As the senator ushered me to his inner sanctum, I caught the flavor and memory of thirty years prior in Montreal when I had to meet the renowned neurosurgeon Dr. Wilder Penfield under similar circumstances. As a medical student interested in temporal lobe physiology, I had sat up in the night coach from New York to Montreal, killed half a day walking about the city before my appointment, arrived early, and was "stacked" by the secretary in a comfortable leather chair in the medical library where I promptly fell sound asleep, only to be awakened with a loud, it echoes in my head to this day, "Doctor Crawshaw" uttered by the unbelievably tall white-coated man, standing before me with his "thousand minions." I survived, both occasions, but I cannot say I ever get used to it. The senator showed me to a comfortable chair. I came up to speed and we were off.

The senator began immediately by expressing his gratitude to the medical profession for the care and consideration he and his family had received over the years. He was specific in his thanks, citing the care his brother, President Kennedy, had received as well as his father, his sister, his son, and himself. The experiences had left him both with the conviction he had received the best and with the hope that all Americans would be treated as well. He spoke with respect, concluding with a plea that all those in the practice of medicine "will give us the benefit of your judgment, experience, and sense of commitment."

Slowly my eyes grew accustomed to the light, for the windows on the gray January day with its freight of snow did little to add to the one lamp in our corner of the room. The senator sat erect in his straight-backed chair, while Dr. Caper and I were as much at ease as we would permit ourselves in our comfortable, deep-upholstered chairs. The room was warm, overheated, and foreign to my West Coast ways. The senator was in shirt-sleeves, armpits stained with dried sweat from what I later learned was a grueling press conference on the just-announced Supreme Court ruling invalidating the elections fair practice act.

Still tense from the press conference, the senator took a few minutes to unwind. And as in testimony with politicians, he relaxed by giving a mini-speech. Not that what he said was empty rhetoric, far from it, but it was rhetoric, a little high-blown for a two-man audience. He related what I have heard from so many legislators, at all levels of government, and have come to categorize as the legislator lament. "If you people (health professionals) would only get together on the issues prior to testifying before the legislature—" Of course, he and others like him are right; there is little excuse for the bickering, jostling, and power plays, the parochialism, that hospitals, insurance companies, physicians, and the host of protectors of the sick indulge in.

Then, as he relaxed I began to see the man, not the television personality but the individual, and the insight was not pleasant. He had the intense, weary look, the face all horizontal lines, of a man straining against a heavy weight. I had met another rock roller, an "uphill" man, a modern Sisyphus, burdened with the unhappy knowledge that his purpose was larger than himself.

"Senator, permit me to change the subject a bit," I interjected. "I am not so much interested in legislative programs as in the spirit, the fiber of medicine. I am interested in what is happening on the front lines."

I asked what he would be doing if he were wearing a white coat in the practice of medicine and, unlike his secretary who stayed with specifics, he responded in general terms. "Part of the problem is the failure of medicine to accept political responsibility, then to see the other person's political viewpoint, and, finally, accepting responsibility, to accommodate, or adjust to, differing views and programs—it is not particular to a county medical society—I see that it takes a willingness to be involved in the policy making and decision making of medicine as well as the responsibility which goes with it."

He paused to catch his breath, and to focus him I asked him how closely he followed his local bar association, the front line of his profession. He answered directly, "In the limitations of time I try as a lawyer and as a member of the Judiciary Committee to be very much involved in the administrative bar—I meet with the American Bar Association and stay in close contact with the national Bar as well as the state and locals."

Then he returned to the medical profession. "Organized medicine has appeared for too long in the opposition, on issue after issue, and in many respects it has been a blind opposition which has meant that the medical profession's credibility has been compromised. Earnestly, I feel that local doctors need to involve themselves in their organizations, to press forward their views, their concerns. Now that takes sacrifice; sacrifice in time and resources, but it has to be done if we are going to make sense of health policy in this country. Nor do I say this in terms of the medical profession alone but in terms of every profession of our society. Citizens' sacrifice for involvement in our democracy is necessary.

Edmund Burke (1729-1797) said it, 'All that is necessary for evil to overcome good is for good men to remain silent.' If the men and women in the medical profession who have the intelligence, the training, the understanding are going to remain on the sidelines, then health policy is in trouble. We in Washington are limited because we are not getting the input. The expression of concern that the country suffers...."

He mentioned his concern about the unfair burden "defensive medicine" placed on the profession and the conversion of the patient into an adversary.

I asked him about the personal aspect of the patient-doctor relationship and he responded, "A part of the present problems in the delivery of health care stem from the loss of personal association and contact between patients and the health professions. I think we should be working to cope with these problems."

I asked him where compassion might fit into all the evolving grand scheme. Without hesitation he replied, "It is an extraordinarily difficult challenge. It is a very special relationship, a basic part of our whole health delivery system, epitomized in the family physician who is there at birth and sees the child grow to full manhood or womanhood. He is a physician, a counselor, an extension of the family—compassion is a very, very important aspect of our health system which is under pressure with the growth of specialization and the problems determining priorities of resource. Compassion is a central element in our health care system, for me it is absolutely so."

Though not high pitched, the intensity of the senator's response continued, direct and focused, and in hopes of giving scope to his imagination I asked, "If you had three wishes for the health of our country, three magical wishes, what would they be?"

He paused, started, then not so much bemused as beguiled he paused again. As he thought, the room was quiet. Dr. Caper changed his position, leaning forward into the circle of the lamp light.

The senator, obviously satisfied with his thought, began, "First, I would wish that the best is available to people in our society without limitation to those in real need."

"Secondly, I would want assurance that the care would be the best. But then that is still part of my first wish." He did not elaborate.

"Secondly, I wish the country was sensitive to the importance of preventive medicine. By this I mean sensitive to the individual's responsibility for good health habits. Health is not simply a matter of the financial ability to pay for health care, providing money does not remove the very substantial individual responsibility for health."

I interjected, "Much as the constitution does not guarantee us health rights, it guarantees us the right to pursue health."

"Right," he shot back, "I think this means some major kind of change in our whole view of preventive medicine—health education—health discipline. We are very far from that."

"Thirdly, I wish us an understanding of our responsibility to humanity. You know, to the extent that we can provide some relief from suffering and disease to our brothers and sisters around the world."

He paused, "Can I mention one other area that I, er, it's just that those were a tough three."

"You would like a fourth wish? By all means."

He smiled softly— "It is this whole area of bioethics, the moral issues which come with medical progress. I think this area is of enormous importance and consequence and we have not been giving it the kind of thought it deserves. We know the human element is being rapidly altered and thrown into the legal domain. This is enormously distressing, the usurping of the human element."

I fully agreed that moving the ethical questions from the bedside to the courtroom was destructive, and the senator reinforced his concern with the findings revealed at his recent hearings. "Phil (Dr. Caper) can get you the proceedings."

The subjects of medical politics, of communication between organized medicine and legislators, of medicine, and welfare-medicare were touched on before the senator brought our meeting to a close with, "Delighted you came to see me. Let us stay in touch."

Then the door opened on the reception room, necks craned, voices hushed; constituents rushed forward. Dr. Caper and I made off through the crowd and finally I was back in my hotel for a pause to think about what had transpired.

What to make of the encounter? What to relate to frontline fellow physicians? The bare account must stand or fall on its own. Though many may doubt the senator's sincerity, much of what he said, about a philosophy of health care, compassion at the center, acceptable good care for all, individual citizen responsibility for personal health, an informed profession dedicated to developing the best for the community, made sense. What concerned physician could disagree with these goals?

But then there will be those physicians who might see the interview as with a charming devil quoting scripture, a man who says one thing and does another.

I can hear them now. "He is out to relicense and recertify; just to start, then, mark my words, he will have us all marched off to some HMO in the boondocks to spend the rest of our lives filling out government forms." Perhaps they are right, but what a waste to argue the point, for who can read another's motives with certainty?

On the airplane returning to Oregon, an idea gradually emerged which may be useful to fellow physicians. "Senator Kennedy" is more than the man, he is a team. Much as a surgical team may be known by the surgeon, yet represent the collective thought and effort of many bright and dedicated people, so "Senator Kennedy" represents a dedicated legislative team and it would be wise for all politically concerned physicians (approximately 99.8 percent of the profession) to consider that man not as an individual but as a team, to be understood in terms of its different parts.

Not that I can analyze the Kennedy team, but from my brief encounter a few broad generalities emerge. First, unlike Pogo, who met the enemy and found that they was us, the Kennedy team is not us; they are unified in their expectation of change, a change they will participate in bringing about. Succinctly they are "for" not "against."

Second, they work at a number of different levels, if I can judge by the response of the receptionist, Dr. Caper, and the senator. Certainly the receptionist's benignly arrogant knowingness, may be easily matched by the acerbic certainty of more than a few Marcus Welbys loose in the husting.

But unlike that pompous doctor, the receptionist speaks for and to an electorate, not just for and to herself. On the Kennedy team, she represents an attitude that people like to hear. She is there with an answer, no matter how distracting the immediate circumstances may be. She will answer your question, but from what I hear the public does not find this true for doctors. The senator's team answers all its mail and I imagine there is a top sergeant on the team, not necessarily the alert receptionist, who sees that this work gets done. How many doctors' offices answer all the questions thrown their way?

Third, the Kennedy team can coordinate a legislative program with a medical philosophy through the work of Dr. Caper, a capable physician trained at Massachusetts General Hospital, and his full-time physician assistants. Not to judge Dr. Caper's philosophy of medicine, of which I do not know enough since he is diffident to the point of being enigmatic, but I can say he is in there working for change. Granted, if all of us devoted our professional lives to power politics on Capitol Hill the health of the nation would go to hell in a handbasket. But think of the leverage should every physician devote a considered portion of his serious thinking to the dynamics of social problems. It is a leverage the Kennedy team has, which in the words of General Sherman gets them there "firstus with the mostus," and not just on election day.

Fourth, and last, is the charismatic character of the team. They are consistently speaking up for the little guy. They voice the hopes of the deprived, the sick, and the uneducated. The Kennedy team gets more than attention, they get the little guy's respect.

There is more for physicians to learn about the Kennedy team than new ways of hating the senator. There are lessons that I have heard voiced sometimes by organized medicine, sometimes by individual physicians, yet apparently still to be learned by the profession at large:

1. Unity of thought and purpose within the profession.
2. Voiced ideals.
3. Direct communication with the electorate, not through representatives.
4. A consistent, explicit philosophy leading to an implemented strategy of serving not the profession, nor the medical schools, nor the hospitals, nor the insurance companies, but patients!

The one central point I have to pass along to frontline doctors is the reinforced, bone-deep belief that every political statement made by physicians, whether to patients, to legislators, to the media, or to each other should literally begin and end with, "In the interest of patients—" If this be professional treason, I stand condemned.

Endnotes

Reprinted from *Portland Physician* 33(1976): 15-19, with permission.

Powerless Groups

Trust that citizens have for one another is the inner, psychological counterpart to social harmony.
—Jean-Pierre Vernant (1914-)
The Origins of Greek Thought

Most formal educational institutions, in my opinion, obstruct the student in developing the most important trait for working with the mentally ill, compassion. I believe steps can be taken to investigate if not to develop and reinforce the inherent compassion in students. Compassion can be feeling with as well as for another, or as Chekhov put it a "talent for humanity." With this in mind I suggest powerless groups as an essential format in mental health education.

First, to illustrate how education may be as blind as justice in discharging its duties, let me relate a personal experience concerning my education in medical school. I took anatomy in the summer of 1943. Because of the war I was an army enlisted man, as well as a medical student. I studied hard and thought I learned the relationships of a number of organs, muscles, and bones. But what I remember now is not the insertion of the gluteus maximus, but the harassment and burden of power problems inhibiting me as a student. I learned that four humans, myself and three fellow students, could withstand the terror of slowly dismembering a decomposing human body in the stifling heat of an ancient laboratory. In our anatomy course it was grades we were after and if we did not have what it took to sustain our scholastic averages, we were only a few weeks away from the front lines. Our appreciation of ourselves as humans was subliminal, for consciousness was focused on survival.

Do not think that our professors were responsible for the situation. It was the system, and our professors worked hard against the power that ground us down. I remember one fine man who made it a practice of giving the anxious student the opportunity in the weekly anatomy orals to ask and then answer his own questions. If there is a special heaven for teachers he should have no trouble entering, for he had compassion.

It took me twenty years to realize that the real test was to survive, not necessarily as an informed individual but as an understanding one. This was taught me in spite of the educational system, implicitly not explicitly.

Similar problems are present in mental health education. Most students enter the mental health field consciously preoccupied with the power problems of educational systems. As it stands, the students are selected, trained, graded, certified, and then empowered to anoint, inject, or intone. The student is passive with regard to understanding, yet active with regard to a power position. The student is led through courses, then deposited in the community to begin the task of slowly dissecting the sometimes decomposing social apparatus. Generally the young professional is left lonely and helpless with the immense difficulty of seeing things as they are, not as they are supposed to appear. Not that the new practitioner is necessarily unsupervised but the supervision is nearly always from the institution's perspective. Too often, training has left the practitioner without the compassion to see through circumstantial power plays to the patient beyond. The passive student once preoccupied by grades evolves into the passive practitioner interested in job specifications and ratings.

As a director of a small mental health clinic, I became more and more impressed with the failure of formal educational experiences to mobilize and reveal the most valuable resource of the mental health worker—the spirit of compassion. Even the most enlightened of lectures often missed the mark, while discussion groups rarely opened a sustained insight into the human dynamics of psychopathology. Personal supervision, the close one-to-one relationship, did sustain and reinforce considered compassion in the students. But the expense in time, emotion, and money—the necessary cost for maintaining intensive supervision—limited it to the immediate staff.

Inadvertently, another form of mental health education evolved, the powerless group, which divorces itself rather effectively from power struggles. This form of education does not eliminate power relationships, but does minimize them. A common danger that mental health education programs frequently fall into is orienting themselves to a presenting problem as a potential source of social power. Involuntarily, as leaders and teachers react to community demands by enlarging the program's scope, they seek more and more power. Consequently, programs attempt to train "more nurses for schizophrenics," "school counselors for delinquents," and the emphasis shifts within the program from understanding to aggrandizement. Consequently, mental health programs often become wedged between the powers that be and the powers that wish to be.

Powerless groups are intended as a mental health educational vector in order to diminish staff preoccupation with social, economic, and hierarchical power that is part of any system of mental health education.

The Powerless Group

A powerless group is a series of meetings of individuals who do not plan to move to any action program in the context of the meetings, but are willing to discuss in depth their role in the community. They seek consensual validation for their position by considering information, conviction, and feelings of three orders: personal, interpersonal, and hearsay. In defining a powerless group as powerless the emphasis is on the external stance towards the community, for internally the group fosters the power dynamics of an individual group—with leadership, status, and role playing as much expected and accepted as in any other discrete group.

The formation of a powerless group calls upon an individual to recognize a commonality of concern and then invite others, often crossing institutional lines, to meet and discuss the concern. The rules for the group are self-determined, while the goal of the powerless group remains enhancing human understanding in the context of the community. Practically, it holds the interest of those who suffer from institutional discontent yet are not interested in rebellion, that is, most of us.

It is wise also to say what a powerless is *not*: The powerless group is not a therapy group, since it is not intended for personal understanding of the individual as a person, nor is it a sensitivity group, which is again largely directed at increasing personal understanding within the context of the group. A close approximation is Alcoholics Anonymous, a meeting of those who have suffered and speak about their suffering without necessarily analyzing their feelings, yet expecting within the group a degree of consensual validation which reinforces their ability to function. The powerless group is not an educational group, certainly not educational in the sense of the teacher and the taught. There is no educational institutional structure to the powerless group. There are no curricula, tests, grades, certificates, diplomas, nor degrees. If any educational aids are used they are improvised and defined by the group, not by a preexisting institution or leader. It is not a social club with pleasure as a goal, nor does it have any peripheral social meaning as such.

The following three examples of powerless groups evolved out of operational needs without a theoretical perspective. I was involved with each of the three groups in varying capacities.

Group one was drawn from approximately thirty-five staff members of a girls' residential psychiatric care institution. The institution was in the throes of a severe administrative crisis. It was changing basic precepts from custodial to treatment, as well as experiencing considerable change of staff. Powerless meetings were offered, by me, to the members of the institution with the provisions (1) that meetings not be held in the institution as this might inhibit the discussions, (2) that meetings would follow regular timing, 11:30 to 1:00, bimonthly, and (3) that attendance was absolutely voluntary, with no administrative coercion, including tacit.

Individuals who were interested brought their own sack lunches to a mental health clinic six miles away from the institution. There was no agenda for the meetings, which continued for twenty-four months. The attendance varied from a low of five to a high of twenty-five. Participants from the institution included the chief of social work, a number of social workers, social work students, nuns of the religious order that ran the institution, college girls who acted as housemothers and counselors, the business manager, the telephone operator, receptionist, and volunteers. At first, discussions centered on clinical observations of specific patients but with time they enlarged to general problems. Subjects ranged from the runaway, Christmas in an institution, and the troublemaker, to general staff problems, intrastaff rivalry, interprofessional rivalry, and supervisor-supervisee friction, to the ultimate subject, the goals of the institution as perceived by the staff. As the crisis in the institution resolved, the need for the powerless group subsided and by mutual agreement discontinued.

The second group consisted of senior professionals in mental health in the state of Oregon. Its self-imposed structure included three social workers, three psychologists, and three psychiatrists. The group met for dinner one evening a month without an agenda. Occasionally, state representatives and public officials attended meetings as guests. Most group discussion revolved about consensual validation in a power-free environment. In a sense it might be called a gossip or bull session but it was much more than that. It was a place where leaders in the mental health field could check on what the others were thinking about. Though projects were suggested, it appeared the members had adequate access to power-oriented groups elsewhere. As one member said, sitting down to dinner, "What a relief to go to a meeting where I do not have to come up with a program, be on a committee, or raise money." No demands for power were placed on any members. Each paid for their dinner and the organization existed for their needs, not for itself.

Externally the group appeared to be powerful. At one meeting a state senator remarked, "You probably do not realize it but one of the main reasons that mental health legislation fails is the diversity of professional opinion. If you professionals do not get together, how can you expect the legislature to justify spending tax money? However, if you get together, the way you seem to here—nobody can stop you." He saw the group as potentially powerful and with his political mind wondered when it would move into action.

Group three was made up of first-line personnel from the helping agencies of a county of one hundred thousand. This group originated when I, as director of the local mental health clinic, realized that those who appeared to profit most by clinic staffing sessions were visiting first-line helping personnel of the county. Therefore, I wrote the heads of the helping agencies in the county (health, welfare, and the juvenile court) offering to meet with any of their staff who might wish to discuss human problems in our county. The meetings were held on a bimonthly basis, from 11:30 to 1:00, with the participants bringing their sack lunches. The meeting place was the office of the local federal agency for the poor, the Community Action Program, a "neutral" site in the community power structure. Again, attendance was strictly voluntary. Anyone involved in any of the helping agencies was free to come to introduce any subject. A wide range of subjects evolved, discussions of team dynamics, of the psychology of the unwed mother, actual informed discussion between a welfare caseworker and his client at one meeting, presentations by the county fathers on particular helping programs, study of local clinic utilization problems—who does and does not care for care.

Group three's membership included welfare caseworkers, indigent nonprofessionals from the Community Action Program organization, public health nurses, and occasionally members of the sheriff's office, the juvenile authority, and the educational services. The attendance ranged from as few as eight to as many as sixty.

Of all the powerless groups, group three was closest to community power and had the greatest difficulty in finding itself as a powerless group. Calls for action, here and now, repeatedly interrupted the group process. In one of the presentations by an invited county official, he forcefully declared that to be effective the group had, whether it liked it or not, to become a political force. During this discussion many members agreed that the very nature of the beast meant that the group must move to an action-oriented position. Nor was the problem resolved by some members claiming that the group was just an "empty do-nothing, hot-air outfit" (yet they showed up repeatedly to denounce it), while others felt that the value of the group lay in not having to go any place. The struggle around group structure, as contrasted to process, became so intense that a steering committee was appointed by the group, though who and where it was to steer was left undefined. To this observer, it seemed the members were so accustomed to a power orientation that they were confused and could not tolerate the concept of powerlessness.

Results

The three powerless groups described above produced:

1. A specific, unique form of interpersonal interaction characterized by candid observations of social conditions as they are. The interaction seemed to quickly unburden the participant of commonplace preoccupations, offering an opportunity to examine fundamental beliefs in a benign, nonpunishing atmosphere.

2. Continuity of the group that did not appear artificial nor coerced by external sources expecting "power."

3. A unique form of small group dynamics. Though this has not been scientifically evaluated, it appears unusual,

particularly in the way leadership shifted to where it was needed, while initiative sprang directly from need.

Groups have structure and process, as well as an interface with the society within which they exist. Much group structure and process is determined by the interface conditions. The more social and economic power displayed at the interface, the more internal group energy is bound to group response (for example, an infantry squad, where internal dynamics are stereotyped in service to maintaining maximum available force at the interface with larger organizations). Thus mental health organizations' power-oriented programs, including education, counterproductively display their own weakness. Each can quickly generate an establishment, complete with zealots, workers, tag-alongs, and victims, who direct considerable group attention towards the interface. Too often with such programs, a "humanizing" system of mental health education initiates dehumanization in its staff.

Powerless groups should be fostered and studied for their internal dynamics and effectiveness, since they appear to encourage intuition, reflection, conviction, and compassion in contrast to *power* groups which develop logic, orientation, force, and enthusiasm. By their unique internal freedom, powerless groups are a potential tool for revealing and mobilizing the innate compassion of mental health students.

Endnotes

Reprinted from *American Journal of Psychiatry* 125 (#7)(1969). Original title: "Powerless Groups, A Vector in Mental Education."

Friends of Medicine

What keeps us from opening our hearts to our friends is less our mistrust of them than of ourselves.
—François La Rochefoucauld (1613-1680)

Fortunately, the humanity of doctors is more often recognized in their strengths than weaknesses. The doctor is looked to for leadership, forbearance, intelligence, and wisdom, but, unhappily, the expectation is not always fulfilled. The doctor who displays appetites where he is expected to abstain, ignorance when he should know, or weakness when he should be strong, is a persistent problem to patients, colleagues, and society. The experience of Oregon's doctors in meeting this problem through the Friends of Medicine moves from speculation to experience in engaging with dysfunctional doctors.

Beginnings

The Friends of Medicine began in 1968 with a letter from a local doctor to the county medical society. He shared his deep concern for a colleague of many years who appeared to be deteriorating. He gave examples of his colleague's poor medical judgment, his incompetence, his loss of friends and hospital privileges. The writer wondered if a committee existed within the government of medicine to help this man before he took a final plunge into professional oblivion. The letter stirred deep feelings in the society's members and administrative staff.

The horrid and sometimes terrifying experience of standing by to watch a colleague fray his life to shreds was too common; but what could be done? How could we protect him and his patients from his destructive behavior? The letter's clear plea to help the doctor and protect his patients was the beginning of the Friends of Medicine.

The initial group, the Committee of Concern, was led by a doctor, not the author, who well knew the desperate problems that illness and poor judgment had brought down on the heads of fellow doctors. He had spent years as a member of the state board of medical examiners, that window on personal and professional tragedy, and was aware that one in ten of Oregon's doctors appeared before the board during their professional life. He had heard doctors' spouses pleading that their alcoholic husbands be given yet another chance. He knew the dilemma of choosing between depriving isolated rural communities of their only direct medical care and exposing them to the danger and misery of incompetent care. Having lived through all this, he wanted more than discipline for disabled doctors, and the committee crystallized around this wish.

The backgrounds of the members were diverse: a professor of family medicine; a former president of the state medical association; a radiologist; a general practitioner who had served as president of the local medical society; a psychiatrist with the state board of medical licensure; a general practitioner who was the chairman of the state committee on professional care; a psychiatrist interested in the iatrogenic problems of the medical profession; the executive officer of the medical society—an internist interested in developing new modes of communication within the government of medicine; an internist interested in the future planning of the state medical society; a retired ophthalmologist who had served on the Oregon Medical Association's committees for many years; and a surgeon with wide experience in rural medicine.

After considerable discussion a strong consensus developed that no additional medical regulatory bodies were needed in Oregon. The state board of medical licensure, emerging peer review committees in hospitals, and county medical societies appeared to offer more than enough regulators. To a man, the group declined any regulatory punitive role.

Further agreement centered on the need for trust. Success depended on the members understanding their relationship with the group as confidential, and knowing it would remain inviolate. The members expected the records would be minimal, confidential, and inaccessible to all but the record keeper. Cross-checking within the profession and, worse, gossip could undermine an already weak man or woman. The committee decided to remain independent of all other medical and governmental organizations while carefully examining its membership for conflicts of interest and information. At this point, the member who was also a member of the state board of medical licensure resigned, promising to rejoin once free of any conflict of interest.

Growth

In eight years the organization grew, if not flourished, as its work unfolded as an educational institution with conferences, lectures, and research fostering enlightened consideration for the plight of the disabled doctor. Persistent emphasis was placed on ensuring that the disabled doctor was not condemned out of hand but understood as a person in need. Special attention was devoted to recognizing and treating the drug- and alcohol-dependent doctor, including a statewide conference on alcoholism to which doctors of national prominence in treating these problems were invited. The chronic problem of doctors' reluctance to act as their brother's keeper was repeatedly addressed through articles and lectures.

The state medical society's auxiliary, the spouses' organization, was encouraged to develop techniques in detecting and helping the family of the disabled doctor. They undertook an extensive and confidential investigation of family life among the state's doctors, touching on the time spent at home, satisfactions and dissatisfactions, the consumption of alcohol, and the presence of recognized yet unresolved problems. The survey findings galvanized them into reaching out to the dysfunctional "medical" family.

Aims

A conference on the disabled doctor sponsored by the Oregon Medical Association served as an example of our increasing skill in educating ourselves. The conference ran for three days, over a weekend, focusing on physician support systems. The first day was limited to members of the Friends of Medicine, who prepared themselves to lead small group discussions. Approximately 150 doctors and spouses participated in the discussions during the next two days.

The conference goals included: (1) increased awareness among professionals of the problems of the disabled doctor, with an enhanced referral system; (2) increased coordination of support systems; (3) research into specific problems; and (4) improved quality of care for patients/ physicians.

The second day focused on defining the incompetent physician as intellectually, morally, and emotionally impaired. Through candid discussion the conference uncovered values for judging impaired doctors.

Sources of support for the disabled doctor came next. The list included: (1) Oregon Board of Medical Examiners; (2) medical school; (3) hospital staffs; (4) hospital administrators; (5) medical societies—general and specialty; (6) professional service review organization; (7) Friends of Medicine; (8) other health professions (nurses, psychologists); (9) the doctor's family; and (10) medical society auxiliaries.

In addition to conferences and education, the Friends of Medicine aimed at developing research. A study of an epidemic of suicides among a discrete group of doctors was targeted. In two years, eight physicians on probation with the state board of medical licenses had committed suicide, and two others had made serious suicidal attempts. This represented an exceptionally high death rate, about 150 times the expected figure. The Friends of Medicine encouraged a team of psychologists, psychiatrists, and medical sociologists to uncover the cause or causes of this tragedy.

The Friends of Medicine also acted by helping disabled doctors through an informal network of senior doctors. When a doctor considered himself in trouble or was recognized by a colleague as struggling with an overwhelming personal problem, he could confidentially contact anyone in the "network." The message passed to the leader of the Friends of

Medicine, who judged the best approach, often by discussion with a small group of the Friends. Then, working with the disabled doctor himself, and his friends and family, the members set to work mobilizing professional and financial resources of the medical community.

Sometimes securing a less demanding position for an overextended doctor while offering an opportunity for supervision in an understanding and less threatening assignment made the difference. Helping a destitute doctor, reduced to accepting state welfare, find sustaining work commensurate with his reduced ability restored dignity, self-esteem, and productivity. In other cases, where psychiatric help was indicated for an emotionally disturbed doctor, a referral was the beginning of recovery.

Certainly not all doctors followed recommendations, but the disabled doctor is often profoundly grateful that someone cares. The Friends of Medicine were repeatedly successful in making the doctor aware of a problem before a disaster occurred. The disabled doctor was relieved of professional loneliness, a common accompaniment to slipping downhill.

Because of the sensitive nature of the direct work with disabled doctors, the Friends of Medicine abandoned recordkeeping. Consequently, no recorded experiences remain for statistical evaluation. The general impression of years of work is that the effort of the Friends of Medicine resulted in a discernible improvement in the doctors' service to patients in Oregon.

Increasingly, controls are placed on the practice of medicine to ensure the quality of health care. Most controls are intended to detect, rehabilitate, or eliminate the disabled doctor. Unfortunately, most of these controls are formal and coercive rather than informal and trusting. Throwing the book at a doctor in difficulty should never be confused with offering a lifeline.

The Friends of Medicine was an organization of doctors that attempted to detect, in an informal and confidential way, the disabled doctor at an early point. It then aimed to rehabilitate the doctor with minimal loss of self-esteem, professional status, and service to community. The Friends of Medicine had some success, both through direct service and by increasing the profession's awareness of the social and psychological problems of the disabled doctor. As other institutions followed the lead in helping the doctor in distress, the Friends of Medicine quietly withdrew from the scene.

Endnotes

Reprinted, with permission, from *British Medical Journal* 2(6186, 1979): 372-373, the BMJ Publishing Group, and from *Portland Physician* 28 #10(1973):6-8.

The Patient-Physician Covenant

The tree is known by its fruit.
—Matthew 12:33

Medicine is, at its center, a moral enterprise grounded in a covenant of trust. This covenant obliges physicians to be competent and to use their competence in the patient's best interests. Physicians, therefore, are both intellectually and morally obliged to act as advocates for the sick wherever their welfare is threatened and for their health at all times.

Today this covenant of trust is seriously threatened. From within, there is growing legitimation of the physician's materialistic self-interest; from without, for-profit forces press the physician into the role of commercial agent to enhance the profitability of health care organizations. Such distortions of the physician's responsibility degrade the patient-physician relationship that is the central element and structure of clinical care. To capitulate to these alterations of the trust relationship is to significantly alter the physician's role as healer, carer, helper, and advocate for the sick and for the health of all.

By its traditions and very nature, medicine is a special kind of human activity—one that cannot be pursued effectively without the virtues of humility, honesty, intellectual integrity, compassion, and effacement of excessive self-interest. These traits mark physicians as members of a moral community dedicated to something other than its own self-interest.

Our first obligation must be to serve the good of those persons who seek our help and trust us to provide it. Physicians, as physicians, are not, and must never be, commercial entrepreneurs, gateclosers, or agents of fiscal policy that runs counter to our trust. Any defection from primacy of the patient's well-being places the patient at risk by treatment that may compromise quality of or access to medical care.

We believe the medical profession must reaffirm the primacy of its obligation to the patient through national, state, and local professional societies; our academic, research, and hospital organizations; and especially through personal behavior. As advocates for the promotion of health and support of the sick, we are called upon to discuss, defend, and promulgate medical care by every ethical means available. Only by caring and advocating for the patient can the integrity of our profession be affirmed. Thus we honor our covenant of trust with patients.

Endnotes

Reprinted from *Journal of the American Medical Association* 273(1995): 1553, with permission. Coauthors: D.E. Rogers, E.D. Pellegrino, R.J. Bulger, G.D. Lundberg, L.R. Bristow, C.K. Cassel, and J.A. Barondess.

The Soul of Medicine

Hence the soul must be a substance in the sense of the form of a natural body having life potentially within it.
—Aristotle (383-322 B.C.)
On the Soul

Medical talk of soul, often seen as arcane, airy speculation, can lead to practical clinical insights and behaviors. Comparing medical thinking in the recent past, the distant past, and today should enhance appreciation of the role of the soul of medicine. By comparing how practitioners thought then and think now, greater certainty can be had in judging the essence of our profession today. Then from a renewed vision of what we are about, the soul of medicine, we can explore a strategic approach for our mission in the daily practice of medicine, or so I hope to convince hands-on practitioners.

Background from the Last Century

Sir William Osler, our esteemed teacher, offers a sure beginning when considering our profession's search for identity. He, in particular, would rise to the challenge of identifying who we are and what we are about. In fact, Osler's last lecture, "The New Science and the Old Humanism," addresses this question poignantly.[1] It was a brave address for, though he does not mention it, his beloved only child, Revere, serving as a British artillery officer in World War I, had been killed at the front the year before. Osler's grief is transmuted, as a complete physician's should be, into reflections on what is best for survivors. He addresses his audience realistically, not optimistically, as practical men and women facing "changed conditions with the reinforcement of hope or with the strong resolution of despair."

Osler cites the phenomenal changes brought about in his lifetime by progress in science. These developments amazed him much as advances in nuclear physics and computers amaze us. He does homage to the undeniable benefits mankind owes to science. Then, on a somber note, he reports how scientists became part of the national hysteria of World War I, recently paralleled, although largely unremarked, by medical scientists and their organizations who irrationally pursued academic sanctions.[2] Where contemporary scientists supply "smart" bombs and nuclear weapons, Osler focuses on the development of toxic gas and aerial bombing as scientific weapons of destruction. Aware of the horrifying scope of man-made violence he acknowledges physicians' culpability for contributing to a misguided sense of humanity.

With stark courage Osler challenges the scholars of Oxford University by calling the academic world to question. In measured words he underlines liberal education's failure to forge a clear ethical path for the medical profession into the twentieth century.

For Osler the profession's central problem, which I believe to be ours as well, is clarifying and declaring our relevant and inclusive principles of practice. In a word, the Hippocratic oath no longer suffices for him, nor for us, as adequate foundation in determining who we practitioners are and how we should but serve patients.

Osler proposed a nineteenth-century dynamic of medical practice— the humane balance of art and science. Osler's vision of the complete physician wisely balancing medical science with clinical art failed to anticipate the world in the twenty-first century in which we practice. His dynamic no longer rings true for us.

Today the dynamic of medical practice is so far askew it is difficult to appreciate that art once balanced with science. Today practitioners are preoccupied with science, medical advances, or economics, corporatization of health care delivery. Physicians no longer have a functional concept of the art of medicine. To understand the present dislocation, our professional development and thinking must be reexamined. We must take up Osler's challenge to reconsider the essence of our profession, the soul of medicine.

Present Thinking

A major reason for the profession's present reluctance to examine our soul may be traced to the emergence of experimental clinical medicine. In 1616, with Harvey's demonstration of the circulation of blood, medical thinking began to shift to a new paradigm. Scholastic deduction from philosophical hypothesis gave way to inductive reasoning based on experimentally validated evidence, the scientific method. At first imperceptibly, physicians reoriented their thinking; some 350 years later the scientific method brought universal acceptance of transmission of infection by germs and viruses, not bad air.

Like most methods, however, the scientific one supporting medical science has its shortcomings, if not flaws. Brilliant in describing specific outcomes, the scientific method is deficient in attributing human values to its findings. The scientific method fine-tunes the practitioner's thinking, asking for quantities while ignoring qualities. Measurements are sought—what is the cholesterol level, the partial pressure of blood gases, the degree of malignancy of a tumor—before, and sometimes to the exclusion of, the experienced meaning of the illness to the patient.

Implacably, pointed questions of medical science also narrow practitioners' vision to ever diminishing units of matter, organs, cells, and molecules. The "agreed upon fact" becomes the fulcrum of clinical thinking about the illness, while willy-nilly leaving the patient on the periphery. Following medical science's lead, present-day medical practice focuses on the physical findings, offering minimal perspective on the patient as a person, the community as a community, or the world as a human experience.

In contrast, the ancients postulated the primary life principle, the soul, as their central "agreed upon fact" from which they deduced a theory of therapeutics focusing on the actual life of the patient. Though the Hippocratic theory of therapeutics with its calibrations of diet and daily routine towards reestablishing health equilibrium to the patient's humors has little or no substance for us, the approach did frame useful questions for physicians to relate to patients as sick fellow human beings. Thus Hippocrates brought epilepsy under the aegis of medicine and into a world shared by doctor and patient, by construing it as a secular not sacred disease. The ancient theory of medicine—valuing the patient as an individual with soul—remains so powerful that two thousand years later the medical profession, perforce, respects the Hippocratic oath, narrow and misty window that it is, when searching for first principles of ethical behavior for the twenty-first century.

As curiosity about soul served the Hippocratic practitioner, so a revived curiosity about the soul of medicine may serve present-day practitioners in thinking out fundamental causes of our professional dis-ease. Searching questions are needed, not about fire and vapors, the ancient's approach to metabolism and pulmonary function, but about the medical profession's role in preauthorized surgery, malpractice insurance, managed care, the business of medicine, and the growing angst of patients.

Granted, miraculous medicine pours forth from an incredible cornucopia of medical science, yet it eschews clarifying first principles of practice. Today scientific reductionist philosophy offers no comfort and little direction to a practitioner contending with our complex and threatening world. Unlike ancient medicine, scientific medicine does not speak to the growing experiential distance between patient and doctor.

One confounding result of the depersonalized philosophy of science is physicians' loss of practical control over important aspects of patient care. Hypertrophied medical science permits, if not encourages, the control of clinical service shifting from the aegis of doctors to nonmedical personnel. Motivated as the new medical stewards of care are by the discrete goals of their particular service, they impose themselves, sometimes between doctor and patient. Significant areas of medical economics, health administration, professional discipline, and clinical support services recede from doctors' control. Resulting confusion generates acute social and political conflicts for doctors in serving patients' needs. Nor can exaggerated claims for science's powers to cure be expected to correct the profession's problem of diminishing leadership in serving patients.

Expanded Thinking

Reflection reveals that the concept of "soul" can be as meaningful to medical practice as is the concept of "mind." Who can question that a soulless profession would be any less flawed than a mindless one? Yet it should be emphasized that transferring the concept of soul from individual human beings as the ancients conceived it, to a social organization, the medical profession, was not a literary sleight of hand, a clutter of words confounding a confusion of meaning. In common parlance, speaking of the soul of a people or nation carries the meaning of the essence of that group's being and individuality. Thus the soul of medicine speaks for the profession's essence, its ethos.

Clinical application of the concept of soul starts with metaphysics, a study defined by Aristotle as the reality that exists above and beyond the material world. A simple example should make this clear. Danish community nurses have set themselves the task of clarifying the "invisible" work of caring. They seek to make the "invisible" world of caring recognizable to their larger world, the bureaucratic health delivery system dominating their professional lives. They do not believe every professional act of caring for a patient can be measured in physical, budgetary, or administrative terms. For them much of authentic caring lies outside cookbook prescription, passed over by the systems analyst, "invisible" to administrative eyes, "intangible" to budget makers.

In the United States the "invisible" work of caring lies behind the dissatisfaction with the RB-RVS (Resource Based–Relative Value Scale), the federal government's regulations for physician reimbursement. The fulcrum of the contention hinges on reimbursement for "cognitive" contributions (medical caring) versus physical manipulation (surgical curing). Although a feeble approach to consideration of basic principles, it is an honest beginning for a contemporary search for soul in medicine.

Beyond RB-RVS and similar machinations, physicians must be crystal clear on what we are about in caring for patients. Despite increasing cultural, ethical, and economic pressure, we must avoid engaging in politics as politicians. Expedient as it may seem, direct political action by doctors is an unlikely means of solving our dislocations or defining our role. Political power, as much as any other power, corrupts—as it inevitably becomes self-serving.

Simply put, the public's belief in the profession's dedication to patient care diminishes proportionally to the profession's aggrandizement of political power and conspicuous wealth. This relationship appears in surveys that report the U.S. public's confidence in the medical profession dropped from 72 percent in 1963 to 37 percent in 1981, a level which flatly extends to the present.[3]

Like the Danish nurses, we need to be about the business of discussing and developing a common language for explaining medicine's "invisible" work in caring for patients. The operational word is "invisible." However, what may be "invisible" to purblind eyes can be "seen" when examined with a vision of the soul of medicine.

From Antiquity

A brief review of past attempts by physicians and scientists to locate the soul is instructive in understanding first principles of medicine. For

Hippocrates (460-377 B.C.) the soul existed within the body of the patient without specific location.[4] Incidentally, in keeping with the "invisible" in medicine, Hippocrates notes, "Without doubt no man who sees only with his eyes can know anything of what has been described here [in the art of medicine]."[5]

Hippocrates' contemporaries were more specific in locating the soul. Aristotle (384-322 B.C.), the first great scientist, centered the soul in the heart, while his teacher, Plato (428-348 B.C.), located it in the brain, going so far as postulating it having three elements: rational, passionate, and spiritual.

Soul searching preoccupied medical minds down through the ages. Galen (138-201 A.D.) staunchly maintained that the soul was situated in the brain. Just as strongly, Avicenna (980-1037) described it seated in the heart while five hundred years later Argenterius (1513-1572) vouched for its location in the heart,[6] and Descartes (1596-1650) located the soul in the pineal gland.[7]

Though experimental investigation has largely displaced learned conjecture, discussion of the soul has never been abandoned by medical science. Under the soul's Greek name, psyche, its study survives today. Psychology continues the learned discussion led by Sigmund Freud (1856-1939) in his analysis of the inner world of man and Carl Jung (1875-1961) in his studies of the collective unconscious. Freud's description of a tripartite psyche with id, ego, and superego bears remarkable similarity to Plato's tripartite soul. Presently, psychoanalysts reappraise their philosophical foundations, postulating an "autonomous self," an "innate organizing principle,"[8] while neuropsychologists avidly seek the location of psyche, often identified as "mind," "consciousness," or "intentionality," among the molecules of the nervous system. However, in general medicine, as new metaphors support theories of therapeutics, collegial discussion of soul wanes.

The Soul of Medicine Today

The location of the soul of medicine remains a relevant question when examining what Thomas Kuhn describes as a paradigm shift, a new order of recognition of observed facts.[9] The prevailing paradigm, the reductionistic materialism of science, falters in explaining disparate social, economic, and ethical phenomena related to the treatment of patients, leaving a palpable void in the thinking of practitioners. The void, that unacceptable professional gap that is recognized as patienthood, the state of being a patient, and what is done about patienthood manifests itself as widespread angst among physicians. A new paradigm is needed to meet the issue.

The concept of the soul of medicine points, as other paradigms do not, toward functional solutions. It challenges us to lift our eyes from the patient's chart and with broad vision seek solutions in worlds beyond the research laboratory. But how to construct such a paradigm, which according to the ancients must come from understanding our essence, our ethos?

Much as a man writes an unconscious autobiography in the stubs of his checkbook so a profession inadvertently describes its soul with its sworn values. Thus medical oaths, a form of cultural DNA, can be signposts pointing to the location of the soul of the profession.

Interestingly, the ethical direction indicated by medical oaths has shifted in the last fifty years. At graduation ceremonies the classical Hippocratic oath no longer predominates with its emphasis on professional solidarity and paternalistic attitude towards patients. More than half of North American medical schools replaced the classical Hippocratic oath with contemporary modifications, new oaths, prayers, and covenants.[10] They include the Ohio State version of the Hippocratic oath, the Geneva oath, the Prayer of Maimonides, and the Clouser covenant as well as many idiosyncratic medical oaths. Values reach out beyond autonomous professional power as healing is valued as a shared responsibility of doctor, patient, and community.

The revisions and additions to oaths and covenants express new values and new directions, hinting at a changing ethos. Evolving medical covenants demonstrate the shift by no longer characterizing the graduate as a discrete solo practitioner but rather as a collaborating physician, a proactive member of a community. Democratically, covenants include the audience in the oath-taking ceremony with group responses, declarations, and joint swearing of the covenant. Here is evidence that the soul of medicine is moving beyond the halls of academe to where the profession and the public intersect, the shared space between the doctor and the patient, the patient-doctor relationship.[11]

Surprising corroboration of soul shifting to the patient-doctor relationship is found in Armstrong's study in the medical literature of how practitioners refer to patients.[12] He searched thirty-five consecutive years of the *British Journal of Venereal Diseases* for examples of doctors' attitudes towards patients, documenting changes.

His investigation starts with the autocratic medical attitudes of 1931, "What a lot of valuable time could be saved if our patients could be taught that all we want to hear from them is an account of their symptoms, as concise as possible, in chronological order." Doctors' interest in the psychological aspects of practice first appears in 1948 with reference to the patient who disagrees with a treatment regime, pejoratively referred to as a "contemporary defaulter." In 1953 the British Medical Association Venereologist Group Committee study of "defaulter" behavior broadened the psychological understanding of their management: "the whole patient must be studied as well as his infected tissues."

By 1957 Balint published his classic text on the patient-as-subject calling for doctors to understand patients' behaviors and reactions to the illness and doctor as well as the illness itself.[13] In 1966 formal analysis of patient-doctor interaction enters the medical literature. In 1976, it has been reported, practitioners were being asked to understand the whole patient, the whole life of the patient. This shift in the profession's perception of its role offers circumstantial evidence of where the soul of medicine should now be sought.

Further evidence for locating the soul of medicine at the intersection of the profession and the public comes from two inadvertent experiments, the Health Decisions movement and the Mini-Internship Program. Both offer open forums for the public and the profession to mutually consider evolving patient-doctor relationships.

The Mini-Internship Program originated in Oregon in 1975 to bring local community leaders directly into the world of medicine. Lay people, frocked in white coats, spend two days at the side of busy practitioners much as medical interns do.[14] The clinical experience is preceded and followed by intense group discussions, first laying out the ground rules of confidentiality, later supporting an intimate exchange of concerns and values between doctors and the mini-interns. The Mini-Internship Program was extended nationally with the sponsorship of the American Medical Association.

The Health Decisions movement, with a wider approach, conducts statewide community meetings for the public to discuss, with the help of doctors, tough issues concerning health care and its delivery.[15, 16] The movement spread from Oregon to twenty-one other states with thousands of community meetings focused on critical medical life-and-death issues.

A characteristic pattern of response emerges from these open encounters between the public and the profession. As citizens express their personal values for prudent, effective medical care, doctors respond with their values. Together, with alternating tension and conciliation, they openly investigate shared concerns in the pursuit of informed, compassionate care.

As the meetings approach a common goal through shared values, an unusually strong sense of mutual reinforcement emerges. The degree of heightened commonality is difficult to appreciate for those who have not participated. At times, especially in the mini-internships, the exchanges end in clearly validated consensus. This does not imply that negative feelings or contrary ideas are absent. Rather, dissension is repeatedly worked through by returning to shared values—first principles of the patient-doctor relationship. Thus citizens and doctors unconsciously locate the soul of modern medicine through the vitality of their deliberations.

The soul of medicine can also be located by means of "soul therapy," psychotherapy, where the ultimate source of healing does not lie in mood-altering medications nor behavioral prescriptions but in the experience of shared personal suffering. With co-passion the essence of the patient is touched by the essence of the therapist. Consequently, the soul of medicine's healing bond can be located within the intimate disclosures and understanding interpretations shared through patient-doctor trust.

The assembled evidence offers a plausible hypothesis: the soul of medicine exists within and about the patient-doctor relationship to be discovered in the act of participating in the patient's suffering. Based on psychology rather than anatomy, the soul of medicine can be located in the space halfway between a suffering patient and a caring physician.

Persuasive Conjecture

Should the hypothesis that the soul of medicine exists in the caring patient-doctor relationship be accepted by concerned practitioners, a widening perspective opens on our possible ethical, social, civic, political, and economic behaviors. Stimulated by a renewed paradigm we can fashion imaginative means for recovering diminished public respect and curtailed professional autonomy in service to patients. Simply put, our future as a vital profession lies in considering how we resonate with the soul of medicine alive in the patient-doctor relationship.

Strengthened with an understanding of our essence we can then deliberately join our professional behaviors to universals, linking the patient-doctor relationship to our economic, scientific, civic, and ethical actions. Such is the path to Osler's goal of a unified, science-based, compassionate understanding of who we are and what we are about.

The Faculties of Soul

How do practical applications follow from our accepted universal? As the first mover of medical practice, the soul of medicine operates through its faculties. While these faculties originate within and are motivated by the same source, the soul of medicine, the faculties manifest themselves as apparently independent activities of medical practice. Individually, each faculty is associated with a discrete body of medical knowledge, language, rules, and traditions. Collectively, they are the immanent powers manifest in the practitioner's behavior in wise service to patients.

It is not necessary to return to Plato to understand the four faculties of the soul of medicine to be intellectual, economic, social, and aesthetic. It may take a leap of imagination to accept the immutable presence of these four faculties in every patient-doctor relationship, but for better or worse, active practitioners intuitively recognize these in their daily clinical behavior.

The intellectual faculty of soul, scientific knowledge and medical skills, looms large in clinical practice. Based on reason, this faculty embraces the whole of biomedical knowledge, the science of medicine. The aesthetic faculty, or art of medicine, works through the human element of charity, faith, and hope to insure that the patient's emotional and spiritual life is recognized, never ignored.[17] The social, or communitarian, faculty encompasses the societal strictures of tradition, law, licensing, and certification, holding doctors accountable to patient, government, and society. Finally, the economic faculty, in former days known as the nutritive faculty, deals with the metabolism of resources that inevitably accompanies the care of patients.

In a development Osler never anticipated, the faculties of soul have grown imperceptibly to the point that they can assume autonomous identities as specialized systems within and about the health delivery establishment. Where the nineteenth-century doctor exemplified in his person all of medicine's faculties of soul, today's practitioner looks to surrogates, aides, and stewards to assume the multiplicity of professional responsibilities that accompany the four faculties of medical soul.

Through expediency or neglect, practitioners have relinquished significant degrees of authority over the faculties of soul, first to assistants and, to surrogates. In turn the surrogates refashion the power of the faculties into independent systems or domains. Frequently, these systems of financing, administration, and bioethics are dominated by nonmedical experts, some friendly stewards, others imperious autocrats. Whether in cooperation with the doctor or not, stewards of the delivery establishment have turned the power of the faculties of soul into a thing unto itself— distanced from the patient-doctor relationship, severed from the needs of patients.

A cursory definition of the surrogates and their roles proves enlightening. The ultimate arbiters of the medical knowledge domain have become the biomedical research scientists, empowered by detailed knowledge of pathological processes to outrank less authoritative practitioners. Thus the bench scientist can preempt clinicians' definition of quality care.

The aesthetic domain belongs to the bioethicists who, as physician surrogates, cultivate a burgeoning academic discipline, while professing to know best the clinical questions to ask and thus, by implication, the proper answers to modern ethical dilemmas.

The economic domain is dominated by business managers, bookkeepers, accountants, managed carers prepared in the name of efficiency to control funds and resources of clinical medicine.

The social, or communitarian, domain is overseen by regulators, lawyers, and government officials, famous for trampled confidentiality, insensitive encounters, unworkable red tape, and diminished vision, transacted in the name of some parochially greater good.

With the physician's diminishing professional autonomy, the four domains increasingly answer to themselves rather than to the patient's advocate. Consequently, physicians must strive for a new dynamic countering the self-serving hegemony of institutional domains by centering our contributions to the health care delivery system on the patient's need for compassionate care. Patently, Osler's concept of twofold balancing of medical science with medical art proves inadequate to the times. Today we must develop a fourfold dynamic of medical practice capable of properly monitoring and balancing the four semi-autonomous faculties. No small task, but possible.

Opportunities

Possessing a tool is never to be confused with skill in using it. As tools, the faculties of the soul of medicine offer opportunities for their skillful use. To ensure that no harm is done by the surrogate leaders of the four domains, "the physician's apprentices," a higher order of tools, the conceptual faculties of the soul of medicine, must prevail. These tools apply for stewards of the domains of health delivery *only* as they express the soul of medicine. Physicians must learn to translate and to apply the information resulting from "faculty" tools in a manner that is understandable, or at least acceptable, to their surrogates. Anything less and patients become endangered.

Predictably, the present struggle for the control of health care will intensify. Who should control the faculties of medicine—physicians or the stewards of the domains? When confronting the experts of the domains, practitioners discover their strongest ally to be patients. Incredible as it may sound, the practitioner, empowered by the concept of the soul of medicine, can involve the patient in a shared dynamic, not the dynamic between science and the art of medicine but the dynamic of balancing the four faculties of the soul of medicine. What could be more practical than practitioners and patients fashioning new instruments for the patient-doctor relationship, instruments for pursuing the "invisible" work of caring?

Practically, the control of the faculties of the soul of medicine belongs to those who develop them. Though the odds may be poor that our harried profession will embrace the philosophy of the soul of medicine sufficiently to contain the spread of destructive scientism, with its rituals of reason, we have successfully faced and overcome more obscure and daunting challenges. To move forward, physicians need open, organized, sustained collegial discussion centering on who we are and what our first principles should be in the twenty-first century. Only as we examine our hearts do we encompass the burgeoning world of health care and remain respected patient advocates.

Let us be about these reflections and discussions. Then, with the conviction that the essence of medicine exists in the patient-doctor relationship, we can take the important step of prudently addressing our medical, social, and economic technology.

Remembering Osler's admonitions, we address the future by drawing on our profession's past. We do this without expectation of deep understanding or support from others. We rise by pulling at our bootstraps. We grow professionally by judiciously nurturing ourselves on a diet of "reinforced hope or resolution of despair." Thus we must live in touch with the "invisible" soul of medicine.

Endnotes

From *Transactions of the College of Medicine of South Africa*, July-December 1993, 58-63, with permission.

1. W. Osler, *The Old Humanities and the New Science In a Way of Life* (New York: Dover Publications, 1951), 8-33.
2. R. Crawshaw, "Academic Sanction: Targeting South African Science," *Journal of the American Medical Association* 262(1989):1499-1503. "Academic Sanction" appears in part 8 of *Compassion's Way*.
3. S. Lipset and W. Schneider, *The Confidence Gap* (New York: The Free Press, 1981), 48.
4. *Hippocrates*, trans. W.H.S. Jones, Loeb Classic Library, v.4, p.239 (Cambridge: Harvard University Press, 1969).
5. *Hippocrates*, op. cit, p.209.
6. O. Temkin, *Galensim* (New York: Cornell University Press, 1972).
7. "Descartes" in *Encyclopedia Britannica,* Macropaedia, v.5, p.601 (Chicago: University of Chicago, 1974).
8. S.C. Averill, Introduction to "The Autonomous Self" by John D. Sutherland, *Bulletin of the Menninger Clinic* 57(1): 3-32.
9. T. Kuhn, *The Structure of Scientific Revolution,* In International Encyclopedia of Unified Science, v.2, no.2, ch. X. (Chicago: University of Chicago Press, 1970).
10. R. Crawshaw, "Contemporary Use of Medical Oaths," *Journal of Chronic Diseases* 23(1970): 144-150.
11. W.F. May, *Code and Covenant of Philanthropy and Contract* (MIT Press, 1977.)
12. D. Armstrong, "The Doctor-Patient Relationship: 1930-80," in *The Problem of Medical Knowledge,* Eds. P. Wright and A. Teacher (Edinburgh: Edinburgh University Press, 1982).
13. M. Balint, *The Doctor, His Patient and the Illness* (London: Pitman Publishing, 1957).
14. R. Crawshaw, "Mini-Internships: An Experience in Health-Care Delivery for Community Leaders," *New England Journal of Medicine* 309(20 Oct 1983): 992-94. This essay can be found in part 10 of *Compassion's Way.*
15. B. Jennings, "A Grassroots Movement in Bioethics," *Hastings Center Report,* Special Suppl., June/July 1988.
16. R. Crawshaw, M. Garland, B. Hines, and C. Lobitz, "Oregon Health

Decisions, An Experiment with Informed Community Consent," *Journal of the American Medical Association* 254(22): 3213-3216.
17. K. Menninger, M. Mayman, and P. Pruyser, *The Vital Balance* (New York: Viking Press, 1963), 357.

The Humanitarian Imperative and the Practice of Medicine

It is not what a lawyer tells me I may do; but what humanity, reason and justice, tell me I ought to do.

—Edmund Burke (1729-1797)
Speech at County Meeting
Buckinghamshire, England 1784

There is a great and growing turmoil boiling within health delivery systems, locally and globally ancient philosophical conflicts fueled by preemptive scientific thinking. One of the serious casualties of this struggle for control of mankind's future is the humanitarian imperative—the intuitive belief of vital human beings that they are privileged to contribute as they can to the spirit and well-being of the community of man.

Numerous examples of this philosophical discontent are found in the list of inadvertent counterproductive reactions that accompanied the introduction of science into the healing arts. The political, social, and economic restraints on medical care constitute a doleful documentation that needs little amplification. Personal care withers with specialization and bureaucratization of the medical practitioner. The conversion of the intensive-care patient into a "laboratory" whose human condition is measured by dials and test reports is universally recognized as a mixed blessing, saving lives too often at the expense of humanity.

Until recently the value of medical progress went unquestioned even in economic terms. The cost/benefit ratio of science relative to the spirit of mankind, a pressing philosophical question, surfaces in few minds. Questioning the value of medical science is a non sequitur for the scientist who by a lifetime dedication to science has invested his spirit in his pursuit; for the healthy layman it is too abstruse to compete with a thousand closer concerns; for the sick layman intent upon recovery it is absurd; for the health professional, caught up in pressing daily routines, it is an ivory-tower conceit. Yet for all the participants in health services the question exists, What is the price in human spirit paid for by unquestioned compliance with technology's demands? A philosophy of values is essential, fearfully important, for only with the deep understanding that philosophy offers in a scientific age can the spirit of man mature and grow in dignity and strength.

Understanding the untoward effects of science demands an appreciation of the prescientific world and the system of thinking that Sir Francis Bacon changed with inductive reasoning. Though it may be impossible to imagine bow-and-arrow technology, slave labor, and witch doctor therapeutics as acceptable culture, it is essential to understand ancient society if only to mark the effects of the science revolution. Granting that prescientific people did not see themselves as unredeemed primitives but as competent human beings deeply concerned with survival and immortality, preoccupied with the meaning of life much as present-day people are, we can gauge the change brought about by science not so much as a miraculous transformation of mentality but as a particular focusing of human thought and consequent behavior. The increasing focus on material life, science, has acted to restrict man's understanding of himself. Emphasis on things, technology, has gradually shifted mankind's attention from the spiritual to preoccupation with the material elements of life. The assumption that each of us is a human being, an unknowable soul existing in infinity, gives way to a belief that man is a machine, a complex technological device.

The Mechanistic Influence of Descartes

The genius of this change, and consequently for the present turmoil in worldwide health delivery that endangers the expression of the humanitarian imperative, is René Descartes. He did it with a simple phrase, *cogito, ergo sum,* I think, therefore I am. Such a seemingly innocuous statement yet one so threatening to the spirit of man! For Descartes this conceptualized life and all that he experienced from that point onward became simply a function of thinking. The universe, whether the path of stars through the heavens or the circulation of blood through the body, became a closed system encompassed by the mind of man. Nature was interpreted as a great machine that accumulated data would describe and control. Man's experience was considered reducible to measurable data to be graphed in ways Descartes pioneered. Thus mankind was seduced into believing it would become all knowing. Science had become the way to ultimate knowledge.

However, the point is neither to develop a history of medical scientific thought nor to cultivate a destructive Luddite attitude. Rather the stress is on the radical change in man's understanding of himself. This amounted to no longer conceiving of man as a social animal but as a mechanical one, a wonderfully complex automan.

Descartes's thinking also imparted mathematical sense with the graph, with x a function of y. It proved a tool of inestimable value in visualizing and extending the limits of mathematics, leading to calculus, while underpinning the quantitative mentality of the Enlightenment. However, Descartes's focus on measurable quantities metaphorically made x, the universe, a function of y, the coordinates of scientific measurement. Unfortunately, like Gulliver in Lilliput, mankind has since been pinned down on this larger graph that yields limitless data but little wisdom leading to the meaning of an individual human in an infinite universe.

Armed, since Enlightenment, with the concept of the universe as a construct of the human mind, scientists have accumulated knowledge at an ever accelerating rate. Today, augmented by the computer, the generation of knowledge proceeds at a reckless pace, sometimes referred to as infoglut. Simultaneously, dominant societies of our culture act as economic machines spinning out goods and services. Descartes's concept has grown political into a totalitarian ideology, in which science, the measurement of data, is the supreme, overriding value. The preeminence of quantifiable ideas and consequent technical power has crowded out cultivation of the philosophy of man—the love of wisdom—and consideration of its handmaiden, the humanitarian imperative.

An example of the unchallenged, growing power of science over humanitarian custom was the medical policy of the Soviet Union whereby physicians were not permitted to inform dying patients of their actual prognosis. Officially, all health professionals were required to be "optimistic" under every circumstance, which explains the policy as simple public relations—much as flight attendants on commercial airplanes are trained to smile and reassure the passengers should the flight become bumpy. However, a profounder logic of science was at work, for the Soviet Union prided itself on being scientific, the professed basis of Marxist dialectical materialism, in all its policies, medical as well as political. The Soviet government promised that, like science, ultimately it had all the answers, including, difficult as it may be to imagine, science-based immortality. Personal dying became a "non-event" for totalitarian science by fiat and went unrecognized in the Soviet patient-doctor relationship. Thus science triumphed over the death of a human being by declaring death of the individual valueless for the individual, the doctor, and society.

Descartes's thinking had minimal impact on his own era, for then his clockwork conceptualization of the universe was treated as heresy. Theistic thinking, in religious dogma and metaphysical speculation, of the day maintained man was created and functioned strictly in accordance with divine will, the extreme opposite of scientism.

For generations Descartes's idea was a philosopher's toy seldom impinging upon the rest of mankind, until, under the impact of the industrial revolution and the triumph of mechanical technology, a new culture emerged. Then the conceptualizer of the new culture, the industrial entrepreneur, unleashed the full power of Descartes's depersonalized world view.

As the industrial revolution generated economic power, social power flowed to those "in the know." Superior knowledge made the informed man "more" than the uninformed man. But spiritual and ethical thinking have not made one man "more" than another in the immediate give-and-take of daily life. Yet humanitarian thinking has gradually lost potency in competition with preponderant scientific materialism, particularly as materialism rewards mankind with "things."

The Influence of Science on Medical Training

The preemptive impact of science on the behavior and training of health professionals has grown during the last forty years. Though modern medicine may be dated as arising in the 1880s with the scientific understanding of infection and bacteriology, only in post-World War II did the training of physicians begin to fracture along "scientific" lines. Then, as the growing body of scientific knowledge proved more than any one individual might master, the initial four-year course of medical school was supplemented with years of specialized study, devoted to developing in the physician increasingly detailed concepts of the organs and organ functions along lines of Descartes's mechanical man. Medical specialization has continued its division into finer subspecialties, with the medical student becoming a physician who becomes an internist who becomes a cardiologist who becomes a pediatric cardiologist, until the explicit rewards of professional life drift further and further from the personal life problems of patients.

Now the medical profession itself reflects the general loss of the humanitarian imperative. There is no training, scientific or otherwise, to reintegrate the divisions of the profession into a unified identifiable whole. Rather, diverse treatments, generating esoteric scientific jargons, widen the gaps between specialties until physicians refer and exchange patients among themselves as bearers of organs. Physicians have increasing implicit difficulty communicating about the original central unifying concern of the profession, the concern for a particular human being—the Humanitarian Imperative.

Terrible as it may be, the training, rewards, and collegial reinforcement of modern physicians seriously diminished *official* space for human values. Though the art of medicine may be espoused, it lacks a place in the medical school curriculum, in the programs of continuing medical education, in the language of physicians, and, most importantly, in physicians' thinking.

Where the Eskimo may have 117 different words to describe snow in all its variety, the modern U.S. physician with 268 national medical specialty organizations and 125 medical schools has but one word for human suffering: stress—a word borrowed from engineering to express the breaking point of metal. Patently, medicine's humanitarian imperative treads a lonely path bereft of philosophical support for collective understanding.

Much as nature is reputed to abhor a vacuum, the present philosophy of science shrinks from the individual, the statistical non-series. For science the subjective unity of an individual remains an expression of "unknowability." Seen through such a prism, each individual represents an infinity of ignorance, a sample impossible to conceptualize into a statistically significant fact and hence scientifically "unthinkable." Certainly the individual has juices and organs which may be treated in quantifiable fashion, blood counts, urine flows, heartbeats, but scientific thinking can never acknowledge the whole as greater than the sum of its parts. Today we come to the inevitable conclusion that the humanitarian imperative is in bondage to the present concept of material things, to science. Today man exists for medical science only as he is quantifiable and can be fitted to a graph.

The Future of the Humanitarian Imperative

Science, like fire, makes an excellent servant and an evil master. To retain the humanitarian imperative, a humanism that allows meaning for the doctor and the patient larger than the view through an ophthalmoscope, the medical practitioner must not become antiscientific in reasoning but attain to suprascientific thinking. Reflection offers the observing practitioner the humility of recognizing that the view through the ophthalmoscope, the sound through the stethoscope, is always partial—that the patient is more than the sum of the practitioner's scientific measurements. Further, such a humble view privileges the concerned physician to go further, to observe through the practitioner's experience of human suffering the suffering of the patient—a humanitarian contribution to the community of man.

To nurture the humanitarian imperative, the medical practitioner seeks contact with human beings, not organs of human beings or representatives of human beings. The physician engages with the patient in a discourse that does not deny science but affirms humanness. By using science as a mental process and not as an ideology, the physician discovers not only his or her self, but connection with fellow men and women—shared commonality. The physician can venture beyond dependency on science and risk encountering the unknowable other. Caring physicians find meaning in human beings, not in things. It is then that genuine caring takes place.

The intimately shared experience is the necessary vehicle for a caring patient-doctor relationship. Intuitively, human beings deeply believe this true, an imperative. Despite any distance our culture's technology may place between individuals, the truth remains that as each recognizes and acts on the privilege of deep sharing the sharers grow as human beings.

Epiview

There is but one test of a good life: that the man shall continue to grow difficult about his own behavior.
—Robert Louis Stevenson (1883-1886)

Epiview

If a single theme threads through this quest of compassion it is the singularity of the compassionate experience. Unlike faith, secure with its overarching inclusiveness and hope bearing conscious promise, the balm of compassion without preemptive call or anticipatory preparation passes in and out of life in a wholly unique manner, a manifestation of grace unbidden.

How is it that the substance of compassion is so elusive? Is it simply that compassion has no meaning beyond personal experience? Certainly, its singularity exists unbounded by the constraints of reason. The fact of time and tyranny of circumstance mandate that compassion is a once-or-never experience. Made of shared feeling, the compassion experienced is indeterminant process from beginning to end. No two compassionate experiences can ever match.

Compassion flows between two people, occasionally; perhaps more may be involved, but occasionally. Compassion's process lacks, in fact abhors, structure, concrete form. Much as the experience of grace, the compassionate experience is uniquely spontaneous, foreign to expectation, alien to preparation. Capturing compassion as a concept is as productive as netting butterflies in a snowstorm.

Compassion is a validation of the individual, a self originating in childhood. Then circumstances "danced" together in a now inconceivable openness, with unexpected encounters no more than variations on an orchestrated theme of wondrous acceptance. The child plucks a blade of grass the better to examine its color against the deeper green of an overhanging tree, to discover the leaf's rough texture and sharp edges with a stroke against the cheek, to taste its bitterness with a lick and a chew, to measure its slim size against a meadow of stalks, and then, suddenly, secure in "knowing," the child casts aside the blade of grass. However, the leaf is never gone, remaining a most personal possession, a memory, an instant of beauty lived as self. The leaf may vividly reappear, for some, when recaptured by an artistic genius such as Walt Whitman in *Leaves of Grass*. For most, childhood's memories lie waiting somewhere short of consciousness, waiting to endow some future experience, such as the hauntingly sweet fragrance of new mown hay, a preconscious apprehension of life's beauty.

Compassion flows in the stream of aesthetics rather than the cascade of reason. The reasonable mind in its dutiful search for certainty might lead one to believe that there is a thing, compassion. The reasonable mind holds that *the compassion thing* is there for scientific measurement or literary criticism. Once captured and civilized through experiments, sermons, seminars, and books, *the compassion thing* may be harnessed to utilitarian progress. The temptation to believe in this bland muddle of nonexistent *things* seduces us to play the part of Polonius, mouthing empty words as a disguise, our willful denial of pain, our avoidance of the heart's perception of human suffering, with the experience of compassion.

The essence of the stunning scarlet of an autumn leaf, the indulgent smile that goes with patting a tail-wagging dog, suppressed tears for a sick child, the somber pause at the bedside of a dying patient, is a singular unity defying dissection. Rendered by the analytic mind, compassion crumbles into semantic disorder, the death of an experienced known, perhaps a small death, perhaps a great death, but, ironically, the soul-death of the analyst. No matter how keen, full feeling, and attentive the student, compassion can not be taught. What may be learned, and I have tried to communicate this lesson, is awareness of yourself as the necessary part of something immeasurable, unknowably vast yet invariably redeeming.

Our world is real not virtual. The leaves of life sprout about us, the emotions of our universe course in our veins. The experience of compassion does not pass from the lighted world to the retina inwardly, but from the enlightened heart outwardly as we venture to reach something more than ourself reflected. The secret, if there can be such a secret, is understanding compassion as an experience that lies just beyond finite limits as we, ineptly as we may, extend ourselves, beyond our means, our observations, our predictable lives to share a greater being.

To value yet another facet of compassion, it is an epiphany appearing as an experience informed by a prior personal history, revealing that sharing is not a transition from, to, or between others but an unfolding of latent profundity from within.

Certainly, compassion is not love, bound by a thousand loyalties and allegiances, ever negotiating peace with its inevitable counterpart, hate. Love enables and sustains our capacity to experience compassion, but curiosity, whose counterpart is ignorance, the emptiness of death, is the essential comrade of compassion. Despite the crushing burden of ignorance, curiosity leaps over infatuation or rancor; thus curiosity commingles that which is within us with that which is outside of us to make ourselves part of *our* world.

The rational mind approaches the heart's process of compassion with the wholly irrational phenomenon of insight. Suddenly overwhelmed with a flood of new knowledge, facts, and ideas, many of which have lain fallow, the conscious mind is ignited by an unexpected spark and in a flash rearranges disparate thoughts into a new and recognizable whole. Though more a flood of grace than a flash of wisdom bestows the revaluation that you are a vital part of the suffering and joy of the universe—or so I have come to believe.

Chartres
and the
Accidental Pilgrim

Chartres and the Accidental Pilgrim

But, dear reader, you do not know me as I have come to know me. To better inform you, let me take you far down my path to compassion with a tale of my later wanderings leading to the heart of me.

Pilgrims have no choice, for the bearings of their compass are set within them long before they dream of a New Jerusalem. So I learned as an accidental pilgrim on an "architectural" exploration of the sacred relic of faith and beauty, Notre-Dame de Chartres.

I was drawn to the cathedral by my interest in the early Middle Ages. Here lies modern man's first renaissance, the nascent awakening from the six hundred years of the Dark Ages. In a relatively few years, before the vise of feudalism and the crush of Church dogma again closed minds, there was an awakening of humanity with the birth of chivalry during the first Crusade, a flowering of learning accompanying the inception of the first universities, establishment of common law through the Magna Carta, and most dramatic, that explosion of community creativity, the cathedral.

A Sunday pause in work at Paris afforded opportunity to fulfill a long held wish to visit the queen of cathedrals. Rising early on a brisk, scarf-about-the-neck spring morning, I set out on the sixty-mile pilgrimage with an eerie venture into the Parisian underground.

After the drowsy functionary at the Solférino Metro station slid me a ticket to Gare Montparnasse I nimbly took the stairs down through a labyrinth of tunnels to the train platform. As I came to a stop at its edge, the departing echo of my footsteps announced a profound silence.

I am alone, all alone, existential alone, in a neon-lit, tile-lined, poster-plastered crypt of modern technology. There is no one there, no one on my side of the tracks nor on the other. There is no one in the station. Time passes without a sound, no movement of air, no indication of life. I remain fixed, planted like a seed, deep underground, awaiting germination, a lonely soul alert for any prospect of life.

A distant rumble finally reaches my ears. A faint breath of air stirs from the dark face of the tunnel. The rumble grows to the metallic clash of a train rushing into the empty chamber, the motorman hidden in his dark compartment, an indistinguishable latter-day Charon.

As the train slowed, it was readily apparent that all its cars were empty. Obviously, Parisians do not make much use of the Metro early Sunday morning. When a door slid open before me, I hesitated, immobilized by more than a traveler's predictable confusion. For a flash I wondered if, perhaps, the train's destination could be Hades. Then I was inside my private Metro car which swiftly bore me to the railroad station where, through further labyrinths leading up and out, I discovered in the semi-darkness what must be fellow human beings, newspaper-covered bodies of sleeping homeless. Hell proves closer than the twelfth century.

The train to Chartres is as alive as a circus. The spring sunlight pours in through the windows on frolicking day-trippers tossing their rucksacks about, families, complete with prancing children in their Sunday best, off for to visit the relatives, a passel of overly dressed women juggling gossip, back and forth, about who knows what. There is even a bicycle club complete with the members' equipment.

Before the first sight of the spires of Chartres cathedral appeared in the distance, most of the passengers had left the train at intermediate stops. Once detrained, you do not have to ask the way to the cathedral, for much as a queen on her throne that most beautiful of creations does not beckon from above the house tops but dispassionately awaits the pilgrim's progress towards homage.

The way up the hill breaks into a square before the cathedral where a soaring divinity of stone is set off against a milling humanity of the faithful, hurrying past wheelchaired cripples selling boughs of myrtle. It was Palm Sunday and myrtle serves the French for the palm leaves that graced Jesus' entrance into ancient Jerusalem. Hurrying, late but not too late, parishioners, drawing with them their children and elderly, made for the Royal Portal. The service had already begun.

I paused briefly before the austere guardians of the Royal Portal, the Elders of Israel who, in elongated human form turned holy by the chisel of an early-day Mondrian, fixed their gaze over me, scanned the distance, prepared to forbid entrance to greater heathens of belief and spirit than me. A few steps through the rough wooden vestibule, the passageway commoners must use, I discovered myself purblind in the subdued light of the nave. As I waited for my eyes to accommodate, the first impression of the cathedral came from my feet, the feel of massive blocks, everlastingly solid in their foundation yet cobbled and creased by ages of wear. Gradually, as from the bottom of the sea, my vision reached up through an immediate night to a heavenly dawn playing over a vast expanse of man-fashioned stone. High above, the huge clerestory illuminates a symphony of granite with the soft glow of pervasive, incarnate power.

Slowly I made my way to a place among the kneeling faithful. From there the elevated altar at the transept can be seen with the bishop in resplendent scarlet, surrounded by his retinue of priests and canons, conducting the holy service. The air vibrates with an ancient chant as clouds of incense ascend towards the vault. Candles flicker in every corner, burning since the cathedral's day of dedication, proclaiming the presence of past souls, joined in our ritual of belief.

As the service progressed, parishioners about me rose in turn to move toward the altar. I, a heathen, joined the penitent in line, awaiting my turn to accept a fragment of the host from a scowling priest, a swarthy man with sharp Andalusian features. Prayers and a response culminated in a grand recessional, the celebration of the Church triumphant, close enough to touch and then out into the Bishop's keep.

As the cathedral emptied I began, as it were, a private service, saying my "architectural" beads with a first-eyed inspection of the cathedral's wonders. To better understand the encyclopedia of fact and art around me, I carried with me Henry Adams's *Mont Saint Michel and Chartres* (Boston: Houghton Mifflin, 1963). This most complete guide to the form and spirit about me served as Psalter.

The three-story high, glassed walls of the Ambulatory dance to the tune of the morning sun pouring through with every shade and nuance of color, a vibrant celebration of a multitude of biblical tales. Even more captivating is the mark of enterprise and commitment left by twelfth-century artisans. Diminutive figured masons emerge from the sparkle of bright glass fragments, still at work sculpting royal figures. Glassmakers and carpenters pursue their trades with tongs and hammers. Bakers bear baskets of French bread.

Here lies an explanation of why such a monumental undertaking was accomplished in thirty years. Unlike modern attempts at cathedral building such as Barcelona's Temple of the Holy Family, which after ninety years of intermittent effort remains a pathetic shell of steel spires and incomplete concrete, more a monument to spiritual distraction and material preoccupation than consecration of higher vision, the people of twelfth-century Chartres sacrificed until it hurt in a prodigious labor of committed unity. Each worker, from master architect to peasant harnessed to quarried block, consciously participated in a spirit reaching beyond their personal world.

After a cursory ramble of the Ambulatory with its plenitude of magnificent windows, I passed on to study the divine geometry of the Rose windows, North and South. This calls for proper positioning. There is no danger of a foreshortened view. Too close and the deep-seated panes become partially obscured by their framing, too far away and detail is lost. Reversing a chair at the inner lip of the North transept, to face away from the altar and towards the color freighted rose, allows a fully relaxed view while encouraging systematic study.

The North Rose, the "Rose de France," is the gift of a Queen, Blanche of Castille, who defied the nobles of the land in fashioning the Kingdom of France for her son, the sainted King Louis. Her signature appears on the glass as a golden fleur-de-lis. Saint Ann occupies the center pane with the seated Virgin in the uppermost pane. Saint Ann is surrounded, in the geometry of Fibonacci's series that governs so many of nature's displays, such as the serried petals of the sunflower, the whorls on a pine cone, by a host of doves and angels within a larger constellation of biblical worthies. Together, they form a vast blue flame of passion scintillating over a bed of hot, glowing coals of faith.

Henry Adams makes much of the femininity of the North Rose, contrasting it with the masculinity of the South, even speaking of the hostility between the Roses. With sharpened curiosity I searched carefully for evidence of this conflicting style. The conflict I discovered proved quite different and entirely surprising.

Moving to the South Rose calls for no more than reversing a first row chair in the South transept. I am astonished to find how the morning sunlight has turned the South Rose into an eye-shattering enormity of jewels. There in the center, an Apocalyptic Christ sits astride an emerald throne, hands raised, the epitome of foreboding final doom. About him circle luminous guardian angels while beyond, the twenty-four elders of the Apocalypse stare forth, a fierce array of judges for the guilty to fear.

My attention is drawn to the inferior lancets that fill the large space beneath the Rose and the portal below. Here a series of windows, heavy with giant contorted figures of men astride men, is divided by the figure of the Virgin and her infant standing, not sitting, apparently caught between warring parties.

Henry Adams, recalling an interpretation of medieval scholars, explains the lancets as depicting the Apostles on the shoulders of the Israelite, a metaphor of the Old Testament supporting the New. But, for me, that interpretation fails to ring true. I know of no biblical reference, in fact or metaphor, to any such positioning of ancient religious leaders. Matthew astride Isaiah, Mark on Daniel, John on Ezekiel, and Luke burdening Jeremiah. The Apostles, wide-eyed and tenaciously gripping the hair of their mounts, appear not so much as riders to a greater glory but as wrestlers struggling for advantage, ripping scalps from losers. Like Adams, I see them as grotesque warriors astride battle chargers radiating a sense of violence.

The worrisome lancets brought a new and unhappy idea to mind, a world of strife. Asking myself what the creators of the windows might have had in mind prompted a monstrous answer— a thinly disguised memorial to violence. Is not the South Rose a propitiation for the horror of the Albigensian Crusade?

Though I was stunned by the concept of emblazoned evil in a cathedral, the facts fitted. Commencing in 1093, the Albigensian Crusade executed the three-way pact between a militant Pope Innocent the Third, an arrogant and ungovernable aristocracy of Northern French nobles, and the ever lurking Devil. The Pope let loose an indulged lust to annihilate by promising the Dukes of France all the wealth and land they could plunder from the Cathar and Waldensian Christians of southern France, the Midi, who refused obeisance to a corrupt church. The Pope was gratified with their extermination. The nobles reveled in their plundered riches. The Devil's portion came with the initiation of the Inquisition which, with religious faith transmuted into physical terror, ensured for centuries a march of innocents, offered up in barbaric sacrifice by the Church to humiliation, poverty, torture, prison, and fiery death.

CHARTRES AND THE ACCIDENTAL PILGRIM

Together, Pope, nobles, and Satan gave evidence that the sharpest sword is whetted by a prayer.

Certainly not as obvious an example of Christian pillage of Christians as the four bronze horses looted from Constantinople to adorn the portico of the Basilica of St. Mark's in Venice, before my eyes the "Rose de Dreux" insensibly transformed into a celebration of worldly conquest. Though no documents remain, circumstantial evidence stands that sometime prior to 1225 the Duke de Dreux contracted for the South Rose window and paid with more than thirty pieces of martyred Christians' silver. This grim conclusion loaded a charge in my mind, trigger cocked, for I still failed to understand my pilgrim's role to what was unfolding before me.

Thinking, enough of these malignant imaginings, with relief I changed my position to another under the nave, taking with me a savor of self-righteous arrogance at having solved to my satisfaction the mystery of the Rose of Dreux. How easily I suffer the pride of discovering the mote in another's eye. Once again seated in my original pew I looked up and forward to the central windows above the choir. They proved the means of making me into a wholly penitent pilgrim.

There, far above the worldly crowd, in the precise pivot of the center window, Notre-Dame de Chartres sits upon her throne, embracing her cherished infant, afloat in the celestial blue of heaven, a soul-calming view of sustaining care. Carefully, I read Adams's words as he describes a thirteenth-century service:

> Her quiet masculine strength enchants us most. Pierre Mauclerc and Phillipe Hupel and their men-at-arms are afraid of her, the Bishop himself is never quite at his ease in her presence; but to the peasants, and beggars, and the people in trouble, this sense of calm is better than active sympathy. People who suffer beyond the formulas of expression—who are

> crushed in silence, and beyond pain—want no display of emotion—no bleeding hearts—no weeping at the foot of the cross—no hysterics—no phrases! They want to see God, and know that He is watching over his own. How many women are there, in this mass of thirteenth-century supplicants who have lost their children? Probably nearly all, for the death rate is very high in the conditions of Medieval life. (p.194)

I paused as memories of duty on the obstetrical wards of Bellevue Hospital came echoing back. Again, I heard the cries of women in protracted labor, "Mamma mia," "Mother, Mother of God, save me!"

Adams continues:

> There are thousands of such women here, for it is precisely this class who come most; and probably every one of them look up to Mary in her great window, and has felt the actual certainty, as though she saw with her own eyes—there in heaven, while she looked—with her own lost child playing with the Christ-child on her knee. (p.194)

I could go no further as a flood of my past overwhelmed me. My mother had lost such a child, Chicky. Before I was born, seventy-six years ago, my four-year-old sister came in from play with a cough only to die two days later of diphtheria. I was born two years after the tragedy, and as my grief stricken mother repeatedly told me, I was her one and only child, the answer to God's prayer. Tears welled up in my eyes. Tears of grief for my mother, my sister, and myself.

I knew Chicky. I knew her too well as the child I was born to replace. Her picture hung fixed over my parents' bed, haunting my childhood. Many the time, even as a wee lad, I was called to that darkened room, "Ralphie, fetch the witch hazel." As a postulant in a ritual of caring, I administered a cloth, dipped in that precious balm, to the brow of my migraine-crippled mother. Overwhelmed by memory, I sobbed. I sobbed and sobbed.

Crying brings little notice to the pilgrim at Chartres. I know because the faithful passed me by without a whit of attention. For a long time I sat, gradually making sense of my feelings and thoughts, pulling myself together.

Chicky had sent me to Chartres, as surely as she had sent me to medical school, as surely as she had set me on a lifelong quest for compassion. I have an angel, perhaps a guardian, certainly a demanding angel, before whom I am ever judged. Judged I was, for I too have stolen from the Christians to build my "Dreux Rose." I was crying as a penitent seeking redemption.

Awareness paralyzed me. My life took on a profound deception, for I sought always to appear as an unusually dutiful son. Seldom, if ever, have I acknowledged my revulsion at my mother's prolonged grief, her exploitive, anguish-fashioned life, particularly as her appeals relentlessly followed me, close to the point of madness, through most of my adult years. I did my duty with more than a measure of well-concealed hate for the woman who bore me. Only Chicky knew how much counterfeit care, perfunctory attention, I gave my mother and have given suffering others, for I molded much of what appears as concern out of reluctant duty, devoid of love. Nor is this conscious insincerity but rather, less than full-hearted compassion for suffering others. Titled clinical objectivity, my flaw carries with it a professional dispensation, the received sin of a physician.

Leaning forward I plucked a sprig of trodden myrtle from the pavement, my palmer's badge for the journey home. Without another glance about I rose from the pew and slowly made my way to the railroad station, not alone, but certain of Chicky pointing the way for this child of God. Who is it that can live a life of the spirit and yet believe the pilgrim chooses his pilgrimage?

Index

A

academic sanction 397–410, 442–443, 605
　defined 398
acceptance 73, 102–103, 194. *See also* consciousness; mercy
accountability
　of physicians 118–121, 122–126, 132–133, 143–154, 260, 313, 330–338, 346–347, 466–471, 480–486, 603–604, 613–614. *See also* civic medicine; community mental health; courage; history: of medicine; patient-doctor relationship; values
　personal 61, 103, 130–138. *See also* choice; honesty
acknowledgment of responsibility 103–104
　defined 103
advance directives 198. *See also* health care delivery: and patient choice
American Health Decisions 517–521, 521–532
apartheid 179–196, 382–383, 397–410, 442. *See also* freedom, slavery
awareness
　of others 89–90
　of self 105, 199. *See also* choice; education

B

bioethics. *See* medical ethics
book reviews
　Corrupted Land, The 130–138
　Doctor Stories, The 259–261
　Psychiatrist for a Troubled World, A 290–294
　Witness to War 275–277

C

caring
　art of 47–53, 62–71, 100–107, 225–229, 351–360
　dedication to 92, 223–224, 259–261, 261–265, 265–272, 272–275, 275–277, 278–280, 281–285, 285–290, 290–294, 579–582
　limits of 271–272, 351–360, 486–491
　unaccountable 532–544, 544–550. *See also* healing; identity:physician's; medical humanism; oath taking; patient-doctor relationship; vocation
character
　development of 87–92, 101
　of physician 47–53, 107, 115–117, 142, 261–265, 265–272, 272–275, 278–280, 290–294, 435, 448
　strength 103, 107, 143–154. *See also* choice; honesty; soul
charity 53–62, 72–75, 348–351, 472–480
choice 85–87, 88–90, 136–137, 198, 281–282. *See also* courage; health care delivery; humanism; identity; medical ethics; medical humanism; oath taking; values; vocation
civic medicine 196–199, 292, 499–503, 503–508, 508–516, 521–532, 603–604
　defined 499
co-suffering (sostradanya) 145, 267–271
community mental health 330, 338–345, 348–351, 369–383, 445, 547–548, 592–598. *See also* accountability: of physicians; medical ethics
　defined 333
consciousness 53–62, 100–107, 142, 225–229, 272. *See also* choice; humanism

corruption 57, 130–138, 308–311, 325–330, 330–338, 411–419, 532–544, 608. *See also* accountability; honesty; suffering: circumstances: -denial, -ignorance; vocation

courage 112, 136–137, 138–143, 154–158. *See also* choice; fellow feeling; oppression; values

cruelty. *See* suffering: circumstances: ignorance

culture
   dynamics of 89, 130–138, 143–154, 172–179, 179–196, 235–237
   shock 161–164
      defined 163

curiosity 53, 58, 72, 102, 125, 143–144, 196–199, 287, 343, 363, 377, 381, 395, 406, 411, 504, 533, 534, 583, 606, 627. *See also* courage; suffering: meaning

D

denial. *See* suffering: circumstances

deontology. *See* oath taking: Soviet

dignity 61, 87–92, 153, 240–244, 278–280, 310–311, 314, 395–397, 442–448, 472–480, 617–622. *See also* medical humanism; values

doctor-patient relationship. *See* patient-doctor relationship

doubt. *See* healing: process; identity; oath taking

E

education
   of community leaders 499–503, 503–508
   of medical students 90, 225–229, 237–240, 308–311, 393
   of public 67–68, 198, 230–231, 233–240, 530–531, 589. *See also* caring; character: of physician; civic medicine; community mental health; health care delivery; identity; medical humanism; patient-doctor relationship; values

ethics. *See* medical ethics

F

feelings
   anger 56, 217–218, 338–345
   disgust 53–62
   gratitude 53–62, 165–167, 215–218, 490
   guilt 53–62, 118–121, 131–132, 308–311
   hate 133, 179–196, 215–218, 229–232, 442–448
   love 57, 93–95, 107, 272, 274
   rage 56, 140–141, 179–196, 229–232, 443–445. *See also* forgiveness; heart; suffering

fellow feeling 165–167, 179–196, 198–199, 420–436, 472–480, 606–616. *See also* heart; humanitarian imperative

film reviews
   3 Women 455–465
   Betrayal 127–129
   Fellini's *Satyricon* 43–47
   Gandhi 255
   Great Santini, The 569–578
   Nicholas and Alexandra 207–213
   Saving Private Ryan 96–99
   Shoah 383–388
   Welfare 303–308

forgiveness 57, 69–70, 72–75, 107, 192–194

free speech 283, 357, 396–397, 429. *See also* oppression

freedom 61, 94, 273, 521–532, 544. *See also* dignity; oppression

G

greed 58, 86, 87–88, 182–183, 346–347, 446. *See also* slavery

H

healing
   future of 579–582, 603–604, 604–617, 617–622
   process 100–107, 143–154. *See also* caring; patient-doctor relationship; soul

health care delivery
  managed care 52, 196–197, 225, 265, 335–336, 351–360, 395–397, 508–516
    defined 509
  patient choice 197–198, 236–237, 311–319, 381–383
  reform 196–199, 311–319, 508–516, 521–532
  systems 226–228, 308–311, 319–325, 351–360, 395–397, 411–419, 548, 579–582. *See also* civic medicine; education; medical ethics; patient-doctor relationship: and trust; suffering: circumstances: -denial, -ignorance, -power misused
Health Decisions movement 611
heart 62–71, 100–106, 179–196, 233–240, 265–272, 472–480, 486–491, 544–550. *See also* fellow feeling; forgiveness
Hippocratic oath. *See* oath taking
history
  from Chinese perspective 172–179
  government welfare 59, 472–480
  of medical oaths 115–117, 122–126
  of medicine 229–232, 276, 334, 369–383, 420–436, 508–516, 551–561, 604–617, 617–622. *See also* community mental health; humanism; oppression
honesty 83–87, 288, 532–544, 544–550, 592–598, 603
hope 244–248, 259–261, 472–480, 604–617. *See also* heart; oath taking: personal medical code; oppression: and physician heroes
Humanism 89–90
  defined 89
humanism 88–91, 233–240. *See also* choice; humanitarian imperative; medical humanism
  defined 89
humanitarian imperative 233–240, 281–285, 589, 617–622. *See also* medical humanism
  defined 238
humility. *See* identity: physician's

I
identity
  medical profession's 274–275, 420–436, 551–561, 583–592, 603–604, 604–617
  personal 83–87, 100–106, 136–137, 240–244. *See also* healing; soul; suffering: circumstances: happenings; suffering: meaning
  physician's 62–71, 100–107, 115, 142–143, 154–158, 167–172, 229–232, 311–319, 603–604. *See also* civic medicine; healing; humanitarian imperative; vocation
ignorance. *See* suffering: circumstances
impaired physicians 346–347, 389–395, 480–486, 598–602. *See also* physician suicide
integrity. *See* medical ethics

J
judgment. *See* character; choice; identity; values

L
leprosy 62–71, 282, 486–491
listening 165–167, 179–196, 419, 466–471, 472–480. *See also* patient-doctor relationship
loneliness. *See* suffering: experience
lying 127–129, 532–544. *See also* corruption

M
Marco Polo syndrome 173, 179
meaning. *See* suffering
medical ethics 125, 132–133, 260, 265, 319–325, 325–330, 351–360, 369–383, 442–448, 466–471, 543, 547, 590, 603–604. *See also* accountability; community mental health; medical humanism; oath taking; patient-doctor relationship; suffering: circumstances
medical humanism 87–92, 233–240, 617–622. *See also* healing; identity; patient-doctor relationship
  defined 89

medical technology 87–88, 319–325, 466–471, 472–480, 504, 579–582. *See also* health care delivery; identity; suffering: meaning
mercy 72–75, 472–480

O

oath taking
  Hippocratic oath 115–117, 118–121, 532, 604–617
  personal medical code 122–126
  Soviet 143–144, 267–268. *See also* identity: physician's; medical ethics
oppression
  and bureaucracy 395–397, 411–419
  and physician heroes 261–265, 265–272, 272–275, 275–277, 278–280, 281–285, 285–290, 290–294, 500–501
  and poverty 53–55, 61–62, 62–71, 162, 279, 351–360, 486–491. *See also* apartheid; suffering: circumstances; values
Oregon Health Decisions 198, 351, 396, 513, 520, 526, 527, 528
Oregon Health Plan 351–360, 396–397, 519–521, 528–529. *See also* health care delivery: reform
osmology 47–53. *See also* patient-doctor relationship: power in

P

patient-doctor relationship
  ambivalence in 215–218, 229–232
  bonding in 104, 213–215
  elements of 81, 100–107
  listening 232, 233–240, 244–248, 259–261, 265–272
  power in 100, 229–232, 579–582, 583–592
  respect 83–87, 105–106, 125, 215–217, 224, 240–244
  sharing in 83–87, 219–224, 259–261. *See also* caring; dignity; healing; identity; oath taking
  trust in 225–229, 311–319, 603–604, 610
physician suicide 333, 389–395. *See also* impaired physicians
Post Aromatic Stress Syndrome 195–196
post traumatic stress syndrome and shell shock. *See* caring: limits of
poverty. *See* oppression

R

reflection. *See* suffering: meaning
religion and faith 106, 124, 148–149, 165–167, 177–178, 261–265, 267, 272–274, 312, 318, 319–320, 324, 378, 433–434, 472–480, 487–488, 490, 595, 613. *See also* charity; science
respect. *See* humanism; patient-doctor relationship

S

science
  and religion 261–265
  limits of 72–75, 100, 120, 125–126. *See also* academic sanction; caring: art of; medical technology; suffering: circumstances: healing
slavery 369–383, 618, 622. *See also* apartheid; freedom
sostradanya. *See* co-suffering
soul 100–107, 179–196, 472–480. *See also* character; healing; heart; identity; values
suffering
  circumstances
    denial 58–59, 319–325, 325–330, 330–338, 351–360, 472–480, 480–486
    happenings 62–71, 83–87, 90, 93–95, 101
    ignorance 369–383, 389–395, 395–397, 420–436, 437–442, 532–544, 544–550
    power misused 397–410, 411–419, 442–448, 466–471
  denial 338–345
  experience
    despair 73–75, 179–196, 284
    fear 53–62, 100–107, 138–143, 179–196, 224, 229–232, 242, 272, 275–276, 311–319
    grief 105–106, 242–243, 265
    hopelessness 125–126, 179–196
    loneliness 100–107, 154–158, 224, 242, 265–272

INDEX 645

suffering,
  experience, continued
    loss 58, 100–107, 128, 218, 242–243, 265, 311–319
    misery 100–107, 214–215
    sorrow 74–75, 95, 104, 179–196, 265–272
  meaning
    for physicians 115, 141–143, 544–550
    from reflection 72–75, 142, 289–290, 472–480, 550
    personal 101–103, 106, 141, 153, 233–240. *See also* education; healing; identity; impaired physicians; suffering: circumstances: healing

V

values
  human 196–199, 240–244, 276, 308–311, 472–480, 604–617
  institutional 130–137, 466–471, 480–486
  personal 83–87, 106–107, 136–137, 162, 312–313. *See also* accountability; freedom
vice. *See* corruption
virtue 133–137, 281, 472–480, 603–604. *See also* courage; healing
vocation 311–319, 472–480, 499–503, 532–544, 551–561, 603–604, 604–617. *See also* civic medicine; identity: medical profession's

---

People and Places
Underlined page numbers denote epigraphs

Acworth Leprosy Hospital 62
Addison, Joseph 109
Aristophanes 225
Aristotle 604, 610

Behrhorst, Carroll Dean Henry 278–280
Bethune, Norman 234, 277
Blake, William 442
Bombay Leprosy Project 67
Bunyan, John 346
Burke, Edmund 617
Burton, Robert 389

Camus, Albert 87
Cavafy 249
Chartres, Cathedral of 631–639
Chekhov, Anton 124, 152, 265–272, 412
Chernoblynsky, Norm 145, 153
Chesterton, G.K. 361
Chiles, John 132
Clements, Charles 275–277
Confucius 172
Cooper, Peter 136
Crashaw, Richard 213

Damien, Father 71, 487–488, 490
Dante 449, 486
de Tocqueville, Alexis 521
Descartes, René 609, 618–620
Dewey, John 544, 579
Dharavi slum 62–68
Drake, Daniel, M.D. 159
Duomo, cathedral of Florence 333
Durant, Will and Ariel 122

Einstein, Albert 118
Emerson, Ralph Waldo 13, 303
Erasmus 420

Fanon, Frantz 252, 277, 382
Frost, Robert 77, 240
Funk, C.E. 154

Ganapati, R. 62, 67–69
Gandhi, Mohandas 255, 255–258, 281
German Leprosy Relief Society 67
Goldsmith, Oliver 244
Gregg, Alan 60–61, 348

Hammarskjöld, Dag 411
Hawthorne, Nathaniel 201

People and Places, continued

Hippocrates 52, 115, 123, <u>290</u>, 609
Hung Hsiu-Ch'uan 177

James, William <u>130</u>

Kafka, Franz <u>480</u>
Kaufman, H. 116–117
Kennedy, Edward 583–592

La Rochefoucauld, François <u>598</u>
Larrey, D.J. 277
Lemercier, Gregoire 549
Lippmann, Walter <u>583</u>
Lowell, James Russell <u>154</u>

Maimonides, Moses <u>261</u>, 261–265, 610
Marat, J.P. 277
Marcus Aurelius Antoninus <u>115</u>
Martial <u>43</u>
Martin-Ibanez, Felix <u>278</u>
Mencken, H.L. <u>397</u>
Menninger, Karl A. 285–290, 549, <u>563</u>
Menninger, William 58, 290–294
Meredith, George <u>127</u>
Milgram, Stanley 134, 334
Mill, John Stuart <u>503</u>
Milton, John <u>338</u>
Molière <u>215</u>
Molokai 71, 486

Osler, William 91, 105, 142, 327, <u>466</u>, <u>551</u>, 604–605
Ovid <u>319</u>

Pandya, Shubhada 62–66, 71
Paracelsus 51, <u>285</u>, 500

Paton, Alan <u>179</u>
Penfield, Wilder 60, 586
Petronius 43
Pirandello, Luigi <u>219</u>
Plato 610
Pogo <u>517</u>

Reed, Thomas 136
Rizal, José <u>272</u>, 272–275
Rockefeller Foundation 60
Roe, Rt. Hon. Mrs. Marion 352
Rush, Benjamin 136, 277, 500, 501, 578

Schweitzer, Albert <u>207</u>, 549
Servetus 500
Shakespeare, William <u>47</u>, <u>72</u>, <u>196</u>, <u>455</u>
Snow, C.P. <u>351</u>
Spengler, Oswald <u>308</u>
Spiro, Howard 536–537
Stevenson, Robert Louis 88, <u>532</u>, <u>623</u>
Sun Yat-sen 252
Swift, Jonathan <u>437</u>

Tennyson, Alfred, Lord <u>83</u>
Thoreau, Henry David <u>17</u>, <u>53</u>, <u>233</u>, <u>265</u>, 533
Twain, Mark <u>369</u>

Venice 72–73
Vernant, Jean-Pierre <u>592</u>
Virchow, Rudolf <u>499</u>, 500, 501

Whitman, Walt <u>93</u>
Wilde, Oscar 80, <u>100</u>, <u>295</u>
Williams, William Carlos <u>259</u>, 259–261